MILLER'S ANESTHESIA REVIEW

Fourth Edition

MILLER'S ANESTHESIA REVIEW

Lorraine M. Sdrales, MD

Associate Professor and Vice Chair
Department of Anesthesiology
Cedars-Sinai Medical Center
Los Angeles, California

Manuel C. Pardo, Jr., MD

Professor and Vice Chair for Education
Department of Anesthesia and Perioperative Care
University of California San Francisco
San Francisco, California

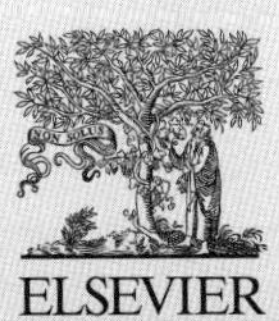

ELSEVIER

Elsevier
1600 John F. Kennedy Blvd.
Ste 1800
Philadelphia, PA 19103-2899

MILLER'S ANESTHESIA REVIEW, FOURTH EDITION ISBN: 978-0-443-11286-7

International Standard Book Number: 978-0-443-11286-7

Executive Content Strategist: Kayla Wolfe
Senior Content Development Specialist: Ann R. Anderson
Publishing Services Manager: Deepthi Unni
Project Manager: Nayagi Anandan
Design Direction: Ryan Cook

Printed in India

Last digit is the print number: 9 8 7 6 5 4 3 2 1

CONTRIBUTORS

Christopher R. Abrecht, MD
Associate Professor
Department of Anesthesia and Perioperative Care
University of California San Francisco
San Francisco, California

Ashish Agrawal, MD
Associate Professor
Department of Anesthesia and Perioperative Care
University of California San Francisco
San Francisco, California

Laura K. Berenstain, MD
Volunteer Professor of Clinical Anesthesiology
Department of Anesthesiology
University of Cincinnati College of Medicine
Cincinnati, Ohio

Jeanna D. Blitz, MD, FASA
Associate Professor
Department of Anesthesiology
Wake Forest University School of Medicine
Winston-Salem, North Carolina

Michael P. Bokoch, MD, PhD
Associate Professor
Department of Anesthesia and Perioperative Care
University of California San Francisco
San Francisco, California

Emilee Borgmeier, MD
Assistant Professor
Department of Anesthesiology
University of Utah
Salt Lake City, Utah

Matthias R. Braehler, MD, PhD
Professor
Department of Anesthesia and Perioperative Care
University of California San Francisco
San Francisco, California

Kristine Breyer, MD
Professor
Department of Anesthesia and Perioperative Care
University of California San Francisco
San Francisco, California

Richard Brull, MD, FRCPC
Professor
Department of Anesthesiology and Pain Medicine
University of Toronto
Toronto, Ontario, Canada

Tyler Seth Chernin, BSc, MD
Associate Professor
Department of Anesthesia and Perioperative Care
University of California San Francisco
San Francisco, California

Frances Chung, MBBS, MD, FRCPC
Professor
Department of Anesthesiology
University of Toronto
Toronto, Ontario, Canada

Hemra Cil, MD
Assistant Professor
Department of Anesthesia and Perioperative Care
University of California San Francisco
San Francisco, California

Daniel C. Cook, MD
Assistant Professor
Department of Anesthesiology
Weill Cornell Medicine
New York, New York

Wilson Cui, MD, PhD
Associate Professor
Department of Anesthesia and Perioperative Care
University of California San Francisco
San Francisco, California

Michael Curtis, MD
Cardiothoracic Anesthesiologist
Department of Anesthesiology
Stanford Healthcare
Pleasanton, California

Ryan Paul Davis, MD
Clinical Assistant Professor
Department of Anesthesiology
University of Michigan
Ann Arbor, Michigan

Andrew James Deacon, B Biomed Sci (Hons), MBBS, FANZCA
Staff Specialist
Department of Anaesthesia and Pain Medicine
The Canberra Hospital
Garran, ACT, Australia

Jennifer DeCou, MD
Associate Professor
Department of Anesthesiology
University of Utah
Salt Lake City, Utah

Anne L. Donovan, MD
Professor
Department of Anesthesia and Perioperative Care
University of California San Francisco
San Francisco, California

Talmage D. Egan, BA, MD, FASA
Professor and Chair
Department of Anesthesiology, Perioperative and Pain Medicine
Spencer Fox Eccles School of Medicine at the University of Utah
Salt Lake City, Utah

David Furgiuele, MD, FASA
Assistant Professor
Department of Anesthesiology, Perioperative Care and Pain Medicine
NYU Grossman School of Medicine
New York, New York

Katrina Gabriel-Ramos, MD, DPBA
Assistant Professor
Department of Anesthesia and Perioperative Care
University of California San Francisco
San Francisco, California

Seema Gandhi, MD, MBBS
Professor
Department of Anesthesia and Perioperative Care
University of California San Francisco
San Francisco, California

Steven Gayer, MD, MBA, FASA
Professor of Anesthesiology and Ophthalmology
Department of Anesthesiology, Perioperative Medicine, and Critical Care
University of Miami Miller School of Medicine
Miami, Florida

Sarah Gebauer, BA, MD
Partner
Elk River Anesthesia Associates
Yampa Valley Medical Center
Steamboat Springs, Colorado

David B. Glick, MD, MBA
Ronald F. Albrecht Professor of Anesthesiology and Department Head
Department of Anesthesiology
University of Illinois College of Medicine
Chicago, Illinois

Kasi Goodwin, MD
Assistant Professor
Department of Anesthesiology, Perioperative and Pain Medicine
Spencer Fox Eccles School of Medicine at the University of Utah
Salt Lake City, Utah

Erin A. Gottlieb, MD, MHCM
Associate Professor
Department of Surgery and Perioperative Care
The University of Texas at Austin Dell Medical School
Austin, Texas

Andrew T. Gray, MD, PhD
Professor
Department of Anesthesia and Perioperative Care
University of California San Francisco
San Francisco, California

Sarah Greene, MD
Staff Physician
Department of Anesthesia and Perioperative Care
University of California San Francisco
San Francisco, California

Hugh C. Hemmings Jr., MD, PhD
Professor and Chair
Senior Associate Dean for Research
Department of Anesthesiology and Pharmacology
Weill Cornell Medicine
New York, New York

David W. Hewson, BSc (Hons), MBBS, PGCert, FHEA, FRCA, PhD
Associate Professor
Department of Anaesthesia and Perioperative Medicine
University of Nottingham
Honorary Consultant Anaesthetist
Department of Anaesthesia and Critical Care
Queen's Medical Centre, Nottingham University Hospitals NHS Trust
Nottingham, United Kingdom

Lindsey Huddleston, MD
Associate Professor
Department of Anesthesia and Perioperative Care
University of California San Francisco
San Francisco, California

Andrew Infosino, MD
Professor
Department of Anesthesia and Perioperative Care
University of California San Francisco
San Francisco, California

Ken B. Johnson, MD
Professor
Department of Anesthesiology
University of Utah
Salt Lake City, Utah

Jeremy Juang, MD, PhD
Associate Professor
Department of Anesthesia and Perioperative Care
University of California San Francisco
San Francisco, California

Carolyn Kloepping, MD
Assistant Professor
Department of Anesthesia and Perioperative Care
University of California San Francisco
San Francisco, California

Martin Krause, MD
Associate Professor
Department of Anesthesiology
University of California San Diego
San Diego, California

Benn Morrie Lancman, MBBS, MHumFac, FANZCA
Specialist Anaesthesiologist
Department of Anaesthesia and Perioperative Medicine
Trauma Consultant, Department of Surgery
Alfred Health
Specialist Anaesthetist
Department of Anaesthesia, Perioperative and Pain Medicine
Peter MacCallum Cancer Centre
Melbourne, Victoria, Australia

Chanhung Lee, MD, PhD
Professor
Department of Anesthesia and Perioperative Care
University of California San Francisco
San Francisco, California

Matthieu Legrand, MD, PhD
Professor
Department of Anesthesia and Perioperative Care
University of California San Francisco
San Francisco, California

Brian P. Lemkuil, MD
Professor
Department of Anesthesiology
University of California San Diego
San Diego, California

Cynthia A. Lien, MD
Professor
Department of Anesthesiology
Medical College of Wisconsin
Milwaukee, Wisconsin

Maytinee Lilaonitkul, MBBS, MRCP, FRCA
Associate Professor
Department of Anesthesia and Perioperative Care
University of California San Francisco
San Francisco, California

Meng-Chen Vanessa Lin, DO
Acting Assistant Professor
Department of Anesthesiology and Pain Medicine
University of Washington
Seattle, Washington

Linda L. Liu, MD
Professor
Department of Anesthesia and Perioperative Care
University of California San Francisco
San Francisco, California

Alan J.R. Macfarlane, BSc (Hons), MBChB, MRCP, FRCA, EDRA
Consultant Anaesthetist
Department of Anaesthesia
Glasgow Royal Infirmary
Honorary Professor
Department of Anaesthesia, Critical Care and Pain Medicine
University of Glasgow
Glasgow, United Kingdom

Genevieve Manahan, MD
Assistant Professor
Department of Anesthesia and Perioperative Care
University of California San Francisco
San Francisco, California

Solmaz Poorsattar Manuel, MD
Associate Professor
Department of Anesthesia and Perioperative Care
University of California San Francisco
San Francisco, California

Mitchell H. Marshall, MD, FASA
Professor
Department of Anesthesiology, Perioperative Care, and Pain Medicine
NYU Grossman School of Medicine
New York, New York

Dylan Masters, MD
Assistant Professor
Department of Anesthesia and Perioperative Care
University of California San Francisco
San Francisco, California

Nathalia Mavignier, MD
Research Scholar
Department of Anesthesia and Perioperative Care
University of California San Francisco
San Francisco, California

Mary Ellen McCann, MD, MPH
Senior Associate in Anesthesia
Department of Anesthesiology, Critical Care and Pain Medicine
Boston Children's Hospital
Associate Professor of Anaesthesia
Department of Anaesthesia
Harvard Medical School
Boston, Massachusetts

Grace C. McCarthy, MD
Assistant Professor
Department of Anesthesiology
Duke University Health System
Durham, North Carolina
Staff Anesthesiologist
Veterans Affairs Health System
Durham, North Carolina

Matthew D. McEvoy, MD
Professor of Anesthesiology and Surgery
Vice Chair for Perioperative Medicine
Department of Anesthesiology
Vanderbilt University Medical Center
Nashville, Tennessee

Nicholas V. Mendez, MD
Assistant Professor
Department of Anesthesia and Perioperative Care
University of California San Francisco
San Francisco, California

Ilan Mizrahi, MD
Instructor
Department of Anaesthesia
Harvard Medical School
Anesthetist
Department of Anesthesia, Critical Care, and Pain Medicine
Massachusetts General Hospital
Boston, Massachusetts

Howard D. Palte, MBChB, FCA(SA)
Professor
Department of Anesthesiology
University of Miami
Miami, Florida

Anup Pamnani, MD
Assistant Professor
Department of Anesthesiology
Weill Cornell Medical College
New York, New York

Ameya Pappu, MBBS, DNB
Clinical Fellow
Department of Anesthesia and Pain Management
Toronto Western Hospital, University of Toronto
Toronto, Ontario

Manuel C. Pardo Jr., MD
Professor and Vice Chair for Education
Department of Anesthesia and Perioperative Care
University of California San Francisco
San Francisco, California

Piyush Patel, MD
Professor
Department of Anesthesiology
University of California San Diego
Chief, Anesthesia Service
Jennifer Moreno VA Medical Center San Diego
San Diego, California

Sophia Poorsattar, MD
Assistant Professor
Department of Anesthesiology and Perioperative Medicine
University of California Los Angeles
Los Angeles, California

Amreen Savanna Rahman, MD
Assistant Professor
Department of Anesthesia and Perioperative Care
University of California San Francisco
San Francisco, California

Mark D. Rollins, MD, PhD
Professor
Department of Anesthesiology and Perioperative Medicine
Mayo Clinic
Rochester, Minnesota

Andrew D. Rosenberg, MD
Professor and Dorothy Reaves Spatz MD Chair
Department of Anesthesiology, Perioperative Care and Pain Medicine
NYU Grossman School of Medicine
New York, New York

Elliot S. Schwartz, MD
Assistant Professor
Department of Anesthesiology
Cedars-Sinai Medical Center
Los Angeles, California

Lorraine M. Sdrales, MD
Associate Professor and Vice Chair
Department of Anesthesiology
Cedars-Sinai Medical Center
Los Angeles, California

Alper Sen, MD
Research Associate
Department of Anesthesiology
The University of Utah
Salt Lake City, Utah

David Shimabukuro, MDCM
Professor
Department of Anesthesia and Perioperative Care
University of California San Francisco
San Francisco, California

Mandeep Singh, MBBS, MD, MSc, FRCPC
Associate Professor
Department of Anesthesiology and Pain Medicine
University of Toronto
Toronto, Ontario, Canada

Jina Lee Sinskey, MD, FASA
Associate Professor
Department of Anesthesia and Perioperative Care
University of California San Francisco
San Francisco, California

Peter Douglas Slinger, MD, FRCPC
Professor
Department of Anesthesia
University of Toronto
Toronto, Ontario, Canada

Sulpicio G. Soriano, MD
Professor
Department of Anaesthesia
Harvard Medical School
Endowed Chair in Pediatric Neuroanesthesia
Anesthesiology, Perioperative and Pain Medicine
Boston Children's Hospital
Boston, Massachusetts

Randolph H. Steadman, MD, MS
Carole Walter Looke Centennial Chair
Department of Anesthesiology and Critical Care
Houston Methodist Hospital
Houston, Texas

Erica J. Stein, MD
Professor
Department of Anesthesiology
The Ohio State University
Columbus, Ohio

Marc P. Steurer, MD, MHA, FASA, DESA
Professor and Associate Chair
Department of Anesthesia and Perioperative Care
University of California San Francisco
San Francisco, California

Kristina R. Sullivan, MD
Professor and Associate Chair for Education
Department of Anesthesia and Perioperative Care
University of California San Francisco
San Francisco, California

Gina Heyue Sun, MD
Fellow, Critical Care Medicine
Department of Anesthesia and Perioperative Care
University of California San Francisco
San Francisco, California

James Szocik, MD
Associate Professor
Department of Anesthesiology
University of Michigan
Ann Arbor, Michigan

Kevin K. Tremper, PhD, MD
Professor
Department of Anesthesiology
University of Michigan
Ann Arbor, Michigan

Christine Warrick, MD
Associate Professor
Department of Anesthesiology
University of Utah
Salt Lake City, Utah

Stephen D. Weston, MD
Associate Professor
Department of Anesthesia and Perioperative Care
University of California San Francisco
San Francisco, California

Victor W. Xia, MD
Professor
Department of Anesthesiology
University of California Los Angeles
Los Angeles, California

Edward Yap, MD
Senior Physician
Department of Anesthesia
The Permanente Medical Group
San Francisco, California
Volunteer Assistant Professor
Department of Anesthesia and Perioperative Care
University of California San Francisco
San Francisco, California

Albert Yen, MD
Assistant Professor
Department of Anesthesia and Perioperative Care
University of California San Francisco
San Francisco, California

PREFACE

The first edition of *Miller's Anesthesia Review* was published in 2001 to fulfill the need for a question-and-answer style review of basic anesthesia principles. The goal was a book that would allow anesthesia learners at every level to participate actively in their own learning.

This fourth edition of *Miller's Anesthesia Review* is a companion book to the eighth edition of *Miller's Basics of Anesthesia*. The two books have matching chapters and are organized in a logical progression from basic anesthesia principles and concepts to more complex issues. In most chapters, the author is the same for the corresponding chapters in *Miller's Basics of Anesthesia* and *Miller's Anesthesia Review*. This is the first edition of *Miller's Anesthesia Review* without Dr. Ronald D. Miller as a co-editor. Dr. Sdrales was honored to collaborate with Dr. Miller on prior editions and welcomes Dr. Manuel C. Pardo, Jr. (the current editor of *Miller's Basics of Anesthesia*) as a co-editor.

This edition of *Miller's Anesthesia Review* features a new style and format. Each chapter begins with a bulleted, outline-style summary that is designed for efficient information transfer. After the outline, a series of questions-and-answers follow, designed to enhance recall and understanding of the key concepts. Question styles include short-answer essays, entering information in a table, or annotating graphics-based information. Page number references are provided at the end of each answer, referring the reader to the eighth edition of *Miller's Basics of Anesthesia*, where further information on the given topic can be found.

As with *Miller's Basics of Anesthesia*, this edition of *Miller's Anesthesia Review* has added four new chapters that reflect the expanding practice of anesthesia: Clinician Well-Being, Perioperative Point-of-Care Ultrasound, Environmental Impact of Anesthetics, and Perioperative Medicine. The remaining chapters have been extensively edited to challenge the reader and to provide up-to-date information on evolving concepts in anesthesia.

There are several ways this study guide can be used. Early anesthesia learners may use it for self-study to solidify information previously read. Anesthesia learners at every level may use it to prepare for specific clinical situations that they may face on a subspecialty rotation or with given cases on a particular day. *Miller's Anesthesia Review* can serve as a study guide for group study in which learners are required to answer questions on specific topics. Similarly, faculty may use the study guide to quiz learners verbally in a coherent, progressive manner in formal or informal settings. Finally, anesthesia providers in practice may find the study guide useful to refresh their knowledge base and to review information and concepts that have evolved since their training. Our intention is that *Miller's Anesthesia Review* will facilitate the learning and retention of current fundamental anesthesia concepts necessary for a solid knowledge base and clinical competence.

We are thankful to the authors of the current and previous editions of *Anesthesia Review*. We also acknowledge Elsevier, our publisher, and their staff. Special thanks to Executive Content Strategist, Kayla Wolfe, Senior Content Development Specialist, Ann Ruzycka Anderson, and Project Manager, Nayagi Anandan.

Lorraine M. Sdrales
Manuel C. Pardo, Jr.

CONTENTS

Chapter

1 SCOPE OF ANESTHESIA PRACTICE

Manuel C. Pardo, Jr.

INTRODUCTION

- Surgery without anesthesia was a painful, dangerous experience, limiting the types of surgery that could be performed
- Requirements for advances in surgery
  - Improved ability to relieve pain during the procedure
  - Ability to manage physiologic changes during and after surgery
- 19th century – discovery of ether as a general anesthetic
- Initial scope of anesthesia practice limited to the operating room
- Specialty advanced beyond the surgical suite to encompass the entire course of perioperative care

ANESTHESIOLOGY AS A MULTIDISCIPLINARY SPECIALTY

- In the US, formal specialty certification of anesthesiologists offered by the American Board of Anesthesiology (ABA)
- ABA also offers subspecialty certification
  - Critical care medicine
  - Pain medicine
  - Hospice and palliative medicine
  - Sleep medicine
  - Pediatric anesthesiology
  - Neurocritical care
  - Adult cardiac anesthesiology
- American Society of Anesthesiologists (ASA) is the largest professional society for anesthesiologists
  - More than 100 committees and editorial boards dedicated to all anesthesia subspecialties and aspects of anesthesia practice
- Many additional anesthesiology professional societies reflect the multidisciplinary nature of the field

PERIOPERATIVE PATIENT CARE

- Scope of hospital-based anesthesia care includes
  - Preoperative unit
  - Regional anesthesia service
  - Postanesthesia care unit
  - Operating room
  - Nonoperating room location
  - Intensive care unit
  - Hospital ward–based services
    - Acute pain service
    - Perioperative medicine service
    - Palliative care service
    - Point-of-care ultrasound service
- Outpatient anesthesia care includes
  - Ambulatory surgery center
  - Preoperative evaluation clinic
  - Pain medicine clinic

ANESTHESIA WORKFORCE

- US anesthesia workforce
  - Physician anesthesiologists
  - Certified registered nurse anesthetists (CRNAs)
  - Certified anesthesiologist assistants (CAAs)
    - Can practice in 18 US jurisdictions
- States have different requirements for scope of practice and supervision
- US anesthesia workforce challenges
  - Expanded breadth of anesthesia services
  - Demand for anesthesia service exceeds supply.
    - Increased population growth
    - Aging of population
  - Only modest growth in number of anesthesia providers
- Changes in anesthesia practice models
  - Consolidation of community practices
  - Acquisition of smaller practices into regional and national anesthesia or multispecialty groups
  - Physicians becoming employees of a hospital or medical foundation
- Transition to value-based care

TRAINING AND CERTIFICATION IN ANESTHESIOLOGY

- US physician anesthesiologists
  - Bachelor's degree
  - Doctor of Medicine or Doctor of Osteopathy degree
  - 4 Years of supervised residency experience
    - Year 1: fundamental clinical skills of medicine
    - Years 2–4: clinical anesthesia training including required subspecialty rotations in obstetric anesthesia, pediatric anesthesia, cardiothoracic anesthesia, neuroanesthesia, preoperative medicine, postanesthesia care, regional anesthesia and pain management, critical care medicine
- CRNAs
  - Bachelor's degree
  - Registration as professional nurse in US or its territories
  - Minimum 1-year full-time equivalent experience as critical care registered nurse
  - By 1998, all accredited nurse anesthesia programs offered master's-level education, minimum 24 months of full-time study
  - After 2022, all accredited programs were required to offer doctoral degrees, typically minimum 36 months of full-time study
- Anesthesia assistants
  - Bachelor's degree
  - Premedical course work
  - 27 months of master's-level education in accredited program

QUALITY AND SAFETY

- Clinical anesthesia practice recognized as a model for quality and safety in medicine
- ASA develops and implements standards, practice guidelines, practice advisories, and alerts
- Anesthesia Patient Safety Foundation (APSF) publishes APSF Newsletter dedicated to safety issues

VALUE-BASED CARE

- US health care spending represents 19.7% of gross domestic product.
- Alternative payment models designed to incentivize value
  - Value defined as outcome (or quality) divided by cost
  - Institute of Medicine quality domains: safety, efficacy, patient-centered, timely, efficient, equitable
  - Value-based payment model: compensation based on outcomes (merit-based) rather than specific services provided
- Enhanced recovery after surgery (ERAS)
  - Perioperative care protocols designed to optimize care
  - Designed around specific types of surgery (e.g., colorectal, arthroplasty, hepatobiliary)
  - Goal to reduce complications, costs, length of stay
- Perioperative surgical home model
  - Coordinated system of perioperative care, with physician-led interdisciplinary team
  - Centered on patient experience, including tracking and improving patient outcomes, decreasing costs, increasing provider satisfaction

FUTURE OF ANESTHESIA CARE

- Advances in clinical management and new drugs and technologies have transformed clinical practice.
- Future will require
  - New models of care with expanded scope of practice
  - Identification of opportunities to improve quality and safety across the entire continuum of care
  - Improved access to care and addressing health care disparities

Clinical Pearls – APSF Perioperative Patient Safety Priorities

1. Culture of safety
2. Teamwork
3. Clinical deterioration
4. Nonoperating room anesthesia
5. Perioperative brain health
6. Opioid-related harm
7. Medication safety
8. Infectious diseases
9. Clinician safety
10. Airway management

QUESTIONS

INTRODUCTION

1. When was ether first used successfully as an anesthetic agent?

PERIOPERATIVE PATIENT CARE

2. How has the scope of anesthesia practice evolved in the past 10–15 years?
3. What roles can anesthesiologists play in health system leadership?

ANESTHESIA WORKFORCE

4. What is the anesthesia care team model in the US?
5. What are the causes of current workforce challenges in anesthesiology?

TRAINING AND CERTIFICATION IN ANESTHESIOLOGY

6. What certification pathways are available to different anesthesia providers in the US after their training is complete?

VALUE-BASED CARE

7. What is the Medicare Merit-based Incentive Payment System (MIPS)?
8. How can a patient's episode of surgical care be used to improve their health beyond the surgical condition?

ANSWERS

INTRODUCTION

1. The first use of a general anesthetic agent occurred in 1842 – the administration of ether by physician Crawford Long in Georgia. However, Dr. Long did not publish his experience until 1849. Dentist William T.G. Morton is credited with the first public demonstration of ether anesthesia administration on October 16, 1846, a date now called "Ether Day." (3)

PERIOPERATIVE PATIENT CARE

2. The scope of anesthesia practice has evolved to focus on improved patient outcomes and quality of care. Anesthesiologists have increased participation in perioperative patient evaluation and management, going beyond preoperative clinics to include the broader concept of perioperative medicine. Increased attention to postoperative outcomes has led to more collaboration between surgeons and anesthesiologists, resulting in the development of multidisciplinary enhanced recovery pathways and of care models such as the perioperative surgical home. (4)
3. In addition to department-specific roles, anesthesiologists are well positioned to assume leadership roles such as perioperative medical directors, chief quality officers, and other administrative positions related to perioperative care and health system management. (4)

ANESTHESIA WORKFORCE

4. The anesthesia care team is defined as care led by a physician anesthesiologist who directs or supervises care by qualified anesthesia personnel. Qualified anesthesia personnel include CRNAs, resident physicians or fellows, and CAAs. The care team practice model is the most common in most states. Other models include anesthesia care provided solely by physician anesthesiologists. In 22 states, governors have opted out of the Medicare requirement for physician supervision of nurse anesthetists, allowing independent CRNA practice. However, individual hospitals and health systems make the decisions regarding the practice of anesthesia. (6)
5. In the US, the demand for anesthesia service far exceeds the supply. While there is modest growth in the number of new anesthesia providers each year, the increasing demand for anesthesia care reflects population growth and aging of the population (largest growth in those aged 65 years or older). (6)

TRAINING AND CERTIFICATION IN ANESTHESIOLOGY

6. After completing an Accreditation Council for Graduate Medical Education (ACGME)-accredited residency program, anesthesia residents can obtain certification from the American Board of Anesthesiology (ABA) through a series of three exams. The BASIC exam can be taken at the end of postgraduate year (PGY)-2 (CA-1) year, whereas the ADVANCED and APPLIED exams can be taken after residency completion. The APPLIED exam includes a standardized oral examination and an objective structured clinical examination. Anesthesiologists who complete additional fellowship training after residency may be eligible for subspecialty certification by the ABA in one of seven areas. Graduates of accredited CRNA programs are eligible to take the National Certification Examination of the National Board of Certification and Recertification for Nurse Anesthetists. Graduates of accredited CAA programs are eligible for the Certifying Examination for Anesthesiologist Assistants. (7)

VALUE-BASED CARE

7. Medicare created the Quality Payment Program (QPP) in 2017 as a value-based payment program. One pathway, the MIPS, requires anesthesia practices to report quality measures that will result in payment adjustments based on performance. Payment adjustments can be neutral, negative, or positive. (8)

8. See below figure outlines an approach to consider the entire perioperative continuum of care as an opportunity to proactively improve health. This approach goes beyond use of the preoperative evaluation merely to gather information and includes the use of evidence-based approaches in all phases of care. (9)

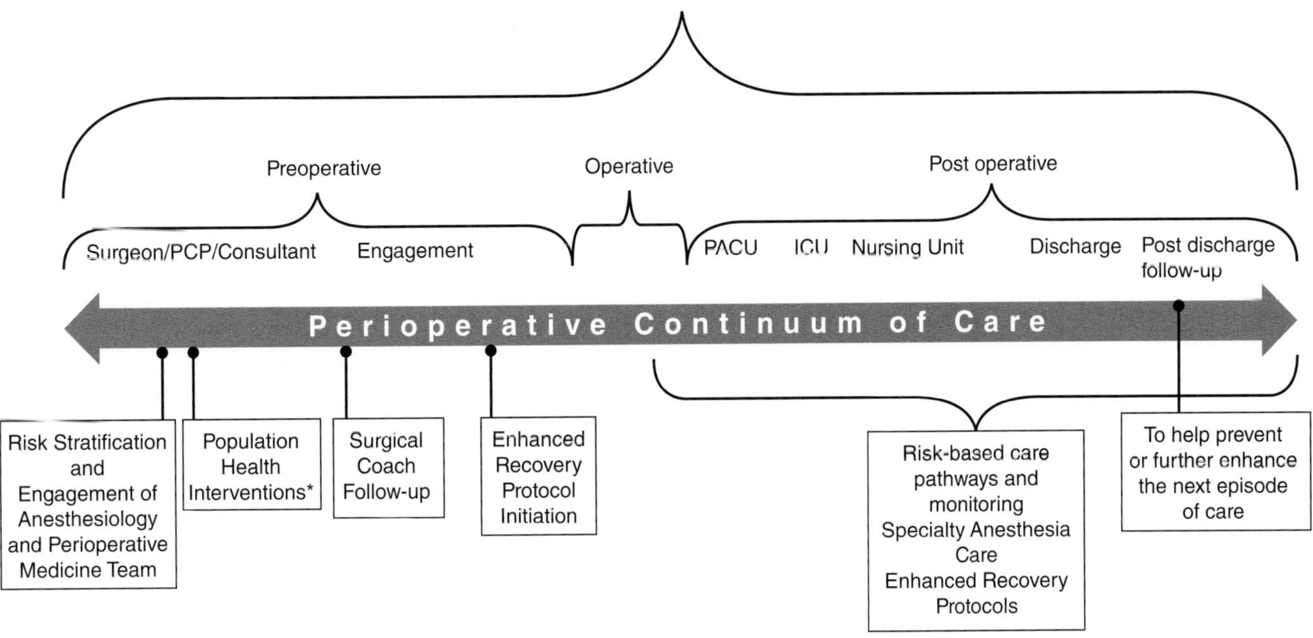

From Mahajan A, Esper SA, Cole DJ, et al. Anesthesiologists' role in value-based perioperative care and healthcare transformation. Anesthesiology. 2021;134[4]:526–540. COPD, chronic obstructive pulmonary disorder; ICU, intensive care unit; PACU, postanesthesia care unit; PCP, primary care physician.

Chapter

2 LEARNING ANESTHESIA

Kristina R. Sullivan and Manuel C. Pardo, Jr.

INTRODUCTION

- Challenges of learning perioperative anesthesia care
  - Increasing quantity of literature
  - Need for increased level of knowledge
  - Need for variety of patient care experiences throughout training
- In addition to clinical care, modalities used to facilitate learning include
  - Problem-based learning
  - E-learning (multiple types)
  - Hands-on task trainers
  - Mannequin-based patient simulation
  - Standardized patient sessions
- Aspects of anesthesia practice developed during training
  - Flexible patient care routines
  - Factual and theoretical knowledge
  - Manual/procedural skills
  - Ability to adapt to dynamic situations

COMPETENCIES, MILESTONES, AND ENTRUSTABLE PROFESSIONAL ACTIVITIES

- Accreditation Council for Graduate Medical Education (ACGME) six core competencies
  - Patient care
  - Medical knowledge
  - Professionalism
  - Interpersonal and communication skills
  - Systems-based practice
  - Practice-based learning and improvement
- Milestones
  - A framework of skill acquisition that includes
    - Description of expected behavior that progresses by levels
    - The complexity of the patient and surgical procedure
    - Level of supervision needed by the trainee
- Entrustable professional activities (EPAs)
  - Another approach to advance competency-based assessment
  - Task or responsibility that trainees are entrusted to perform without supervision once relevant competencies are attained

STRUCTURED APPROACH TO ANESTHESIA CARE

- Three phases of anesthesia care
  - Preoperative
    - Preoperative evaluation
    - Preparing the operating room (equipment, medications)
  - Intraoperative
    - General anesthesia, regional anesthesia, or monitored anesthesia care
  - Postoperative
    - Disposition (postanesthesia care unit [PACU], intensive care unit [ICU], ward, home)

Important Clinical Decisions in Each Phase of Anesthesia Care

Preoperative phase
- Choice of anesthesia based on preoperative evaluation and proposed surgery
  - Need for preoperative procedures to prepare for surgery (e.g., monitoring, regional block)
- Premedication

Intraoperative phase
- Type of anesthesia, including all medications and equipment required
- Whether additional monitors are needed
- What vascular access is required during surgery

Postoperative phase
- Immediate postoperative destination (PACU vs. ICU)
- Postoperative analgesia plan

LEARNING STRATEGIES

- Foundation of clinical training is supervised direct patient care.
- Other learning modalities
  - Independent reading

        - Basic textbooks
        - Selected portions of comprehensive textbooks
        - Review books
        - Anesthesia specialty journals
        - General medical journals
    - Lectures (in-person or virtual)
    - Simulations
        - Task-based simulators
            - Laryngoscopy and tracheal intubation
            - Fiberoptic tracheal intubation and bronchoscopy
            - Intravenous (IV) catheter placement
            - Point-of-care ultrasound trainer (e.g., for regional blocks, echocardiography)
        - Mannequin-based crisis management scenarios
    - Web-based resources
        - Online learning modules
        - Podcasts and videocasts

Learning Orientation

- Performance orientation
    - Trainee with a goal of validating their abilities
- Learning orientation
    - Trainee with a goal of increasing mastery
- Growth mindset theory
    - Orientation to learning is influenced by an individual's beliefs about their intelligence and abilities
    - Growth mindset features
        - Belief that intelligence and abilities are not fixed and can be developed
        - Embracing challenges
        - Viewing effort as necessary for success
        - Considering feedback as important for ongoing learning

Cognitive Load

- Cognitive load theory
    - New information must be processed by the working memory, which has limited capacity.
    - Working memory faces three types of cognitive load:
        - Intrinsic load
            - The load associated with the task itself
            - Related to the degree of difficulty of the material and the expertise of the person processing the information
        - Extraneous load
            - Load imposed that is not necessary to learning the information
        - Germane load
            - Load imposed by the learner's use of strategies to organize and process information
            - May be viewed as a learner's level of concentration devoted to learning

QUESTIONS

COMPETENCIES, MILESTONES, AND ENTRUSTABLE PROFESSIONAL ACTIVITIES

1. What is a "milestone" in the context of skill acquisition in learning anesthesia? Contrast the Level 1 and Level 4 anesthesia resident milestones for patient care competency in perioperative care and management in the table.

	Level 1	Level 4
Anesthesia plan		
Pain management plan		
Impact of anesthesia beyond perioperative period		

2. What is an entrustable professional activity (EPA)? For the EPA listed below, describe the competencies involved, milestones addressed, and potential entrustment decisions.

Task	Induction of anesthesia for a fasted ASA 2 patient without a known difficult airway
Competencies involved	
Milestones addressed	
Entrustment decisions	

STRUCTURED APPROACH TO ANESTHESIA CARE

3. When managing an intraoperative anesthetic, what information influences clinical decisions for changes in management? How are intraoperative decisions made?

LEARNING STRATEGIES

4. What is the "flipped classroom" teaching method?
5. Describe some learning goals that could be set for a beginning anesthesia learner scheduled to care for an adult who will undergo laparoscopic appendectomy for ruptured appendicitis.
6. What is the growth mindset theory? What are the potential benefits of this mindset?
7. What is the cognitive load theory? How can instructors facilitate learning using this theory?

ANSWERS

COMPETENCIES, MILESTONES, AND ENTRUSTABLE PROFESSIONAL ACTIVITIES

1. A milestone is a description of clinical skills that includes a behavioral description, complexity of the patient or procedure, and level of supervision required. (11, 12)

	Level 1	Level 4
Anesthesia plan	Identifies the components of an anesthesia plan	Develops an anesthesia plan for patients with multiple, uncontrolled comorbidities who is undergoing complicated procedures
Pain management plan	Identifies the components of a pain management plan	Implements the anesthesia plan for patients with complex pain history and polypharmacy
Impact of anesthesia beyond the perioperative period	Identifies the potential impact of anesthesia beyond intraoperative period	Implements the anesthesia plan to mitigate the long-term impact of anesthesia

2. An entrustable professional activity (EPA) is a clinical task or responsibility that trainees are entrusted to perform without supervision once relevant competencies are attained. (12)

Task	Induction of anesthesia for a fasted ASA 2 patient without a known difficult airway
Competencies involved	Medical knowledge, patient care, interpersonal and communication skills
Milestones addressed	Perioperative care and management, application and interpretation of monitors, intraoperative care, airway management
Entrustment decisions	Performed by supervisor and observed by trainee, direct supervision (supervisor talked trainee through activity), reactive supervision (supervisor directed trainee from time to time), supervisor available if needed, performed independently by trainee

STRUCTURED APPROACH TO ANESTHESIA CARE

3. The information streams used to make intraoperative decisions include observing the surgical field, physiological monitors, and communications with the surgical and nursing teams. The cycle of mental activity includes observation, decision making, action, and repeated evaluation. The significance of each observation can change over the course of the procedure. See below figure depicts a model of the anesthesia professional's complex process of intraoperative decision making. (14, 15)

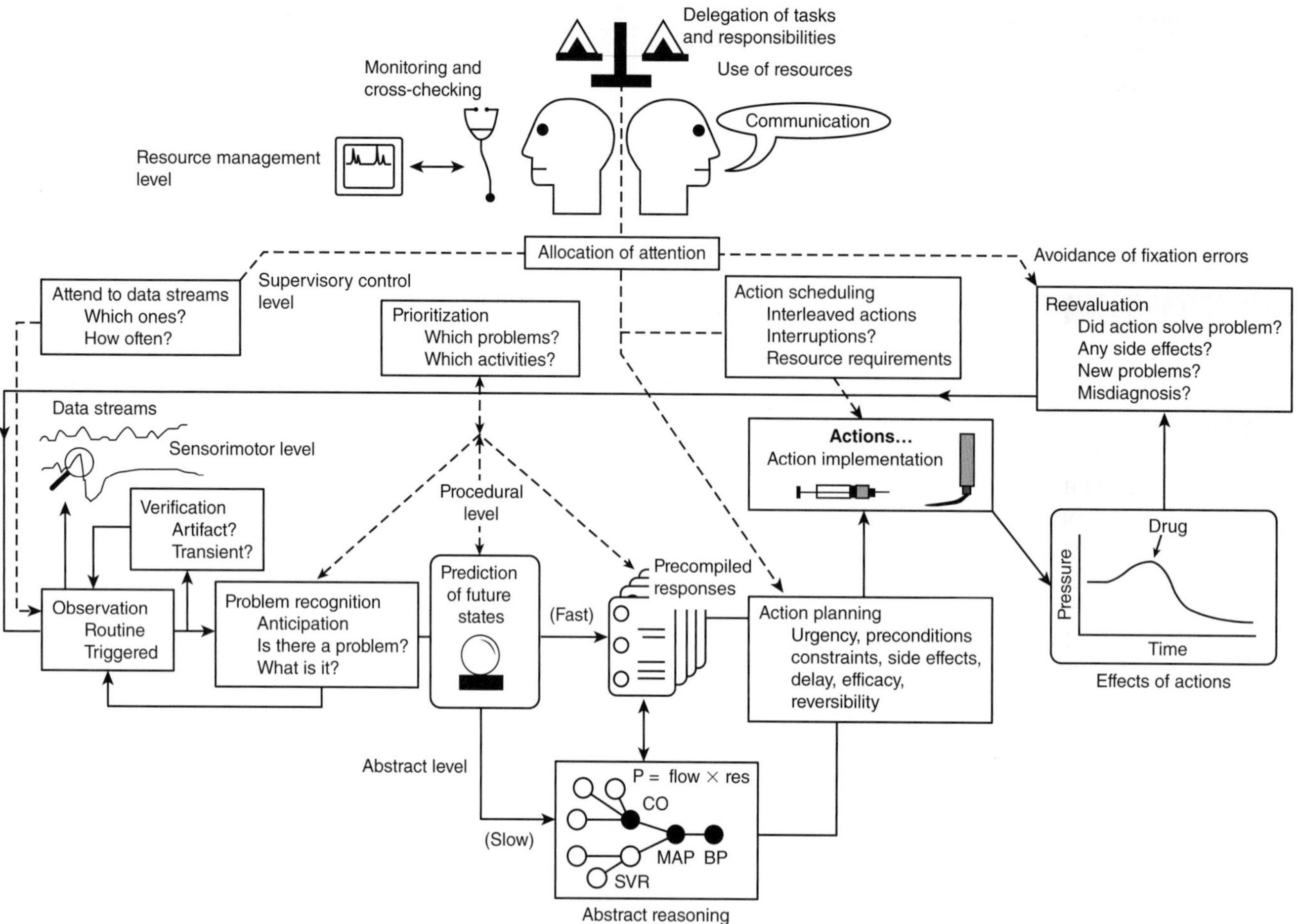

The primary loop (heavy black arrows) of observation, decision, action, and reevaluation is controlled by higher levels of supervisory control (allocation of attention) and resource management. BP, blood pressure; CO, cardiac output; MAP, mean arterial pressure; P, pressure; res, resistance; SVR, systemic vascular resistance. From Gaba DM, Fish KJ, Howard SK, et al. Crisis Management in Anesthesiology, 2nd ed. Philadephia: Saunders; 2014.

LEARNING STRATEGIES

4. The flipped classroom method involves a preassigned learning activity before an in-person or synchronous group discussion. A common approach is to assign learners a web-based resource to review before an in-class active learning session based on its content. (15)
5. Learning goals for a new anesthesia learner could be related to procedural tasks required for patient care, such as IV placement or airway management. Cognitive goals could include understanding the clinical presentation of complications during laparoscopic surgery such as CO_2 embolism or the potential complications of appendicitis such as peritonitis and sepsis. (16)
6. The key belief of the growth mindset is that people can develop their abilities. Growth mindset theory has been most thoroughly studied in primary and secondary schools. Individuals with a growth mindset focus on mastery of their learning goals rather than on their performance. Other features of a growth mindset include embracing challenges and viewing effort as necessary for success. Potential benefits include helping health professional students be more receptive to feedback, supporting the relationship between learners and educators. (16)
7. Cognitive load theory suggests that new information must be processed by the working memory, which has limited capacity. Using this theory, instructors have several ways to facilitate learning. One approach is to teach at the level and expertise of the learner, thereby decreasing intrinsic load. Another approach is to remove content or other interruptions that are not pertinent to the task, decreasing extraneous load. A third approach is to encourage strategies that allow for processing of information in an efficient manner, optimizing germane load. (17)

Chapter

3 CLINICIAN WELL-BEING

Jina Lee Sinskey and Laura K. Berenstain

INTRODUCTION

- Clinician well-being is a critical issue due to widespread clinician burnout.
  - Requires a combination of individual strategies and systems-level solutions
- Interventions to prevent burnout are more effective than those that address burnout after it has occurred.

DEFINING TERMS

Burnout

- Definition: an occupational phenomenon rather than an individual mental health diagnosis (WHO ICD-11)
  - Three key dimensions of burnout: emotional exhaustion, depersonalization, and a diminished sense of personal accomplishment
- Burnout rates in U.S. anesthesiologists and anesthesiology trainees: 51% to 59%
- Negative consequences of burnout: patient care, clinician workforce and healthcare system costs, clinicians' own health and safety

Resilience

- Definition: ability of both individuals and social groups to withstand, adapt, recover, or even grow from adversity, stress, or trauma
- Resilience is a continuous, dynamic state that can be nurtured and trained.

Moral Injury

- Definition: lasting negative effects on an individual's conscience or moral compass when that person perpetrates, fails to prevent, or witnesses acts that transgress one's own deeply held moral beliefs and expectations
- Moral injury in medicine: distress that clinicians experience when they are unable to provide high-quality patient care due to factors beyond their control

Well-Being

- Definition: presence of positive emotions, absence of negative emotions, satisfaction with life, fulfillment, engagement, and positive functioning
  - Well-being is not simply the absence of burnout.
- Eight dimensions of well-being
  - External: social, occupational, financial, environmental
  - Internal: emotional, spiritual, intellectual, physical
- Drivers of clinician well-being can be organized into a hierarchy of needs: basics, safety, respect, appreciation, heal patients, and contribute.

WHY WELL-BEING IS IMPORTANT

- Burnout among physicians is significantly higher than among other U.S. workers even after adjustments for work hours, age, and gender.
  - Perfectionism, self-doubt, inability to delegate, and high levels of commitment can contribute to emotional exhaustion.
  - Maslach suggested the best workers are more predisposed to burnout.
- Chronic occupational stress is linked to neurobiological findings.
  - High levels of norepinephrine and dopamine are released in the brain with uncontrollable stress impairing higher-order functions.
  - Controllable stressors do not result in the same changes.
- Professionalism, teamwork, and patient safety suffer as a result of burnout.
  - Studies show a relationship between burnout and an increased incidence of self-perceived errors and suboptimal patient care.
- Physician turnover due to burnout has a negative financial impact on health care systems.
- The AMA has outlined five arguments for supporting well-being: moral and ethical, business, recognition, regulatory, and tragedy.

FACTORS AFFECTING CLINICIAN WELL-BEING

Individual Factors

- Factors unique to anesthesiology have been shown to result in a higher risk for burnout than in other specialties.
- A 2021 survey of American Society of Anesthesiologists (ASA) members showed 59% at high risk of burnout.
- Physicians have a lower rate of satisfaction with work–life integration than the general U.S. working population.
- Self-valuation accounts for differences in rates of burnout between male and female physicians.

Organizational Level

- Importance of a supportive work environment
  - Perceived lack of support at work is strongly associated with a high risk for burnout in attending anesthesiologists.
- Areas of worklife model
  - Provides an organizational context of burnout
  - Six areas of worklife: workload, control, reward, community, fairness, values
  - The degree of mismatch existing in these six areas is predictive of burnout.
- Importance of culture
  - The culture of medical training often drives clinicians toward the initial stages of burnout by encouraging certain behaviors.
  - Organizational culture can affect factors perceived to be individual in nature (e.g., work–life integration).

Societal Level

- National Academy of Medicine goals for eliminating clinician burnout and enhancing professional well-being
  - Create positive work environments
  - Create positive learning environments
  - Reduce administrative burden
  - Enable technology solutions
  - Provide support to clinicians and learners
  - Invest in research
- Clinicians are reluctant to seek help for mental health conditions.
  - Mental health–related stigma and structural issues can affect ability to practice medicine (e.g., medical licensure).
- The COVID-19 pandemic exacerbated existing clinician burnout.
- Need for inclusive environments to foster professional well-being in medicine
  - Must acknowledge and address that structural racism and health inequities exist in medicine and the medical community
  - Microaggressions: everyday slights, insults, putdowns, invalidations, and offensive behaviors experienced by members of a marginalized group
  - Microinterventions: can nurture an environment of diversity, equity, and inclusion by providing support and affirmation to individuals targeted by microaggressions

MENTAL HEALTH

Fatigue Mitigation

- Definition of fatigue: mental and physical exhaustion and tiredness
- Sleep-related impairment: associated with decreased professional fulfillment, increased burnout, increased self-reported medical errors
- Potential strategies for fatigue mitigation: scheduling interventions (e.g., 16-hour vs. 24-hour shifts), strategic naps, use of bright lights in clinical settings if feasible

Substance Use Disorders

- Substance use disorders are a serious issue in the anesthesia workplace with potentially devastating consequences.
- Unique risks of substance use disorders in the anesthesia workplace
  - Ease of access to venous cannulation equipment
  - Ease of access to potent drugs with abuse potential
  - Proficiency with intravenous cannulation and familiarity with potent drugs with abuse potential
- Incidence of substance use disorders in practicing anesthesiologists and anesthesiology residents: 1% to 2%
  - High risk of relapse in both groups
- Substance use disorders can prove fatal.
  - Nearly 20% of physicians with a substance use disorder died of a substance use disorder–related cause in a study of practicing anesthesiologists.
- Behavioral changes are seen in affected individuals.
- Treatment
  - Referral to an inpatient facility that specializes in the treatment of healthcare professionals
  - Includes detoxification, monitored abstinence, intensive education, exposure to self-help groups, and psychotherapy
- Reentry into clinical practice
  - Must be carefully planned with appropriate staging and monitoring to mitigate the risk of relapse

Depression

- Burnout is a process that can begin with exhaustion and end in despair.
- Burnout and major depressive disorder (MDD) can share symptoms of anhedonia, fatigue, impaired concentration, and changes in appetite and sleep.
    - Burnout is described as a workplace phenomenon.
    - MDD is a clinical disorder with diagnostic criteria defined by the American Psychiatric Association.
    - Distinction between the two is important to avoid delay in treating clinicians with MDD.
- Burnout, depression, and suicidal ideation are frequent among anesthesiology residents.
- Depression is linked to patient safety.
    - Physicians with depression are more likely to experience suboptimal functioning and report medical errors.

Suicide

- Physicians have the highest suicide rate of any profession.
    - Females physicians are at greater risk than male physicians.
- Risk factors
    - Fatigue
    - Isolation
    - Complaints of bullying
    - Aging
    - Perfectionism
    - Reluctance to seek help
- Physicians are more likely to commit suicide because of a job-related problem.
- The National Suicide Prevention Lifeline is available at 1-800-273-8255 (updated in 2020 to a three-digit nationwide number - 988).

INTERVENTIONS TO IMPROVE WELL-BEING

Personal Strategies

- Anesthesiology poses challenges to personal well-being and resiliency strategies.
    - Nutrition, hydration, exercise, and sleep are basic self-care cornerstones.
    - Resiliency-related factors include self-monitoring, setting limits, promotion of social engagement, and capacity for mindfulness.
    - "Best" resiliency strategies are unique to each person.
    - Success in developing resiliency is related to the sustainability of choices.
- Physicians with burnout often have difficulty being "present."
    - Physicians are often obsessed with the past or anxious about the future.
    - Mindfulness facilitates self-reflection and can decrease anxiety by promoting nonjudgmental awareness of the moment.
    - Mindfulness practices have been shown to reduce negative affect system activity in the amygdala.
- If we do not care for ourselves, we cannot effectively care for others.
    - Self-compassion is also associated with compassion toward others.

Systemic Approaches

- National approaches
    - The National Academy of Medicine (NAM) has put forth recommendations for addressing clinician well-being using a systems approach.
    - The ACGME includes well-being requirements for all accredited residency and fellowship programs.
    - The ASA website provides practical resources for clinician well-being.
- Peer support
    - Most anesthesia providers will be involved in a medical error or adverse event.
    - Common emotions: guilt, anxiety, reliving of the episode
    - The term "second victim" refers to health care professionals who are injured by the same errors as their patients who were harmed.
    - Trajectory of second victim: dropping out, surviving, or thriving
    - Peer support programs can provide social support after critical events.
- Well-being education can include small-group discussions and simulations.
    - A study of facilitated small-group discussions showed reduced depersonalization and increased meaning and engagement in work.
- Coaching is distinct from other workplace interventions.
    - Coaching is a relationship of equals that explores personal and professional issues.
    - It can be used for individual, leadership, or team enhancement.
    - A 6-month coaching study showed a 17% decreased in burnout in the intervention group and a 4% increase in the control group.
- Organizational structure to support well-being is encouraged by NAM.
- An integrative model for wellness-centered leadership was proposed in 2021 with three key elements.
    - Leaders care about people always, and leadership is transformational rather than transactional.

  - Cultivation of individual and team relationships
  - Inspire change through intrinsic motivators, values, and professional development

Policies to Support Well-Being

- The NAM Action Collaborative on Clinician Well-Being and Resilience seeks to elevate evidence-based multidisciplinary solutions for clinical well-being challenges.
- The Dr. Lorna Breen Health Care Provider Protection Act was passed in 2021.
  - The Secretary of Health and Human Services will establish evidence-based education and awareness campaigns encouraging health care professionals to seek support and treatment for mental health concerns.

Clinician Well-Being

- Efforts to enhance clinician well-being require a combination of individual strategies and systems-level solutions.
- Burnout is an occupational phenomenon rather than an individual mental health diagnosis (WHO ICD-11).
- Perfectionism, self-doubt, inability to delegate, and high levels of commitment can contribute to emotional exhaustion.
- Professionalism, teamwork, and patient safety suffer as a result of burnout.
- Perceived lack of support at work is strongly associated with a high risk for burnout in attending anesthesiologists.
- Factors unique to anesthesiology have been shown to result in a higher risk for burnout than in other specialties.
- National efforts to address clinician well-being include the NAM Action Collaborative on Clinician Well-Being and Resilience and the Dr. Lorna Breen Health Care Provider Protection Act.

QUESTIONS

DEFINING TERMS

1. In the following table, specify definitions of the following terms related to clinician well-being.

Term	Definition
Burnout	
Resilience	
Moral injury	
Well-being	

WHY WELL-BEING IS IMPORTANT

2. What personal characteristics in physicians contribute to burnout?
3. What are the negative consequences of physician burnout?

FACTORS AFFECTING CLINICIAN WELL-BEING

4. What factors have been independently associated with lower work–life integration scores?
5. What factors are associated with a lower risk of burnout in anesthesiology trainees?
6. The National Academy of Medicine has advocated for a systems approach to clinician well-being. List the National Academy of Medicine's six goals for Eliminating Clinician Burnout and Enhancing Professional Well-Being.

MENTAL HEALTH

7. List behavioral changes described in anesthesiologists with substance use disorders.
8. How do burnout and major depressive disorder differ?

INTERVENTIONS TO IMPROVE WELL-BEING

9. In the following table, list personal strategies, systemic approaches, and policies to support and enhance clinician well-being.

Personal strategies	
Systemic approaches	
Policies to support well-being	

10. Most anesthesia providers will be involved in a medical error or adverse event during their career. Define the term "second victim" and three paths for second victims.

ANSWERS

INTRODUCTION

1. The following table includes definitions of commonly used clinician well-being terms. (18–19)

Term	Definition
Burnout	An occupational phenomenon rather than an individual mental health diagnosis Three key dimensions of burnout: emotional exhaustion, depersonalization, and a diminished sense of personal accomplishment
Resilience	Ability of both individuals and social groups to withstand, adapt, recover, or even grow from adversity, stress, or trauma
Moral injury	Lasting negative effects on an individual's conscience or moral compass when that person perpetrates, fails to prevent, or witnesses acts that transgress one's own deeply held moral beliefs and expectations
Well-being	Presence of positive emotions, absence of negative emotions, satisfaction with life, fulfillment, engagement, and positive functioning Well-being is not simply the absence of burnout

WHY WELL-BEING IS IMPORTANT

2. Perfectionism, self-doubt, inability to delegate, and high levels of commitment are personal characteristics in physicians that contribute to burnout. (19)
3. Professionalism, teamwork, and patient safety can all suffer as a result of burnout. Health systems suffer negative financial consequences as a result of physician turnover. (19)

FACTORS AFFECTING CLINICIAN WELL-BEING

4. Female gender, age between 35 and 44 years, working more hours/week, and certain medical specialties including anesthesiology are independently associated with lower work–life integration scores. (22)
5. A survey of anesthesiology trainees found that factors associated with a lower risk of burnout include perceived workplace resource availability, perceived ability to maintain work-life balance, and having a strong social support system. (22)
6. The National Academy of Medicine's six goals for Eliminating Clinician Burnout and Enhancing Professional Well-Being include: (1) create positive work environments, (2) create positive learning environments, (3) reduce administrative burden, (4) enable technology solutions, (5) provide support to clinicians and learners, (6) invest in research. (23)

MENTAL HEALTH

7. Behavioral changes described in affected anesthesiologists include withdrawal from family and friends, mood swings, increased episodes of anger, irritability, and hostility, spending more time at the hospital (even when off duty), volunteering for extra call, refusing relief for lunch or coffee breaks, requesting frequent bathroom breaks, and signing out increasing amounts of opioids or quantities inappropriate for the given case. (23–24)
8. Although they can share symptoms of anhedonia, fatigue, impaired concentration, fatigue, and changes in appetite and sleep, burnout is defined as a workplace phenomenon. Major depressive disorder is a clinical disorder with diagnostic criteria published by the American Psychiatric Association. (24)

INTERVENTIONS TO IMPROVE WELL-BEING

9. Clinician well-being requires interventions on multiple levels. The following table describes personal strategies, systemic approaches, and policies to support and enhance clinician well-being. (23–26)

Personal strategies	Self-care: nutrition, hydration, exercise, and sleep are basic self-care cornerstones Resiliency-related factors: self-monitoring, setting limits, promotion of social engagement, and capacity for mindfulness Self-compassion
Systemic approaches	National approaches: National Academy of Medicine, ACGME, and ASA Peer support, well-being education, coaching, wellness-centered leadership
Policies to support well-being	The NAM Action Collaborative on Clinician Well-Being and Resilience, the Dr. Lorna Breen Health Care Provider Protection Act

10. The term "second victim" refers to health care professionals who are injured by the same errors as their patients who are harmed. Second victims tend to migrate toward one of three paths: dropping out, surviving, or thriving. Many institutions have formal peer support programs in place to provide social support after critical events, and peer support can and should also be made available outside of specific critical events. (25)

Chapter

4 BASIC PHARMACOLOGIC PRINCIPLES

Jennifer DeCou, Alper Sen, and Ken B. Johnson

INTRODUCTION

Overview of Pharmacokinetic and Pharmacodynamic Concepts
Pharmacokinetic concepts ▪ Volumes of distribution ▪ Drug clearance ▪ Transfer of drugs between plasma and tissues ▪ Binding of drugs to circulating plasma proteins ▪ Physiologic processes that determine pharmacokinetics ▪ Mathematical models used to relate dose to concentration Pharmacodynamic concepts ▪ The concentration–drug effect relationship ▪ Drug–drug interactions

PHARMACOKINETIC PRINCIPLES

- *Pharmacokinetics* describes the relationship between drug dose and drug concentration in plasma or at the site of drug effect over time.
  - "What the body does to the drug"
  - Governed by absorption, distribution, and elimination (metabolism and excretion)
- Intravenously (IV) administered drugs
  - Absorption is not relevant.
  - Time course of the drug is a function of distribution volume and clearance.
- Measured plasma drug concentrations over time
  - Mathematical formulas are applied.
  - Used to create pharmacokinetic parameters

Fundamental Pharmacokinetic Concepts

Volume of Distribution

- *Distribution volume* is the volume within which a drug distributes throughout blood and peripheral tissues.
  - Estimated using the relationship between dose and concentration
  - Concentration (mg/L) = dose (mg) ÷ volume of distribution (L)
  - Distribution volumes are intrinsic to a person, regardless of the drug.
- *Clearance* is the fraction of the distribution volume cleared of drug over time.
  - It is a constant.
  - Described in units of flow (L/min)
  - Begins as soon as a drug is injected into the body
  - Estimates for distribution volume must consider concomitant clearance.
- *Elimination* describes the rate of drug removal from the body.
  - It is not constant.
  - Described in units of drug per time (mg/min)
  - Elimination = clearance × plasma drug concentration
- Central and peripheral volumes of distribution after IV administration
  - Central volume refers to plasma volume.
  - Peripheral volume is tissue volume.
    - Size of peripheral volume represents the drug's solubility in tissue.
    - The more soluble a drug is in tissue, the larger the peripheral volume of distribution.
- Binding of drugs to proteins in blood and peripheral tissues
  - Further increases the volume of distribution
  - Total volume of distribution can be larger than central + tissue volume.
  - Example: fentanyl has an apparent distribution volume of 4 L/kg
- Volume of distribution is not constant over time.
  - Initially may be only the central volume before distributing to peripheral tissues
  - Rate of drug movement to various tissues is modeled with rate constants.

- Peripheral tissue distribution versus elimination after drug administration
  - Initially, drug movement into peripheral tissues can exceed the amount eliminated.
  - Later, the drug amount eliminated can exceed the amount in the peripheral tissues.
  - Example: IV propofol bolus
    - 0 to 4 minutes: distribution to peripheral tissues exceeds elimination
    - After 4 minutes: elimination exceeds distribution to peripheral tissues

Clearance

- Clearance describes the rate of drug removal from the plasma.
  - Described in units of volume per time (L/min)
  - Two processes: systemic and intercompartmental
- Systemic clearance
  - Permanently removes drug from the body
  - Elimination of parent molecule or transformation into metabolites
- Intercompartmental clearance
  - Moves drug between plasma and peripheral tissue
- Clearance provides a single number to describe the decay in drug concentration.
  - Is dependent on the elimination rate and concentration at a given time
  - Can be estimated by the equation Clearance = Q × ER
    - Q = organ blood flow
    - ER = extraction ratio of the drug
- Total clearance is the sum of clearance by each of the metabolic organs (e.g., kidneys, liver, and other tissues).

Examples of Hepatic Clearance: Propofol vs. Alfentanil

Propofol
- Extraction ratio is nearly 1.
- Liver has tremendous metabolic capacity for the drug.
- Change in liver blood flow produces nearly proportional change in clearance.
- Clearance is dependent on liver blood flow: "flow-limited."

Alfentanil
- Extraction ratio is very low.
- Clearance is limited by the liver's capacity to take up and metabolize drug.
- Change in liver blood flow has little impact on clearance.
- Clearance is independent of liver blood flow: "capacity-limited."

Front-End Kinetics

- *Front-end kinetics* describes drug behavior immediately after IV administration.
  - Influenced by
    - How rapidly drug moves into peripheral tissues
    - Elimination
  - Used to describe peak plasma concentrations after a bolus injection
  - Used to characterize speed of onset and duration of action (e.g., induction agents)

Compartmental Pharmacokinetic Models

- No physiologic correlate
- *One-compartment model* represents a single volume and a single clearance.
- *Two- or three-compartment models* represent central + peripheral volume(s).
  - The sum of all the volumes is the volume of distribution at steady state (Vdss).
  - *Central or metabolic clearance* represents drug leaving from the central volume.
  - *Intercompartmental clearance* is clearance from central and peripheral volumes.

Mammillary Three-Compartment Model

Drug administration

I

V_2 Rapidly equilibrating compartment	k_{12} ← / → k_{21}	V_1 Central compartment	k_{13} → / ← k_{31}	V_3 Slowly equilibrating compartment

k_{10}

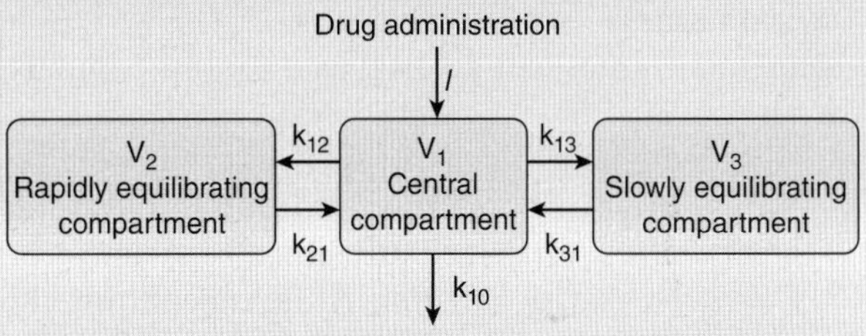

- Central compartment (tank) with peripheral compartments (tanks) connected to it
  - Right: slowly equilibrating peripheral compartment
  - Middle: central compartment (plasma)
  - Left: rapidly equilibrating peripheral compartment
- Compartments (tanks) are connected by intercompartmental clearance (horizontal pipes).
- Drain from central compartment represents metabolic clearance.
- Representations
  - Tanks: volume = volume of compartment, height = concentration of drug
  - Pipes: cross-sectional area = intercompartmental or metabolic clearance

Multicompartment Models

- Plasma concentration over time after IV bolus has characteristic curve.
  - Rapid-distribution phase
    - Immediately after injection
    - Very rapid movement from plasma to rapidly equilibrating tissues
  - Slow-distribution phase
    - Movement of drug to more slowly equilibrating tissues
    - Return of drug to plasma from the more rapidly equilibrating tissues

- Terminal (elimination) phase
  - Decreasing drug due to elimination of drug from the body
  - Drug returns from rapid- and slow-distribution volumes to plasma and is permanently removed by metabolism or excretion.
  - Plasma drug concentration is lower than tissue concentrations.
  - Relative portion of drug in plasma and peripheral volumes of distribution remains constant.
  - Log-linear phase whose slope correlates with the terminal half-life of the drug

Back-End Kinetics

- *Back-end kinetics* describes IV drug behavior when administered as a continuous infusion.
  - Plasma concentration decreases over time once terminated.
  - Predicts time to reach a certain concentration once infusion is terminated
  - Decrement times are a function of infusion duration.
  - Decrement times reflect accumulation in peripheral tissues.
- Decrement times can be used as a tool to compare drugs.
  - 50% decrement times of two drugs may be similar after a short infusion duration but differ greatly after prolonged infusions.
  - *Context-sensitive half-time* is the time required for plasma drug concentrations to decrease by 50%.
    - Once an infusion is terminated
    - *Context-sensitive* refers to infusion duration.
    - *Half-time* refers to a drug's 50% decrement time.

Biophase

- *Biophase* is the time delay between changes in plasma concentration and drug effect.
  - Time required for a drug to diffuse from plasma to site of action and elicit its effect
  - *Hysteresis* describes the lag between drug plasma concentration and effect.
- *Half-life* is a conventional pharmacokinetic term that is not useful in describing the behavior of IV or inhaled anesthetic drugs.

PHARMACODYNAMIC PRINCIPLES

- *Pharmacodynamics* describes the relationship between drug concentration and pharmacologic effects.
  - "What the drug does to the body"
- Plasma drug levels and a selected drug effect are measured simultaneously.
  - Data can be collected from several individuals.
  - Mathematical formulas are applied.
  - Used to create modes of concentration–effect relationships
- Sigmoid curves are used to describe concentration–effect relationships.
  - C_{50} is the concentration at which there is a 50% probability of drug effect.
  - *Gamma* is a pharmacodynamic parameter that represents the slope of the curve.

Potency and Efficacy

- *Potency* describes the amount of drug required to elicit an effect.
  - C_{50} is used to describe potency.
    - High potency: concentration–effect curve of drug is shifted to the left (small C_{50})
    - Low potency: concentration–effect relationship of a drug shifted to the right (large C_{50})
- *Efficacy* is a measure of drug effectiveness once it occupies a receptor.
  - *Full agonists* are drugs that achieve maximal effect.
  - *Partial agonists* are drugs that have a less-than-maximal effect.

Anesthetic Drug Interactions

- *Anesthetic drug interactions* describes the relationship between drugs from one class of anesthetics (e.g., opioids) and drugs from another class of anesthetics (e.g., sedatives).
- Characterized as
  - *Additive:* overall effect is the sum of the two individual effects
  - *Antagonistic:* overall effect is less than if the drug combination was additive
  - *Synergistic:* overall effect is greater than if the drug combination was additive

Examples of Synergistic Drug Interactions in Anesthesia

- When an opioid is coadministered with a sedative-hypnotic (e.g., potent inhaled agent or a sedative such as propofol)
- Analgesia is more profound with a hypnotic than by itself.
- Hypnosis is more profound with an analgesic than by itself.

- *Response surface models* are used to predict a specific drug effect from a combination of drugs.
  - Mathematical models that characterize anesthetic drug interactions
  - Represented as a three-dimensional or topographic plot

SPECIAL POPULATIONS

Patient Demographic and Medical History Considerations for Selecting the Correct Anesthetic Dose
▪ Age ▪ Body habitus ▪ Gender ▪ Chronic exposure to opioids, benzodiazepines, or alcohol ▪ Presence of heart, lung, kidney, or liver disease ▪ Extent of blood loss or dehydration

- Some patient characteristics have been studied, whereas others are more difficult to assess.

Influence of Obesity on Anesthetic Drugs

- Manufacturer dosing recommendations are often scaled to kilograms of actual (total body weight TBW).
- Using mg/kg dosing in obese patients risks administering an excessive dose.
- Several weight scalars have been developed to avoid excessive dosing or underdosing.
  - Each scalar has an associated equation.
  - Goal is to match dosing regimens for what is required for normal-sized patients.
  - Used in place of TBW for both bolus and continuous infusion dosing

Common Weight Scalars
▪ Ideal body weight ▪ Corrected body weight ▪ Lean body mass ▪ Fat-free mass ▪ Modified fat-free mass

Propofol

- Volume of distribution
  - Blood distributes more to nonadipose than to adipose tissues.
  - Higher peak plasma drug concentrations are seen when using mg/kg dosing.
- Clearance
  - Increased because of increased liver volume and liver blood flow
- Suggested dosing scalars for propofol
  - Lean body mass (LBM) for bolus dosing
  - Corrected body weight (CBW) for infusions
    - Some reports suggest this may underdose morbidly obese patients.

Other Sedatives

- Limited information is available (e.g., midazolam, ketamine, etomidate, barbiturates).
  - Boluses should probably be based on TBW to avoid inadequate effect.
  - Continuous infusion rates should be dosed to ideal body weight (IBW).
- For dexmedetomidine, fat-free mass (FFM) scalar may be better choice for bolus dosing.
  - Dosing by TBW can lead to excessive sedation and lower oxygen saturations.

Remifentanil

- Distribution volume and clearance are similar in lean and obese patients.
- Suggested dosing scalars are FFM or IBW.
  - Dosing by LBM results in underdosing.
  - Dosing by TBW results in excessive dosing.

Fentanyl

- Pharmacokinetic models tend to overestimate fentanyl concentrations with increasing body weight.
- *Pharmacokinetic mass* is a modified weight used to improve predictive models for fentanyl.

Other Opioids

- Impact of obesity on drug behavior is not well-defined.

Inhaled Anesthetics

- Prolonged emergence due to accumulation in adipose tissue is not confirmed.
  - Blood flow to adipose tissue decreases with increasing obesity.
  - The time required to fill adipose tissue with volatile anesthetics is long.

Influence of Increasing Age on Anesthetic Drug Pharmacology

- Patient's age should be considered when developing an anesthetic plan.
- Elderly patients generally require less drug to achieve desired anesthetic effect.
  - Examples of analysis to achieve the same effect in 80-year-olds as in 20-year-olds
    - The remifentanil dose should be reduced by 55%.
    - The propofol dose should be reduced by 65%.
- Mechanisms unclear but many possibilities
  - Decreased cardiac output with slower circulation times and higher peak concentrations
  - Decreased drug delivery to metabolic organs and reduced clearance
  - Smaller volume of distribution
  - Other comorbid conditions
    - Anesthesia providers should consider a patient's "physiologic" age.
    - If no significant comorbidities, good exercise tolerance, and normal body habitus, a substantial reduction in anesthetic dosing may not be necessary.

QUESTIONS

PHARMACOKINETIC PRINCIPLES

1. Define pharmacokinetics. What are the fundamental processes that govern pharmacokinetics?
2. What are two properties of a drug that influence its distribution to peripheral tissues?
3. What is the difference between a drug's context-sensitive half-time and a drug's half-life?
4. What is biophase?

PHARMACODYNAMIC PRINCIPLES

5. Define pharmacodynamics.
6. What are drug potency and drug efficacy?
7. What is an anesthetic drug interaction?

SPECIAL POPULATIONS

8. How does using total body weight (mg/kg) affect plasma drug concentrations in obese patients compared to lean patients with less adipose tissue?
9. Do volatile anesthetics accumulate more in obese patients than in lean patients, prolonging emergence in obese patients?
10. How does age influence the dosing of intravenous drugs in elderly patients?

ANSWERS

PHARMACOKINETIC PRINCIPLES

1. Pharmacokinetics describes the relationship between drug dose and drug plasma concentrations. It can be thought of as "what the body does to the drug." Fundamental processes that govern pharmacokinetics are absorption, distribution, and elimination (metabolism and excretion). Absorption does not play a role in intravenously administered anesthetic drugs. (31)

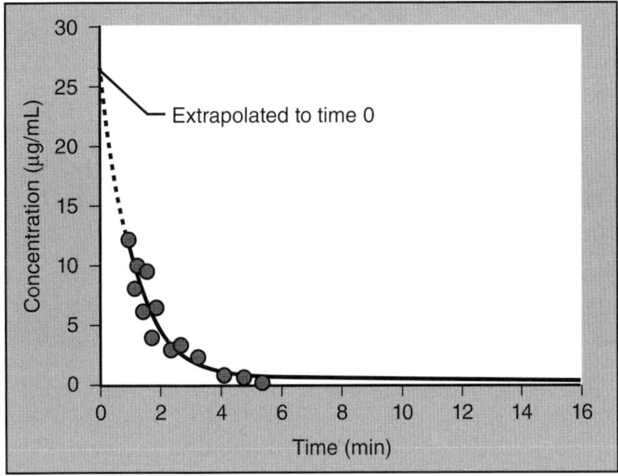

Illustration of a pharmacokinetic analysis. The black dots represent measured plasma drug concentrations over time following a bolus of a drug. The black line represents a pharmacokinetic model. It is a mathematical equation fit to the measured concentrations. The dotted line represents an extrapolation of the mathematical equation to time 0.

2. Two properties of a drug that influence its distribution to peripheral tissues are its solubility and drug binding. The more soluble a drug and the more it binds to peripheral tissues, the greater the total volume of distribution. (32–33)
3. *Context-sensitive half-time* is a term used to describe drug behavior once a continuous infusion of an anesthetic drug is turned off. It is defined as the time required for the plasma concentration to drop by 50% in the context of the infusion duration. *Half-life* is a term used to describe drug behavior of all types of drugs. It is defined as the time required for a drug plasma concentration to decrease by 50%. This term is not very useful in describing the behavior of intravenous or inhaled anesthetic drugs. (38–40)
4. *Biophase* is the time delay between changes in plasma concentration and drug effect. It accounts for the time required for a drug to diffuse from the plasma to the site of action plus the time required to elicit a drug effect. An increase in drug effect lags behind an increase in plasma drug concentrations. The opposite holds true for decreasing plasma concentrations. Pharmacokinetic models are modified to account for this lag time with a predicted "effect site" concentration. (39)

PHARMACODYNAMIC PRINCIPLES

5. Pharmacodynamics is the relationship between drug concentration and pharmacologic effect. It can be thought of as "what the drug does to the body." A pharmacodynamic model describes the relationship between drug concentration (typically the effect site concentration) and drug effect. The relationship is often described by a sigmoid curve, as shown in the figure below. At low concentrations, there is no effect. This segment of the curve is flat. At high concentrations, there is no increase in maximal effect with increasing drug concentrations.

This segment of the curve is also flat. In between, the curve has an increasing slope that tracks the rise in drug effect with the rise in drug concentration. (40–42)

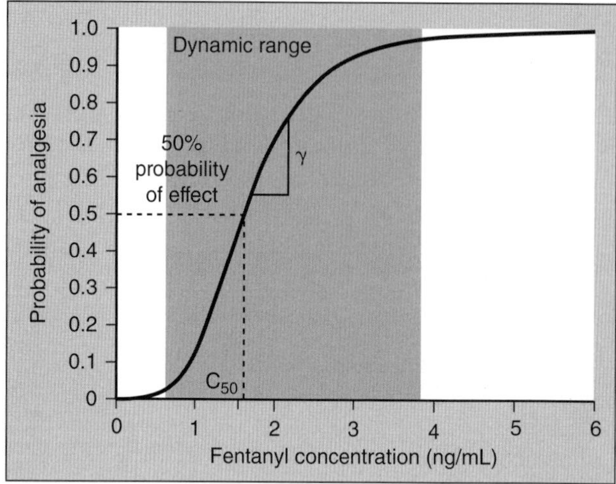

Illustration of a pharmacodynamic model. The gray area represents the dynamic range, the concentration range where changes in concentration lead to a change in effect. Concentrations above or below the dynamic range do not lead to changes in drug effect. The C_{50} represents the concentration associated with 50% probability of effect. Gamma (γ) represents the slope of the curve in the dynamic range.

6. Potency describes the amount of drug required to elicit an effect. C_{50}, which is the effect-site concentration associated with a 50% probability of drug effect, is utilized as a metric for the comparison of potency between drugs. Efficacy describes the effectiveness of a drug to elicit an action when attached to a receptor. Drugs that achieve maximal effect are known as full agonists, and those with an effect less than maximal are known as partial agonists. (42)
7. Anesthetic drug interactions describe the relationship between drugs from one class of anesthetics (e.g., opioids) and drugs from another class of anesthetics (e.g., sedatives). Interactions between opioids and inhaled agents or propofol are primarily synergistic, meaning analgesia is more profound with a hypnotic than by itself; hypnosis is more profound with an analgesic than by itself. (42–43)

SPECIAL POPULATIONS

8. Dosing obese patients with total body weight results in increased plasma drug concentrations due to blood flow distributing more drug to nonadipose tissues than to adipose tissues. (46)
9. Contrary to perception, volatile anesthetics do not accumulate more in obese patients than in lean patients, and emergence in obese patients has not been confirmed to be prolonged. Blood flow to adipose tissue decreases with increasing obesity. In addition, the time required to fill adipose tissue with enough volatile anesthetic to significantly prolong emergence is much longer than the duration of most anesthetics. (48)
10. Both pharmacokinetics and pharmacodynamics are altered with age. In elderly patients, a decrease in cardiac output slows drug circulation and decreases perfusion of metabolic organs. This results in higher peak plasma drug concentrations and decreased clearance. Smaller doses of most intravenous anesthetic drugs are needed in elderly patients to produce the same effect noted in younger patients. (48–49)

Chapter

5 CLINICAL CARDIAC AND PULMONARY PHYSIOLOGY

Gina Heyue Sun

HEMODYNAMICS

Arterial Blood Pressure

- Hypertension and hypotension commonly encountered during anesthesia care
- Hypertension
  - Chronic systemic hypertension may need treatment.
- Hypotension
  - Ranges from mild and clinically insignificant, to major and life-threatening
  - Heart and brain are at greatest risk, then kidneys, liver, and lungs.

Intraoperative Hypotension and Patient Outcomes

- Increased postoperative morbidity and mortality with even 5 minutes' duration of:
  - Systolic blood pressure [SBP] <70 mmHg
  - Diastolic blood pressure [DBP] <30 mmHg
  - Mean arterial pressure [MAP] <50 mmHg
- Increased risk of acute kidney injury in higher-risk patients
- Increased risk of myocardial injury after noncardiac surgery

Physiologic Approach to Hypotension

- Mean arterial pressure (MAP) calculation
  - MAP = SVR × CO
    - SVR is the systemic vascular resistance.
    - CO is the cardiac output.
- Pulse pressure (PP) = SBP – DBP
  - PP created by addition of stroke volume (SV) to DBP within a compliant vascular system
    - The aorta is responsible for most of the compliance in the vascular tree.
    - Increased PP can occur with increased stroke volume.
    - Most common cause of increased PP is poor aortic compliance related to aging

Systemic Vascular Resistance

- Systemic vascular resistance calculation
  - SVR = 80 × (MAP – CVP)/CO
    - CVP is the central venous pressure.
    - Factor 80 converts mmHg units into dyne/s/cm^5.
  - Measuring CVP and CO
    - PA catheter measurements, but not immediately available in all settings
- Causes of decreased SVR during anesthesia care
  - Most drugs administered during general and neuraxial anesthesia
  - Pathologic conditions
    - Sepsis, anaphylaxis, spinal shock, reperfusion of ischemic organs
- Anatomy/physiology of SVR
  - Poiseuille's law
    - Resistance is inversely proportional to the fourth power of the radius of a vessel.
    - Small vessels should provide most resistance.
  - Capillaries—smallest vessels, but so many are arranged in parallel
    - Parallel arrangement reduces its contribution to SVR.
  - Arterioles—provide most of the resistance in the arterial tree

Cardiac Output

- Cardiac output
  - Defined as amount of blood pumped by the heart in 1 minute
    - Blood flow from the right and left sides of the heart are equal.
    - Exception is certain congenital heart malformations.
  - CO = HR × SV
    - SV is the stroke volume (net amount of blood ejected by the heart in one cycle).
- CO measurement methods
  - PA catheter
  - Transesophageal echo
  - Esophageal Doppler
  - Pulse contour analysis

- Cardiac index
  - Defined as CO/BSA
    - BSA is body surface area in square meters.
  - Commonly used index because normal CO changes according to body size

Heart Rate

- Tachycardia and bradycardia
  - Both can cause hypotension if CO is decreased.
  - Tachycardia may result in insufficient time for LV filling.
  - Bradycardia may enhance ventricular filling to a certain extent.
  - Excessively slow HR results in inadequate CO (especially with stiff ventricle).
- Heart rhythm
  - Loss of sinus rhythm and atrial contraction lead to decreased preload.
  - Impact more prominent in patient with poorly compliant ventricles

Ejection Fraction and Stroke Volume

- Ejection fraction (EF)
  - Percentage of ventricular blood volume pumped by the heart in a single contraction
  - EF = SV/EDV
    - SV is stroke volume.
    - EDV is end-diastolic volume.
  - EF 55-70% is normal.
    - Does not differ with body size
- Stroke volume
  - Determined by preload, afterload, and contractility

Preload

- Preload definitions
  - Amount of cardiac muscle "stretch" before contraction
  - Clinically defined as the end-diastolic volume of the heart
- Measurement
  - TEE or PA catheter
    - Can measure left atrial pressure, pulmonary capillary wedge pressure, or pulmonary artery diastolic pressure
  - CVP
    - Left heart filling pressures correlate with measured right heart filling pressures in patients with normal cardiac function without pulmonary disease.
- Ventricular compliance curves
  - Display the relationship between pressure and volume of the heart, as shown in the figure below
- Frank-Starling mechanism
  - Describes the increased pumping action of the heart with increased filling to an ideal volume

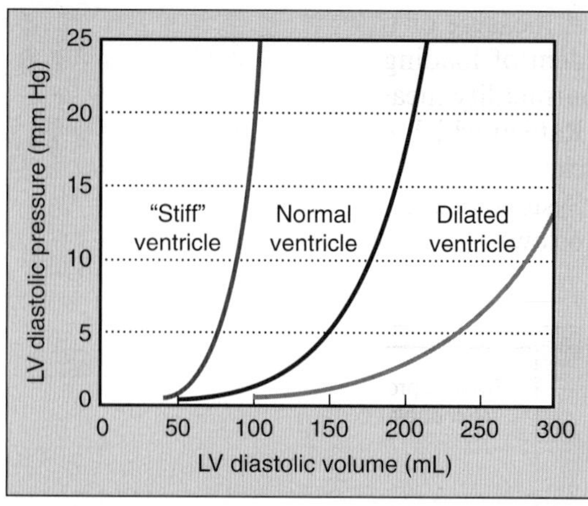

The Pressure-Volume Relationship of the Left Ventricle in Diastole. The pressure–volume relationship of the heart in diastole is shown in the compliance curves plotting left ventricular (LV) diastolic volume versus pressure. The "stiff" heart shows a steeper rise of pressure with increased volume than the normal heart. The dilated ventricle shows a much more compliant curve.

    - Achievement of ideal preload results in increased contraction necessary to eject added ventricular volume, resulting in larger stroke volume.
    - Small increases in preload may have dramatic effects on stroke volume and cardiac output.
  - As filling pressures progressively increase, little additional benefit in SV is derived from increases in preload.
  - Lower contractility or higher SVR shifts the Frank-Starling curve rightward and downward.
- Causes of low preload
  - Absolute
    - Hypovolemia (e.g., hemorrhage, fluid losses)
  - Relative
    - Venodilation (e.g., general or neuraxial anesthesia)
    - Obstruction (e.g., tension pneumothorax, pericardial tamponade)
    - RV failure causing interventricular septum shift and decreased LV filling (e.g., pulmonary embolism)

Using Systolic Pressure Variation (SPV) or Pulse Pressure Variation (PPV) to Assess Preload

- Useful to identify hypovolemia
- More sensitive and specific indicators of volume responsiveness compared to CVP
- Not reliable when using low tidal volume ventilation
  - Especially when lung compliance is low
- *Tidal volume challenge* describes temporarily increasing tidal volume to assess fluid responsiveness.

Contractility

- Contractility definitions
  - Inotropic state of heart

  - A measure of the force of contraction independent of loading conditions
- Contractility measurement
  - Rate at which pressure develops in cardiac ventricles (dP/dT)
  - Systolic pressure-volume relationships (see figure below)

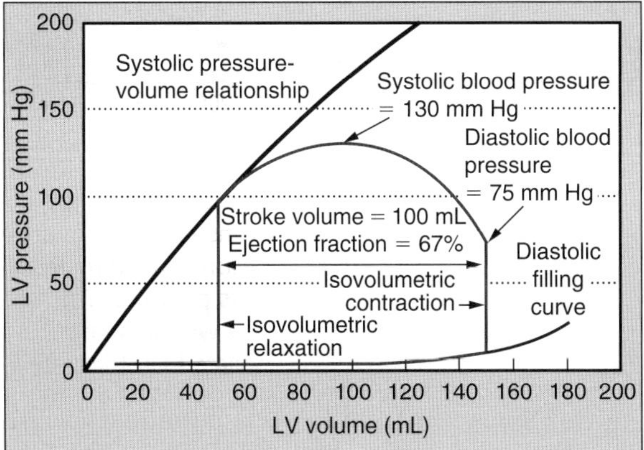

The Ventricular Pressure-Volume Loop. The closed loop (red line) shows a typical cardiac cycle. Diastolic filling occurs along the typical diastolic curve from a volume of 50 mL to an end-diastolic volume (EDV) of 150 mL. Isovolumetric contraction increases the pressure in the left ventricle (LV) until it reaches the pressure in the aorta (at diastolic blood pressure) and the aortic valve opens. The LV then ejects blood, and volume decreases. Pressure in the LV and aorta reaches a peak at some point during ejection (systolic blood pressure), and the pressure then drops until the point at which the aortic valve closes (roughly the dicrotic notch). The LV relaxes without changing volume (isovolumetric relaxation). When the pressure decreases below left atrial pressure, the mitral valve opens, and diastolic filling begins. The plot shows a normal cycle, and the stroke volume (SV) is 100 mL, ejection fraction (EF) is SV/EDV = 67%, and blood pressure is 130/75 mmHg. The systolic pressure–volume relationship (black line) can be constructed from a family of curves under different loading conditions (i.e., different preload) and reflects the inotropic state of the heart.

- Conditions associated with decreased myocardial contractility
  - Myocardial ischemia or previous myocardial infarction
  - Cardiomyopathy
  - Anesthetic drugs
  - Valvular heart disease

Afterload

- Afterload definition
  - Resistance to ejection of blood from the LV
  - Largely determined by SVR and myocardial wall stress
- Wall stress
  - Described using the law of Laplace
    - Wall stress = ventricular transmural pressure × radius / (2 × ventricular wall thickness)
- High SVR
  - Increases cardiac filling pressures
    - Increases wall stress and may contribute to myocardial ischemia
- Low SVR
  - Improves SV by allowing more emptying and increases CO
  - With the same venous return, heart does not fill to the same EDV, resulting in lower LV filling pressures.
- Optimal SVR
  - The SVR at which filling pressures allow the ventricle to operate on the most efficient portion of the Starling curve while not providing excessive afterload

CARDIAC REFLEXES

- Peripheral and central receptor systems that detect various physiologic states
- Brainstem integration of the input
- Neurohumoral output to the heart and vascular system

Autonomic Nervous System

- Sympathetic nervous system (SNS) and parasympathetic nervous system (PNS) efferents innervate the sinoatrial (SA) and atrioventricular (AV) nodes.
  - SNS stimulation
    - Increases HR and contractility through activation of β_1 receptors
  - PNS stimulation
    - Slows HR through activation of muscarinic acetylcholine receptors in the SA and AV nodes
  - PNS suppression
    - Contributes to increased HR

Baroreceptors

- Baroreceptor reflex
  - Receptors: carotid sinus and aortic arch
  - Activation: increased blood pressure that stimulates stretch receptors
  - Afferent: through vagus and glossopharyngeal nerves
  - Response: increased PNS stimulation decreases HR and vasodilates
  - Additional notes
    - Carotid sinus reflex can be used to produce vagal stimulation that can terminate supraventricular tachycardia (SVT).
    - The sensitivity of baroreceptors to changes in blood pressure is significantly altered by chronic hypertension.

- Atrial stretch (Bainbridge reflex)
  - Response: increases heart rate
  - Additional notes
    - The increase in HR may help match CO to venous return.
- Ventricular stretch (Bezold-Jarisch reflex)
  - Response: decreases heart rate and causes peripheral and coronary vasodilation
  - Additional notes
    - Implicated in a range of conditions such as myocardial ischemia, thrombolysis, revascularization, and syncope
- Chemoreceptor reflex
  - Receptors: carotid body and aortic body
  - Activation: arterial hypoxemia
  - Response: SNS stimulation
  - Additional notes
    - Profound hypoxemia can result in bradycardia, possibly through central mechanisms.
- Other reflexes causing bradycardia
  - Oculocardiac reflex: in response to increased ocular pressure
  - Cushing reflex: in response to increased intracranial pressure
  - In response to stretch of abdominal viscera
- Anesthetic effects
  - Many anesthetics blunt cardiac reflexes in a dose-dependent fashion.
    - Decreased SNS responses to hypotension

CORONARY BLOOD FLOW

- Cardiac oxygen supply
  - Heart extracts a larger percentage of oxygen than any other vascular bed.
    - Up to 70%, compared to 25% for the body as a whole
    - Cannot increase O_2 extraction in cases of threatened O_2 supply
  - Coronary arteries vasodilate to increase flow as the primary compensatory mechanism.
- Coronary reserve
  - The ability of coronary vessels to increase flow
  - Determined by endogenous regulators of blood flow
    - E.g., adenosine, nitric oxide, and adrenergic stimulation
  - Compensatory vasodilation in coronary artery stenosis
    - Can maintain blood flow until about 90% stenosis, when coronary reserve is exhausted
- LV perfusion
  - LV is perfused predominantly during diastole.
    - Myocardial wall tension in systole can completely stop blood flow in the subendocardium.
  - Coronary perfusion pressure (CPP) = arterial diastolic BP – LV end-diastolic pressure (LVEDP).
    - Elevated LVEDP (e.g., decompensated heart failure) can compromise coronary perfusion.
- RV perfusion
  - RV is perfused during both systole and diastole.
    - Lower RV intramural pressure throughout the cardiac cycle

PULMONARY CIRCULATION

- Pulmonary circulation components
  - RV, PA, pulmonary capillary bed, and pulmonary veins
- Bronchial circulation components
  - Bronchial arteries
    - Supply oxygen and nutrients to the lungs
  - Bronchial veins
    - Return deoxygenated blood to the RA (via azygous vein) and LA (via pulmonary vein)
    - Bronchial venous blood draining to the LA is a source of physiologic right-to-left shunt

Pulmonary Artery Pressure

- Pulmonary artery pressure (PAP)
  - Much lower than systemic pressure because of low pulmonary vascular resistance (PVR)
- Pulmonary circulation receives entire CO (like systemic circulation)
  - Pulmonary vascular resistance (PVR) must adapt to different conditions

Pulmonary Vascular Resistance

- Model for describing pulmonary response to increases in PAP and CO
  - Results in distention and recruitment of capillaries
  - This increases cross-sectional area and decreases PVR.
- Reciprocal changes between CO and PVR
  - Maintain constant PAP over a wide range of CO in nonpathologic states
- Alveolar distention impact on pulmonary blood flow
  - Large lung volumes
    - Compresses intraalveolar vessels (increases resistance)
    - Recruits extraalveolar vessels (lowers resistance)
  - Small lung volumes
    - Opposite effect with intraalveolar and extraalveolar vessels
    - PVR increase at small lung volumes diverts blood from collapsed alveoli.
  - PVR can increase at both large and small lung volumes.
  - PVR is lowest at functional residual capacity.

- Sympathetic nervous system (SNS) impact on pulmonary blood flow
  - SNS stimulation causes pulmonary vasoconstriction.
  - Effect is minimal compared to the systemic circulation in which neurohormonal influence regulates vascular tone.

Treating Pulmonary Hypertension

- Effective treatment is challenging.
- Classes of medication therapy
  - Inhaled nitric oxide
  - Phosphodiesterase inhibitors
  - Prostacyclin analogs
  - Guanylate cyclase stimulators
  - Endothelin receptor antagonists

Hypoxic Pulmonary Vasoconstriction

- Hypoxic pulmonary vasoconstriction (HPV) is the pulmonary vascular response to low alveolar oxygen partial pressure (P_AO_2).
- Physiologic impact
  - Improves gas exchange
    - Diverts blood away from poorly ventilated areas
    - Decreases shunt fraction
  - During one-lung ventilation, HPV may play a role in the resolution of hypoxemia.
  - Global alveolar hypoxia can cause significant HPV, increasing PAP
    - Examples include apnea, high altitudes.
- Anesthetics and other drugs
  - Inhaled anesthetics impair HPV at higher doses.
  - Calcium channel blockers may blunt HPV in the setting of preexisting V/Q mismatch.
  - Propofol and opioids have no effect.

Pulmonary Emboli

- Pulmonary emboli increase overall resistance through the pulmonary vasculature.
- Types of emboli include clots, air, fat, CO_2, and amniotic fluid.

Arteriolar Thickening

- Conditions associated with arteriolar thickening
  - Primary pulmonary hypertension
    - Idiopathic arteriolar hyperplasia
  - Congenital heart disease (certain types)
  - Cirrhosis (portopulmonary hypertension)

Zones of the Lung

- Impact of gravity on pulmonary vascular system
  - Gravity causes pressure change in the pulmonary vascular system.
  - Every 20 cm change in height produces a 15 mmHg pressure difference.
- West's zones of the lung
  - Zone 1: airway pressure > pulmonary arterial and venous pressure
    - No blood flow despite ventilation
    - Normally does not exist, but with PPV or low PA pressures (e.g., anesthesia, blood loss), zone 1 may develop
  - Zone 2: pulmonary arterial pressure > airway pressure > pulmonary venous pressure
    - Flow is proportional to the difference between PA and airway pressures.
  - Zone 3: pulmonary arterial and venous pressure > airway pressure
    - Flow is proportional to the difference between pulmonary arterial and venous pressure.

Pulmonary Edema

- Lung intravascular fluid balance determinants
  - Cardiogenic (hydrostatic) pulmonary edema
    - Occurs when left-heart filling pressures exceed 20 mmHg
    - Patients with chronic left heart failure may tolerate higher pressures.
  - Noncardiogenic (permeability) pulmonary edema
    - Occurs when increased pulmonary capillary permeability leads to protein-rich fluid in the interstitium and alveoli
    - Direct lung injury (e.g., pneumonia, inhalational injury)
    - Indirect lung injury (e.g., sepsis, acute pancreatitis, severe trauma, blood transfusions)

PULMONARY GAS EXCHANGE

Oxygen

- Arterial hypoxemia
  - Low partial pressure of oxygen in arterial blood (PaO_2)
    - Defined as $PaO_2 < 60$ mmHg
    - Can be relative to expected based on the inspired oxygen concentration (FiO_2)
  - Reflects pulmonary gas exchange
- Hypoxia
  - Low O_2 content in tissues
  - Reflects circulatory factors
- Consequences of hypoxemia
  - Mild to moderate levels of hypoxemia can be well tolerated.
  - Severe, prolonged hypoxemia is associated with permanent neurologic injury.

Measurements of Oxygenation

- Oxyhemoglobin dissociation curve
  - PaO_2 and SaO_2 are related through this curve as noted in figure below

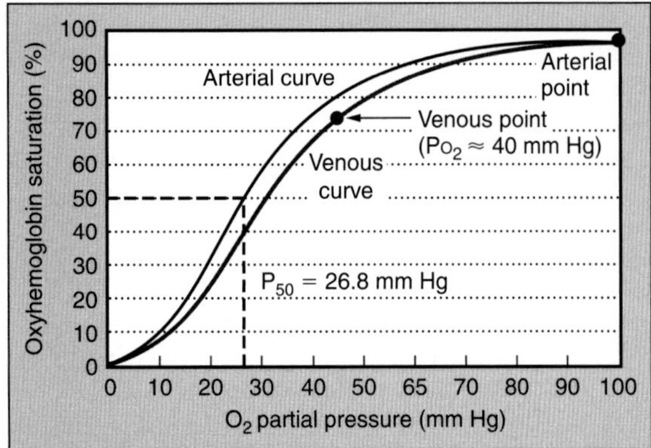

The Oxyhemoglobin Dissociation Curve. The oxyhemoglobin dissociation curve is S-shaped and relates oxygen partial pressure to the oxyhemoglobin saturation. A typical arterial curve is shown in the upper curve. The higher PCO_2 and the lower pH of venous blood cause a rightward shift of the curve and facilitate unloading of oxygen in the tissues (lower curve). Normal adult P_{50}, the Po_2 at which hemoglobin is 50% saturated, is shown (26.8 mmHg). Normal PaO_2 of about 100 mmHg results in an SaO_2 of about 98%. Normal PvO_2 is about 40 mmHg, resulting in a saturation of about 75%.

- Rightward shift of dissociation curve
  - Allows larger amounts of O_2 to dissociate from hemoglobin in the tissues
  - Causes: lower pH, increased CO_2, higher temperature, and increased 2,3-diphosphoglycerate
- Leftward shift of dissociation curve
  - Increases the affinity of hemoglobin for O_2 and decreases offloading into tissues
  - Causes: higher pH, decreased CO_2, lower temperature, and decreased 2,3-diphosphoglycerate
  - Note that fetal hemoglobin is also intrinsically left-shifted.

- Arterial oxygen content (CaO_2)
  - Two components of arterial oxygen content
    - O_2 bound to hemoglobin (vast majority)
    - O_2 dissolved in plasma
  - $CaO_2 = SaO_2 (Hb \times 1.39) + 0.003 (PaO_2)$
    - The capacity of hemoglobin (Hb) for O_2 is 1.39 mL of O_2 per gram of Hb fully saturated.
    - O_2 solubility in blood is 0.003 mL O_2/dL/mmHg.
  - Dissolved oxygen can be clinically significant with FiO_2 100% and with hyperbaric oxygen.
- Multiwavelength pulse oximetry
  - Newer blood gas machine oximeters now measure methemoglobin (MetHb) and carboxyhemoglobin (COHb).
    - This allows for the measurement of the true SaO_2, or *fractional saturation.*
  - Functional saturation
    - Defined as % of oxyhemoglobin saturation relative to Hb available to bind O_2
    - Functional saturation = $HbO_2/(Hb + HbO_2)$
  - Fractional saturation
    - Calculated relative to *all* hemoglobin
    - Fractional saturation = $HbO_2/(Hb + HbO_2 + MetHb + COHb)$

Determinants of Alveolar Oxygen Partial Pressure

- Alveolar gas equation
  - Describes transfer of O_2 from environment to alveoli
  - $P_AO_2 = FiO_2 \times (P_B - P_{H2O}) - PCO_2/R$
    - P_B is the barometric pressure.
    - P_{H2O} is the vapor pressure of water (47 mmHg at normal body temperature).
    - R is the respiratory quotient (ratio of CO_2 production to O_2 consumption, approx. 0.8).
  - FiO_2 and hypoventilation
    - Increased FiO_2 can mask the adverse effects of hypoventilation
    - Example: with 30% FiO_2, pulse oximeter saturation may remain normal despite $PaCO_2$ 70 mmHg.
- Calculating the time for SaO_2 to decrement during apnea
  - Apnea occurs commonly after induction of anesthesia.
    - Maximizing storage of oxygen in the lung is important to delay arterial hypoxemia.
    - Apnea during anesthesia occurs at FRC.
    - In contrast, voluntary breath-hold occurs at total lung capacity.
  - Safe apnea time (minutes) = FRC × end-tidal $O_2\%/VO_2$
    - FRC is 30 mL/kg, VO_2 is O_2 consumption (at rest, typically 3.5 mL/kg/min)
    - When breathing room air, hypoxemia develops within 30 seconds.
    - When breathing 100% oxygen, might take 7 minutes to reach SaO_2 90%
  - Hypoxemia during apnea
    - Hypoxemia begins when enough alveoli have collapsed and intrapulmonary shunt develops, not simply when oxygen stores have become depleted.
    - Obese patients have higher oxygen consumption and develop hypoxemia with apnea more rapidly.

Venous Admixture

- Describes physiologic causes of arterial hypoxemia for which P_AO_2 is normal
- A-a gradient
  - Reflects venous admixture
  - Normal A-a gradient is 5 to 10 mmHg but increases with age.
    - A-a gradient is most useful on room air.
  - The P/F ratio (PaO_2/FiO_2) is a simple and useful measurement of oxygenation.
    - More consistent at high FiO_2

- Isoshunt diagrams
  - An approach to quantitate oxygenation issues
  - Integrates effects of shunting, supplemental O_2, and oxyhemoglobin dissociation curve (see figure below)

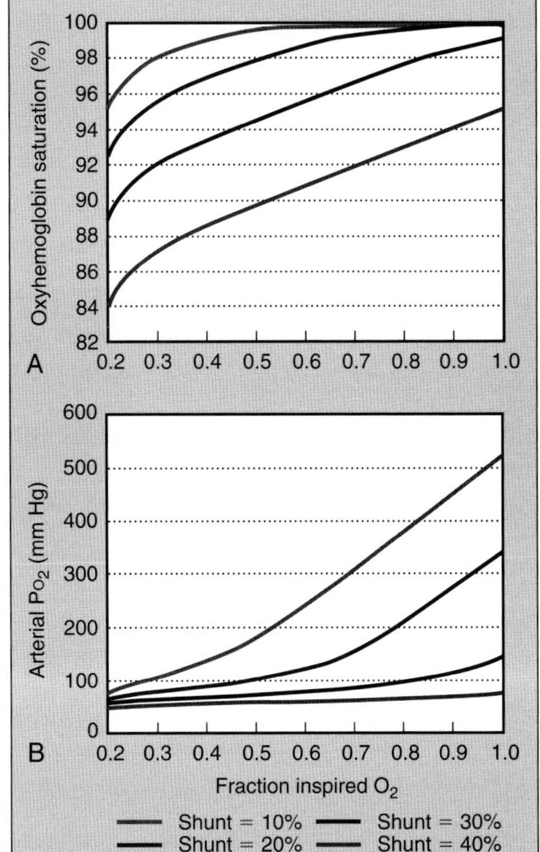

Effect of Varying Shunt Fraction and FiO_2 on Oxygenation. The effect of intrapulmonary shunting and FiO_2 on PaO_2 (A) and SaO_2 (B) is shown graphically at shunt fractions from 10% (mild) to 40% (severe). Assumed values for these calculations are hemoglobin, 14 g/dL; $PaCO_2$, 40 mmHg; arterial-to-venous oxygen content difference, 4 mL O_2/dL; and sea-level atmospheric pressure, 760 mmHg. Increased FiO_2 still substantially improves oxygenation at high shunt fractions but is unable to fully correct it.

- Intrapulmonary shunt
  - An important cause of elevated A-a gradient and hypoxemia
  - Mechanism of hypoxemia
    - Mixed venous blood not exposed to alveolar gas mixes with blood from normal areas of lung, leading to lower PaO_2.
    - Occurs when alveoli are not ventilated (e.g., atelectasis) or when alveoli are fluid-filled (e.g., pneumonia, pulmonary edema)
  - $Qs/Qt = (Cc'O_2 - CaO_2)/(Cc'O_2 - CvO_2)$ calculates the shunt fraction (Qs/Qt)
    - C is the oxygen content.
    - c′ is the end-capillary blood.
    - a is the arterial blood, and v is the mixed venous blood.
- Ventilation-perfusion (V/Q) mismatch
  - Disparity between the amount of ventilation and perfusion in various alveoli
  - Impact of administering 100% oxygen on V/Q mismatch
    - In poorly ventilated alveoli: can achieve a PaO_2 on the plateau of the oxyhemoglobin dissociation curve
    - With a large (e.g., 40%) intrapulmonary shunt: leads to minimal improvement because it only adds more O_2 to normal perfused alveoli (see figure above)
- Diffusion impairment
  - Occurs when equilibrium has not been reached between the PO_2 in the alveolus and PO_2 in pulmonary capillary blood
    - Rarely occurs clinically, even in patients with limited diffusing capacity
    - Example: high-altitude exercise, due to lower PO_2 and rapid transit time of blood through pulmonary capillaries
- Venous oxygen saturation (SvO_2)
  - SvO_2 can be an important contributor to hypoxemia when a large intrapulmonary shunt is present.
    - Lower SvO_2 results in a mixture having lower PaO_2.
  - Causes of lower SvO_2
    - Low cardiac output, anemia, hypoxemia, shivering, agitation
  - Causes of higher SvO_2
    - High cardiac output, sepsis (disrupted cellular metabolism), hemoconcentration, hyperoxia, sedation, paralysis
  - Shunt fraction may be underestimated in patients with sepsis.

Carbon Dioxide

- Carbon dioxide in the body
  - Produced in the tissues
  - Carried in blood
    - As bicarbonate
    - As dissolved gas
    - Bound to Hb as carbaminohemoglobin (small amount)
- Carbon dioxide dissociation curve is linear (unlike oxyhemoglobin dissociation curve).

Hypercapnia

- Effects of hypercapnia
  - New-onset hypercapnia may indicate respiratory difficulty or oversedation.

- Severe hypercapnia ($PaCO_2 > 80$ mmHg) may cause CO_2 narcosis.
  - Can contribute to delayed awakening from anesthesia
- May indicate impending respiratory failure
  - If so, arterial hypoxemia and anoxia can rapidly ensue.

Organ Systems Affected by Hypercapnia

- Heart
  - Coronary artery vasodilation
  - Decreased cardiac contractility
- Lungs
  - Pulmonary vasoconstriction
  - Right-shift of oxyhemoglobin dissociation curve
- Central nervous system
  - Somnolence
  - Cerebral vasodilation
- Kidneys
  - Bicarbonate reabsorption

Determinants of Arterial Carbon Dioxide Partial Pressure

- $PaCO_2$ is a balance of CO_2 production and removal.
- Can be expressed by an alveolar CO_2 equation
  - $PaCO_2 = k \times VCO_2/V_A$
    - k is a constant (0.863) that corrects units.
    - VCO_2 is carbon dioxide production.
    - V_A is alveolar ventilation.
- Rebreathing
  - Anesthesia circuits may permit rebreathing.
  - Causes of high inspired PCO_2 concentrations
    - Exhausted CO_2 absorbents
    - Malfunctioning expiratory valves on anesthesia machine
    - Certain transport breathing circuits
- Increased CO_2 production
  - Fever
  - Systemic absorption of CO_2 during laparoscopy
  - Malignant hyperthermia
  - Thyroid storm
  - Limb tourniquet release
  - Administration of IV sodium bicarbonate (converted into CO_2)
- Increased dead space
  - Refers to areas of lung receiving ventilation that do not participate in gas exchange
  - Types of dead space
    - Anatomic: areas of tracheobronchial tree that are not involved in gas exchange
    - Alveolar: alveoli that are not involved in gas exchange due to lack of blood flow
    - Physiologic (total) dead space = anatomic + alveolar dead space
  - Examples
    - Lung disease (cystic fibrosis, emphysema)
    - Pulmonary embolism
    - Decreased PA pressure (hemorrhagic shock, which increases zone 1 through decreased arterial pressure)
    - Increased airway pressure (positive pressure ventilation/PEEP, which increases zone 1 through increased airway pressure)
  - Dead space (Vd/Vt) calculation
    - $Vd/Vt = (PaCO_2 - P_ECO_2)/PaCO_2$
    - P_ECO_2 is the mixed-expired CO_2.
    - Some physiologic dead space (25%–30%) is considered normal since anatomic dead space is always present.
  - $PaCO_2$-P_{ETCO_2} gradient
    - Useful indicator of the presence of alveolar dead space
    - $PaCO_2$-P_{ETCO_2} gradient will change as $PaCO_2$ changes with hyperventilation or hypoventilation, even when dead space is constant.
- Hypoventilation
  - Decreased minute ventilation is the most important and common cause of hypercapnia.
    - Decreased tidal volume, respiratory rate, or both
    - If alveolar ventilation decreases by half, $PaCO_2$ approximately doubles.
  - $PaCO_2$ changes during apnea.
    - During the first minute of apnea, $PaCO_2$ increases from a normal of 40 mmHg to 46 mmHg (with normal $PvCO_2$).
    - After the first minute, $PaCO_2$ rises more slowly as CO_2 production is added to blood (~3 mmHg/min).

Differential Diagnosis of Increased Arterial Carbon Dioxide Partial Pressure

- Analysis of increased $PaCO_2$ values
  - Clinical assessment of minute ventilation
  - Capnography
    - Can easily detect rebreathing
  - Measurement of arterial blood gases
    - Comparison of end-tidal PCO_2 with $PaCO_2$
    - Can identify abnormal alveolar dead space
    - Can be used to infer abnormal CO_2 production
- Significant abnormalities of CO_2 physiology can be masked by increased minute ventilation.
  - Can compensate for substantial increases in dead space and CO_2 production

PULMONARY MECHANICS

Static Properties

- Lung is composed of elastic tissue that stretches under pressure.

- Surface tension
  - Plays significant role in lung compliance because of air–fluid interface in alveoli
  - Surface tension decreased by surfactant production by the lung
    - Stabilizes small alveoli, which would otherwise collapse
- Chest wall
  - Has its own compliance curve
  - Chest wall tends to collapse.
- Balance between chest wall and lungs
  - At FRC, the tendency is for the chest wall to expand.
  - Balanced by the tendency for the lungs to collapse due to elastic recoil

Dynamic Properties and Airway Resistance

- Airway resistance
  - Mainly determined by airway radius
- Factors influencing airway resistance
  - Radius of airways
  - Smooth muscle tone
    - Altered by bronchospasm, inflammation of airways
  - Foreign bodies
  - Compression of airways
  - Turbulent gas flow
  - Anesthesia equipment
- Spontaneous ventilation
  - Negative pressure transmitted from the intrapleural pressure keeps the small airways open.
  - Pleural pressure becomes less negative in certain conditions (e.g., emphysema).
    - Small airway resistance is increased.
    - Dynamic compression occurs during exhalation.
- Positive-pressure ventilation
  - Increased resistance in breathing circuit or patient airways manifests as elevated airway pressures.
    - Flow through increased resistance leads to pressure change.
  - Distinguishing airway resistance from static compliance is useful for evaluating high peak airway pressures.
    - Perform an inspiratory hold to remove the pressure contribution from gas flow/airway resistance.
    - While ventilation is paused, airway pressure decreases toward a plateau pressure.

CONTROL OF BREATHING

Central Integration and Rhythm Generation

- Brainstem areas generate respiratory rhythm.
- Processes afferent information and provides efferent output to respiratory muscles

Central Chemoreceptors

- Ventrolateral medullary surface receptors respond to changes in pH and $PaCO_2$.
  - CO_2 is in rapid equilibrium with carbonic acid.
    - Immediately affects local pH around central chemoreceptors
    - Described clinically as CO_2 responsive chemoreceptors
- Blood-brain barrier
  - Protects central chemoreceptors from rapid changes in metabolic pH

Peripheral Chemoreceptors

- Carotid bodies
  - The primary peripheral chemoreceptors in humans
  - Aortic bodies have no significant role as chemoreceptors.
- Conditions stimulating carotid bodies
  - Low PO_2
  - High PCO_2
  - Low pH
    - Unlike the central chemoreceptors, metabolic acids immediately affect peripheral chemoreceptors.
- Sensitivity of peripheral chemoreceptors
  - Because of high blood flow, peripheral chemoreceptors are very sensitive.
  - Rapid response rates to changes in arterial (not venous) blood values

Hypercapnic Ventilatory Response

- Impact of hypercapnia on ventilatory response
  - Ventilation increases dramatically as $PaCO_2$ is increased in a linear fashion as noted in the figure below.
  - At high PO_2, most of this response results from central chemoreceptors.
  - At room air, about one-third of this response results from peripheral chemoreceptors.
- Apneic threshold
  - Defined as the $PaCO_2$ at which ventilation is zero
  - As CO_2 rises, ventilation returns and stabilizes at a $PaCO_2$ setpoint that is about 5 mmHg higher.
- Peripheral chemoreceptors compared to central chemoreceptors
  - Peripheral chemoreceptors respond faster than central chemoreceptors.
  - Slower brainstem response takes about 5 minutes to reach 90% of steady-state ventilation.

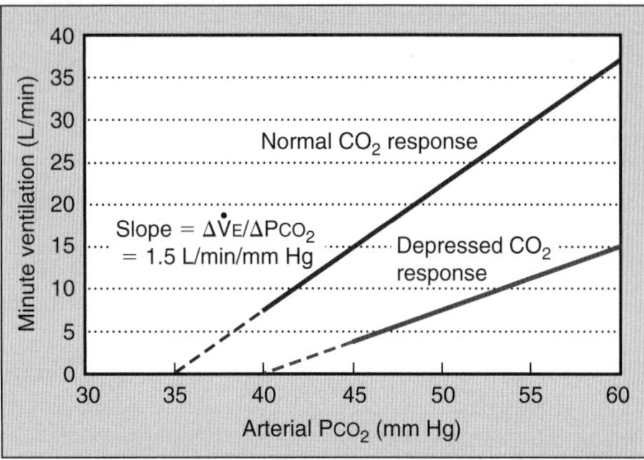

The Hypercapnic Ventilatory Response. The hypercapnic ventilatory response (HCVR) is measured as the slope of the plot of PCO_2 versus minute ventilation (VE). End-tidal PCO_2 is usually substituted for $PaCO_2$ for clinical studies. The apneic threshold is the PCO_2 at which ventilation is zero. It can be extrapolated from the curve, but it is difficult to measure in awake volunteers, although it is easy to observe in patients under general anesthesia. A depressed carbon dioxide response results from opioids, which lower the slope and raise the apneic threshold.

Hypoxic Ventilatory Response

- Impact of hypoxemia on ventilatory response
  - Ventilation increases as PaO_2 and SaO_2 decrease due to stimulation of peripheral chemoreceptors.
    - The response is rapid, taking only seconds to appear (in contrast to the response to hypercapnia).
  - The central response to hypoxemia paradoxically results in decreased minute ventilation, called hypoxic ventilatory decline (HVD).
- Prolonged arterial hypoxemia
  - Ventilation rises to an initial peak (reflecting rapid peripheral chemoreceptor response).
  - Then, ventilation decreases to an intermediate plateau in 15 to 20 minutes (reflecting slower addition of HVD).
- Hypoxemia and hypercapnia have synergistic effects on the carotid body.
  - The response to hypoxemia is much larger with higher $PaCO_2$ levels and dramatically less with lower $PaCO_2$ levels.

Effects of Anesthesia

- Opioids, sedative-hypnotics, and volatile anesthetics
  - All have dose-dependent depressant effects on ventilation.
  - Decrease both hypoxic and hypercapnic ventilatory responses
  - Most depressant effects exerted in the central integratory area

Disorders of Ventilatory Control

- Neonates with a history of prematurity and post-conceptual age <60 weeks
  - May have episodes of apnea after anesthesia
  - Sudden infant death syndrome may be due to immature ventilatory control.
- Patients who are morbidly obese or have sleep apnea
  - Exhibit problems with ventilatory control
- Central hypoventilation syndrome (CHS), formerly known as Ondine's curse
  - Results in profound hypoventilation during sleep and anesthesia
  - Caused by blunting of hypoxic and hypercapnic ventilatory responses
- Periodic breathing
  - Breathing pattern in which sequential breaths are separated by apneic episodes
  - Occurs during drug-induced sedation
  - Mechanism: most likely occurs when peripheral chemoreceptors are activated by mild hypoxemia

Identifying the Cause of Respiratory Failure

- Stepwise approach
  - Differentiate between hypoxemic, hypercarbic, or mixed etiologies.
  - Focus on whether issue is external or intrinsic to patient.
  - Assess for presence of dead space or shunt.

INTEGRATION OF THE HEART AND LUNGS

Supply and Delivery

- Fick equation
  - $VO_2 = CO \times (CaO_2 - CvO_2)$
    - VO_2 is oxygen consumption.
    - CaO_2 is the arterial oxygen content.
    - CvO_2 is the mixed venous oxygen content.
    - CO is the cardiac output
  - Highlights relationship between the heart and lungs

Oxygen Delivery

- Oxygen delivery (DO_2)
  - Defined as total amount of oxygen supplied to the tissues
  - $DO_2 = CO \times CaO_2$
- Oxygen content (CaO_2)
  - Can be limited by anemia or hypoxemia
  - Increased cardiac output can compensate to maintain oxygen delivery.

Oxygen Extraction

- Oxygen extraction
  - Defined as oxygen removed from blood by tissues to meet metabolic demand
- Mixed venous O_2 saturation (SvO_2)
  - Normal value is 75%.
  - If tissues extract more oxygen, SvO_2 decreases.
  - Increasing FiO_2 will increase SvO_2 even though the extraction by tissues has not changed.
- Arteriovenous O_2 content difference ($AVDO_2$)
  - Defined as ($CaO_2 - CvO_2$)
  - Independent of changes in FiO_2
  - Impact of anemia
    - $AVDO_2$ decreases
    - Mechanism: extracting the same percentage of O_2 means extracting less total O_2 due to lower Hb concentration
- The most reliable measure of oxygen extraction is the calculated O_2 extraction ratio.
  - O_2 extraction = $(CaO_2 - CvO_2)/CaO_2$

Anemia

- Anemia
  - Threatens the oxygen supply
- Adaptations to anemia
  - Body can increase CO or extract more oxygen.
  - Normal physiologic conditions
    - CO increases to maintain DO_2.
  - During anesthesia with a blunted HR response
    - Increased O_2 extraction is a more important mechanism of compensation.

Metabolic Demand

- Increased O_2 consumption in response to increased metabolic demand
  - Usual response is increased CO and O_2 extraction.
  - During anesthesia
    - Relatively constant and low O_2 consumption
  - During recovery from anesthesia
    - May have significant increases in metabolic demand (shivering, early ambulation)
  - Requires increased minute ventilation for increased oxygen needs and to eliminate extra CO_2 produced

Mechanical Relationships

- Cardiac and respiratory system mechanical relationships
  - Shared location in the thoracic cavity
- Lung recruitment maneuver or prone positioning
  - If heart is in underfilled state, can impede venous return and lead to hemodynamic compromise
- Positive pressure ventilation
  - Can improve V/Q matching in lung units
  - Can increase RV afterload
  - Can decrease LV afterload through reduction in LV wall stress

QUESTIONS

HEMODYNAMICS

1. Describe pulse pressure and how it changes from the proximal to distal parts of the vascular tree.
2. Describe differences between the RV and the LV in relation to the tolerance of preload and afterload.
3. Which measurements from a PA catheter reading are directly measured versus calculated?

CARDIAC REFLEXES

4. A patient is receiving general anesthesia for a Roux-en-Y gastric bypass. The surgeon asks for a 30-second "breath-hold" at 50 cmH_2O. During this maneuver, the patient becomes bradycardic to the 30s. What is the most likely explanation of this phenomenon?

CORONARY BLOOD FLOW

5. What are the main determinants of myocardial oxygen demand? Describe why tachycardia is detrimental in ischemic heart disease.

PULMONARY CIRCULATION

6. What are the main contributors to a physiologic right-to-left shunt leading to venous admixture?
7. At what lung volume is the pulmonary vascular resistance the lowest? At what lung volume is the airway resistance the lowest?

PULMONARY GAS EXCHANGE

8. A patient is receiving transfusion of 1 unit of packed red blood cells that has been stored in the blood bank for 2 weeks. What is the expected level of 2,3-diphosphoglycerate (DPG) compared to freshly donated blood?
9. After several minutes of preoxygenation, an 80-kg patient has an end-tidal O_2 reading of 80% and oxygen saturation of 100%. After induction of anesthesia, the patient develops apnea. How long will it take for the patient's oxygen saturation to fall below 90%?

PULMONARY MECHANICS

10. What is the difference between static and dynamic compliance? Describe the differential diagnosis of high airway pressure during mechanical ventilation.

CONTROL OF BREATHING

11. Describe the normal hypercapnic ventilatory response. What is the apneic threshold?

ANSWERS

HEMODYNAMICS

1. The pulse pressure (PP) is the difference between the systolic and diastolic pressure. PP varies throughout the vascular tree due to differences in vessel stiffness and wave reflections. The morphology of an arterial waveform changes with increased distance from the aorta: the systolic peak becomes higher, the diastolic trough becomes lower, and the PP therefore becomes wider. This is largely due to distal pressure amplification, where pressure waves from the aorta travel down to higher resistance arteriolar beds and are reflected proximally. PP is normally at least 25% of the systolic BP. A low PP may represent a low stroke volume state such as hypovolemic or cardiogenic shock. PP may increase with exercise or underlying states with high vascular resistance. (52)
2. The LV is a thicker-walled cavity that tolerates high afterload rather well compared to the much thinner-walled RV, which cannot easily generate high enough ventricular systolic pressures to overcome high pulmonary artery pressures. A prime example of this is seen in acute pulmonary embolus where even moderate elevations in pulmonary vascular resistance can lead to RV dilation and failure, whereas acute increases in aortic pressure generally do not cause immediate LV failure. On the other hand, the RV tolerates preload better than the LV, likely due to its higher muscle compliance. For example, RV function appears to be preserved in patients with longstanding volume overload secondary to moderate to severe tricuspid regurgitation. However, severe RV overload shifts the interventricular septum toward the LV and decreases filling of the left heart, leading to low cardiac output. (54–55)
3. PA catheter values may be directly measured or calculated. Direct measurements include RA pressure, PA pressure, PA wedge pressure, mixed venous saturation, and core temperature. The cardiac output via thermodilution method is estimated by injecting a known volume of indicator fluid into the RA port and measuring the change in blood temperature at the distal pulmonary artery port. The area under the temperature-time curve is inversely proportional to the flow rate in the pulmonary artery. Furthermore, reported SVR and PVR are calculated values, not directly measured. (52)

CARDIAC REFLEXES

4. The bradycardia and likely resulting hypotension seen in this scenario can be explained by the Bezold-Jarisch reflex, in which noxious ventricular stimuli sensed by LV chemoreceptors and mechanoreceptors lead to vagal activation and induce a triad of bradycardia, hypotension, and coronary vasodilation. The high intrathoracic pressure impaired venous return, and while often this can lead to reflex tachycardia, in some cases of profound hypovolemia, this cardioprotective mechanism is thought to allow a reduction in oxygen consumption (via bradycardia, reduced afterload) and restoration of myocardial perfusion (via coronary vasodilation). (55)

CORONARY BLOOD FLOW

5. Heart rate is the most important factor that affects myocardial oxygen demand. In addition to increasing contractility (which can exacerbate a low supply-to-demand ratio), tachycardia reduces diastolic filling time, leading to lower cardiac output as well as decreased time for coronary perfusion to the LV. The majority (75%) of LV perfusion from the coronary arteries occurs during diastole. Other major determinants of myocardial oxygen demand include afterload and wall tension. Wall tension is affected by high afterload according to the Law of Laplace, as the myocardium must generate greater systolic pressure. (54–56)

PULMONARY CIRCULATION

6. There are two major anatomical physiologic shunt sources leading to venous admixture: bronchial veins and Thebesian veins. Bronchial veins supply the bronchial walls with oxygenated blood and then subsequently are drained into the pulmonary veins. The Thebesian veins are small valveless veins in all four chambers of the heart that drain deoxygenated blood from the inner myocardium directly into the corresponding chamber, with left-sided ones contributing to a physiologic shunt. (56, 60)

7. The pulmonary vascular resistance is lowest at functional residual capacity (FRC). This is due to the opposing effects of lung volume on alveolar and extra-alveolar blood vessels. At small lung volumes, the alveolar capillaries are not compressed by the air sacs and have lower resistance, whereas the extra-alveolar parenchymal vessels are compressed. As the alveoli fill during inspiration, the opposite occurs whereby the small alveolar capillaries become compressed and have higher resistance, while the extra-alveolar vessels are enlarged due to radial traction. The alveolar and extra-alveolar PVR are added together to result in a U-shaped cumulative PVR curve, where the PVR is lowest at FRC and highest at residual volume (RV) and total lung capacity (TLC). On the other hand, airway resistance is lowest at total lung capacity and highest at residual volume since higher lung volumes lead to alveolar traction that keeps the airways open. (56–57, 64–65)

PULMONARY GAS EXCHANGE

8. Stored red blood cells have a marked decrease in 2,3-DPG levels even after 24 hours in cold storage, and the entire 2,3-DPG supply is virtually depleted after about two weeks. This leads to a shift of the oxyhemoglobin dissociation curve to the left and may cause impaired oxygen delivery. Once transfused, there is in vivo recovery of 2,3-DPG which may take several hours to several days. (58)
9. The safe apnea time (i.e., time to desaturate to $SpO_2 < 90\%$), can be estimated by the equation FRC × ETO_2/ VO_2, where ETO_2 is the end-tidal oxygen concentration and VO_2 is the expected oxygen consumption (around 3.5 mL/kg/min in the average adult). For an 80-kg patient, the FRC is 30 mL/kg × 80 kg = 2400 mL. End-tidal O_2 concentration of 80% means that there is 1920 mL of oxygen in the reservoir. Therefore with average O_2 consumption rates, the time to use this 1920 mL oxygen tank would be 6.8 minutes. However, higher oxygen consumption rates can occur in patients with obesity, fever, sepsis, and other hypermetabolic states. In addition, the estimated time does not account for the carbon dioxide rise that occurs with apnea and which also occupies space in the alveoli. (60)

PULMONARY MECHANICS

10. There are two types of compliance involved in the respiratory system: static and dynamic. Static compliance describes the change in volume divided by the change in pressure when there is no airflow, such as during an inspiratory hold maneuver (called plateau pressure or $P_{plateau}$). Static compliance = tidal volume/ ($P_{plateau}$ – PEEP). Dynamic compliance, on the other hand, describes change in volume divided by change in pressure during normal breathing (using the peak inspiratory pressure or PIP). Dynamic compliance is always lower than static compliance because airway resistance increases with increasing airflow. Dynamic compliance = tidal volume/(PIP – PEEP). When high airway pressures are encountered during mechanical ventilation, first assess whether there is both high peak pressure and plateau pressure (indicating primarily a compliance problem), or whether there is a high peak pressure but normal plateau pressure (indicating more of an airway resistance problem). The differential diagnosis for reduced respiratory system compliance includes decreased lung compliance (e.g., pulmonary edema or consolidation, ARDS, large pleural effusions or pneumothorax, auto-PEEP) and decreased chest wall compliance (e.g., morbid obesity, abdominal distension or massive ascites, kyphoscoliosis, inadequate anesthesia). The differential for increased respiratory system resistance includes increased flow rates and causes of increased airway resistance (e.g., bronchospasm, secretions or mucus plugging, endotracheal tube kinking or biting, pooling of condensed water in the circuit, small endotracheal tube). (64–65)

CONTROL OF BREATHING

11. As $PaCO_2$ increases, ventilation increases dramatically. In the awake state, a 1 mmHg rise in $PaCO_2$ is associated with a 1.5 L/min increase in ventilation. As $PaCO_2$ continues to increase, the rise in minute ventilation is eventually limited to the maximal minute ventilation. With decreases in $PaCO_2$ below resting levels, the minute ventilation does not decrease to zero because of a drive to breathe related to wakefulness. However, during anesthesia, a decrease in $PaCO_2$ (e.g., from assisted mechanical ventilation) can reach a value at which ventilation stops: the apneic threshold. (66)

Chapter

6 AUTONOMIC NERVOUS SYSTEM

David B. Glick and Erica J. Stein

- The autonomic nervous system (ANS) controls involuntary activities of the body outside consciousness.
  - Primitive: its characteristics are largely preserved across all mammalian species.
  - Essential: oversees responses to immediate life-threatening challenges and the body's vital maintenance needs.

Branches of the Autonomic Nervous System

The sympathetic nervous system
- Controls the "fight-or-flight" response
- Redistribution of blood flow from the viscera to skeletal muscle
- Increased cardiac output

The parasympathetic nervous system
- Oversees the body's maintenance needs
- Examples include digestion and genitourinary function

ANATOMY OF THE AUTONOMIC NERVOUS SYSTEM

The Sympathetic Nervous System

- Originates from T1–L2 or L3 of the spinal cord
  - The cell bodies of these neurons lie in the spinal gray matter.
  - The nerve fibers extend to paired ganglia.
    - Sympathetic chains lie immediately lateral to the vertebral column or extend to unpaired distal plexuses (e.g., the celiac and mesenteric plexuses).
- Preganglionic sympathetic fibers synapse at the ganglion of the level of their origin and can course up and down the paired ganglia.
  - A sympathetic response can be amplified and diffuse.
- The postganglionic neurons run a long course to innervate the target effector organs.
- Preganglionic sympathetic nerve releases acetylcholine (ACh).
  - ACh binds to nicotinic cholinergic receptor on the postganglionic nerve.
- Postganglionic nerve releases norepinephrine at the synapse with the target organ.
  - Other classic neurotransmitters of SNS include epinephrine and dopamine.
  - Cotransmitters, such as adenosine triphosphate (ATP) and neuropeptide Y, modulate sympathetic activity.
- Receptors
  - The α_1-, β_1-, β_2-, and β-receptors are postsynaptic, adrenergic.
    - Bind norepinephrine and epinephrine
  - The α_2-receptor is presynaptic.
    - Binds norepinephrine
    - Binding decreases subsequent norepinephrine release (negative feedback).
  - D_1 (postsynaptic) and D_2 (presynaptic) receptors
    - Bind dopamine
- Sympathetic neurotransmitters are synthesized from tyrosine.

Sympathetic Nervous System Neurotransmitter Synthesis

In the postganglionic nerve ending:
- Tyrosine to dihydroxyphenylalanine (DOPA)
  - Rate-limiting step
  - Catalyzed by the enzyme tyrosine hydroxylase
- DOPA to dopamine
- Dopamine to norepinephrine

In the adrenal medulla:
- Norepinephrine is methylated to epinephrine.

- Neurotransmitters are stored in vesicles until the postganglionic nerve is stimulated.
  - The vesicles merge with the cell membrane and release their contents into the synapse.
    - Only 1% of the total stored norepinephrine is released with each depolarization, leaving a tremendous functional reserve.
  - The released norepinephrine binds to the presynaptic and postsynaptic adrenergic receptors.
  - The postsynaptic receptors then activate secondary messenger systems in the postsynaptic cell via G protein–linked activity.

- Norepinephrine is then released from these receptors and mostly taken up at the presynaptic nerve terminal and transported to storage vesicles for reuse.
- Norepinephrine that escapes this reuptake process and goes into the circulation is metabolized by either the monoamine oxidase (MAO) or catechol-*O*-methyltransferase (COMT) enzyme in the blood, liver, or kidney.

The Parasympathetic Nervous System

- Arises from cranial nerves III, VII, IX, and X and from sacral segments S1–S4
- Parasympathetic nervous system (PNS) ganglia are in close proximity to (or even within) their target organs.
- Preganglionic parasympathetic nerve terminals release ACh.
  - ACh binds to nicotinic cholinergic receptor on the postganglionic nerve.
- Postganglionic nerve releases ACh at the synapse with the target organ.
  - The ACh receptors of the target organ are muscarinic receptors.
  - Muscarinic receptors are coupled to G proteins and secondary messenger systems.
  - ACh is rapidly inactivated within the synapse by the cholinesterase enzyme.

ADRENERGIC PHARMACOLOGY

Endogenous Catecholamines

Norepinephrine

- The primary adrenergic neurotransmitter; binds to α- and β-receptors
- Primary use: increase in systemic vascular resistance due to its α_1-adrenergic effects
  - Short-acting (half-life is 2.5 minutes), usually given as a continuous infusion
    - Starting rates of 3 μg/min or more and titrated to the desired effect
  - Reflex bradycardia often results.
  - Vasoconstricts the pulmonary, renal, mesenteric, and peripheral circulations
    - Infusions must be carefully monitored to prevent injury to vital organs.
    - Prolonged infusions can cause ischemia in the fingers and toes.
  - Endocrine and metabolic effects include increased levels of blood glucose, lactate, and free fatty acids.

Epinephrine

- Binds to α- and β-adrenergic receptors
  - Therapeutic effects of epinephrine are positive inotropy, chronotropy, and enhanced conduction in the heart (β_1), smooth muscle relaxation in the vasculature and bronchial tree (β_2), and vasoconstriction (α_1).
    - The predominant effect depends on the dose administered.
    - Endocrine and metabolic effects include increased levels of blood glucose, lactate, and free fatty acids.
- Exogenous epinephrine is used intravenously to treat life-threatening events.
  - 1 mg can be given for cardiovascular collapse, asystole, ventricular fibrillation, pulseless electrical activity, or anaphylactic shock.
  - Vasoconstricts the peripheral vasculature to maintain myocardial and cerebral perfusion
- Used locally to decrease local anesthetic systemic absorption and reduce surgical blood loss
- Continuous infusion administration in less acute circumstances
  - Individual responses to epinephrine vary.
  - Titrate to effect while monitoring the patient for signs of compromised renal, cerebral, or myocardial perfusion.
    - Rates of 1 to 2 μg/min: primarily stimulates β_2-receptors and decreases airway resistance and vascular tone
    - Rates of 2 to 10 μg/min: increases heart rate, contractility, and conduction through the atrioventricular node
    - Doses >10 μg/min: α_1-adrenergic effects predominate, resulting in generalized vasoconstriction, which can lead to reflex bradycardia.
- Aerosol administration to treat severe croup or airway edema
- Subcutaneous administration to treat bronchospasm
  - Doses of 300 μg every 20 minutes with a maximum of three doses
  - Treats bronchospasm two ways
    - Direct effect as a bronchodilator
    - Stabilizes mast cells to decrease their release of antigen-induced bronchospastic substances (as may occur during anaphylaxis)
- Interaction with halothane
  - Epinephrine decreases the refractory period of the myocardium.
  - Risk of arrhythmias during halothane anesthesia is increased when epinephrine is given.
  - The risk of arrhythmias seems to be less in children but increases with hypocapnia.

Dopamine

- Binds to α- and β-receptors, as well as dopaminergic receptors
- Acts directly and indirectly by stimulating norepinephrine release from storage vesicles
- Uniquely able to improve blood flow through the renal and mesenteric beds in shock states by binding to postjunctional D_1 receptors

- Rapid metabolism by MAO and COMT (half-life = 1 minute) requires it be given as a continuous infusion.
  - Rates of 0.5 to 2.0 μg/kg/min: D_1 receptors are stimulated, and renal and mesenteric beds are dilated.
  - Rates of 2 to 10 μg/kg/min: β_1-receptors are stimulated, and cardiac contractility and cardiac output are increased.
  - Doses ≥10 μg/kg/min: predominant α_1-receptor binding causing marked generalized constriction of the vasculature, negating any benefit to renal perfusion
- Routine use for patients in shock is questionable.
  - No beneficial effect on renal function has been shown.
  - May increase mortality risk and the incidence of arrhythmic events

Synthetic Catecholamines

Isoproterenol

- Binds to β-receptors: β_1-adrenergic stimulation is greater than β_2-adrenergic effects.
- Half-life ranges from 2.5 to 5 minutes (no reuptake into the adrenergic nerve endings).
- Adverse effects include tachycardia and arrhythmias.
  - No longer part of the advanced cardiac life support (ACLS) protocols
- Principal uses
  - Chronotropic drug after cardiac transplantation
  - Initiates atrial fibrillation or other arrhythmias during cardiac electrophysiology ablation procedures
- May cause vasodilation by β_2-adrenergic stimulation with larger doses

Dobutamine

- A synthetic analog of dopamine; predominantly β_1-adrenergic effects
- Comparison with other agents
  - Inotropy is more than chronotropy and less of a β_2-type effect than isoproterenol.
  - Less of an α_1-type effect than norepinephrine
  - No endogenous norepinephrine release or dopamine receptor stimulation like dopamine
- Potentially useful in patients with congestive heart failure (CHF) or myocardial infarction complicated by low cardiac output since it directly stimulates β_1-receptors
  - Doses <20 μg/kg/min usually do not produce tachycardia.
  - Does not rely on endogenous norepinephrine stores for its effects, making it useful in catecholamine-depleted states such as chronic CHF
- Prolonged treatment with dobutamine causes downregulation of β-adrenergic receptors.
  - Tolerance and even tachyphylaxis may occur after 3 days.
  - Intermittent infusions of dobutamine can avoid this effect.
- No controlled trials have demonstrated improved survival.

Fenoldopam

- Selective D_1 agonist; potent vasodilator that enhances renal blood flow and diuresis
  - Clinical studies on its use as a nephroprotective agent have provided mixed results.
- Approved for intravenous treatment of severe hypertension at infusion rates of 0.1 to 0.8 μg/kg/min
  - Peak effect takes 15 minutes.
  - Alternative to sodium nitroprusside with fewer side effects (e.g., no thiocyanate toxicity, rebound effect, or coronary steal) and improved renal function

Noncatecholamine Sympathomimetic Amines

- Most noncatecholamine sympathomimetic amines act at α- and β-receptors.
  - Directly via binding of the drug by adrenergic receptors
  - Indirectly through the release of endogenous norepinephrine stores
- Mephentermine and metaraminol are rarely used currently.

Ephedrine

- Increases arterial blood pressure and has a positive inotropic effect
- Tachyphylaxis may develop as norepinephrine stores are depleted.
  - Repeat doses in life-threatening events (instead of switching to epinephrine) may contribute to morbidity.
- Used as a pressor in hypotensive pregnant patients
  - Phenylephrine is now the preferred treatment for hypotension in the parturient because of a decreased risk of fetal acidosis.
- Helpful in treating moderate hypotension, particularly if accompanied by bradycardia
  - Usual dose is 2.5 to 10 mg (intravenously) or 25 to 50 mg (intramuscularly).

SELECTIVE α-ADRENERGIC RECEPTOR AGONISTS

α_1-Adrenergic Agonists

Phenylephrine

- Selective α_1-agonist
- Principal uses
  - For peripheral vasoconstriction when cardiac output is adequate (e.g., in the hypotension that may accompany spinal anesthesia)

- To maintain afterload in patients with aortic stenosis whose coronary perfusion is compromised by a decline in systemic vascular resistance
- As a mydriatic and nasal decongestant
  - Topically to prepare nares for nasotracheal intubation (often with local anesthetics)
- Rapid onset and duration of action (5–10 minutes) when given intravenously
  - Can be given as a bolus (40–100 μg) or as an infusion (starting rate 10–20 μg/min)
- Larger doses (up to 1 mg) may lead to conversion of supraventricular tachycardia to sinus rhythm through reflex action.
  - This treatment option is not part of current ACLS algorithms.

α_2-Adrenergic Agonists

- Primary effect is sympatholytic.
  - Stimulates prejunctional inhibitory α_2-receptors to reduce peripheral norepinephrine release
- Traditional use is as antihypertensive drugs.
- Anesthetic applications based on sedative, anxiolytic, and analgesic properties

Clonidine

- Selective agonist for α_2-receptors; prototypical drug of this class
- Antihypertensive effects: central and peripheral attenuation of sympathetic outflow
  - Transdermal patch is available if a patient cannot take clonidine orally.
  - Withdrawal may precipitate a hypertensive crisis
  - Labetalol is used to treat clonidine withdrawal syndrome.
- Anesthesia adjuvant: can reduce IV or inhaled anesthetic requirements in general or regional anesthetic technique
- Chronic pain uses
  - As analgesic adjuncts to local anesthetics and opioids (also for acute pain)
  - In epidural for the treatment of intractable pain
  - For patients with reflex sympathetic dystrophy and neuropathic pain syndromes
- Perioperative use was thought to decrease myocardial infarction and perioperative mortality rates in patients who had vascular surgery.
  - A large 2014 randomized trial of perioperative clonidine did not show a reduction in death or nonfatal myocardial infarction within 30 days of noncardiac surgery.

Dexmedetomidine

- Selective for α_2-receptors
- Clinical effect is short; distribution half-life is less than 5 minutes (half-life = 2.3 hours).
  - Available as an IV solution with usual dosing of 0.3 to 0.7 μg/kg/h
  - Can also give an initial dose of 1 μg/kg over 10 minutes
- Dose-dependent decreases in heart rate, cardiac output, and circulating catecholamines
- Increases sedation, analgesia, and amnesia; decreases inhaled anesthetic need, and minor impact on respiratory depression
  - Useful for awake fiberoptic intubation
  - Decreases the need for opioids for perioperative management of obese patients with obstructive sleep apnea

β_2-ADRENERGIC RECEPTOR AGONISTS

- Treats asthma in lower doses
  - Large doses can cause severe side effects related to β_1-adrenergic stimulation.
  - Commonly used agonists include metaproterenol (Alupent, Metaprel), terbutaline (Brethine, Bricanyl), and albuterol (Proventil, Ventolin).
- Arrests premature labor
  - Ritodrine (Yutopar) has been marketed for this purpose.
  - β_1-Adrenergic adverse effects are common, especially when given IV.

α-ADRENERGIC RECEPTOR ANTAGONISTS

- Have long been used as antihypertensive drugs
- Side effects of marked orthostatic hypotension and fluid retention make them less popular.

Phenoxybenzamine

- The prototypical α_1-adrenergic antagonist (though it also has α_2-antagonist effects)
- Irreversibly binds α_1-receptors; new receptors must be synthesized before complete recovery.
- Decreases peripheral resistance and increases cardiac output
- Adverse effect is orthostatic hypotension.
  - Syncope can result from rapid movement from the supine to standing position.
- Nasal stuffiness is another adverse effect.
- Most common use is for the treatment of catecholamine-secreting pheochromocytomas.
  - Establishes a "chemical sympathectomy" preoperatively, making arterial blood pressure less labile during surgery
  - If exogenous sympathomimetics are given after α_1-blockade, their vasoconstrictive effects are inhibited.
- Recommended treatment for a phenoxybenzamine overdose is a norepinephrine infusion.
  - Some receptors remain free of the drug.
  - Vasopressin may also be effective in this setting.

Prazosin

- Potent selective α_1-blocker
  - Antagonizes the vasoconstrictor effects of norepinephrine and epinephrine
- Orthostatic hypotension is a major problem.
- Improves lipid profiles by lowering low-density lipoprotein levels and raising the level of high-density lipoproteins
- Starting dose is 0.5 to 1 mg given at bedtime due to the risk of orthostatic hypotension.
- Doxazosin (Cardura) and terazosin (Hytrin) have pharmacologic effects similar to those of prazosin but have longer pharmacokinetic half-lives.
- Used for the preoperative preparation of patients with pheochromocytomas
  - Much less costly than phenoxybenzamine
  - Modest intraoperative hypertensive episodes are more common because the antagonism is competitive instead of permanent.
- Agents such as tamsulosin (Flomax) show selectivity for the α_{1A}-receptor subtype.
  - Effective in the treatment of benign prostatic hyperplasia
  - Lacks the hypotensive effects seen with nonselective α_1-blockers

Yohimbine

- α_2-Antagonist; increases the release of norepinephrine
- Little clinical utility in anesthesia

β-ADRENERGIC ANTAGONISTS

- Clinical indications include ischemic heart disease, postinfarction management, arrhythmias, hypertrophic cardiomyopathy, hypertension, heart failure, migraine prophylaxis, thyrotoxicosis, and glaucoma.
  - Reverses ventricular remodeling and reduces mortality rate in patients with heart failure and reduced ejection fraction
- Perioperative use was thought to improve survival by decreasing the surgical stress response.
  - A large study of oral metoprolol started on day of surgery and continuing for 30 days (POISE trial) demonstrated increased mortality rate in the β-blocker group.
  - Subsequently found to prevent nonfatal myocardial infarctions but increase the rate of death, hypotension, bradycardia, and stroke
- The 2014 American College of Cardiology/American Heart Association (ACC/AHA) guideline recommends that patients on chronic β-blocker therapy undergoing noncardiac surgery continue therapy perioperatively, but β-blocker therapy should not be started on day of surgery.
- β-Adrenergic blockers in anesthetic practice (propranolol, metoprolol, labetalol, and esmolol) have IV formulations and well-characterized effects.
  - Vary in cardioselectivity and duration of action
  - Nonselective β-blockers act at the β_1- and β_2-receptors.
- Cardioselective β_1-receptor blockade decreases the velocity of atrioventricular conduction, heart rate, and cardiac contractility.
  - The release of renin by the juxtaglomerular apparatus and lipolysis at adipocytes also decreases.
  - At larger doses, selectivity for β_1-receptors is lost, and β_2-receptors are also blocked.
    - Potential for bronchoconstriction, peripheral vasoconstriction, and decreased glycogenolysis

Adverse Effects of β-Adrenergic Blockade

- Cardiac: life-threatening bradycardia (even asystole) and decreased contractility may precipitate heart failure in patients with compromised cardiac function.
- Pulmonary: can exacerbate bronchospastic lung disease, such that β_2-blockade may be fatal
- Endocrine: long-term use of β-antagonists in patients with diabetes mellitus is relatively contraindicated.
  - Warning signs of hypoglycemia (tachycardia and tremor) can be masked.
  - Compensatory glycogenolysis is blunted.
- Patients with pheochromocytomas should avoid the use of β-blockers to avoid worsening of hypertension unless α-receptors have already been blocked.
- Overdose of β-blocking drugs may be treated with atropine.
  - Isoproterenol, dobutamine, or glucagon along with cardiac pacing may be required to maintain adequate rate of contraction.
- Undesirable drug interactions
  - Verapamil: rate and contractility effects of verapamil are additive to those of β-blockers.
  - Digoxin: combined with β-blockers can have powerful effects on heart rate and conduction and should be used with special care.

Specific β-Adrenergic Blockers

Propranolol

- Prototypical, nonselective β-blocking drug
- Highly lipid soluble and extensively metabolized in the liver
  - Metabolism varies greatly from patient to patient.
  - Clearance of the drug can be affected by liver disease or altered hepatic blood flow.
- Available in an IV form and was initially given as either a bolus or an infusion
  - Infusions of propranolol have largely been supplanted by the shorter-acting esmolol.
  - Bolus doses of 0.1 mg/kg may be given; typically initiated at 0.25 to 0.5 mg and titrated to effect.

- Clinical use
  - Efficacious in vasospastic disorders, perhaps due to shifting of the oxyhemoglobin dissociation curve to the right
  - To mitigate tachycardia in hyperthyroidism
    - Also inhibits the peripheral conversion of T_4 thyroid hormone to the more active T_3 hormone

Metoprolol

- Cardioselective β-blocker; approved to treat angina pectoris and acute myocardial infarction
- No dosing adjustments are necessary in patients with liver failure.
- Oral dosage is 100 to 200 mg/day once or twice daily for hypertension and twice daily for angina pectoris.
- Intravenous dosing is 2.5 to 5 mg every 2 to 5 minutes up to a total dose of 15 mg, with titration to heart rate and blood pressure.

Labetalol

- Competitive antagonist at the α_1- and β-adrenergic receptors
- Metabolized by the liver, its clearance is affected by hepatic perfusion.
- Intravenous dosing is in 5- to 10-mg doses every 5 minutes, or infuse up to 2 mg/min.
- Clinical use
  - Effective in the treatment of patients with aortic dissection and in hypertensive emergencies
  - For postoperative hypertension in patients with coronary artery disease
    - Vasodilation is not accompanied by tachycardia.
  - Treats hypertension in pregnancy on a long-term basis and in acute situations
    - Uterine blood flow is not affected, even with significant reductions in blood pressure.

Esmolol

- Esmolol is cardioselective with a uniquely short half-life of 9 to 10 minutes.
- Hydrolyzed by bloodborne esterases
  - Peak effects of loading dose within 5 to 10 minutes; diminish in 20 to 30 minutes
  - If continuous use is needed, the longer-lasting β-blocker metoprolol can replace it.
- Can be given as a bolus (0.5 mg/kg) or as an infusion.
  - To treat supraventricular tachycardia, bolus 500 μg/kg over 1 minute, followed by an infusion of 50 μg/kg/min for 4 minute.
    - If the heart rate is not controlled, repeat the loading dose followed by a 4-minute infusion of 100 μg/kg/min.
    - If needed, repeat the sequence with the infusion increased in 50-μg/kg/min increments up to 300 μg/kg/min.
- Clinical use
  - When β-blockade of short duration is desired, particularly in anesthesia practice
  - In critically ill patients in whom the adverse effects of bradycardia, heart failure, or hypotension may require rapid drug withdrawal
  - To treat intraoperative and postoperative hypertension and tachycardia

CHOLINERGIC PHARMACOLOGY

- There is a relative paucity of drugs that affect cholinergic transmission.
- Direct cholinergic agents are used to treat glaucoma (topical) or to restore gastrointestinal or urinary function.
- Anticholinergic agents (muscarinic antagonists) and anticholinesterases are used in anesthesia practice.

Muscarinic Antagonists

- Competitive antagonists with neurally released ACh for access to muscarinic cholinoceptors
- Effects are faster heart rate, sedation, and dry mouth.
  - Quaternary ammonium compounds (e.g., glycopyrrolate) do not readily cross the blood–brain barrier and have few actions on the CNS.
- Among these drugs, there is no significant specificity of action, but there are some quantitative differences in effect.
- Clinical use
  - Anesthetic premedication to decrease secretions and prevent harmful vagal reflexes
    - Especially in some pediatric and otorhinolaryngologic cases
    - For planned fiberoptic intubation
  - As prophylaxis for postoperative nausea and vomiting (scopolamine patch)
  - To block the adverse muscarinic effects (bradycardia) of the anticholinesterase drugs used to reverse neuromuscular blockade
    - Glycopyrrolate has a longer duration of action than atropine and has largely replaced it for this purpose.
- Adverse effects
  - CNS side effects for those with tertiary structure that cross the blood–brain barrier
    - Atropine (large doses of 1–2 mg) or scopolamine
    - Symptoms include delusions and delirium.
    - Treated with physostigmine, an anticholinesterase that crosses the blood–brain barrier
  - Eye, bladder, skin, and psychological effects can be associated with scopolamine patch.

Cholinesterase Inhibitors

- Impair the inactivation of ACh by the cholinesterase enzyme and sustain cholinergic agonism at nicotinic and muscarinic receptors
- Clinical use (most used are physostigmine, neostigmine, pyridostigmine, and edrophonium)
  - Reverse neuromuscular blockade
  - Treat myasthenia gravis
  - Stimulate intestinal function
  - Applied topically to the eye as a miotic
- Adverse effects
  - Most prominent side effect is bradycardia.
  - Impairs the function of the pseudocholinesterase enzyme
  - One topical drug (echothiophate iodide) irreversibly binds cholinesterase and can interfere with the metabolism of succinylcholine.

QUESTIONS

1. What are the two branches of the autonomic nervous system, and what are the primary actions of each of these branches?
2. Draw a schematic diagram of the parasympathetic and sympathetic nervous systems. For each include the preganglionic nerve fiber, the postganglionic nerve fiber, and the receptor types on the postganglionic nerve fiber and end organ.
3. What are two differences between the preganglionic fibers of the sympathetic nervous system (SNS) and the preganglionic fibers of the parasympathetic nervous system (PNS)?
4. What are the neurotransmitters and receptors of the autonomic nervous system (ANS)?
5. Where are the sympathetic neurotransmitters synthesized, and what is the rate-limiting step in their synthesis?
6. What happens to norepinephrine after it is released from the presynaptic and postsynaptic adrenergic receptors?
7. What happens to ACh after it is released from the muscarinic receptors of the PNS back into the postganglionic synapse?
8. For each of the following, indicate what the adrenergic effect is at the effector organ and which receptor (α_1, α_2, β_1, or β_2) primarily mediates the response.

Effector Organ/Effect	Adrenergic Response	Receptor Involved
Heart rate		
Force of contraction		
Arteries		
Veins		
Vessels to skeletal muscle		
Bronchial tree		
Splenic capsule		
Gastrointestinal tract		
Insulin release from pancreas		
Liver glycogenolysis		

9. What effect does the administration of exogenous epinephrine have on blood glucose, lactate, and free fatty acid levels?
10. What is the mechanism behind epinephrine's efficacy in treating cases of anaphylaxis?
11. To which receptors does dopamine bind? What are its primary effects at doses of 0.5 to 2 μg/kg/min, 2 to 10 μg/kg/min, and >10 μg/kg/min?
12. What effects make dobutamine a useful agent in patients with severe congestive heart failure? What are dobutamine's shortcomings in this setting?
13. What are ephedrine's *direct* and *indirect* actions?
14. Why should repeated doses of ephedrine be avoided in life-threatening circumstances (such as the hypotension that accompanies a high spinal)?
15. Describe the pharmacologic action and clinical effects of dexmedetomidine.
16. What are the two principal clinical uses for β_2-adrenergic agonists?
17. What is the primary use, and what are the common side effects of α_1-adrenergic antagonists?
18. Name nine clinical indications for β-blocker therapy.
19. What are the current ACC/AHA recommendations for the perioperative administration of β-blockers in patients undergoing noncardiac surgeries?
20. How are the pharmacologic effects of labetalol different from those of the other intravenous β-adrenergic blocking agents?
21. What accounts for the relatively short (9–10 minutes) half-life of esmolol?
22. Which of the muscarinic antagonists has no sedative effects, and why?

ANSWERS

1. The two branches of the autonomic nervous system are the sympathetic nervous system (SNS) and the parasympathetic nervous system (PNS). The primary function of the SNS is to control the "fight-or-flight" response (increasing cardiac output and redistributing blood flow from the viscera to the skeletal muscles), whereas the PNS is primarily responsible for the body's maintenance needs (e.g., digestion and genitourinary functions). (69)
2. The figure below is a schematic diagram of the parasympathetic and sympathetic nervous systems. (71)

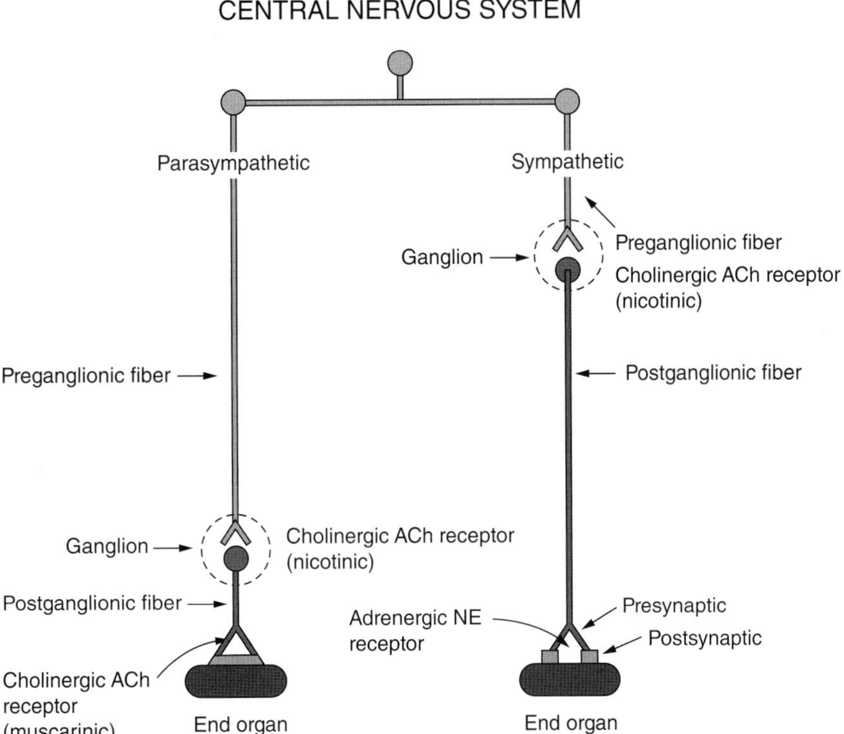

Schematic diagram of the peripheral autonomic nervous system. Preganglionic fibers and postganglionic fibers of the parasympathetic nervous system release acetylcholine (ACh) as the neurotransmitter. Postganglionic fibers of the sympathetic nervous system release norepinephrine (NE) as the neurotransmitter (exceptions are fibers to sweat glands, which release ACh). (From Lawson NW, Wallfisch HK. Cardiovascular pharmacology: a new look at the pressors. In Stoelting RK, Barash J, eds. *Advances in Anesthesia*. Chicago: Year Book Medical Publishers; 1986:195–270.)

3. There are two differences between the preganglionic fibers of the SNS and the preganglionic fibers of the PNS. First, the cell bodies of the preganglionic neurons of the SNS reside in the spinal gray matter in the thoracolumbar region (T1-L2 or L3), while the neurons of the PNS arise from cranial nerves III, VII, IX, and X and sacral segments S1-S4. Second, the preganglionic fibers of the SNS are relatively short as the SNS ganglia are either adjacent to the vertebral column in the paired sympathetic chains or in the unpaired midline sympathetic plexuses (celiac, superior mesenteric, and inferior mesenteric). The preganglionic parasympathetic nerve fibers, on the other hand, are quite long, extending all the way to their target organs before reaching the parasympathetic ganglia. (69–72)
4. The neurotransmitter released by the preganglionic neurons of the SNS is acetylcholine (ACh). It binds to nicotinic receptors on the postganglionic neuron. The postganglionic neurons of the SNS release norepinephrine that is bound by adrenergic receptors (α_1, α_2, β_1, β_2, and β_3) on the end organ. Like the SNS, the preganglionic neurons of the PNS release ACh that is bound to nicotinic receptors on the postganglionic neurons. The postganglionic PNS neurons release ACh that is bound to muscarinic receptors on the end organ. (71–72)
5. The sympathetic neurotransmitters norepinephrine, epinephrine, and dopamine are synthesized in the postganglionic sympathetic nerve ending. The rate-limiting step in their synthesis is the transformation of tyrosine to dihydroxyphenylalanine (DOPA), which is catalyzed by the enzyme tyrosine hydroxylase. (71)

6. The vast majority of the norepinephrine released back into the synapse is taken up at the presynaptic nerve terminal and transported to storage vesicles for reuse. The norepinephrine that escapes the reuptake process makes its way into the bloodstream, where it is metabolized by the enzyme monoamine oxidase (MAO) or catechol-*O*-methyltransferase (COMT) in the blood, liver, or kidney. (71)
7. ACh released from the muscarinic receptors back into the synapse is rapidly broken down into choline and acetate in a reaction catalyzed by acetylcholinesterase. (72)
8. The table below indicates what the adrenergic effect is at the effector organ and which receptor (α_1, α_2, β_1, or β_2) primarily mediates the response. (75)

Effector Organ/Effect	Adrenergic Response	Receptor Involved
Heart rate	Increase	β_1
Force of contraction	Increase	β_1
Arteries	Vasoconstriction	α_1
Veins	Vasoconstriction	α_2
Vessels to skeletal muscle	Vasodilation	β_2
Bronchial tree	Bronchodilation	β_2
Splenic capsule	Contraction	α_1
Uterus	Contraction	α_1
Gastrointestinal tract	Relaxation	α_2
Insulin release from pancreas	Decrease	α_2
Liver glycogenolysis	Increase	α_1

9. Intravenous administration of exogenous epinephrine causes blood glucose, lactate, and free fatty acid levels to rise. (72)
10. Epinephrine treats anaphylaxis by stabilizing mast cells, which truncates the anaphylactic response. (73)
11. Dopamine binds α, β, and dopamine receptors. At infusion rates of 0.5 to 2 μg/kg/min, the renal and mesenteric vessels are dilated. At 2-10 μg/kg/min, cardiac contractility and cardiac output are increased. At >10 μg/kg/min, there is marked generalized vasoconstriction (even of the renal and mesenteric vessels). (74)
12. Dobutamine can increase cardiac output via its β_1-mediated inotropic effects and its β_2-mediated vasodilatory effects. The issue with dobutamine therapy in the setting of congestive heart failure is that after 3 days of therapy, tolerance and/or tachyphylaxis can develop due to the downregulation of β-adrenergic receptors. While dobutamine does increase cardiac output, there are no controlled studies demonstrating improved survival in heart failure patients on dobutamine therapy. (75)
13. Ephedrine's direct effect results from the drug's binding to α- and β- adrenergic receptors. Its indirect effects are the result of its ability to cause the release of endogenous norepinephrine stores. Tachyphylaxis to ephedrine's indirect effects can develop as endogenous norepinephrine stores are exhausted. (76)
14. Evidence from closed claims analysis of unexpected cardiac arrest during spinal anesthesia suggested that there was increased mortality when repeated doses of ephedrine were given in life-threatening circumstances instead of switching early on to epinephrine as the resuscitative agent. (76)
15. Dexmedetomidine is an α_2-agonist. It binds to the α_2-receptors that are located on the presynaptic sympathetic nerve ending. Its clinical effects include sedation, analgesia, and amnesia. It also decreases heart rate, cardiac output, oral secretions, and circulating catecholamine levels. (77)
16. β_2-Adrenergic agonists are used to treat asthma (metaproterenol, terbutaline, and albuterol) and to arrest premature labor (ritodrine). All of these agents lose their β_2-selectivity at higher doses with resultant β_1-adrenergic stimulation. (77)
17. α_1-Adrenergic receptor antagonists are rarely used antihypertensive agents because of their unattractive side effect profile. These side effects include orthostatic hypotension, fluid retention, and nasal stuffiness. They are, however, the agents of choice for creating a chemical sympathectomy prior to surgical excision of a pheochromocytoma. (77–78)

18. Clinical indications for β-adrenergic blockade include ischemic heart disease, postinfarction management, arrhythmias, hypertrophic cardiomyopathy, hypertension, heart failure, migraine prophylaxis, thyrotoxicosis, and glaucoma. (78)
19. The 2014 ACC/AHA Guideline on Perioperative Cardiovascular Evaluation and Management of Patients Undergoing Noncardiac Surgery recommends that patients on chronic β-blocker therapy continue their β-blockers in the perioperative setting but that new β-blocker therapy should not be initiated on the day of surgery. (78)
20. Labetalol's pharmacologic effects are different from other intravenous β-adrenergic blocking agents because, in addition to labetalol's antagonism of β-adrenergic activity, it is also a competitive antagonist at the α_1-receptors. As a result, it is commonly used to treat patients with aortic dissections or hypertensive emergencies. (79)
21. Esmolol is hydrolyzed by bloodborne esterases, which accounts for its short half-life. Its short half-life makes it especially useful in intensive care unit or operating room settings, where the β-adrenergic blockade might need to be stopped abruptly if the patient's hemodynamic status changes. (79)
22. Glycopyrrolate is a muscarinic antagonist without sedative effects because its quaternary structure renders it too large to cross the blood–brain barrier. The CNS side effects of the other muscarinic antagonists (atropine and scopolamine) are treated with physostigmine, an anticholinesterase that can cross the blood–brain barrier. (80)

Chapter

7 INHALED ANESTHETICS

Daniel C. Cook and Hugh C. Hemmings, Jr.

HISTORY

- Diethyl ether administered at the first public demonstration of inhaled anesthesia
- Performed at Massachusetts General Hospital on October 16, 1846

CHEMICAL AND PHYSICAL PROPERTIES

Molecular Structures

- The most widely used volatile anesthetics are all halogenated ethers.
- Halothane is a polyhalogenated alkane
- Halogen atom substitution determines the pharmacokinetic and metabolic profiles of volatile anesthetics.
  - Desflurane and sevoflurane have only fluorine substitutions.
  - This contributes to their relatively rapid uptake and elimination.
- Nitrous oxide (N_2O) is a commonly used low-potency anesthetic gas.
- Xenon is a noble gas that can produce general anesthesia.
  - Seldomly used due to its high cost and difficult procurement and delivery
  - May have specific applications as a neuroprotectant

Physical Properties

Physicochemical Properties of Inhaled Anesthetics

- Partial pressure—Pressure contributed by one individual gas to the total pressure of a gas mixture
- Vapor pressure—Partial pressure exerted by the gaseous phase of a chemical in equilibrium with its liquid phase
- Solubility—Amount of gas that can be homogeneously dissolved into a liquid
  - Dissolved concentration is directly proportional to the partial pressure of the gas, $C = kP$, and the solubility constant, k, is temperature dependent.
- Partition coefficient—Ratio of concentrations at equilibrium of a solute dissolved in two different solvents

- Modern potent inhaled anesthetics are liquids at standard temperature and pressure.
- "Volatile" anesthetics are delivered as vapors.
- Vapor pressure quantifies the propensity of a liquid to evaporate.

How Vapor Pressure Influences Desflurane Handling

- Desflurane has a relatively high vapor pressure at room temperature.
  - Boiling point is 22.8°C (73°F)
- Unique bottle design and vaporizer filling mechanism
- Bottle is designed to avoid opening.
  - Prevents rapid evaporation of the agent
  - Protects against pollution of the procedural area

UPTAKE AND DISTRIBUTION IN THE BODY

Vaporizers

- Potent, volatile anesthetics use a variable bypass vaporizer to deliver a precise concentration.
  - Gas in vaporizer splits into two paths in a specific ratio.
  - One path bypasses, while the other gets saturated with anesthetic.
  - Desired concentration (volume %) results from the remixing of gases.
  - The volatile anesthetic is diluted into the fresh gas flow of the anesthesia machine.
- Desflurane requires a unique vaporizer design that heats and pressurizes the anesthetic.
  - The vapor is injected in controlled volumes into the fresh gas flow.

Anesthetic Circuit

- Time is required to reach steady-state gas concentration within the anesthesia circuit for delivery to the patient.
- This time constant of the circuit (τ) is determined by the fresh gas flow (FGF) and the circuit volume (Vc) with the equation $t = Vc/FGF$.

Partition Coefficients

- The solubility of an inhaled anesthetic in different tissues determines its uptake and distribution.
- Blood:gas partition coefficient is the solubility of greatest relevance to pharmacokinetics.
  - This coefficient describes uptake of anesthetic from the alveoli to the pulmonary capillaries.
- At steady state, the partial pressures in the alveoli, blood, and brain are the same.
  - The concentrations in each of these compartments will be different.
  - The lower the solubility, the lower is the concentration in blood for a given partial pressure.

Clinical Importance of Anesthetic Solubility

The solubility of an inhaled anesthetic is the physical property primarily responsible for the pharmacokinetic profile of the drug.

Gas Exchange

- Partial pressure gradient from alveolar gas to pulmonary capillary blood drives anesthetic uptake.
- Rate of induction is dependent on how quickly alveolar anesthetic concentration (F_A) matches the inhaled concentration (F_I).
- Anesthetics with lower solubility reach an F_A:F_I ratio of 1 more quickly.
  - This explains their quicker induction profile.
- Increasing delivery of anesthetic gas to the alveolus speeds induction.
- Rate of induction is impacted by multiple patient factors.

Determinants of Rate of Induction With Inhaled Anesthetics

- Induction with inhaled anesthetics is determined by the partial pressure gradient across the alveolar membrane.
- Anesthesia provider-related factors
  - Influence the delivery of anesthetic gas to the alveoli
  - Higher fresh gas flow, anesthetic concentration, and alveolar ventilation all increase the rate of induction.
- Patient factors
  - Increased cardiac output causes increased pulmonary capillary blood flow and decreases the rate of induction.
  - Dead space ventilation and right-to-left shunts decrease the rate of induction.

Concentration Effect and Second Gas Effect

- Nitrous oxide is administered in substantially higher concentrations than volatile anesthetics.
  - Uptake of nitrous oxide from alveoli reduces alveolar volume and concentrates remaining alveolar gases.
- The *concentration effect* describes the relative increase in remaining alveolar nitrous oxide as alveolar volume decreases with nitrous oxide uptake.
  - This explains the more rapid uptake of nitrous oxide at higher compared to lower concentrations.

Impact of the Concentration Effect on Rate of Induction

The concentration effect is responsible for the more rapid induction of nitrous oxide compared to desflurane, despite having nearly equal blood:gas partition coefficients.

- The *second gas effect* describes the increase in uptake of an inhaled anesthetic coadministered with nitrous oxide.
  - The rapid uptake of nitrous oxide reduces alveolar volume and concentrates the remaining alveolar gases.
  - This increases the partial pressure gradient of the second inhaled anesthetic.

MINIMUM ALVEOLAR CONCENTRATION (MAC)

Definition of Inhaled Anesthetic Potency

Potency of inhaled anesthetics is quantified and compared between agents as *minimum alveolar concentration* (MAC), the concentration required to prevent movement in 50% of a population in response to a surgical stimulus.

- Quantifies the relative potency of inhaled anesthetics based on patient immobility
- Standard deviation of MAC is ~10% of its mean value.
  - Preventing movement in 67% of patients (1 SD above the mean) requires 1.1 MAC.
- MAC is approximately additive between agents.
  - A mixture of 0.5 MAC of sevoflurane and 0.5 isoflurane would have a combined potency of 1 MAC.
- Other definitions of MAC exist, which are related to the standard definition by a multiplicative factor.
  - MAC-amnesia is about one-fourth MAC.
  - MAC-awake is about one-third MAC.
  - MAC blunted autonomic response (BAR) is about 1.5 times MAC.
- MAC is impacted by patient characteristics, disease states, and other medications.
  - MAC is increased (i.e., anesthetic potency is reduced) by acute stimulant intoxication, chronic alcohol or benzodiazepine use, hypernatremia, hyperthermia, and having red hair.

- MAC is decreased (i.e., anesthetic potency is increased) by acute central nervous system (CNS) depressant intoxication, chronic stimulant use, hypothermia, hyponatremia, pregnancy, anemia, advancing age, and other commonly used medicines in anesthesia, such as local anesthetics, opioids, benzodiazepines, and α_2-adrenergic agonists.

MECHANISMS

Molecular Mechanisms

- Various molecular targets of inhaled anesthetics have been identified as possibly contributing to their effects.
  - Among the most promising molecular mechanisms are modulation of ligand- and voltage-gated ion channels.
  - Complexes in the mitochondrial electron transport chain, exocytotic proteins, and other proteins might also contribute.
- Direct effects on the lipid bilayer are unlikely to contribute to anesthetic action, though lipophilicity of inhaled anesthetics influences their ability to access and bind to proteins.

Neuronal Network Mechanisms

- Loss of consciousness due to inhaled anesthetics likely results from disrupted neuronal communication and connectivity between brain regions
- Immobility from volatile anesthetics is largely by direct effect on the spinal cord and not the brain

ORGAN SYSTEM EFFECTS

Central Nervous System

- Progressive inhibition of neuronal function leads to stereotypic electroencephalography (EEG) patterns.
  - Beta power decreases, while alpha and delta powers increase.
  - Excessive anesthetic concentrations produce burst suppression and ultimately an isoelectric EEG.
- Depression of neuronal function decreases cerebral blood flow by decreasing cerebral metabolic rate for oxygen ($CMRO_2$).
- Direct vasodilation opposes this effect above 1 MAC, thereby increasing intracranial pressure.
- Cerebral autoregulation is inhibited above 1.5 MAC.

Clinical Relevance of EEG Changes Due to Inhaled Anesthesia

Stereotypic changes in electrophysiologic activity of the brain under anesthesia underlie the use of processed EEG for brain state monitoring of patients receiving inhaled anesthesia.

Cardiovascular System

- Hypotension is primarily caused by reduced systemic vascular resistance (SVR) and inhibition of the baroreceptor reflex.
- Myocardial contractility decreases at supraclinical concentrations.
- Cardiac output is generally preserved.
- QT segment is prolonged due to ion channel effects in the heart.
- Tachycardia is caused most prominently by desflurane due to its vagolytic effect.
- Halothane can cause sinus bradycardia and can predispose to ventricular tachycardia.

Effect of Volatile Anesthetics on Blood Pressure

All volatile anesthetics cause hypotension by decreasing SVR and inhibiting the baroreceptor reflex.

Pulmonary System

- Respiratory rate is increased.
- Tidal volume is decreased.
- The respiratory drive in response to oxygen and carbon dioxide are affected.
  - Hypoxic ventilatory response (HVR) is suppressed at low doses and is abolished at surgical doses.
  - Central chemoreceptor response is strongly inhibited but not abolished.
  - Patients administered volatile anesthetics are reliant on $PaCO_2$ to stimulate ventilation.
- Mucociliary function is inhibited.
- Volatile anesthetics are bronchodilators through smooth muscle relaxation.
- Hypoxic pulmonary vasoconstriction is diminished in a dose-dependent manner.

Effect of Volatile Anesthetics on Respiratory Drive

Volatile anesthetics inhibit the ventilatory response to hypoxia and hypercarbia, contributing to respiratory depression.

Renal System

- Methoxyflurane metabolism caused excessive plasma fluoride levels and contributed to high-output renal failure, which led to its discontinuation.
- Sevoflurane breakdown by alkaline carbon dioxide absorbents produces compound A and nephrotoxicity in animal models.
  - Compound A has not led to kidney injury in humans.
- Volatile anesthetics produce ischemic preconditioning of the kidneys in animal models.
- Few data exist to identify if volatile anesthetics are protective or injurious to kidneys.

Hepatic System

- Portal vein blood flow is decreased but hepatic arterial blood flow is maintained or increased.
  - There is a net decrease in hepatic blood flow.
- Halothane hepatitis is fulminant liver failure occurring in 1/15,000 cases.
  - Caused by autoimmune response to trifluoroacetylated compounds as a result of halothane metabolism

Neuromuscular Function

- Volatile anesthetics potentiate the effects of nondepolarizing neuromuscular blockers.
- Noncompetitive antagonism of nicotinic acetylcholine receptors in muscle.
- Inhibits release of acetylcholine from motor neurons.

UNIQUE ISSUES WITH NITROUS OXIDE

- MAC is 104% and MAC-awake is about 0.6 MAC.
  - High concentrations are required for surgical anesthesia.
  - Must be used with other anesthetic agents to achieve general anesthesia
- Diffusion hypoxia can occur during emergence.
  - Partial pressure gradient causes nitrous oxide to diffuse into alveoli.
  - Remaining gases in the alveoli become diluted (including oxygen).
- Nitrous oxide can rapidly expand enclosed gaseous compartments.
  - High partial pressure and solubility compared to nitrogen
  - Examples include pneumothorax, blebs, closed-loop bowel obstruction, and recent ophthalmic procedures with insoluble gases (e.g., sulfur hexafluoride).
- Inhibits methionine synthetase, particularly in patients with vitamin B_{12} deficiency
  - Can precipitate neuropathy and megaloblastic anemia

Effect of Nitrous Oxide on Closed Gaseous Spaces

Nitrous oxide should be avoided under procedural or pathologic conditions involving closed gaseous spaces, since its diffusion can cause significant expansion and increases in pressure.

TOXICITY AND ADVERSE EVENTS

Postoperative Nausea and Vomiting

- Use of inhaled anesthetics increases the risk of postoperative nausea and vomiting.

Malignant Hyperthermia

- Volatile anesthetics or succinylcholine can cause malignant hyperthermia (MH), leading to sustained muscular contraction and rigidity.
  - Manifestations include rhabdomyolysis and hypermetabolic symptoms.
- Caused by mutations in ryanodine receptor 1 (*RyR1*) or dihydropyridine receptor (*CACNA1*)
  - Causes excessive calcium efflux from sarcoplasmic reticulum
- MH is a medical crisis because of its high mortality without treatment.
- MH-triggering drugs should be avoided in patients with a known or suspected family history.
- The specific treatment is dantrolene, an inhibitor of the RyR1 ryanodine receptor.
  - Other management steps limit the hypermetabolic response, such as cooling, bicarbonate administration, hyperventilation with 100% oxygen, and resuscitation with fluids and vasopressors as necessary.

Presenting Signs of Malignant Hyperthermia

- Unexplained increase in temperature or end-tidal CO_2
- Tachycardia
- Lactic acidosis
- Hyperkalemia
- Rhabdomyolysis

Developmental Neurotoxicity

- Inhaled anesthetics cause abnormal widespread apoptosis in developmentally young animal models.
- Brief, single exposures to inhaled anesthetics do not cause developmental impairment in toddlers in large clinical trials.

Concern for Neurocognitive Development in Young Children Receiving Inhaled Anesthesia

The FDA issued a warning that anesthetics, including inhaled anesthetics, can impair cognitive or behavioral development in patients under the age of 3, especially for prolonged or repetitive exposures.

Postoperative Cognitive Dysfunction

- Persistent cognitive impairment following anesthesia is controversial.
- The Perioperative Neurotoxicity Working Group has issued recommendations.
  - Avoid hypotension, hypothermia, and deliriogenic drugs.
  - Monitor end-tidal anesthetic concentrations and processed EEG to minimize drug doses.

Cancer Recurrence and Morbidity

- Volatile anesthesia may cause decreases in recurrence-free survival compared to intravenous anesthesia in patients having cancer surgery, but large trials are needed.

Reactions With Carbon Dioxide Absorbents

- Generation of enough heat to cause fire
  - Results from prolonged reaction in desiccated absorbents with outdated formulations containing strong bases
  - Sevoflurane is at more risk than other volatile anesthetics.
- Carbon monoxide can result from the reaction with volatile anesthetics, especially with desiccated absorbents.
  - Absorbent type increases risk [KOH > NaOH >> $Ba(OH)_2$ > $Ca(OH)_2$].
  - Risk is increased with desflurane and isoflurane.
- Sevoflurane is degraded to compound A by CO_2 absorbent.
  - Compound A is nephrotoxic in animal models, but no human clinical renal toxicity has been demonstrated.

METABOLISM, ELIMINATION, AND RECOVERY

- Isoflurane, sevoflurane, and desflurane are minimally metabolized.
- Termination of their effect is driven by exhaling the drug.
- Context-sensitive half-time is the time for partial pressure in blood to decrease by half.
  - Dependent on duration of administration and tissue solubility
  - Higher solubility increases context-sensitive half-time.
- Hysteresis of inhaled anesthetic concentrations during induction and emergence indicates that less anesthetic is required to maintain anesthesia than induce it, termed *neural inertia.*
  - Demonstrates that consciousness does not depend solely on inhaled anesthesia partial pressure
  - Also depends on neurobiological mechanisms of loss and return of consciousness
- Return of consciousness likely depends on the brain passing through several discrete functional states.

Pharmacokinetics of Elimination of Inhaled Anesthetics

Because currently used inhaled anesthetics are minimally metabolized, elimination is driven by drug exhalation, with the rate depending on the blood:gas partition coefficient and duration of administration.

ENVIRONMENTAL CONSIDERATIONS

- Inhaled anesthetics have deleterious effects by ozone depletion and as greenhouse gases.
- The global warming potentials of inhaled anesthetics are desflurane > nitrous oxide > isoflurane > sevoflurane (considering a 100-year time horizon).

Agent-Specific Environmental Impact of Inhaled Anesthetics

Inhaled anesthetics are greenhouse gases, with sevoflurane exerting the least detrimental effects.

QUESTIONS

CHEMICAL AND PHYSICAL PROPERTIES

1. What are the commonly used inhaled anesthetics?
2. What are the molecular structures of commonly used inhaled anesthetics?
3. Why are some inhaled anesthetics referred to as volatile?
4. How does molecular composition affect pharmacokinetics of volatile anesthesia?
5. Why is vapor pressure an important characteristic of volatile anesthetics?
6. How is solubility of inhaled anesthetics in body compartments quantified?

UPTAKE AND DISTRIBUTION IN THE BODY

7. How are volatile anesthetics added to fresh gas flow for clinical use?
8. How does solubility of inhaled anesthetics impact the rate of anesthetic induction?
9. What are the concentration and second gas effects with nitrous oxide administration?

MINIMUM ALVEOLAR CONCENTRATION (MAC)

10. How are the potencies of inhaled anesthetics quantified and compared?
11. What is the population standard deviation of MAC?
12. What is the MAC of two coadministered inhaled anesthetics?
13. Are there other clinical endpoints used to define MAC?
14. What patient factors influence MAC?
15. What drugs affect MAC?

MECHANISMS

16. What molecular mechanisms are responsible for the effects of volatile anesthetics?
17. What are the network-level effects of volatile anesthetics in the brain?
18. How do volatile anesthetics produce immobility?

ORGAN SYSTEM EFFECTS

19. What changes are observed in electrophysiologic activity of the brain by volatile anesthetics?
20. How do volatile anesthetics impact cerebral blood flow?
21. What is the effect of volatile anesthetics on arterial pressure?
22. How do volatile anesthetics affect cardiac output?
23. How do volatile anesthetics affect the electrophysiology of the heart?
24. How do volatile anesthetics impact minute ventilation?
25. What is the impact of volatile anesthetics on respiratory drive?
26. What is the effect of volatile anesthetics on airway tone?
27. Do volatile anesthetics cause kidney injury?
28. Which anesthetic is linked most consistently to hepatotoxicity?
29. What effect do volatile anesthetics have on hepatic blood flow?
30. What is the effect of volatile anesthetics on neuromuscular function?

UNIQUE ISSUES WITH NITROUS OXIDE

31. What are relative contraindications to the use of nitrous oxide?

TOXICITY AND ADVERSE EVENTS

32. Do inhaled anesthetics contribute to postoperative nausea and vomiting (PONV)?
33. What is malignant hyperthermia?
34. How is malignant hyperthermia treated?
35. What are the neuropsychological concerns of administering inhaled anesthesia to young children?
36. Do inhaled anesthetics impact cognitive function?
37. Do inhaled anesthetics impact cancer recurrence?
38. What are adverse events associated with the interaction of volatile anesthetics with carbon dioxide absorbent?

METABOLISM, ELIMINATION, AND RECOVERY

39. How are desflurane, sevoflurane, and isoflurane eliminated?
40. What other factors impact emergence from inhaled anesthesia?

ENVIRONMENTAL CONSIDERATIONS

41. How do inhaled anesthetics impact the environment?

ANSWERS

CHEMICAL AND PHYSICAL PROPERTIES

1. The inhaled anesthetics used most widely today are nitrous oxide and the volatile anesthetics isoflurane, sevoflurane, and desflurane. (83)
2. Isoflurane, sevoflurane, and desflurane are halogenated ethers. Halothane, which is no longer in common use, differs in that it is an alkane. Nitrous oxide is the oxide of nitrogen and has no carbon atoms. (83)

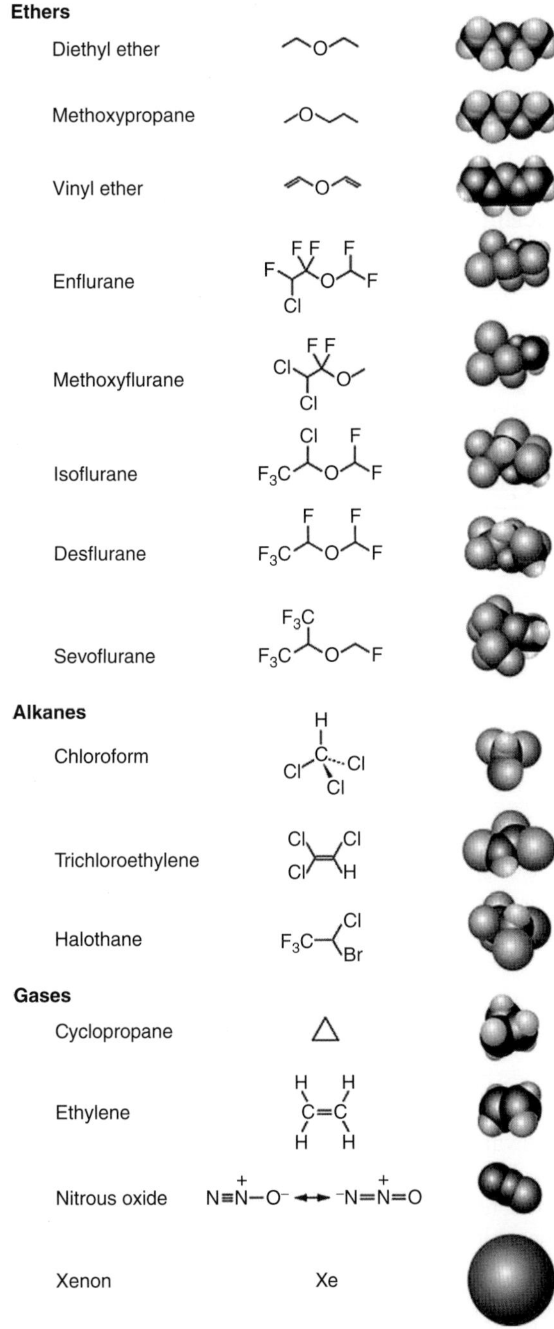

Molecular structures and space-filling models of historical and currently used inhaled anesthetics. Figure depicts the molecular structures and space-filling model of historical and currently used inhaled anesthetics. (From Hudson AE, Hemmings HC Jr. Pharmacokinetics of inhaled anesthetics, Ch. 3. In: Hemmings HC Jr, Egan TD, eds. *Pharmacology and Physiology for Anesthesia: Foundations and Clinical Application*. 2nd ed. Philadelphia: Elsevier; 2019:45.)

3. Volatile anesthetics are inhaled anesthetics that are liquids at standard temperature and pressure but are delivered to patients as gases. Volatility refers to the propensity of a liquid to evaporate. Drugs such as nitrous oxide and xenon, a noble gas, are inhaled anesthetics but exist as gases under standard conditions, so these are classified as gaseous, not volatile, anesthetics. (83)
4. The modern volatile anesthetics are halogenated, which is primarily responsible for the differences in their uptake and elimination. Fluorine substitution, in particular, has been effectively used to improve these characteristics. For instance, desflurane differs from isoflurane only in the replacement of a chlorine atom with fluorine, but desflurane has a drastically different pharmacokinetic profile. (83)
5. Vapor pressure quantifies the propensity of a liquid to evaporate. It is defined as the pressure exerted by a gas within a closed chamber that is in equilibrium with its liquid phase at a given temperature. Chemicals more likely to evaporate will have more gas particles, thus yielding higher vapor pressures. Boiling occurs when vapor pressure exceeds ambient pressure. The vapor pressure of isoflurane (240 mm Hg) and sevoflurane (160 mm Hg) are relatively low, but the vapor pressure of desflurane (669 mm Hg) is near atmospheric pressure (760 mm Hg). This property drives its unique bottle and vaporizer design. (84)
6. Partition coefficients describe the relative solubility of inhaled anesthetics. At equilibrium, the partial pressure of a gas dissolved in two solvents is equal, but the concentrations may differ. The partition coefficient is the ratio of concentrations between two compartments at equilibrium. More soluble inhaled anesthetics have a higher blood:gas partition coefficient. The blood:gas partition coefficient is particularly important to the uptake and, therefore, rate of induction with inhaled anesthetics. The comparative properties of inhaled anesthetics are shown in the table below. (85)

Potencies and physical and pharmacokinetic properties of historical and currently used inhaled anesthetics.

Characteristic	*Halothane*	*Methoxyflurane*	*Isoflurane*	*Sevoflurane*	*Desflurane*	*Nitrous Oxide*	*Xenon*
Partition Coefficients							
Blood–gas	2.54	11	1.46	0.65	0.45	0.46	0.14
Brain–blood	1.9		1.6	1.7	1.3	1.1	
Muscle–blood	3.4		2.9	3.1	2.0	1.2	
Fat–blood	51		45	48	27	2.3	
MAC (age 40)	0.75	0.16	1.28	2.05	6.0	104	0.71
Vapor pressure at 20°C (mm Hg)	244	22.5	240	160	669		
Molecular weight	197.4	165	184.5	200.1	168.0	44.0	131.3
Percent metabolized	15–40	70	0.2	5	0.02		

Adapted from McKay RE. Inhaled anesthetics, Chapter 8. In: *Basics of Anesthesia,* 7th ed. Philadelphia: Elsevier; 2018: 81. Based on Steward A, Allott PR, Cowles AL, et al. Solubility coefficients for inhaled anaesthetics for water, oil, and biological media. *Br J Anaesth.* 1973;45:282–293. Yasuda N, Targ AG, Eger EI. Solubility of I-653, sevoflurane, isoflurane, and halothane in human tissues. *Anesth Analg.* 1989;69:370–373.

UPTAKE AND DISTRIBUTION IN THE BODY

7. Vaporizers allow liquid volatile anesthetics to be converted into gas and added to the fresh gas flow. Most vaporizers use a variable bypass design. For a desired concentration, a defined portion of gas flow is diverted into a chamber saturated with anesthetic vapor and recombines with the bypassed gas. Desflurane uses a different design because the boiling point of desflurane is near normal room temperatures and boiling of anesthetic within the vaporizing chamber would prevent precise output of desflurane. The Tec6 vaporizer for desflurane heats and pressurizes the anesthetic and injects it into the fresh gas to ensure controlled output concentrations. (85)
8. Because partial pressures equilibrate across body compartments, achieving a targeted anesthetic partial pressure in the brain requires reaching that partial pressure in the alveoli. According to Henry's law ($C = kP$), more soluble anesthetics, which have a higher solubility constant k (and higher blood:gas partition coefficient), require a higher anesthetic concentration in the blood to reach the targeted partial pressure. Thus alveolar anesthetic diffuses into pulmonary capillary blood to a greater extent, slowing the rate at which the desired alveolar partial pressure is achieved. Experimentally, this has been demonstrated by comparing the time required for the fractional concentration of alveolar anesthetic (F_A) to reach the targeted concentration being

inhaled by the patient (F_I). More soluble anesthetics require longer for the ratio of F_A:F_I to approach 1, highlighting the impact of solubility on the rate of induction of anesthesia. (87)

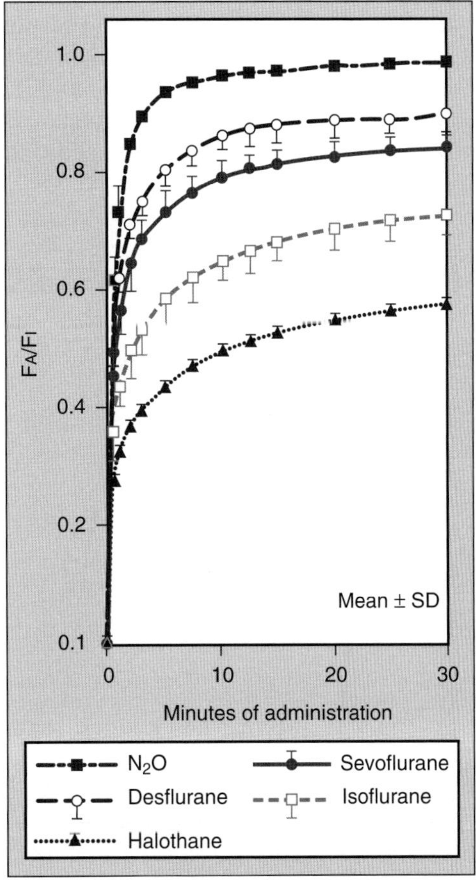

Solubility in blood is the principal property of inhaled anesthetics governing equilibration between alveolar gas and blood, and thereby the rate of induction of anesthesia. FA, Fraction of alveolar gas; FI, fraction of inhaled gas. (From McKay RE. Inhaled anesthetics, Ch. 7. In Pardo M, ed. *Basics of Anesthesia*. 7th ed. Philadelphia: Elsevier; 2018:91, Figure from From Yasuda N, Lockhart SH, Eger EI II, et al. Comparison of kinetics of sevoflurane and isoflurane in humans. Anesth Analg. 1991;72:316-324, used with permission.).

9. Nitrous oxide is used clinically at substantially higher concentrations compared to volatile anesthetics. As nitrous oxide diffuses from alveoli into pulmonary capillary blood, the alveolar volume is appreciably decreased, thereby concentrating the remaining alveolar nitrous oxide and maintaining a higher partial pressure gradient. The increase in the alveolar concentration of nitrous oxide results in an increased rate of anesthetic uptake. The use of nitrous oxide at relatively high concentrations also increases the concentration of coadministered volatile anesthetics as nitrous oxide diffuses from alveoli, decreasing overall alveolar volume. Thus the concentration of nitrous oxide impacts the rate of uptake of a volatile anesthetic. In diffusion hypoxia, the second gas effect is reversed and expired nitrous oxide dilutes alveolar oxygen. (88)

MINIMUM ALVEOLAR CONCENTRATION (MAC)

10. Minimum alveolar concentration (MAC) is used to compare the potencies of inhaled anesthetics. MAC is defined as the concentration of an inhaled anesthetic required to prevent movement of 50% of subjects in a population in response to a surgical stimulus. Anesthetics that are more potent require less of the drug to achieve this endpoint and, hence, have a lower MAC. (88)

11. The standard deviation (SD) of MAC in the population is typically about 10% of MAC. Thus to prevent movement in 95% of the population would require 2 SDs, or 20%, over MAC, equal to 1.2 MAC. (90)
12. MAC is approximately additive. Thus delivering 0.5 MAC isoflurane with 0.5 MAC sevoflurane yields a gas mixture with a combined potency of 1 MAC. (90)
13. MAC-awake is the concentration required for half a population to respond voluntarily to a verbal command. For isoflurane, sevoflurane, and desflurane, MAC-awake is approximately one-third MAC. MAC-amnesia is the concentration required to prevent memory in half of subjects, and it is more variable for different anesthetics but less than MAC-awake. MAC-blunted autonomic response (BAR) is the concentration required for half a population to block the autonomic response (e.g., hypertension, tachycardia) to surgical stimulus; MAC-BAR is about 1.5 times MAC. (90)

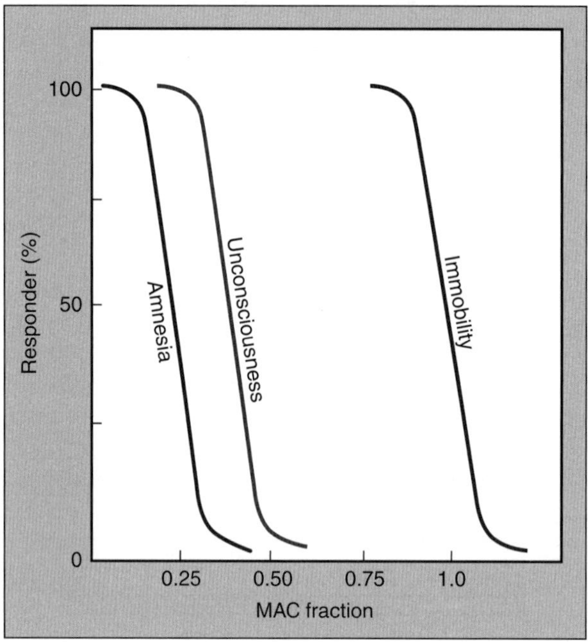

Definition of minimum alveolar concentration (MAC). MAC is defined as the concentration of an inhaled anesthetic required to produce immobility in response to a noxious stimulus in 50% of the population. This definition has been applied to other clinical endpoints, such as amnesia and unconsciousness, in addition to immobility. The steep slope reflects the small population variability in sensitivity to inhaled anesthesia. (From Hudson AE, Herold KF, Hemmings HC Jr. Pharmacology of inhaled anesthetics, Ch. 11. In: Hemmings HC Jr, Egan TD, eds. *Pharmacology and Physiology for Anesthesia: Foundations and Clinical Application.* 2nd ed. Philadelphia: Elsevier; 2019:222).

14. Age is an important factor impacting MAC, which is reported not as a range but as a single value relative to a specific age (typically 40 years of age). For each decade, MAC decreases by 6%; however, this trend is broken for infants. for whom MAC increases until age 6 months. Other important patient factors affecting MAC are pregnancy, which lowers MAC, and red hair, which increases MAC. Certain pathophysiological conditions influence MAC as well. For example, hypothermia, hyponatremia, and anemia decrease MAC, while hyperthermia and hypernatremia increase MAC. (90)
15. Many drugs used commonly by anesthesia providers decrease MAC, such as opioids, benzodiazepines, propofol, etomidate, barbiturates, local anesthetics, and α_2-adrenergic agonists. Other drugs not used in perioperative care can also decrease MAC, such as verapamil and lithium. Acute intoxication with CNS depressants, such as ethanol, decreases MAC, whereas use of stimulants, such as cocaine or amphetamine, increases MAC. Chronic use of these drugs has the opposite effect on MAC. Factors that increase or decrease anesthetic requirements are given in the box below. (90)

Factors affecting minimum alveolar concentration (MAC)

Factors Increasing MAC	Factors Decreasing MAC
Drugs ▪ Amphetamine (acute use) ▪ Cocaine ▪ Ephedrine ▪ Ethanol (chronic use)	Drugs ▪ Propofol ▪ Etomidate ▪ Barbiturates ▪ Benzodiazepines ▪ Ketamine ▪ α_2-Agonists (clonidine, dexmedetomidine) ▪ Ethanol (acute use) ▪ Local anesthetics ▪ Opioids ▪ Amphetamines (chronic use) ▪ Lithium ▪ Verapamil
Age ▪ Highest at age 6 months	Age ▪ Elderly patients
Electrolytes ▪ Hypernatremia ▪ Hyperthermia	Electrolyte disturbance ▪ Hyponatremia
Red hair	Other factors ▪ Anemia (hemoglobin <5 g/dL) ▪ Hypercarbia ▪ Hypothermia ▪ Hypoxia ▪ Pregnancy

From McKay RE. Inhaled anesthetics. Ch. 7. In Pardo M, ed. *Basics of Anesthesia,* 7th ed. Philadelphia, PA: Elsevier; 2018:86.

MECHANISMS

16. The precise molecular mechanisms of volatile anesthetics are not fully understood. The most promising molecular targets are ligand-gated and voltage-gated ion channels of neurons that impact excitability and neurotransmission, such as inhibition of NMDA and AMPA receptors, potentiation of $GABA_A$ receptors, inhibition of voltage-gated sodium channels, and potentiation of potassium channels. The net effect of these mechanisms is inhibition of excitatory and potentiation of inhibitory neurotransmission. Disruption of lipid bilayers was an early hypothesis based on the correlation of anesthetic potency with lipophilicity; however, the abundance of current evidence favors anesthetic interactions with proteins and not lipids as the likely molecular mechanisms. (91)
17. Volatile anesthetics block normal patterns of connectivity between different regions of the CNS that are believed to underlie consciousness. This effect is likely caused by effects on action potential frequency and timing. (92)
18. Volatile anesthetics act directly on targets in the spinal cord to produce immobility. In rodent models, MAC is unchanged by cervical dislocation and lowered by delivering volatile anesthetics directly to the vasculature of the spinal cord. Thus the brain likely does not contribute substantially to immobility. (92)

ORGAN SYSTEM EFFECTS

19. Volatile anesthetics generate stereotypical dose-related changes in electroencephalographic (EEG) patterns. As volatile anesthetic dose is increased, β frequencies (13–25 Hz) decrease as higher amplitude and lower frequency activity, primarily in the α (8–13 Hz) and δ (1–4 Hz) ranges, increases. At doses above 1 MAC, θ (5–8 Hz) frequencies emerge. With doses exceeding 1.3 MAC, burst suppression occurs, and increasing doses ultimately cause an isoelectric EEG. (92)
20. Volatile anesthetics alter the relationship between cerebral blood flow (CBF) and cerebral metabolic rate ($CMRO_2$) since they depress neuronal activity but are also direct vasodilators. Cerebral autoregulation describes the preserved cerebral blood flow over a range of systemic arterial pressures. Volatile anesthetics abolish cerebral autoregulation at concentrations above 1.5 MAC, although sevoflurane better preserves cerebral autoregulation. (94)

21. Volatile anesthetics lower systemic vascular resistance (SVR) in a dose-dependent manner and inhibit the baroreceptor reflex, leading to systemic hypotension. (94)
22. Volatile anesthetics cause agent-specific inhibition of myocardial contractility. This effect is offset in a dose-dependent manner by tachycardia and reduced SVR such that cardiac output is variably but minimally affected. (94)
23. All volatile anesthetics prolong the QT segment. Volatile anesthetics exhibit agent-specific differences in their ability to cause tachycardia. Desflurane, in particular, exerts a vagolytic effect driving tachycardia at higher concentrations or with sudden changes in concentration. (94)
24. Respiratory rate increases with volatile anesthesia, but tidal volume concurrently decreases, resulting in an overall decrease in minute ventilation. (94)
25. Volatile anesthetics potently inhibit the hypoxic ventilatory response (HVR), abolishing the usual increase in minute ventilation resulting from hypoxemia. The peripheral chemoreceptor response to hypercarbia is also severely inhibited, but the central chemoreceptor response is less impacted. (94)
26. Volatile anesthetics are bronchodilators. This effect should not be confused with the agent-specific pungency of inhaled anesthetics, which can precipitate coughing. (95)
27. Metabolism of fluorinated volatile anesthetics increases plasma fluoride levels in an agent-specific manner. Methoxyflurane leads to the highest and most sustained plasma fluoride concentrations, which contributes to high-output renal failure and led to discontinuation of its use for general anesthesia. The other anesthetics are not associated with renal failure. Volatile anesthetics decrease renal blood flow and oxygenation, but, conversely, they cause ischemic preconditioning that might be protective of kidney injury. Besides methoxyflurane, there is no definitive evidence that inhaled anesthetics cause clinically significant nephrotoxicity or renal protection. (95)
28. Halothane causes fulminant hepatoxicity in 1/15,000 cases, resulting from an autoimmune response to trifluoroacetylated adducts of hepatocellular proteins due to halothane metabolism. (95)
29. Volatile anesthetics at concentrations above 1 MAC decrease total hepatic blood flow, driven by effects on portal blood flow, as opposed to hepatic arterial blood flow. (96)
30. Volatile anesthetics potentiate the effect of neuromuscular blockers by noncompetitive antagonism of nicotinic acetylcholine receptors in muscle and possibly by decreasing neurotransmitter release from motor neurons. (96)

UNIQUE ISSUES WITH NITROUS OXIDE

31. Nitrous oxide can rapidly expand a closed, gaseous space because it is used clinically at relatively high partial pressures and it is 30 times more soluble than nitrogen, which therefore diffuses out more slowly. Thus it is prudent to avoid nitrous oxide in patients with pneumothorax, blebs, closed-loop bowel obstruction, recent ophthalmic procedures with insoluble gases (e.g., sulfur hexafluoride), and other clinical conditions characterized by a closed gaseous space. In addition, nitrous oxide inhibits methionine synthetase, thereby contributing to subacute combined degeneration and megaloblastic anemia. Therefore nitrous oxide should be avoided if other risk factors for these conditions are present, such as patients with vitamin B_{12} deficiency. (97)

TOXICITY AND ADVERSE EVENTS

32. Both volatile anesthetics and nitrous oxide increase the risk of PONV in a dose-dependent manner. The additive risk to PONV of nitrous oxide use for less than an hour is low. (97)
33. Malignant hyperthermia (MH) is an autosomal dominant pharmacogenetic disease of mutated ryanodine receptor 1 (*RyR1*) or dihydropyridine calcium channels (*CACNA1*) that causes uncontrolled efflux of calcium from the sarcoplasmic reticulum in response to volatile anesthetics or succinylcholine. The result is sustained muscle contraction and rigidity leading to rhabdomyolysis and hypermetabolic symptoms, including severe hyperthermia, hypercarbia, tachycardia, and lactic acidosis. (98)
34. The primary treatment goal is to identify patients with known or possible MH so the anesthesia plan can be developed to avoid triggering drugs. Anesthesia providers should investigate both the patient's personal and family anesthetic histories. Symptomatic MH is a medical crisis due to high mortality and morbidity without treatment. The specific treatment is dantrolene, an inhibitor of the RyR1 ryanodine receptor. Other measures aim to limit injury caused by hypermetabolism and rhabdomyolysis, such as cooling, hyperventilation, sodium bicarbonate, intravenous fluids, and vasopressor treatment as needed. An important resource is the Malignant Hyperthermia Association of the US (MHAUS), a hotline that provides expert guidance on clinical issues related to MH. (98)

35. Multiple distinct anesthetics, including inhaled anesthetics, exhibit neurotoxicity in animal models, causing abnormal, widespread apoptosis in the brain in early development that is associated with persistent cognitive and behavioral changes. The FDA issued a warning in 2016, updated in 2017, stating that drugs used for general anesthesia or sedation may have detrimental cognitive or behavioral effects if administered to children under 3 years of age repetitively or for durations over 3 hours. Large prospective cohort studies and the GAS study, a randomized trial of spinal or inhaled anesthesia for hernia repair in children under one year of age, suggest that a single, relatively short exposure to inhaled anesthesia does not lead to clinically significant developmental delay or detectable cognitive effects. Additional prospective and randomized studies are required to define the risk of exposure to inhaled anesthesia in this age group, particularly with prolonged or repetitive exposures. (99)
36. Delirium is a syndrome defined by acute fluctuation in attention, awareness, and cognition. Patients over the age of 60 years undergoing major surgery under general anesthesia, including with inhaled anesthetics, experience postoperative delirium at a rate of approximately 20%–40% of cases. Patients with preexisting cognitive impairment are at increased risk. Whether inhaled anesthesia is associated with persistent impairment remains controversial because few prospective randomized studies have compared cognitive outcomes in older adults undergoing surgery with inhaled anesthesia or other approaches. The Perioperative Neurotoxicity Working Group, convened as part of the American Society of Anesthesiologists Brain Health Initiative, recommends monitoring age-adjusted end-tidal MAC concentration and titrating anesthesia to EEG-based intraoperative brain monitoring, among other measures. (100)
37. Large retrospective analyses indicate that regional anesthesia or total intravenous anesthesia may decrease cancer recurrence after surgical resection compared to general anesthesia with volatile anesthetics. However, randomized trials comparing these groups have found no differences in recurrence between these comparators. Additional randomized clinical trials are necessary to determine if volatile anesthetics increase the risk of recurrence and, if so, identify the patient factors or cancer types most susceptible. (100)
38. Carbon monoxide can be generated from the chemical reaction of desiccated absorbent, most readily with KOH or NaOH-based mixtures, and volatile anesthetics, primarily desflurane and isoflurane. Heat generated by exothermic reactions of outdated absorbents has caused fires. Sevoflurane interacts with absorbent to generate compound A, which can be inhaled with rebreathed gas. Though compound A exhibits nephrotoxicity in high doses in animal models, it does not cause clinically significant nephrotoxicity in humans. However, generation of compound A has prompted the FDA to issue a warning to avoid use of fresh gas flows less than 1 L/min and to adjust concentrations such that total delivery does not exceed 2 MAC hours at fresh gas flows less than 2 L/min. (101)

METABOLISM, ELIMINATION, AND RECOVERY

39. Though older volatile anesthetics, such as halothane, are extensively metabolized in the liver by the CYP450 system, desflurane, sevoflurane, and isoflurane are minimally metabolized. Thus elimination occurs primarily by exhalation. Similar to induction, the rate of elimination is driven largely by solubility, i.e. the blood:gas partition coefficient. However, inhaled anesthetics also exhibit context-sensitive half-times, such that the duration of administration affects the rate of elimination. This phenomenon is driven by redistribution of anesthetics to tissues with lesser perfusion, which serve as a depot of anesthesia that must be depleted to lower blood partial pressure. (101)
40. Inhaled anesthetics exhibit hysteresis in the doses required for induction and maintenance of general anesthesia. Lower doses are required to maintain general anesthesia than for induction. Animal studies have shown that mutations affecting the sleep cycle or alertness can impact the degree of hysteresis. Moreover, different discrete EEG states are observed in the process of emergence. Thus regaining consciousness from inhaled anesthesia is not solely dependent on the anesthetic concentration, and there are likely several functional brain states that occur and explain the hysteresis of anesthesia maintenance, termed *neural inertia*. (102)

ENVIRONMENTAL CONSIDERATIONS

41. Inhaled anesthetics cause deleterious atmospheric effects. Nitrous oxide depletes the ozone layer. Both nitrous oxide and volatile anesthetics are greenhouse gases. Due to their variable stability and lifetimes in the atmosphere, the relative global warming potential is desflurane > nitrous oxide > isoflurane > sevoflurane (considering a 100-year time horizon). (104)

Chapter

8 INTRAVENOUS ANESTHETICS

Michael Curtis and Michael P. Bokoch

WHY INTRAVENOUS ANESTHETICS?

- Primary advantage of intravenous (IV) anesthetics (vs. inhaled anesthetics)–ability to rapidly induce hypnosis and provide sufficient depth of anesthesia for laryngoscopy
- Relative disadvantage–current inability to measure the concentration of IV anesthetics at the effect site (i.e., the brain) in real time
  - No equivalent of "minimum alveolar concentration (MAC)" or end-tidal agent monitoring for IV anesthetics
  - Clinician must rely on knowledge of pharmacokinetics, clinical endpoints (e.g., respiratory rate), surrogate monitors (e.g., processed electroencephalogram [EEG]), and clinical experience for optimal and safe use
- IV anesthetics are typically lipophilic and preferentially partition into highly perfused, lipid-rich tissues such as the brain and spinal cord
  - Accounts for rapid onset of action
  - Relatively rapid termination of action (i.e., 5 to 10 minutes) results from redistribution into less-perfused, inactive tissues such as skeletal muscle

GABA$_A$ RECEPTOR AGONISM

- γ-Aminobutyric acid type A (GABA$_A$) receptors
  - Ligand-gated ion channels
  - Activated by the neurotransmitter GABA
  - Conduct inhibitory (hyperpolarizing) chloride currents across the plasma membrane of neurons
- GABA$_A$ receptors are pentameric, with the most common type in the brain being composed of two α, two β, and one γ subunit
- GABA$_A$ receptors are the most common target of IV anesthetics, with four of the anesthetic classes described here (propofol, barbiturates, benzodiazepines, and etomidate) acting as GABA agonists

Primary Receptor Targets for IV Anesthetics

GABA$_A$ agonism	Propofol, barbiturates, benzodiazepines, etomidate
N-Methyl-D-aspartate (NMDA) antagonism	Ketamine
α_2-Adrenergic receptor agonism	Dexmedetomidine

- Despite all acting as GABA agonists, these IV anesthetics manifest different clinical effects due to
  - Heterogeneity of the GABA$_A$ receptor (multiple variations with 19 possible subunits exist in the human genome)
  - Varying location of action (e.g., brain vs. spinal cord)
  - Multiple drug-binding sites on each receptor
    - Benzodiazepines bind to an extracellular portion of the receptor
    - Propofol, barbiturates, and etomidate bind within the transmembrane domain

PROPOFOL

Physical Properties and Pharmacokinetics

- Formulated in an emulsion containing soybean oil, glycerol, and egg lecithin
  - No evidence for cross-reactivity in patients with allergies to egg, soy, or peanut
  - Susceptible to bacterial overgrowth and thus should be discarded within 12 hours of opening
- Although primarily metabolized hepatically, major contributors to plasma clearance also include the kidneys, small intestine, and lungs
  - Rapid clearance explains more complete recovery with less "hangover"
- Hypnotic effect is terminated by redistribution

Continuous Intravenous Infusion

- Ideal for use as continuous infusion due to efficient plasma clearance, rapid metabolism, and slow redistribution back into central compartment
- Context-sensitive half-time remains short even after a prolonged infusion

Pharmacodynamics

- Increases the flow of inhibitory chloride currents via $GABA_A$ receptor agonism

Central Nervous System

- Provides hypnotic action without analgesia
- At high doses, decreases cerebral metabolic rate of oxygen consumption ($CMRO_2$) producing burst suppression on the EEG
- Decreases cerebral blood volume, intracranial pressure (ICP), and intraocular pressure
- Preserves cerebral autoregulation better than higher doses of volatile anesthetics
- Occasionally see excitatory effects such as twitching but is an anticonvulsant

Cardiovascular System

- Profound vasodilation and can blunt the normal baroreflex response (i.e., the normal increase in heart rate in response to hypotension)
- Does not depress myocardial contractility at clinical doses

Respiratory System

- Blunts upper airway reflexes (e.g., gag, laryngospasm) and lower airway reflexes (e.g., bronchospasm) better than etomidate or barbiturates
- Respiratory depression, apnea, and upper airway collapse due to loss of muscle tone
  - Frequently seen with induction doses
  - May occur at sedative doses used during monitored anesthesia care

Other Effects

- Has antiemetic properties
- Propofol infusion syndrome (PRIS)
  - Rare, potentially fatal side effect
  - Usually seen after long-term administration (i.e., >20 hours)
  - Characterized by arrhythmias, metabolic acidosis, rhabdomyolysis, elevated triglycerides, and hyperkalemia

Clinical Uses

- Pain on injection is a common complaint but can be reduced by using larger veins or injecting with fentanyl or lidocaine

Induction and Maintenance of General Anesthesia

- Typical induction doses
  - 1–2.5 mg/kg IV for adults and 2.5–3.5 mg/kg IV for children
  - Morbidly obese patient–doses should be calculated based on lean body weight rather than total body weight
- Typical doses for maintenance of general anesthesia: 100–200 μg/kg/min IV
- Total IV anesthesia (TIVA)
  - Propofol may be used as the sole sedative-hypnotic agent
  - Often combined with opioids because propofol lacks significant analgesic properties
  - In retrospective studies, propofol TIVA may also be associated with better outcomes after cancer surgery compared with volatile anesthetics (not yet supported by prospective studies)

Sedation

- Typical dose for sedation may be lower, in the 25–75 μg/kg/min range
- Useful for sedation in ICU or for procedures in or outside of the operating room

Antiemetic

- Subanesthetic boluses or infusions (e.g., 10–20 mg IV bolus, or 10–20 μg/kg/min IV infusion) may be used for postoperative nausea and vomiting (PONV) treatment
- Full propofol TIVA is associated with less PONV than volatile anesthetics
- Propofol TIVA in the ambulatory setting may not reduce unplanned admissions, postdischarge nausea and vomiting, or cost

BARBITURATES

Pharmacokinetics and Pharmacodynamics

- Barbiturates activate the $GABA_A$ receptor via a transmembrane domain of the pentameric ion channel, allowing for direct opening of the chloride channel in the absence of endogenous GABA molecules (similar to propofol)
- Thiopental and methohexital are alkaline after reconstitution
  - Prevents bacterial overgrowth and extends shelf-life
  - May cause precipitation and tissue injury if mixed with acidic solutions like neuromuscular blocking agents
- Most barbiturates undergo hepatic metabolism, primarily via oxidation, with the resulting metabolites being inactive and excreted in the urine or bile
- Contraindicated in acute intermittent porphyria
  - Barbiturates can stimulate aminolevulinic acid synthetase, which increases the production of porphyrins

- Methohexital is cleared more rapidly by the liver than thiopental and has a shorter elimination half-time, allowing for faster and more complete recovery
- Thiopental recovery after repeated doses or infusion is markedly prolonged due to a long context-sensitive half-life

Central Nervous System

- Central nervous system (CNS) depression in a dose-dependent fashion, ranging from sedation to general anesthesia
- No analgesic effects and may reduce the pain threshold
- Potent cerebral vasoconstrictors, meaning barbiturates can decrease cerebral blood flow (CBF), cerebral blood volume, and ICP
- Decreased $CMRO_2$ up to the point where the EEG becomes isoelectric
- Methohexital activates epileptic foci, facilitating seizure-mapping surgeries or electroconvulsive therapy (ECT)

Cardiovascular System

- Induction doses reduce systemic arterial blood pressure via decreased sympathetic outflow and subsequent peripheral vasodilation
- Generally, cause less hypotension than propofol
- May blunt the baroreceptor reflex and cause negative inotropic effects, but these effects are generally not profound in vivo

Respiratory System

- Respiratory depression via reduced tidal volumes and respiratory rate (similar to propofol)
- Less potent suppression of the laryngeal and cough reflexes (vs. propofol); thus, an inferior choice for instrumenting the airway in the absence of neuromuscular blockade

Side Effects

- Accidental intraarterial injection
  - Significant vasoconstriction, with intense pain and sufficiently severe tissue injury to result in gangrene
  - Damage may be related to barbiturate crystal formation occluding distal, small-diameter arterioles–venous injection likely avoids this issue due to the greater capacity of venodilation
- Subcutaneous injection (extravasation) can similarly result in severe tissue injury, with some recommending injecting 5–10 mL 0.5% lidocaine in an attempt to dilute the barbiturate concentration
- While life-threatening allergic reactions to barbiturates are rare, related histamine release is occasionally seen

Clinical Uses

Induction of Anesthesia

- Administration of thiopental 3–5 mg/kg IV or methohexital 1–1.5 mg/kg IV can induce anesthesia in less than 30 seconds, with some patients reporting a garlic or onion taste during this time
- Rarely useful to maintain general anesthesia due to long context-sensitive half-time
- Methohexital is one of the drugs of choice for ECT as it does not shorten the seizure duration

Neuroprotection

- May be titrated to achieve an isoelectric EEG, which decreases $CMRO_2$ and has been hypothesized to provide neuroprotection from focal cerebral ischemic events (this idea is controversial–and unlikely of benefit for global ischemia, as seen in cardiac arrest)
  - No evidence for improved outcomes in patients with traumatic brain injury
- Barbiturates may be helpful in decreasing ICP
  - Most useful in patients with space-occupying intracranial lesions
- Prolonged infusions used to achieve a "barbiturate coma" can result in immune suppression, electrolyte disturbances, and hypothermia

BENZODIAZEPINES

Pharmacokinetics and Pharmacodynamics

- Benzodiazepine binding to $GABA_A$ receptors
  - Enhances conduction of chloride currents (similar to barbiturates and propofol)
  - Benzodiazepine binding alone is insufficient to fully activate the receptor but rather enhances the ability of endogenous GABA to open the chloride channel
  - Acts almost exclusively on postsynaptic nerve endings in the central nervous system (cerebral cortex)
  - Minimal peripheral effects
- Route of administration may be IV, oral, intramuscular, intranasal, or sublingual
- Midazolam, lorazepam, and diazepam are all highly protein bound
- Metabolism
  - Primarily via oxidation by hepatic cytochrome P450 3A4
  - Exception: lorazepam, which is excreted after single-step conjugation to glucuronic acid
- Midazolam has useful pharmacokinetic properties
  - Twice the affinity for $GABA_A$ receptors as diazepam
  - Shortest context-sensitive half-time of widely available benzodiazepines (excluding remimazolam), making it the most suitable for continuous infusion

- Metabolite (1-hydroxymidazolam) has some sedative effects, but it is typically clinically insignificant except in the cases of renal or hepatic dysfunction or prolonged infusion times

Central Nervous System

- Sedation/hypnosis
- Anterograde (but not retrograde) amnesia
- Anticonvulsant/antiepileptic
- Muscle relaxation (via spinal cord pathways) at larger doses
- Decrease $CMRO_2$ and cerebral blood flow (CBF)
  - Effect is less than with propofol or barbiturates
  - Unable to produce an isoelectric EEG
  - Minimal decrease in ICP in patients with limited intracranial compliance
- No neuroprotective properties

Cardiovascular System

- Minimal changes in blood pressure or heart rate in small doses
- Hypotension (due to peripheral vasodilation) may occur with high doses sufficient to induce general anesthesia, especially with hypovolemia

Respiratory System

- Minimal respiratory depression when given alone
- May result in severe ventilatory depression when coadministered with opioids

Side Effects

- Allergic reactions to benzodiazepines are extremely rare to nonexistent
- Lorazepam and diazepam may be painful on IV or intramuscular (IM) administration due to the propylene glycol solvent (midazolam does not require this and is typically not painful)

Clinical Uses

- The most frequent uses for benzodiazepines include preoperative anxiolytic medication, sedation, induction of anesthesia, and suppression of seizure activity
- Flumazenil is a benzodiazepine reversal agent:
  - Dose of 8–15 µg/kg IV may be used to treat patients experiencing delayed awakening
  - Brief duration of action (approximately 20 minutes), resedation may occur
  - May induce seizures in patients on chronic benzodiazepine therapy

Preoperative Medication and Sedation

- Amnestic, anxiolytic, and sedative effects make them useful preoperatively
- Synergistic effects on respiratory depression when combined with propofol or opioids
- Has more pronounced effects of sedation and amnesia in older persons
- Midazolam premedication
  - 1–2 mg IV–more rapid onset, more intense amnesia, and less postoperative sedation compared with diazepam
  - Useful oral premedication commonly used for children: 0.5 mg/kg orally given 30 minutes before induction of anesthesia
  - Lowers the incidence of PONV
- ICU sedation
  - May be useful as a sedative, use caution in critically ill and mechanically ventilated patients
  - Linked to increased rates of delirium and longer ICU stays compared with propofol and dexmedetomidine

Induction of Anesthesia

- Used infrequently due to both delayed onset of action and slower awakening compared with propofol
- Doses of 0.1–0.3 mg/kg IV of midazolam can be used with the advantage of fewer cardiovascular side effects

Suppression of Seizure Activity

- Efficacy is related to their ability to enhance the inhibitory effects of GABA, especially in the limbic system
- Diazepam 0.1 mg/kg IV usually abolishes seizures from local anesthetics or alcohol withdrawal
- Lorazepam 0.1 mg/kg IV is the treatment of choice for status epilepticus
- Midazolam IM (10 mg for patients >40 kg, 5 mg for those 13–40 kg) can be effective for status epilepticus when there is no IV access

Remimazolam

- New, ultrashort-acting benzodiazepine that is broken down by tissue esterases (analogous to remifentanil), gained FDA approval in 2020
- Several trials have demonstrated safety and utility in procedural sedation, particularly endoscopy
- May cause moderate hemodynamic effects (i.e., increased heart rate and decreased blood pressure)

KETAMINE

Pharmacokinetics and Pharmacodynamics

- Although ketamine has multiple mechanisms of action, the major anesthetic effect is produced by noncompetitive inhibition of the NMDA receptor complex
- Ketamine stereochemistry
  - Conventionally exists as a racemic mixture
  - *S*(+)-Enantiomer is more potent than the *R*(–)-enantiomer

- Recently an $S(+)$-enantiomer–only formulation (esketamine) has been developed and approved by the FDA for treatment of major depression
- Highly lipid soluble with rapid onset of effect
- Metabolism
  - Primarily in the liver via the cytochrome P450 system
  - Norketamine–primary active metabolite
    - One-third the activity of ketamine
    - Further metabolized and excreted in the urine
- Ketamine is the only IV anesthetic with low protein binding (12%)

Central Nervous System

- Unlike other IV anesthetics, ketamine is a cerebral vasodilator
- Increases both CBF and $CMRO_2$
  - Historic literature has emphasized concern for elevated ICP with ketamine administration
  - More recent studies have challenged this notion (especially with controlled ventilation)

CNS Effects of IV Anesthetics

Anesthetic	MAP	ICP	CBF	$CMRO_2$
Propofol / Barbiturates	↓	↓	↓	↓
Etomidate	↔ or ↓	↓	↓	↓
Ketamine	↑, ↔, or ↓	↑ or ↔	↑ or ↔	↑ or ↔

- At low doses, ketamine may facilitate seizures
- At anesthetic doses, can serve as an anticonvulsant when more conventional medications are ineffective
- Produces a characteristic hypnotic state "dissociative anesthesia" with patient's eyes open and slow nystagmus gaze
- Transient, self-resolving psychotomimetic symptoms
  - Vivid dreams, hallucinations, out-of-body experiences, and distorted visual and auditory sensitivity
  - Sense of euphoria explains its potential for abuse
  - Coadministration with a benzodiazepine may limit unpleasant experiences
  - A history of psychosis and schizophrenia is not an absolute contraindication to use of ketamine but should be weighed among risks and benefits

Cardiovascular System

- May cause temporary, but significant, increases in systemic arterial blood pressure, heart rate, and cardiac output
- Central sympathetic and adrenocortical stimulation, as well as inhibition of norepinephrine reuptake
- Effects can be blunted with coadministration with other anesthetics
- Direct myocardial depressant
  - Effect is typically masked by sympathetic stimulation
  - Can be significant and cause instability in critically ill patients with limited cardiovascular or sympathetic reserve

Respiratory System

- Primary advantage of ketamine is that it does not produce significant respiratory depression (i.e., spontaneous breathing is usually maintained)
- Transient apnea and hypoventilation can be seen with rapid, large IV boluses used for induction of anesthesia
- Increased lacrimation and salivation may occur
  - May increase risk of laryngospasm
  - Reduced by premedication with an anticholinergic, like glycopyrrolate
- Relaxes bronchial smooth muscle and may treat severe bronchospasm

Clinical Uses

Induction and Maintenance of Anesthesia

- Induction: 1–2 mg/kg IV or 6 mg/kg IM
- Maintenance
  - Not commonly used this purpose, but ketamine does have a favorable context-sensitive half-life
  - Can be achieved with 30–90 μg/kg/min ketamine alone, or 15–30 μg/kg/min ketamine plus 50–70% nitrous oxide
- Ketamine can also be coadministered with propofol (e.g., "ketofol"), which may minimize the need for supplemental opioids

Analgesia

- Small boluses of ketamine (0.2–0.8 mg/kg IV) can provide analgesia without respiratory suppression
- Subanesthetic infusions (3–5 μg/kg/min) can be used to reduce opioid tolerance and opioid-induced hyperalgesia, although not all studies show a reduction in pain scores
- Chronic pain
  - Moderate evidence exists for the use of ketamine infusions to reduce pain from complex regional pain syndrome (CRPS)
  - Use in other refractory pain conditions such as fibromyalgia, headaches, and phantom limb pain is more controversial

Treatment of Major Depression

- Ketamine has seen significant use as a rapid-onset option for treatment-resistant major depression

- Both IV and intranasal administration showing improved symptoms and sustained effect with repeated administration

ETOMIDATE

Pharmacokinetics and Pharmacodynamics

- Potentiates $GABA_A$ receptor–mediated chloride currents (similar to most other IV anesthetics discussed)
- Metabolism of etomidate is primarily hepatic via ester hydrolysis, with the subsequent inactive metabolites being excreted in the urine and bile
- Highly protein bound (77%), primarily to albumin

Central Nervous System

- Reduces $CMRO_2$ and causes direct cerebral vasoconstriction, resulting in decreased CBF and ICP
- May activate seizure foci and prove helpful in ECT

Cardiovascular System

- Hemodynamic stability is the chief characteristic of IV induction with etomidate
- Hypotension may still occur in the setting of hypovolemia

Hemodynamics during Induction

Effect	Propofol	Etomidate
MAP	↓↓	↔ or ↓
Heart rate	↔ or ↓	↔ or ↑
Systemic vascular resistance	↓↓	↔ or ↓

Respiratory System

- Respiratory depression is less pronounced with etomidate than with barbiturates
- Apnea can still follow rapid IV boluses, and exaggerated suppression can be seen when combined with opioids or inhaled anesthetics

Endocrine System

- Etomidate causes adrenocortical suppression via dose-dependent inhibition of 11β-hydroxylase, which is an enzyme necessary for the conversion of cholesterol to cortisol
- Significant adrenocortical suppression can last for up to 4 to 8 hours after an induction dose of etomidate
- Relative adrenal insufficiency can persist for up to 24 to 48 hours afterward
- The clinical significance of adrenocortical suppression after an IV induction dose of etomidate is controversial
    - Some studies show no changes in subsequent outcomes
    - Other studies show an increased risk of mortality in patients with or at risk of sepsis
    - This effect of etomidate is the principal factor limiting its use
- Development of novel, short-acting etomidate derivatives (e.g., ABP-700) with no adrenocortical side effects is under way

Clinical Uses

- Standard induction doses (0.2–0.3 mg/kg IV) achieve similar onset of unconsciousness as propofol and thiopental, with less postinduction hypotension
    - Useful in patients with compromised myocardial contractility, coronary artery disease, or severe aortic stenosis
- Etomidate is formulated with propylene glycol, which can lead to pain and venous irritation on injection
- Involuntary myoclonus is commonly seen after administration, which is due to the transient imbalance between excitatory and inhibitory signals in the thalamocortical tract
- Etomidate does not provide any analgesia and PONV may be seen more commonly than after use of propofol or thiopental

DEXMEDETOMIDINE

Pharmacokinetics and Pharmacodynamics

- The highly active *S*-enantiomer of medetomidine, dexmedetomidine, works through activation of CNS α_2-adrenergic receptors
- It undergoes rapid hepatic metabolism via *N*-methylation, hydroxylation, and conjugation, with its inactive metabolites being excreted in the urine and bile
- While clearance is high, dexmedetomidine has a significant context-sensitive half-time, increasing from 4 minutes after a 10-minute infusion to 250 minutes after an 8-hour infusion

Central Nervous System

- Hypnosis likely originates from agonism of α_2-adrenergic receptors in the brain (locus ceruleus)
- Analgesic effects arise from spinal cord receptors
- Sedative effect more closely resembles physiologic sleep than other IV anesthetics
    - EEG changes with characteristic "sleep spindles"
    - May activate endogenous sleep pathways
- Decreases CBF, with no significant change in either ICP or $CMRO_2$
- Patients can develop tolerance, with withdrawal symptoms seen after cessation of prolonged infusions

- Seizure foci and evoked potentials are not suppressed, making dexmedetomidine useful for epilepsy and spine surgeries, respectively
- Associated with decreased risk of postoperative cognitive dysfunction
  - For example, reduced delirium in the ICU and the immediate postoperative period
  - Whether long-term cognitive outcomes are influenced remains an area of research

Cardiovascular System

- Bolus or loading doses of dexmedetomidine may produce
  - Transient increases in systemic arterial blood pressure and subsequent reflex bradycardia
  - Caused by increased peripheral vascular resistance (but probably not pulmonary vascular resistance) from peripheral smooth muscle α_2-adrenergic receptors
  - Severe bradycardia, heart block, or even asystole may result from unopposed vagal stimulation, with the response to anticholinergic drugs being unchanged
- Prolonged infusions of dexmedetomidine generally produce
  - Moderate decreases in heart rate and systemic vascular resistance
  - Sympatholysis mediated by central nervous system α_2-adrenergic receptors

Respiratory System

- Minimal depression of the respiratory rate, may cause small to moderate decreases in tidal volume
- May be safely administered through tracheal extubation
- Response to hypercapnia appears unchanged, but the response to hypoxemia is blunted to a similar degree as when propofol is used
- Upper airway obstruction as a result of sedation is still possible and comparable to propofol

Immune System

- Capable of blunting the surgical stress response, similar to epidural anesthesia
- Anti-inflammatory effects possibly play a role in renal, myocardial, and cognitive effects of dexmedetomidine

Clinical Uses

- Sedation
  - Typical sedative infusion dose 0.2-1 μg/kg/hr. May go as high as 1.5 μg/kg/hr for a short time or stimulating procedures (watch for bradycardia).
  - FDA approved in 1999 for sedation in intensive care and procedural settings
  - May reduce the duration of mechanical ventilation, shorten the length of ICU stays, and improve ICU sleep quality
  - No proven mortality benefit
- Adjunct to general anesthesia–decreases both inhaled and IV anesthetic requirements
  - 0.5–1 μg/kg IV loading dose over 10–15 minutes
  - Followed by an infusion of 0.2–0.7 μg/kg/hr
  - Reduces opioid usage and pain scores in some, but not all, settings
  - Extensively used in pediatrics
    - Prevents emergence delirium
    - Does not affect time to extubation or discharge
- Perineural injection–can both improve analgesia and prolong duration of local anesthetics in both neuraxial and peripheral nerve blockade

Dosing for Adjunct Effects of IV Anesthetics

Anesthetic	Adjunct Effect	Dosing
Propofol	Antiemetic	10–20 mg IV bolus, or 10–20 μg/kg/min IV infusion
Ketamine	Analgesia	3–5 μg/kg/min IV infusion
Dexmedetomidine	Sedation/analgesia/antidelirium	0.5–1 μg/kg IV load over 10–15 min, followed by 0.2–0.7 μg/kg/hr IV infusion

QUESTIONS

WHY INTRAVENOUS ANESTHETICS?

1. What are some primary advantages and disadvantages of IV anesthetics over inhaled anesthetics?
2. Complete the following table entering "increased," "decreased," or "unchanged" to describe the effect of the given IV anesthetic.

Effect	Propofol	Thiopental	Midazolam	Ketamine	Etomidate	Dexmedetomidine
SBP						
Heart rate						
SVR						
Ventilation						
Respiratory rate						
Response to CO_2						
CBF						
$CMRO_2$						
ICP						
PONV						

3. Complete the following table entering yes or no to describe the effect of the given IV anesthetic.

Effect	Propofol	Thiopental	Midazolam	Ketamine	Etomidate	Dexmedetomidine
Anticonvulsant						
Anxiolysis						
Analgesia						
Emergence delirium						
Pain on injection						

$GABA_A$ RECEPTOR AGONISM

4. Why do the clinical effects of different $GABA_A$ agonists vary so widely?

PROPOFOL

5. Your patient has an egg allergy; does this serve as a contraindication to the administration of propofol? How about a soy allergy?
6. What is propofol infusion syndrome (PRIS), and what clinical findings should prompt investigation of it?
7. What is the relationship between postoperative nausea and vomiting (PONV) and propofol?

BARBITURATES

8. Why are barbiturates contraindicated for patients with acute intermittent porphyria?
9. What properties of barbiturates make them useful in the treatment of space-occupying intracranial lesions?
10. Name some clinical side effects that may be seen with a barbiturate coma.
11. What are some differences of methohexital from other barbiturates?

BENZODIAZEPINES

12. Describe the effects of benzodiazepine binding to the $GABA_A$ receptor.
13. Why are benzodiazepine infusions typically avoided as sedation for critically ill patients?
14. What is remimazolam? What is another drug that is metabolized by a similar mechanism?
15. How do the CNS effects of benzodiazepines compare with propofol and barbiturates?
16. Match each of the following drugs to the correct plot (A, B, or C) of context-sensitive half-time: propofol, remimazolam, and thiopental.

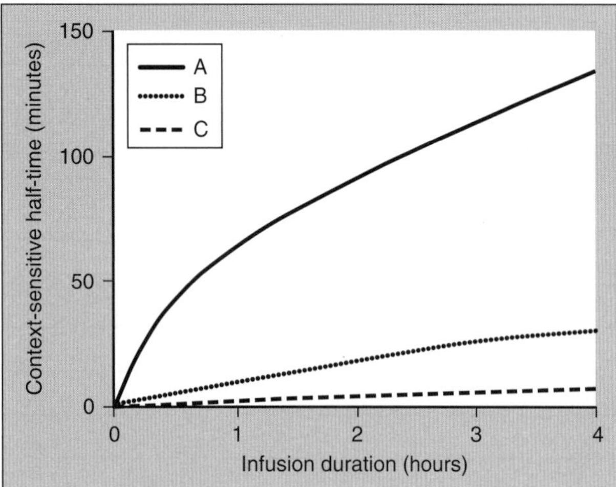

KETAMINE

17. What is the primary mechanism of action of ketamine?
18. In terms of CNS effects, how does ketamine differ from most other IV anesthetics?
19. How does ketamine affect ventilation and the respiratory system?
20. Besides anesthesia, what are some alternative uses of ketamine?

ETOMIDATE

21. What effects might etomidate have on the endocrine system? How long can these effects last?
22. Describe the cardiovascular impact of the administration of etomidate.
23. Besides the induction of anesthesia for surgical operations, what is a common use of etomidate?

DEXMEDETOMIDINE

24. Describe the mechanism of action of dexmedetomidine.
25. What are some effects that one might see after administering a bolus dose of dexmedetomidine?
26. What are some adjunct uses for dexmedetomidine, outside of serving as a patient's primary sedative?
27. What is an advantage of using dexmedetomidine for sedation in the ICU, as opposed to another IV anesthetic?

ANSWERS

WHY INTRAVENOUS ANESTHETICS?

1. The primary advantages of IV anesthetics over their inhaled counterparts include their ability to more rapidly induce hypnosis and provide anesthesia for laryngoscopy. However, the downside to their use is the current inability to measure their concentration at the effect site (e.g., brain) in real time, meaning clinicians must rely on their knowledge of pharmacokinetics, surrogate monitors, and prior experience to effectively use them. (107–108)
2. The effect of each IV anesthetic is described in the table below, with two exceptions. Ketamine may cause direct myocardial depression and hypotension in critically ill or catecholamine-depleted patients, and dexmedetomidine when bolused may increase SVR and blood pressure. (112)

Effect	Propofol	Thiopental	Midazolam	Ketamine	Etomidate	Dexmedetomidine
SBP	Decreased	Decreased	Unchanged to decreased	Increased	Unchanged to decreased	Decreased
Heart rate	Unchanged to decreased	Increased	Unchanged	Increased	Unchanged to decreased	Decreased
SVR	Decreased	Decreased	Unchanged to decreased	Increased	Unchanged to decreased	Decreased
Ventilation	Decreased	Decreased	Unchanged	Unchanged	Unchanged to decreased	Unchanged to decreased
Respiratory rate	Decreased	Decreased	Unchanged to decreased	Unchanged	Unchanged to decreased	Unchanged
Response to CO_2	Decreased	Decreased	Decreased	Unchanged	Decreased	Unchanged
CBF	Decreased	Decreased	Decreased	Increased to unchanged	Decreased	Decreased
$CMRO_2$	Decreased	Decreased	Decreased	Increased to unchanged	Decreased	Unchanged
ICP	Decreased	Decreased	Unchanged	Increased to unchanged	Decreased	Unchanged
PONV	Decreased	Unchanged	Decreased	Unchanged	Increased	Unchanged

3. The effect of each IV anesthetic is described in the table below. (112)

Effect	Propofol	Thiopental	Midazolam	Ketamine	Etomidate	Dexmedetomidine
Anticonvulsant	Yes	Yes	Yes	Yes?	No	No
Anxiolysis	Yes	No	Yes	No	No	Yes
Analgesia	No	No	No	Yes	No	Yes
Emergence delirium	No	No	No	Yes	No	May reduce
Pain on injection	Yes	No	No	No	Yes	No

$GABA_A$ RECEPTOR AGONISM

4. $GABA_A$ agonists exhibit different characteristic effects due to multiple possible binding sites on the pentameric $GABA_A$ receptor (benzodiazepines on the extracellular portion, while propofol, etomidate, and barbiturates bind in the transmembrane domain), varying location of action (e.g., brain vs. spinal cord), and heterogeneity of the $GABA_A$ receptor itself. (109)

PROPOFOL

5. Despite propofol being formulated in an emulsion that includes soybean oil and egg lecithin, there is no evidence for cross-reactivity in patients with egg, soy, or peanut allergies and it can be safely administered to these patients. (110)
6. Propofol infusion syndrome (PRIS) is a rare and potentially fatal side effect of propofol, classically seen after its long-term administration (i.e., >20 hours) as an infusion. It is typically characterized by profound metabolic acidosis, rhabdomyolysis, hyperkalemia, arrhythmias, and elevated triglycerides. (113)
7. Propofol has antiemetic properties, with low-dose infusions (e.g., 25 μg/kg/min) frequently being used as a preventative agent of PONV. (113)

BARBITURATES

8. Barbiturates can stimulate aminolevulinic acid synthetase, increasing the production of porphyrins and potentially precipitating an exacerbation of acute intermittent porphyria. (114)
9. Barbiturates are potent cerebral vasoconstrictors; by reducing cerebral blood flow and cerebral blood volume, they can decrease ICP. These properties are useful for patients undergoing craniotomy for space-occupying lesions. In addition, barbiturates may provide neuroprotection from focal cerebral ischemia, which can occur with surgical retraction during intracranial surgery. (115)
10. A "barbiturate coma" from prolonged infusions can result in immunosuppression, hypothermia, and electrolyte imbalances. (115)
11. Methohexital is unique among barbiturates in that it may decrease the seizure threshold, making it useful for electroconvulsive therapy (ECT). It is also cleared more rapidly by the liver than thiopental and has a shorter elimination half-time, meaning there is a shorter time to recovery from administration. (114)

BENZODIAZEPINES

12. Unlike propofol, etomidate, and barbiturates, a benzodiazepine binding to the $GABA_A$ receptor alone is not sufficient to fully activate the receptor; instead, it only enhances the ability of endogenous GABA to open the chloride channel. (115)
13. Benzodiazepine infusions are frequently avoided as sedation in the critically ill as they have been linked to higher rates of delirium and longer ICU stays compared with propofol and dexmedetomidine. (116)
14. Remimazolam is an ultrashort-acting benzodiazepine that gained FDA approval in 2020 after studies demonstrated its safety and efficacy in procedural sedation. Its short duration of action can be attributed to the fact that it is broken down by tissue esterases, similar to remifentanil. (118)
15. Compared with barbiturates and propofol, benzodiazepines decrease $CMRO_2$ and cerebral blood flow to a lesser degree, with usually minimal change in ICP. Benzodiazepines are also unable to produce an isoelectric EEG when administered as the sole agent. (118)
16. For the graph shown in question 16, A = Thiopental (longest context-sensitive half-time), B = propofol (intermediate), and C = remimazolam (shortest context-sensitive half-time). (110, 114, 118)

KETAMINE

17. Ketamine's anesthetic effect is primarily due to its noncompetitive inhibition of the NMDA receptor, though it does have multiple other mechanisms of action. (118)
18. Unlike the $GABA_A$ agonists in this chapter, ketamine has the potential to increase cerebral blood flow and $CMRO_2$. Historically, there has been concern that ketamine increases ICP, though some recent studies have challenged this notion. (119)
19. One of the advantages of ketamine over other anesthetics is that it does not result in significant respiratory depression, though transient apnea can be seen after large boluses. It also can relax bronchial smooth muscle, making it useful in the treatment of severe bronchospasm. However, it also increases salivation, potentially complicating manipulation of the airway. (119)
20. Alternative uses for ketamine include for treatment-resistant major depression, as well as for some chronic pain syndromes (e.g., complex regional pain syndrome). (119, 120)

ETOMIDATE

21. Etomidate causes adrenocortical suppression via inhibition of 11β-hydroxylase, thus preventing the conversion of cholesterol to cortisol. Significant adrenocortical suppression can be seen for 4 to 8 hours after administration, with relative adrenal insufficiency persisting for up to 24 to 48 hours. (120)
22. Hemodynamic stability on induction of anesthesia is one of the primary advantages of etomidate compared with propofol or barbiturates. However, hypotension can still be seen, especially in the setting of hypovolemia. (120)
23. Etomidate lowers the seizure threshold, making it a useful anesthetic for ECT. (120)

DEXMEDETOMIDINE

24. Dexmedetomidine is an α_2-adrenergic receptor agonist, with activity primarily in the locus ceruleus (CNS) and spinal cord receptors. (121)
25. Bolus doses of dexmedetomidine frequently result in transient increases in systemic arterial blood pressure (due to elevated systemic vascular resistance from activation of peripheral α_2-adrenergic receptors) and subsequent reflex bradycardia. Heart block, or even asystole, can result from unopposed vagal stimulation. (122)
26. Perineural dexmedetomidine can serve as an adjunct analgesic for peripheral nerve blockade, both increasing analgesia and prolonging the duration of nerve blockade. IV dexmedetomidine may act as an aid to prevent emergence delirium, especially in the pediatric population. (122)
27. Studies have shown that dexmedetomidine may reduce the duration of mechanical ventilation, shorten the length of ICU stays, and improve sleep quality in the ICU. However, there has been no proven mortality benefit associated with dexmedetomidine infusions. (122)

Chapter

9 OPIOIDS

Kasi Goodwin and Talmage D. Egan

BASIC PHARMACOLOGY

Structure-Activity

- Opioids are generally
  - Highly soluble weak bases
  - Highly protein bound
  - Largely ionized at physiologic pH
- Physiochemical properties affect clinical behavior, e.g., speed of onset
  - Protein binding
  - Ionized fraction
  - Lipid solubility

Mechanism

- Three classic opioid receptors: mu (μ), kappa (κ), and delta (δ)
- G protein is activated when opioid agonist binds.
  - Effects are primarily inhibitory.
- Therapeutic effects occur at multiple sites.

Sites of Opioid Therapeutic Effects

Dorsal horn of spinal cord
- Inhibits the release of substance P
- Mitigates the transfer of painful sensation to the brain

Brainstem
- Modulates spinal cord transmission through descending inhibitory pathways

Forebrain
- Thought to change the affective response to pain

Metabolism

- Mostly metabolized by the liver
- Some undergo hepatic conjugation and are renally excreted (e.g., morphine).
- Variation in the metabolic pathway can alter the clinical effect (e.g., codeine).

CLINICAL PHARMACOLOGY

Pharmacokinetics

- Pharmacokinetic differences guide the selection and administration of opioids.
  - Pharmacokinetic simulations of effect-site concentrations are helpful.
- Key pharmacokinetic behaviors for bolus injections
  - Latency to peak effect-site concentration (i.e., *bolus front-end kinetics*)
  - Time to clinically relevant decay of concentration (i.e., *bolus back-end kinetics*)
- Key pharmacokinetic behaviors for continuous infusions
  - Time to steady-state concentration after starting (i.e., *infusion front-end kinetics*)
  - Time to clinically relevant decay in concentration after stopping (i.e., *infusion back-end kinetics*)

Pharmacodynamics

Therapeutic Effects
- Analgesia
  - Acts at spinal cord and brain μ receptors
- Sedation
  - All produce dose-dependent drowsiness and sleep
- Suppression of the cough reflex
  - Reduces coughing and "bucking" against an endotracheal tube

Adverse Effects
- Depression of ventilation
  - Alters the relationship between minute volume and arterial pCO_2
    - Reduces the ventilatory response to rising pCO_2
    - Can result in apnea when the arterial pCO_2 is below a certain threshold (*apneic threshold*) see below figure

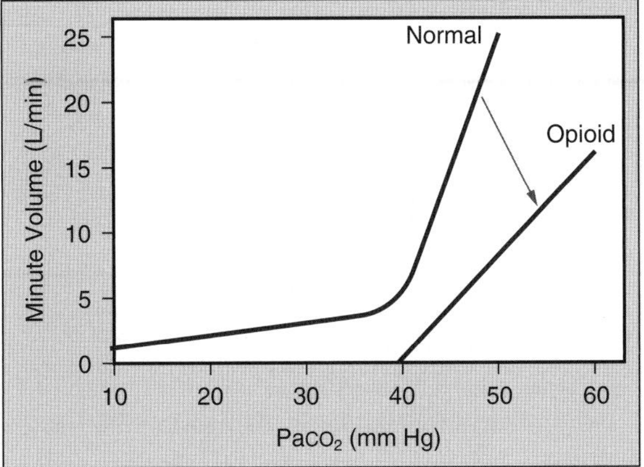

Opioid-induced ventilatory depression study methodology. This method characterizes the relationship between $PaCO_2$ and minute volume. The curve labeled "Normal" represents the expected response of minute volume to rising $PaCO_2$ levels in an awake human. Note the dramatic increase in minute volume as CO_2 tension rises. The curve labeled "Opioid" represents the blunted response of minute volume to rising CO_2 levels after administration of an opioid. Note that the slope of the curve decreases and the curve no longer has a "hockey stick" shape; this means that at physiologic $PaCO_2$ levels, the patient receiving sufficient opioid may be apneic or severely hypoventilatory. (Adapted with permission from Gross J.B.: When you breathe IN you inspire, when you DON'T breathe, you ... expire: new insights regarding opioid-induced ventilatory depression. Anesthesiology 2003; 99: pp. 767-770.)

- Clinical signs
  - Initially decreased respiratory rate
  - With increasing doses, decreases in both respiratory rate and tidal volume

Risk Factors for Opioid-Induced Ventilatory Depression
▪ Large opioid dose ▪ Advanced age ▪ Concomitant use of other central nervous system depressants ▪ Renal insufficiency (e.g., morphine) ▪ Natural sleep

- Cardiovascular physiologic alterations
  - Increase in vagal nerve tone (fentanyl congeners)
  - Vasodilation by depression of brainstem vasomotor centers and by direct effect on vessels
    - Most pronounced in patients with high sympathetic tone
- Muscle rigidity
  - Usually after rapid large bolus administration of fentanyl congeners
  - Can make bag and mask ventilation difficult or impossible
- Nausea and vomiting
  - Chemoreceptor trigger zone stimulation in the area postrema on the floor of the fourth ventricle in the brain
- Pupillary constriction
  - Stimulation of Edinger-Westphal nucleus of oculomotor nerve
  - Occurs in low doses of opioids, even when patient is opioid tolerant
- Tonic contraction of the gastrointestinal smooth muscle
  - Decreases coordinated, peristaltic contractions
  - Delayed gastric emptying
  - Opioid-induced ileus and chronic constipation
- Spasm of sphincter of Oddi
  - False-positive cholangiogram during gallbladder surgery
  - Reversible completely (naloxone) or partially (glucagon)
- Urinary retention
  - Decreased bladder detrusor tone
  - Increased tone of the urinary sphincter
- Depression of cellular immunity
  - Effect of chronic opioid intake
  - Inhibits transcription of interleukin-2 in activated T cells
  - Impaired wound healing, perioperative infections, and cancer recurrence are possible.
- CNS adaptations requiring escalation in dosing to control pain
  - *Tolerance*: decrease in analgesic response over time
  - *Opioid-induced hyperalgesia*: increased pain response to noxious stimuli while undergoing opioid treatment

Drug Interactions

- Pharmacokinetic drug interactions
  - One drug influences the concentration of another.
    - Example is increased opioid concentration when combined with propofol infusion.
- Pharmacodynamic drug interactions
  - One drug influences the effect of another.
  - Synergistic effect of opioids with other sedatives
    - Example is the reduction of the minimum alveolar concentration when opioids are combined with volatile anesthetics.

Specific Populations

Hepatic Failure

- Liver failure must be severe to have a major impact on opioid pharmacokinetics.
- Patients with hepatic encephalopathy are vulnerable to opioid sedative effects.

Kidney Failure
- Clinically important when active metabolites accumulate
  - Morphine 6-glucuronide (M6G)
    - Potent analgesic effects
    - Can cause respiratory depression
  - Normeperidine
    - Analgesic effects
    - Excitatory CNS effects including anxiety, myoclonus, and seizures

Gender
- Morphine in women is more potent with a slower onset of action.

Age
- Increased potency
- Decreased clearance and central volume of distribution
- Substantial opioid dose reduction is usually necessary in elderly patients.

Obesity
- Pharmacokinetics are more related to lean body mass than total body weight.

Unique Features of Individual Opioids

Codeine
- Codeine is a prodrug.
- Converted to morphine by the liver microsomal isoform CYP2D6.
  - Patients lacking CYP2D6 activity have no therapeutic response to codeine.
  - Patients with *CYP2D6* gene duplications can exhibit excessive therapeutic and adverse effects from codeine.
    - Special risk to nursing babies of mothers with this genetic abnormality

Morphine
- Associated with histamine release
- Slow onset time risking "stacking" of doses
- M6G is only 10% of morphine's metabolism but contributes to its analgesic effects.

Fentanyl
- Can be delivered via intravenous, transdermal, transmucosal, transnasal, and transpulmonary routes

Alfentanil
- Short-half life after single bolus injection
- Effect can be prolonged after continuous infusion

Sufentanil
- Most potent opioid commonly used in anesthesia practice
- Absolute doses used are much smaller compared with other opioids.
  - Sufentanil dose is a 1000-fold less than morphine dose.

Remifentanil
- Very short-acting opioid
- Quickly achieves steady-state and easily titratable as continuous infusion
- Loses its μ receptor agonist activity upon ester hydrolysis

Opioid Agonist-Antagonists and Pure Antagonists

Properties of Opioid Agonist-Antagonists

- Analgesics with a "ceiling effect"
- Lower potential for ventilatory depression than pure agonists
- Perceived lower abuse potential than pure agonists
- Used for the treatment of chronic pain
- Used for the treatment of opioid use disorder
- Some degree of competitive antagonism when administered with full agonists

Tramadol
- Centrally acting analgesic
  - Moderate μ receptor and weak κ and δ receptor affinity
- Antagonist activity at the 5-HT and nicotinic acetylcholine receptors
  - With other serotonin medications risks serotonin syndrome, CNS excitability, and seizures

Buprenorphine
- Very potent with high affinity for μ receptor
- Moderate doses treat chronic pain.
- Higher doses can antagonize the effects of other opioids.
  - The treatment of acute-on-chronic pain can be difficult.
- Can be administered sublingually, transdermally, or parenterally
- Buprenorphine is playing an increasing role in the treatment of opioid use disorders (OUDs).

Nalbuphine
- Can use as a sole agent for sedation with less ventilatory depression
- Can use to reverse ventilatory depression in opioid overdose while maintaining some analgesia

Naloxone/Naltrexone
- Naloxone is an injectable μ antagonist
  - Used in the reversal of opioid overdose and to treat opioid-induced pruritus
  - Has many negative effects (e.g., tachycardia, hypertension, seizures)
  - Duration of action is shorter than for most opioids.
  - Nasal spray and autoinjector preparations are designed for laypersons.
- Naltrexone is a longer-acting μ antagonist.
  - Oral, injectable, and implantable forms
  - Used in long-term management of opioid addiction

CLINICAL APPLICATION

Key Questions to Address When Selecting the Appropriate Opioid

- How quickly must the desired opioid effect be achieved?
- How long must the opioid effect be maintained?
- How critical is it that opioid-induced ventilatory depression or sedation dissipate quickly?
- Is the capability to raise and lower the level of opioid effect quickly during the anesthetic critical?
- Will there be significant pain postoperatively that will require opioid treatment?

EMERGING DEVELOPMENTS

Opioid Abuse Epidemic

- Abuse of prescription and illicit opioids has skyrocketed in the United States.
  - Death and OUD have resulted
- This has led to increased focus on improved opioid stewardship.
  - CDC has issued guidelines for opioid prescribing.
  - Increased interest in "multimodal general anesthesia"

Multimodal General Anesthesia (and Opioid-Free Anesthesia)

- Synergism typically results when anesthetic drugs of different mechanisms are administered together.
  - Includes opioids, α_2-agonists, local anesthetics, and *N*-methyl-D-aspartate (NMDA) antagonists
- Opioid-free anesthesia aims to decrease (or eliminate) perioperative opioids.
  - This approach is controversial.
- The impact of minimizing perioperative opioids on OUD is unclear.

Biased μ-Receptor Agonists

- Two distinct transduction pathways mediate opioid effects.
  - G protein–coupled pathway: analgesic, reward, and pleasure effects
  - Beta-arrestin pathway mediates respiratory depression and gastrointestinal effects.
- Biased opioids are full agonists of the G protein pathway.
  - Preserved analgesic effects with less constipation or ventilatory depression
  - Oliceridine is a biased agonist recently approved by the U.S. Food and Drug Administration.
  - The role of biased opioids is still emerging.

QUESTIONS

BASIC PHARMACOLOGY

1. What is the mechanism of action of opioids?
2. Describe the locations and classes of opioid receptors.
3. Which opioids have active metabolites?

CLINICAL PHARMACOLOGY

4. What are the four key pharmacokinetic behaviors of opioids?
5. What properties of an opioid affect its latency time to peak effect (i.e., bolus front-end kinetics) after a bolus injection?
6. Describe a clinical example of how an opioid bolus latency time to peak effect would influence patient-controlled analgesia (PCA) dosing.
7. What are some therapeutic effects of opioids?
8. What are the effects of opioids on ventilation?
9. What is an example of a pharmacokinetic drug interaction of opioids?
10. What is an example of a pharmacodynamic drug interaction of opioids?
11. What are some considerations of using opioids in patients with kidney failure?
12. How does the onset time of morphine compare with the other opioids? What are some potential drawbacks of the administration of morphine?
13. How does fentanyl compare with morphine with regard to its effect-site equilibration time? What is the potency of fentanyl relative to morphine?
14. How are the effects of fentanyl terminated? How does the context-sensitive half-time of fentanyl compare with other opioids?
15. What are some clinical uses of remifentanil?
16. By what mechanism do opioid agonists/antagonists work?
17. What role does the opioid antagonist naloxone play in clinical practice? What are some adverse effects of naloxone?
18. What role does the opioid antagonist naltrexone play in clinical practice?

CLINICAL APPLICATION

19. What are some common clinical indications for the use of opioids in anesthesia practice?
20. What is the basis of opioid selection in different clinical situations?

ANSWERS

BASIC PHARMACOLOGY

1. Opioids exert their effects through their agonist actions at the opioid receptors. The main action of opioids appears to be through the interaction with G proteins, resulting in inhibition of the activity of adenylate cyclase and increasing potassium conductance. This ultimately results in hyperpolarization of the cell and leads to a suppression of synaptic transmission. (126)
2. Opioid receptors are located in various tissues throughout the central nervous system (CNS) and exert their therapeutic effects at multiple sites. They inhibit the release of substance P from primary sensory neurons in the dorsal horn of the spinal cord, mitigating the transfer of painful sensations to the brain. Opioid actions in the brainstem modulate nociceptive transmission in the dorsal horn of the spinal cord through descending inhibitory pathways. Three classic opioid receptors have been identified: μ, κ, and δ. More recently, a fourth opioid receptor ligand, ORL1, has also been identified, but its function is quite different from that of the classic opioid receptors. Although the existence of opioid receptor subtypes has been proposed, it is not clear from molecular biology techniques that distinct genes code for them. (127)
3. Both meperidine and morphine have active metabolites that can accumulate in renal failure, and thus these drugs must be used with caution in this patient population. Genetic variations in codeine metabolism can also affect clinical drug effect. (127)

CLINICAL PHARMACOLOGY

4. The four key pharmacokinetic behaviors of opioids are (1) latency to peak effect site concentration after bolus injection (i.e., bolus front-end kinetics), (2) time to clinically relevant decay of concentration after bolus injection (i.e., bolus back-end kinetics), (3) time to steady-state concentration after starting a continuous infusion (i.e., infusion front-end kinetics), and (4) time to clinically relevant decay in concentration after stopping a continuous infusion (i.e., infusion back-end kinetics). (127–128)
5. The latency time to peak effect (bolus front-end kinetics) of common intravenous opioids after administering a bolus is influenced by the opioid's ionization and lipid solubility. Opioids that are un-ionized, unbound, and have high lipid solubility rapidly equilibrate to the effect site. The time-to-peak effect is also influenced by the amount of drug administered in the initial bolus. (128)
6. Front-end kinetics of fentanyl make it well suited for patient-controlled analgesia (PCA) use. In contrast to morphine, the peak effect of a fentanyl bolus is manifest before a typical PCA lockout period has elapsed, thus mitigating the "dose-stacking" problem. (128)
7. Pain relief is the primary therapeutic effect of opioid analgesics. Additionally, in the operative setting, opioid effects of drowsiness, decreased airway irritability, and attenuation of the cough reflex are considered therapeutic benefits. (130)
8. All the μ-receptor agonist opioids produce a dose-dependent depression of ventilation. This is reflected by an increase in the resting $Pa{CO_2}$, an increase in the apneic threshold, a decrease in the responsiveness to the ventilatory stimulant effects of carbon dioxide, and a decrease in the hypoxic ventilatory drive. The administration of opioids affects the rate of breathing and the tidal volume. The respiratory rate is typically slowed and insufficiently compensated by an increase in the tidal volume. Consequently, the minute ventilation is decreased. (131)
9. A pharmacokinetic drug interaction is one in which the administration of a drug influences the concentration of another administered drug. An example of this occurs when opioids are administered concurrently with a continuous propofol infusion. Opioid concentrations may be higher when administered with a continuous propofol infusion than they are when the same dose is administered alone. This may be due in part to the hemodynamic changes (i.e., decreased hepatic blood flow) induced by propofol. (132)
10. A pharmacodynamic drug interaction is one in which the administration of a drug influences the effect of another drug. The most common and most important pharmacodynamic drug interaction of opioids is their synergistic effect when administered with sedatives. Opioids also synergistically reduce the MAC of volatile anesthetics. This opioid-induced MAC reduction can be substantial, by up to 75% or more. (132)
11. Kidney failure has major clinical relevance when administering morphine and meperidine. Two metabolites of morphine, morphine-3-glucuronide, and morphine-6-glucuronide (M3G and M6G), are excreted via the

kidney. M3G is inactive, but M6G is an analgesic whose potency approaches that of morphine. Life-threatening respiratory depression can develop in patients with renal failure administered morphine as a result of very high levels of M6G. Normeperidine is the main metabolite of meperidine and is excreted through the kidney. Normeperidine has analgesic and excitatory central nervous system (CNS) effects. The manifestations of normeperidine CNS toxicity include anxiety, tremulousness, myoclonus, and frank seizures. For most other opioids, kidney failure has minimal clinical importance. (133–134)

12. Morphine is the prototype opioid to which other opioids are compared. Because of its low lipid solubility and almost completely ionized form at physiologic pH, morphine has a prolonged latency to peak effect because of its slow penetration of the CNS. At steady-state concentrations, its ventilatory depressive effects are indistinguishable from other opioids. Unfortunately, its pharmacology predisposes patients to delayed respiratory depression as well as potential dose stacking when administered by PCA. (135)
13. Fentanyl administered intravenously has a more rapid onset and shorter duration of action than morphine. This reflects in part its greater lipid solubility. The effect-site equilibration time of fentanyl is approximately 6 minutes. Its shorter duration of action is reflective of its rapid redistribution to inactive tissue sites, leading to a rapid decrease in the plasma concentration. Fentanyl is 75 to 125 times more potent than morphine. (135)
14. The effects of fentanyl are terminated through its redistribution to inactive tissue sites and through metabolism by the liver. The expected duration of action is reflected in the context-sensitive half-time (CSHT). Fentanyl's CSHT increases significantly over time, making fentanyl less suitable for cases in which a rapid decline in opioid effect after stopping a continuous infusion is desirable. Conversely, if an opioid effect is desired after stopping a continuous infusion (e.g., for postoperative analgesia), fentanyl may be a suitable choice. (135)
15. The most common clinical application of remifentanil is for TIVA, when combined with propofol. It is also useful as a bolus injection when rapid effect and recovery are desired, in surgical cases that have rapidly fluctuating anesthetic requirements, when a "large-dose" opioid technique is advantageous but the patient will not be mechanically ventilated postoperatively, or during monitored anesthetic care when a brief "pulse" of opioid effect may help the patient tolerate local anesthetic infiltration. (135)
16. Opioid agonists/antagonists are partial μ-receptor agonists while simultaneously serving as competitive antagonists at μ receptors and other opioid receptors. (136)
17. Naloxone is an intravenous complete opioid antagonist used to emergently reverse opioid-induced ventilatory depression. In smaller doses, naloxone can be used during the emergence of anesthesia to restore adequate ventilatory effort. Another clinical use of naloxone is for the treatment of opioid-induced pruritus. Some adverse effects of naloxone include precipitation of acute opioid withdrawal syndrome, nausea, vomiting, tachycardia, hypertension, seizures, and pulmonary edema. (136)
18. Naltrexone is available orally as an additive to orally administered opioids and is used as a deterrent to opioid abuse. (137)

CLINICAL APPLICATION

19. Opioids have been used in various clinical areas of anesthesia. To increase the safety of opioid use for postoperative pain control, they can be delivered by a PCA machine. Opioids can be combined with other drugs and techniques to decrease pain as well. Another common indication of opioid use is for "balanced anesthesia," where opioids are primarily used for MAC reducing properties, thereby minimizing the direct myocardial depression and other untoward hemodynamic effects of the volatile anesthetics. Total intravenous anesthesia can be achieved when opioids are administered in combination with propofol infusions. (137)
20. Pharmacokinetic differences between opioids are the main consideration in selecting them for appropriate purpose. All μ agonists are equally efficacious when given in equipotent doses. Among key elements when selecting an opioid for administration is the desired time of onset, the duration of effect, and potential side effects. Side effects for consideration in the perioperative domain include sedation, respiratory depression, and intestinal ileus. (137)

Chapter

10 LOCAL ANESTHETICS

Elliot S. Schwartz

HISTORY

- Chemical structure
  - Local anesthetics are weak bases with a lipophilic aromatic ring and a hydrophilic amino group.
  - Classified into two groups: esters and amides
  - Classification is determined by the bond between the lipophilic and hydrophilic groups (either an ester or an amide bond).
- Esters
  - First clinical use of a local anesthetic was in the 1880s with cocaine.
  - Examples: cocaine, procaine, chloroprocaine, and tetracaine
  - Undergo hydrolysis by plasma esterases
- Amides
  - Advantages over esters include stability and reduced incidence of allergic reactions.
  - Lidocaine was the first amide and was introduced in 1948.
  - Examples: lidocaine, mepivacaine, prilocaine, bupivacaine, and ropivacaine
  - Metabolized by hepatic enzymes

Distinguishing Between an Ester and an Amide

As a shortcut, look at the generic name. If it contains two of the letter "i," then it is an amide (e.g., lidocaine, mepivacaine). If it contains a single letter "i," then it is an ester (e.g., cocaine, tetracaine).

NERVE CONDUCTION

- Resting membrane potential
  - A resting axon has a negative potential of –90 mV across its membrane with the inside negative relative to the extracellular fluid.
  - The negative potential is generated by relative ion concentrations.
    - Outward transport of sodium ions
    - Inward transport of potassium ions
    - Greater membrane permeability to potassium ions relative to sodium ions allows potassium cations to leak out.
- Action potential
  - Excitation increases the membrane permeability to sodium ions.
  - Positively charged sodium ions rapidly enter the axon, causing a large upswing in membrane potential.
  - An action potential is triggered once a critical potential is reached (threshold potential), and a wave of depolarization is propagated down the nerve.
- Classification of nerve fibers
  - Fiber diameter
    - Larger diameter correlates with more rapid conduction velocity.
  - Presence or absence of myelin
    - Myelinated
      - Each axon is encased in multiple membranous wrappings formed by one Schwann cell.
      - Forces current to flow through periodic interruptions in the myelin (nodes of Ranvier), increasing conduction velocity
      - Myelinated fibers are relatively more susceptible to local anesthetics.
    - Unmyelinated
      - Slower conduction velocity
  - Functions: proprioception, touch, pressure, pain, temperature, large motor, small motor
- Types of nerve fibers
  - Type A fibers: larger diameter, myelinated, faster conduction velocity
  - Type B fibers: smaller diameter, myelinated
  - Type C fibers: smallest diameter, unmyelinated, slowest conduction velocity

Calculation of Concentration

How is concentration in mg/mL determined?

- A 1% solution of lidocaine means there is 1 g/100 mL, which equals 10 mg/mL.
- As a shortcut, move the decimal over to the right by one place (e.g., 2% lidocaine = 20 mg/mL or 0.5% bupivacaine = 5 mg/mL).

LOCAL ANESTHETIC ACTIONS ON SODIUM CHANNELS

- Mechanism of action: block sodium ion influx through voltage-gated sodium channels
  - Binding site to the sodium channel is intracellular.
  - Decreases the rate of depolarization in response to excitation
  - Prevents achievement of the threshold potential and therefore prevents the firing of an action potential
  - "Frequency-dependent" block describes the intensification of a block with more frequent rates of nerve firing.

pH, Net Charge, and Lipid Solubility

- Local anesthetics exist in equilibrium at physiologic pH in uncharged and charged forms.
  - Uncharged base form (unprotonated, hydrophobic) can readily diffuse across the neural membrane.
  - Charged form (protonated, hydrophilic) can bind to the receptor within the axoplasm.
  - Pathway
    - Uncharged form penetrates neural membrane.
    - Ionizes to charged form in the axoplasm
    - Binds to the sodium channel in its charged form
- Onset of action
  - Correlates with a lower pKa of the local anesthetic
    - The pKa is the pH at which the concentrations of the uncharged and charged forms are equal.
    - The lower the pKa of a local anesthetic (closer to physiologic pH of 7.4), the greater is the fraction of the uncharged form, which readily diffuses across the lipid membrane.
    - Example: pKa of lidocaine is 7.9 and pKa of bupivacaine is 8.1. Lidocaine has a faster onset than bupivacaine.
    - Notable exception: chloroprocaine has a high pKa (8.7) but a very rapid onset because it is administered at very high concentrations.
  - Increasing the solution's pH (e.g., by adding bicarbonate) speeds onset time by increasing the uncharged fraction.
    - The effect is most pronounced when bicarbonate is added to formulations of premixed lidocaine and epinephrine (which are packaged at a much lower pH than solutions of plain lidocaine).
  - Lower pH environments (acidosis associated with infection, inflammation, ischemia) slow onset time and negatively affect the quality of the local anesthesia.
- Potency
  - Correlates with increased lipid solubility, i.e., tissue penetration of the local anesthetic
  - Example: bupivacaine is far more lipophilic than lidocaine, and about four times as potent as lidocaine.
- Duration of action
  - Correlates with higher protein binding and increased lipid solubility, which trap the local anesthetic within the nerve

DIFFERENTIAL LOCAL ANESTHETIC BLOCKADE

- Differential blockade is the clinical observation that local anesthetics block various nerve functions with different sensitivities in a concentration-dependent manner.
  - For example, an epidural with dilute concentrations of local anesthetic could produce autonomic blockade and analgesia with relative sparing of motor strength.

SPREAD OF LOCAL ANESTHESIA AFTER INJECTION

- Local anesthetics diffuse across barriers down their concentration gradient after injection.
- Nerve fibers on outer surface (mantle) are blocked before fibers at innermost layers (core).
  - Outer mantle fibers generally innervate more proximal structures.
  - Proximal anesthesia can precede distal anesthesia.
- Anatomic location of autonomic, sensory, and motor nerve fibers within mixed peripheral nerves explains the sequence of onset and recovery from local anesthesia.
  - Autonomic effects can precede sensory effects and, last, muscle weakness.

PHARMACOKINETICS

- Systemic absorption competes with drug entry into nerves at target site.
- Peak plasma concentration from systemic absorption:
  - Increases with higher blood flow at the site of injection
  - Increases with decreased systemic clearance (e.g., liver disease or CHF)
  - Decreases for drugs with high lipophilicity or protein binding
  - Decreases with vasoconstriction at injection site (e.g., addition of epinephrine)

Plasma Uptake of Local Anesthetic After Regional Anesthetic Procedures
Intercostal > Caudal > Epidural > Brachial plexus > Lower extremity

Local Anesthetic Vasoactivity

- Local anesthetics can cause vasodilation via blockade of vascular smooth muscles and indirectly via blockade of sympathetic fibers.
- Clinical effect of adding vasoconstrictors to local anesthetics (e.g., epinephrine) is variable among local anesthetics and different blocks.
  - For example, spinal tetracaine significantly increases spinal cord perfusion. Consequently, the effect on duration with addition of epinephrine is more pronounced with spinal tetracaine.

Metabolism

- Esters undergo hydrolysis by plasma esterases.
  - Patients with pseudocholinesterase deficiency may have prolonged systemic clearance.
- Amides are metabolized by hepatic microsomal enzymes.
  - Plasma clearance parallels hepatic blood flow.

Additives

- Epinephrine
  - Causes local vasoconstriction, decreases systemic absorption, and may decrease potential of systemic toxicity
  - Variably prolongs nerve block
    - The effect on prolonging duration tends to be more pronounced with shorter-acting agents that cause relatively more vasodilation.
  - Marker for inadvertent intravascular injection (tachycardia and hypertension)
  - Decreases local bleeding with infiltration
  - Contraindicated in areas that lack collateral flow (e.g., digit blocks)
  - Consider dose reduction or avoiding in certain patient populations (e.g., ischemic heart disease).
- Other additives that can be used to prolong analgesia of peripheral nerve blocks include α_2-agonists (clonidine, dexmedetomidine), opioids (buprenorphine), antiinflammatories (dexamethasone), and NMDA receptor blockers (magnesium).

ADVERSE EFFECTS

Systemic Toxicity

- Local anesthetic systemic toxicity (LAST) is caused by excessive plasma concentration following inadvertent intravascular injection (most common cause) or absorption from injection site
- Increased risk: higher dose, high blood-flow injection site (e.g., intercostal block), absence of vasoconstrictor, and patient comorbidities affecting plasma clearance (e.g., liver or cardiac disease)

Techniques to Reduce the Risk of LAST

- Restrict total dose (use weight-based recommendations as a guide)
- Fractional dosing (administer 3–5 mL at intervals while monitoring)
- Frequent aspiration (to monitor for intravascular injection)
- Addition of epinephrine (to serve as an intravascular marker)
- Ultrasound guidance (reduces risk by visualizing needle tip and decreasing dose)
- Avoidance of heavy sedation or general anesthesia (permits monitoring for early CNS symptoms)

Central Nervous System (CNS) Toxicity

- CNS symptoms of toxicity can occur before cardiovascular signs.
- CNS toxicity classic progression: circumoral numbness, metallic taste, facial tingling, restlessness, vertigo, tinnitus, slurred speech, seizures, coma
- Treatment is supportive, benzodiazepines can be used for seizures.

Cardiovascular System Toxicity

- Hypotension (relaxation of arteriolar vascular smooth muscle), myocardial depression (prolonged PR and widened QRS intervals), cardiac arrest
- Ratio of the dose causing cardiovascular collapse to the dose causing seizures for lidocaine is about double the calculated ratio for bupivacaine.
  - Bupivacaine is considered more cardiotoxic than lidocaine.

Lipid Resuscitation

- Lipid emulsion (20%) infusion is used to treat local anesthetic systemic toxicity
  - Lipids may extract local anesthetic from the circulation, effectively reducing the plasma concentration ("lipid sink").
  - Intravenous bolus of 1.5 mL/kg over 2 to 3 minutes (100 mL if >70 kg) followed by a continuous infusion at 0.25 mL/kg/min (250 mL over 15–20 min if >70 kg)

Management of LAST
▪ Rare, but potentially fatal; must be recognized and treated promptly ▪ If suspecting LAST, abort injection and call for help. ▪ Maintain oxygenation/ventilation (hypoxia and acidosis worsen LAST). ▪ Treat seizures (typically with benzodiazepines). ▪ Consider early lipid resuscitation. ▪ Consider calling cardiopulmonary bypass team. ▪ Avoid specific medications that can worsen LAST (additional local anesthetics, β-blockers, calcium channel blockers, vasopressin). ▪ If cardiac arrest, reduce epinephrine dose to ≤1 μg/kg.   – Higher epinephrine doses are associated with worse outcomes in animal models.

Local Tissue Toxicity

- All local anesthetics have intrinsic toxicities to nerve and muscle at high enough concentrations and prolonged durations of exposure, though not frequently clinically observed.
- Factors that may increase risk of nerve vulnerability include preexisting nerve injury, metabolic/inflammatory conditions, increased tissue pressure, and systemic hypotension.
- For prolonged infusions, lower concentrations of local anesthetic should be used.

Allergic Reactions

- Adverse reactions that have a true allergic mechanism are rare, comprising <1% of all adverse reactions to local anesthetics.
  - Most reported adverse responses are related to epinephrine absorption/injection (tachycardia, palpitations), vasovagal reactions, or early manifestations of systemic toxicity.

Cross-Sensitivity

- Ester local anesthetics are more likely to cause allergic reaction.
  - Esters produce metabolites related to PABA, a potential trigger of hypersensitivity reactions.
  - Patients with an allergic reaction to an ester can usually receive an amide local anesthetic.
- Allergic reactions can also be provoked by preservatives within commercial formulations of both esters or amides (methylparaben or compounds similar to PABA).
  - Consider using a preservative-free formulation as the initial adverse reaction may have been provoked by the preservative.

Documentation

- Should include clinical signs (e.g., rash, laryngeal edema, hypotension, bronchospasm), serum tryptase, and possibly intradermal testing for confirmation

SPECIFIC LOCAL ANESTHETICS

Amino Esters

Procaine

- Early injectable local anesthetic, primarily for spinal anesthesia
- High incidence of nausea with spinal injection
- Hypersensitivity reactions and instability limited use after lidocaine introduced.

Tetracaine

- Slowly metabolized relative to other esters
- Useful for spinal due to long duration of action
  - Epinephrine with tetracaine may increase risk of transient neurologic symptoms.
- Rarely used for epidurals or peripheral blocks due to slow onset, profound motor blockade, and toxicity risk

Chloroprocaine

- Rapid metabolism in plasma decreases risk of systemic toxicity.
- Fast onset and short duration of epidural anesthesia
  - May impair effectiveness of subsequent dose of epidural bupivacaine or epidural opioids
- Short-duration spinal
  - Historically, preservative in commercial formulation was thought to contribute to neurotoxic injury after intrathecal administration.
  - Intrathecal injections should be bisulfite-free.
- Unique role in pediatric blocks
  - Continuous epidural infusion in neonates/infants
  - Repeat loading dose of epidural or peripheral perineural infusions in which plasma concentrations otherwise would have been nearing toxic range

Amino Amides

Lidocaine

- Versatile and commonly used local anesthetic
- Can cause neurotoxicity (i.e., cauda equina syndrome) when administered for spinal anesthesia
  - Most common mechanism is maldistribution of large doses through small-bore catheters for continuous infusion.
- Transient neurologic symptoms (TNS) limit use as a spinal anesthetic.
  - Clinical presentation: severe pain in buttocks and lower extremities after spinal
    - NOT associated with sensory loss, motor weakness, bowel/bladder dysfunction, or abnormalities on magnetic resonance imaging
    - Manifests 12 to 24 hours after surgery, typically resolved within 3 days (rarely persists beyond 7 days)
  - Risk factors: lithotomy position and outpatient status; highest risk with intrathecal lidocaine or mepivacaine

- First-line treatment: nonsteroidal antiinflammatory drugs (NSAIDs)

Mepivacaine

- Combined piperidine ring of cocaine with xylidine ring of lidocaine
- Similar onset to lidocaine but with less vasodilation and slightly longer duration
- Often used for short-duration spinal anesthesia

Prilocaine

- Rapid metabolism and reduced CNS toxicity relative to lidocaine
- Risk of inducing methemoglobinemia through accumulation of its metabolite ortho-toluidine has limited clinical use.

Bupivacaine

- Long duration of action, slower onset
- High-quality sensory analgesia relative to motor blockade at lower doses
  - This feature established bupivacaine as a popular choice for epidural anesthesia during labor and postoperative pain management.
- Common spinal and epidural anesthetic
- Higher risk of cardiotoxicity resulting in refractory cardiac arrest
  - Bupivacaine only slowly dissociates from voltage-gated sodium channels in cardiac myocytes ("fast-in, slow-out").
  - Preventive measures and early detection techniques for inadvertent intravascular administration are critical.
  - Cardiotoxicity is of no concern when small doses are administered for spinal anesthesia.

Single Enantiomers

Stereochemistry

- Compounds may have the same molecular formula and same sequence of bonds but differ in spatial orientations (stereoisomers).
- Enantiomers: compounds are mirror images but may have different biologic activity.
- Bupivacaine contains equal parts of both enantiomers (racemic mixture).

Ropivacaine

- *S*-Enantiomer only (may have lower cardiac toxicity than the *R*-enantiomer)
  - Favorable interaction with cardiac sodium channels
  - More likely to produce vasoconstriction, reducing systemic uptake
- Slightly less potent (less lipid soluble) than bupivacaine

Levobupivacaine

- *S*-Enantiomer of bupivacaine with similar onset/duration
- Risk of cardiotoxicity is possibly reduced compared with bupivacaine.

Topical Local Anesthetics

- Systemic absorption is rapid and efficient through mucosal surfaces
  - Excessive dosing from nasal, oral, or tracheobronchial mucosa can lead to systemic toxicity, especially in infants and children.
- Keratin layer of intact skin impairs efficient diffusion of local anesthetic.
  - Highly concentrated oil formulations can overcome this barrier.
  - EMLA (eutectic mixture of local anesthetics) cream is a combination of 2.5% lidocaine and 2.5% prilocaine.
    - Used in pediatrics prior to IV placement
    - May take an hour for adequate topical anesthesia

Tumescent Local Anesthesia

- Subcutaneous infusion of large volumes of dilute local anesthetic and epinephrine
- Total dose administered can be eightfold larger than recommended doses for peripheral nerve blockade because of the tumescent technique.
  - Plasma lidocaine concentrations remain in a safe range and can peak 12 hours after administration.
  - Avoid additional doses of local anesthetic over the next day after tumescent administration.

Systemic Local Anesthetics for Acute and Chronic Pain

- Low-dose, brief infusions of intravenous lidocaine may be effective for extended perioperative or neuropathic pain control.

WHEN LOCAL ANESTHESIA FAILS

- Technical failure
  - Local does not reach nerve.
  - Needle placement is not in correct location.
  - Technical failure more likely with blind techniques compared with ultrasound guidance.
- Wrong block (e.g., inadequate coverage of subset of nerves innervating a surgical site)
- Wrong drug (e.g., selection of a short-duration anesthetic for a procedure with significant postoperative pain)
- Anatomic variation
- Biologic variation in local anesthetic responsiveness

   - Ehlers-Danlos syndrome type III shows relative resistance to local anesthetics.
- Infiltrating at a site of infection or inflammation (reduced effectiveness due to local acidosis)
- Tachyphylaxis (tolerance) with repeated dosing or prolonged infusions
- Chronic pain/hyperalgesia: these patients may appear clinically to require larger volumes or concentrations to achieve adequate analgesia.
   - Clinicians should avoid "blaming the patient" for insufficient sensory block caused by a variety of technical or biological factors.

FUTURE LOCAL ANESTHETICS AND CONCLUSIONS

- Site 1 sodium channel blockers
   - Appear to have minimal cardiotoxicity with weaker affinity for the sodium channel subtype in the myocardium
- Liposomal bupivacaine
   - Bupivacaine contained within lipid structure, allowing for slow release of local anesthetic
   - FDA approved in 2011
   - Clinical trials have been mixed, but a recent meta-analysis showed no advantage to using liposomal bupivacaine compared with nonliposomal bupivacaine.
- Active research into sensory-selective blockade (avoiding motor and autonomic blockade) by developing drugs that bind preferentially to specific subtypes of sodium channels on sensory fibers

QUESTIONS

HISTORY

1. Complete the following chart comparing properties of ester and amide local anesthetics. For stability and allergic potential, indicate whether the ester or amide local anesthetic is relatively "lesser" or "greater".

Property	Esters	Amides
Chemical structure		
Clearance		
Stability		
Allergic reactions		

NERVE CONDUCTION

2. Describe the resting membrane potential, threshold potential, and action potential, and their relevance in nerve conduction.
3. What is the composition and function of myelin?
4. Complete the following chart about the properties used to classify nerve fibers. For diameter, use large, medium, and small. For conduction velocity, use fast, intermediate, and slow.

Type	Subtype	Myelinated	Diameter	Conduction Velocity	Function
A	Alpha				
	Beta				
	Gamma				
	Delta				
B					
C					

LOCAL ANESTHETIC ACTIONS ON SODIUM CHANNELS

5. What is the mechanism of action and effect of local anesthetics on nerves?
6. What is the clinical relevance of a local anesthetic's lipid solubility and pKa? Use lidocaine and bupivacaine as examples.
7. How does the local pH in the area of local anesthetic injection affect its onset time?

SPREAD OF LOCAL ANESTHESIA AFTER INJECTION

8. After a peripheral nerve block of an extremity, a clinician notes proximal prior to distal skeletal muscle weakness. What explains this phenomenon?

PHARMACOKINETICS

9. Name some factors that influence the peak plasma concentration of local anesthetic following its injection.
10. What are some factors that affect local vasoactivity after local anesthetic injection?
11. For each of the local anesthetics listed, indicate whether they undergo ester hydrolysis, hepatic metabolism, and/or first-pass pulmonary extraction.

Local Anesthetic	Ester Hydrolysis	Hepatic Metabolism	First-Pass Pulmonary Extraction
Prilocaine			
Levobupivacaine			
Chloroprocaine			
Ropivacaine			
Mepivacaine			
Benzocaine			
Lidocaine			
Procaine			
Bupivacaine			
Tetracaine			

12. How does pseudocholinesterase deficiency affect local anesthetic clearance?
13. What are possible clinical effects of adding epinephrine to an injected local anesthetic solution?
14. A dose of local anesthetic has a label on the vial indicating the epinephrine concentration is 1:200,000. What is the concentration in mcg/mL?

ADVERSE EFFECTS

15. What are some factors that influence the risk of local anesthetic systemic toxicity (LAST)?
16. What are the clinical effects of LAST?
17. What modifications to standard cardiopulmonary resuscitation protocols are recommended when managing cardiac arrest due to LAST?
18. A patient has a documented history of an IgE-mediated reaction to tetracaine. Is it safe to administer lidocaine?

SPECIFIC LOCAL ANESTHETICS

19. List the primary uses, advantages, and drawbacks of each local anesthetic in the table.

Local Anesthetic	Primary Uses	Advantages	Drawbacks
Procaine			
Tetracaine			
Chloroprocaine			
Lidocaine			
Mepivacaine			
Prilocaine			
Bupivacaine			
Ropivacaine			
Levobupivacaine			

20. What are transient neurologic symptoms (TNS), and how are they treated?
21. Which local anesthetics can cause methemoglobinemia, and how is it treated?
22. What is the unique chemical feature of solutions containing ropivacaine or levobupivacaine?
23. When is the peak plasma concentration following tumescent local anesthesia?

FUTURE LOCAL ANESTHETICS AND CONCLUSIONS

24. What is the advantage of liposomal bupivacaine?

ANSWERS

HISTORY

1. Properties of ester and amide local anesthetics are compared in the chart below. (144)

Property	Esters	Amides
Chemical structure	Ester bond	Amide bond
Clearance	Ester hydrolysis	Hepatic metabolism
Stability	Lesser	Greater
Allergic potential	Greater	Lesser

NERVE CONDUCTION

2. The nerve axon membrane potential at rest is –90 mV due to the the energy-dependent transport of sodium out and potassium into the cell, combined with the leak of potassium ions back out through the permeable neural membrane. Nerve excitation increases the membrane's permeability to sodium ions, and sodium ions flow into the axon from the extracellular space. An action potential is a self-propagating wave of depolarization caused by the rapid influx of sodium ions. When the transmembrane potential reaches the threshold potential, the action potential then fires, and the nerve impulse is transmitted down the axon. (144)
3. Myelin is the multiple membranous wrappings from Schwann cells that envelops an axon and forces current to flow between the narrow gaps of adjacent myelinated segments. These gaps are referred to as the nodes of Ranvier. The action potential "jumps" from one node of Ranvier to the next. Myelinated fibers have a faster conduction velocity and have increased susceptibility to local anesthetic blockade by allowing the local anesthetic to pool at the nodes of Ranvier. (144, 145, and 150)
4. The properties used to classify nerve fibers are reflected in the chart below. (145, Table 10-1)

Type	Subtype	Myelinated	Diameter	Conduction Velocity	Function
A	Alpha	Yes	Large	Fast	Proprioception, large motor
	Beta	Yes	Large	Fast	Touch, pressure, small motor
	Gamma	Yes	Medium	Intermediate	Muscle tone
	Delta	Yes	Medium	Intermediate	Pain, temperature, touch
B		Yes	Medium	Intermediate	Preganglionic autonomic
C		No	Small	Slow	Dull pain, temperature, touch

LOCAL ANESTHETIC ACTIONS ON SODIUM CHANNELS

5. Local anesthetics bind to the intracellular portion of voltage-gated sodium channels and change the channel conformation, which blocks the influx of sodium ions. By preventing sodium ions from passing through the sodium channel, the rate of depolarization is decreased, the threshold potential cannot be reached, and an action potential does not fire. (144)
6. The lipid solubility of the local anesthetic correlates with tissue penetration, time to uptake, potency, and duration of action. The pKa describes the propensity of a local anesthetic to exist in charged/uncharged state such that the lower the pKa, the greater the percentage of unionized fraction at a given pH. Bupivacaine is more lipid soluble and more potent than lidocaine. This is reflected in why a peripheral nerve block can achieve surgical density with

0.5% bupivacaine or 2% lidocaine. However, its onset time is slower than lidocaine. The pKa of bupivacaine is 8.1, and the amount of uncharged bupivacaine at physiologic pH of 7.4 is 17%. The pKa of lidocaine is 7.9, and the amount of uncharged lidocaine at physiologic pH is 24%. The higher fraction of uncharged molecules of lidocaine means there are more molecules that can readily diffuse across the neural membrane, making its onset time relatively quicker than bupivacaine when all other factors (technique, dose) are equal. (146 and 149)

7. The pH affects the relative ionized and unionized fraction of local anesthetic. For example, bicarbonate increases the fraction of unionized local anesthetic molecules, thereby decreasing the time to the onset of anesthesia. In contrast, the local acidosis at a site of inflammation, infection, or ischemia increases the time to onset and decreases the quality of the local anesthetic block by increasing the fraction of charged local anesthetic molecules. (146)

SPREAD OF LOCAL ANESTHESIA AFTER INJECTION

8. Diffusion of the local anesthetic along a concentration gradient from the outer surface of the nerve (mantle) to the inner surface (core) can explain the earlier onset of peripheral nerve blockade in the proximal extremity. The outer mantle fibers innervate more proximal structures relative to core nerve fibers, which generally innervate more distal structures. (148)

PHARMACOKINETICS

9. Factors influencing peak plasma concentration include local blood flow at the site of injection (systemic uptake) and drug clearance, vasoactivity, lipohilicity, protein binding, and clearance. (148)
10. Vasoactivity after local anesthetic injection is influenced by direct local anesthetic effect on vascular smooth muscle, sympathetic efferent fibers, and the addition of vasoconstrictors. (148)
11. The table below indicates which local anesthetics are hydrolyzed, metabolized, or extracted. (Table 10.2, 149)

Local Anesthetic	Ester Hydrolysis	Hepatic Metabolism	First-Pass Pulmonary Extractiom
Prilocaine		X	X
Levobupivacaine		X	
Chloroprocaine	X		
Ropivacaine		X	
Mepivacaine		X	
Benzocaine	X		
Lidocaine		X	X
Procaine	X		
Bupivacaine		X	X
Tetracaine	X		

12. Like succinylcholine, ester local anesthetics (procaine, chloroprocaine, and tetracaine) are metabolized by pseudocholinesterase. Although mild or moderate decreases in pseudocholinesterase levels rarely have significant clinical impact, patients who are homozygous for the atypical form of pseudocholinesterase can have a markedly prolonged duration of action. (151)
13. Epinephrine added to an injected local anesthetic solution can cause local vasoconstriction decreasing systemic absorption and potentially systemic toxicity, prolonged duration of effect, serve as marker for inadvertent intravascular injection, and decrease local bleeding. Possible downsides of epinephrine include increasing heart rate and blood pressure in susceptible patients and causing tissue ischemia in areas that lack collateral blood flow (e.g., digit blocks). (151)
14. The concentration of 1:200,000 means 1 gram of epinephrine is dissolved in 200,000 mL of solvent (1 g/200,000 mL = 1000 mg/200,000 mL = 1 mg/200 mL = 1000 mcg/200 mL = 5 mcg/mL). (151)

ADVERSE EFFECTS

15. The risk of LAST is influenced by site of injection, total dose, vasoconstrictors (epinephrine), and patient comorbidities. Inadvertent intravascular injection is the most common cause. (151)
16. Central nervous system manifestations of LAST include circumoral numbness, metallic taste, and facial tingling progressing toward severe CNS signs such as seizures and coma. Cardiovascular findings include profound hypotension, conduction abnormalities (prolonged PR interval, widened QRS complex), and myocardial depression leading to cardiovascular collapse. (151)
17. Modifications by the American Society of Regional Anesthesia (ASRA) to advanced cardiac life support (ACLS) are recommended during resuscitation for LAST including (1) early administration of a 20% lipid emulsion, (2) smaller bolus doses of epinephrine (≤1 mcg/kg), (3) early consideration of cardiopulmonary bypass, and (4) avoidance of particular medications (local anesthetics, β-blockers, calcium blockers, and vasopressin). (152)
18. Yes, it is safe to administer lidocaine to a patient with a documented IgE-mediated reaction to tetracaine. There is no cross-sensitivity between amides and esters. Anaphylactic reactions to any local anesthetic are extremely rare but are more common with esters due to the ester metabolite para-aminobenzoic acid (PABA). However, ester and amide local anesthetics can share a common preservative, such as methylparaben, that can have allergic potential. Consequently, a patient with a prior allergic reaction to an ester local anesthetic may benefit from a formulation of an amide local anesthetic that is preservative-free. (153)

SPECIFIC LOCAL ANESTHETICS

19. The table below lists the primary uses, and some advantages and disadvantages of the given local anesthetic. (Table 10.2, 153–155)

Local Anesthetic	Primary Uses	Advantages	Drawbacks
Procaine	Local, peripheral, spinal	Limited data suggests lesser risk of TNS	Hypersensitivity, instability
Tetracaine	Topical, spinal	Long duration	Slow onset, slow metabolism, risk of toxicity, with epinephrine risk of TNS
Chloroprocaine	Local, IV, peripheral, epidural, spinal	Rapidly metabolized, low toxicity risk, rapid onset, short duration, useful in pediatric patients	Neurotoxicity after intrathecal injection thought to be due to preservative bisulfite
Lidocaine	Topical, local, IV, peripheral, epidural, spinal	Versatile	Neurotoxicity (cauda equina syndrome) with continuous small-bore catheter spinal, TNS
Mepivacaine	Local, peripheral, epidural, spinal	Short-duration spinal anesthesia with less vasodilation than lidocaine	Some risk of TNS
Prilocaine	Topical, local, IV, peripheral, epidural, spinal	Rapid metabolism, reduced toxicity, used topically in EMLA cream	Metabolite ortho-toluidine can accumulate and cause methemoglobinemia
Bupivacaine	Local, peripheral, epidural, spinal	Sensory > motor blockade	Refractory cardiac arrest with inadvertent intravascular injection
Ropivacaine	Local, peripheral, epidural, spinal	Sensory > motor blockade, less cardiotoxic than bupivacaine	Less potent than bupivacaine
Levobupivacaine	Local, peripheral, epidural, spinal	Less cardiotoxic than bupivacaine	Sensory equals motor blockade

20. Transient neurologic symptoms (TNS) are characterized by severe pain of the lower extremities and buttocks within 12 to 24 hours after spinal anesthesia without associated motor weakness or bowel/bladder dysfunction. The symptoms are self-limited (typically 3 days), but it can be excruciatingly painful. Neurotoxicity with severe long-term sequelae (cauda equina syndrome) has been reported. It is associated with administration of lidocaine and mepivacaine, lithotomy position, and outpatient status. NSAIDs are the first-line treatment. (154)
21. Methemoglobinemia has been reported after large doses of prilocaine and topical benzocaine. Prilocaine is used most frequently for topical anesthesia prior to IV placement as part of EMLA cream (lidocaine 2.5%/prilocaine 2.5%). The treatment of methemoglobinemia is 1 to 2 mg/kg of intravenous methylene blue given over 5 minutes. (154)
22. Enantiomers (a class of stereoisomers) are molecules that are mirror images of each other, and they may differ in biologic activity. Bupivacaine is a racemic mixture, meaning it contains equal parts of the two enantiomers. Levobupivacaine and ropivacaine only contain the single *S*(−)-enantiomer of bupivacaine. This single enantiomer solution may not only have a more favorable interaction with cardiac sodium ion channels, but it may also be more likely to produce vasoconstriction (potentially reducing systemic uptake). (143, 155)
23. In tumescent local anesthesia, large volumes of very dilute local anesthetic and epinephrine are injected into subcutaneous tissue until it is firm (tumescent). Total doses of lidocaine as high as 35 to 55 mg/kg are used for this technique, far higher than the usual recommended lidocaine maximum dose of 5 mg/kg (7 mg/kg with epinephrine). Peak plasma concentrations can occur more than 12 hours after injection of tumescent local anesthesia. Although several case series support the safety of this technique when guidelines are followed, toxicity has been reported when other local anesthetics have been administered over the next day. (156)

FUTURE LOCAL ANESTHETICS AND CONCLUSIONS

24. Liposomal bupivacaine was formulated for slow release of the local anesthetic for up to 72 hours after local infiltration, especially after surgical procedures. The administration is uniquely associated with two peaks in the plasma concentrations with the first peak occurring within 1 hour of administration (when free bupivacaine from the injection is systemically absorbed) and the second peak occurring 12 hours later. Outcomes of clinical trials with liposomal bupivacaine has been mixed, and recent meta-analyses have indicated there may be no advantage to using liposomal bupivacaine compared with nonliposomal bupivacaine. (157)

Chapter

11 NEUROMUSCULAR BLOCKING AND REVERSAL AGENTS

Cynthia A. Lien

INTRODUCTION

- Neuromuscular blocking agents (NMBAs) interrupt the transmission of nerve impulses at the neuromuscular junction.
- Classification of NMBAs
  - Mechanism of action: depolarizing and nondepolarizing
  - Duration of action: short, intermediate, and long acting

Clinical Uses

- In the operating room to facilitate endotracheal intubation and optimize surgical conditions
- In other clinical settings to facilitate urgent/emergent intubation and to facilitate mechanical ventilation
- Depth of neuromuscular blockade (NMB) is monitored by muscular response to stimulation of a superficial nerve

Choice of Neuromuscular Blocking Agent

- Choice is based on several different factors, including speed of onset, duration of action, route of elimination, and associated adverse effects.
- Choice is also based on patient-related factors, such as comorbidities, duration of the procedure or surgery, plans for antagonism of residual NMB

THE NEUROMUSCULAR JUNCTION

- Components include
  - Prejunctional motor nerve ending
  - Postjunctional membrane of skeletal muscle separated by a synaptic cleft
- The initiation of neuromuscular transmission occurs via arrival of a stimulus at the nerve terminal causing an influx of calcium ions and subsequent acetylcholine (ACh) release.
- Synchronized release of ACh from synaptic vesicles allows ACh to bind to receptors on the postjunctional membrane, generating an action potential.
- Most of the ACh released in response to neural stimulation is hydrolyzed by acetylcholinesterase at the neuromuscular junction.

Prejunctional Receptors and Release of Acetylcholine

- Cholinergic receptors are found both presynaptically (motor nerve terminal) and postsynaptically.
- Prejunctional receptors modulate the release of ACh into the neuromuscular junction.
  - This occurs through a positive feedback mechanism.
  - They are stimulated by ACh and administration of succinylcholine and neostigmine.
  - They are inhibited by small doses of nondepolarizing NMBAs.

Postjunctional Receptors

- An intrinsic membrane protein with five distinct subunits
- The ACh binding site is located primarily in the two α subunits of the receptor.
- Occupation of one or both α subunits by a nondepolarizing NMBA causes the central ion pore of the ACh receptor to remain closed so that sodium cannot flow into the muscle cell.
- Nondepolarizing NMBAs may also cause channel occlusion.
  - This type of NMB is resistant to drug-enhanced antagonism with anticholinesterases.

Extrajunctional Receptors

- Located throughout the muscle membrane rather than concentrated in the postjunctional aspect of the muscle cell
- Activation is typically suppressed through neural activity.

- Conditions associated with a proliferation of extrajunctional receptors: prolonged inactivity, sepsis, denervation, burn injury, trauma
- When activated, these receptors stay open longer and permit more ions to flow across the muscle cell membrane – resulting in hyperkalemia.

STRUCTURE–ACTIVITY RELATIONSHIPS

- NMBAs are quaternary ammonium compounds with at least one positively charged nitrogen atom that binds to one or both binding sites on the postsynaptic cholinergic receptor.
- NMBAs have structural similarities to ACh.
  - Nondepolarizing NMBAs are either aminosteroid compounds or benzylisoquinolinium compounds.
    - Pancuronium is a bisquaternary aminosteroid.
    - Vecuronium and rocuronium are monoquaternary analogues of pancuronium.

DEPOLARIZING NEUROMUSCULAR BLOCKING AGENTS: SUCCINYLCHOLINE

Characteristics of Blockade

- Succinylcholine (SCh) mimics the action of ACh and produces a sustained depolarization of the postjunctional membrane (*phase I blockade*).
- Because SCh is not a substrate for acetylcholinesterase (it is metabolized by butyrylcholinesterase that is found in the plasma but not the neuromuscular junction), it remains available to bind to ACh receptors until it diffuses away from the neuromuscular junction.
- *Phase II blockade* may develop in response to administration of a large dose of SCh (>3–5 mg/kg) or administration over a prolonged time period.
  - *Phase II blockade* is present when the postjunctional membrane repolarizes but does not respond normally to ACh.
  - Monitoring during *phase II blockade* provides results that are similar to a nondepolarizing block (fade in the train-of-four [TOF] ratio).

Pharmacodynamics

- Potency – ED_{95} 0.3 mg/kg; typical dose for intubation 0.5–1.5 mg/kg
- Onset of NMB—rapid onset, within 30 to 60 seconds
- Duration of action 5 to 10 minutes
- The sustained depolarization produced by SCh administration manifests as generalized skeletal muscle contractions known as *fasciculations*.
- When pretreating with a defasciculating dose of a nondepolarizing NMBA 2 to 4 minutes before SCh administration, the dose of SCh should be increased by 70%.

Metabolism

- Plasma cholinesterase (butyrylcholinesterase, pseudocholinesterase), produced in liver
- Anticholinesterases, such as used for the treatment of myasthenia gravis, may result in prolonged skeletal muscle paralysis after SCh administration.
- Atypical plasma cholinesterase
  - Atypical enzyme cannot hydrolyze ester bonds.
  - Presents clinically as prolonged NMB in otherwise healthy patient after conventional SCh dose
    - Prolonged muscle paralysis lasting 60 to 180 minutes in homozygous patients
    - For patients heterozygous for the atypical enzyme, duration of SCh blockade is 20 minutes.
  - The local anesthetic dibucaine reflects the quality (not quantity) of plasma cholinesterase in patients by testing the percent inhibition of enzyme activity.

Adverse Side Effects

- Cardiac dysrhythmias – bradycardia, junctional rhythm, sinus arrest
- Hyperkalemia
- Myalgias
- Increased intraocular pressure
- Increased intracranial pressure
- Increased intragastric pressure
- Trismus
- Trigger for malignant hyperthermia when combined with volatile anesthetics in susceptible patients

NONDEPOLARIZING NEUROMUSCULAR BLOCKING AGENTS

- Classification
  - Based on structure and duration of action
  - Compete with ACh for binding sites on postjunctional receptors

Pharmacokinetics

- Varies based on structure; processes include:
  - Elimination as unchanged compound through the kidney or liver
  - Enzymatic hydrolysis
  - Spontaneous breakdown
  - Metabolism in the liver
- Influenced by many factors, including hypovolemia, hypothermia, acidosis, hepatic disease, renal disease
- Highly ionized: do not cross blood–brain barrier or placenta

Pharmacodynamic Responses

- Factors affecting onset of NMB include potency, protein binding, clearance, and dose.

- Potentiation by volatile anesthetics, aminoglycosides, local anesthetics, lithium, magnesium, dantrolene
- Diminished effects can be seen with calcium, corticosteroids, some anticonvulsants
- Neuromuscular diseases (e.g., myopathies) are associated with altered responses.
- Electrolyte abnormalities have a varied impact on the pharmacodynamics of NMBAs.

Adverse Effects

- Cardiovascular effects
  - Blockade of muscarinic receptors, histamine release, vagolysis
  - Magnitude depends on underlying patient factors, e.g., hypovolemia
- Critical illness myopathy and polyneuropathy
  - At-risk patients: asthma exacerbation receiving corticosteroids, acute injury, multiple organ system failure requiring prolonged mechanical ventilation
  - Symptoms: quadriparesis with or without areflexia
  - Course of disease: unpredictable but weakness can persist for months
- Hypersensitivity reactions
  - Causative agent for intraoperative anaphylaxis: most commonly aminosteroidal NMBAs
  - Reported severity reaction varies widely.
  - Hypersensitivity vs. anaphylaxis
    - Grading system can be used for intraoperative diagnosis of anaphylaxis.
    - Skin-prick or intradermal testing >4 to 6 weeks after an allergic reaction is gold standard.

Long-Acting Nondepolarizing NMBA: Pancuronium

- Potency: ED_{95} 70 mcg/kg; dose for intubation: 0.08–0.12 mg/kg
- Onset 3 to 5 minutes and duration of action of 1.3 × ED_{95}: 90 minutes
- Metabolism and elimination: primarily urinary elimination (80%), also hepatic deacetylation
- Cardiovascular effects: vagolysis (10–15% increase in BP and HR after intubating dose)

Intermediate-Acting Nondepolarizing NMBAs

- Vecuronium
  - Monoquarternary aminosteroid
  - Potency: ED_{95} 50 mcg/kg; dose for intubation: 0.1–0.2 mg/kg
  - Onset 3 to 5 minutes and duration of action of 2 × ED_{95}: 40 minutes
  - Elimination through the kidneys and metabolism in the liver
- Rocuronium
  - Monoquarternary aminosteroid
  - Potency: ED_{95} 0.3 mg/kg; dose for intubation: 0.6–1.0 mg/kg
  - Onset (fast) 1 to 2 minutes and duration of action of 4 × ED_{95}: 70 minutes
  - Elimination mainly as unchanged compound in the bile, plus 30% renal excretion
- Atracurium
  - Bisquarternary isoquinolinium
  - Potency: ED_{95} 0.25 mg/kg; dose for intubation: 0.5 mg/kg
  - Onset 3 to 5 minutes and duration of action of 2 × ED_{95}:50 minutes
  - Elimination: ester hydrolysis (66%) and Hofmann elimination (33%)
  - Cardiovascular effects: histamine release (flushing, hypotension, and tachycardia), especially with rapid bolus administration of doses > 2 × ED_{95}
- Cisatracurium
  - Bisquarternary isoquinolinium
  - Potency: ED_{95} 50 μg/kg; dose for intubation: 0.1–0.2 mg/kg
  - Onset (slow) 5 to 7 minutes and duration of action of 4 × ED_{95}: 70 minutes
  - Elimination: Hofmann degradation

Short-Acting Nondepolarizing NMBA: Mivacurium

- Benzylisoquinolinium
- Potency: ED_{95} 80 μg/kg; dose for intubation: 0.15–0.25 mg/kg
- Onset 2 to 3 minutes and duration of action of 2 × ED_{95}: 15 minutes
- Enzymatic hydrolysis by plasma cholinesterase
- Cardiovascular effects: histamine release

MONITORING THE EFFECTS OF NONDEPOLARIZING NEUROMUSCULAR BLOCKING AGENTS

Monitoring and Reversal of Neuromuscular Blockade

Quantitative neuromuscular monitoring is the only way to confirm complete recovery of neuromuscular function.

Profound paralysis after NMBA administration can be measured with the post-tetanic count, which can provide an estimate until time to first twitch with TOF monitoring.

The parameters used to determine need, choice, and dose of neuromuscular reversal agents include TOF count, post-tetanic count (if TOF count is 0), and quantitative TOF ratio (when TOF count is 4).

A TOF ratio <0.4 should not be antagonized with neostigmine.

No reversal is required if TOF ratio is >0.9 as determined by a quantitative monitor of a peripheral muscle group.

- Clinical uses
    - Need for administration of additional NMBA and the dose of reversal agent
    - Adequacy of recovery of neuromuscular function
        - Defined as a TOF ratio = 0.9 at the adductor pollicis
- Types of assessment
    - Clinical: inaccurate (e.g., head-lift, grip strength, tidal volume)
    - Qualitative monitoring: tactile or visual "measurement" has inadequate sensitivity
        - Stimulus patterns: single-twitch, TOF, double burst, post-tetanic count
        - TOF ratio based on concept that ACh is depleted by successive stimulations
        - Post-tetanic count quantifies profound depth of NMB (no twitches on TOF).
    - Quantitative monitoring
        - Stimulus patterns: TOF, post-tetanic count
        - Types:
            - Mechanomyography (the gold standard, not clinically available)
            - Electromyography (measures action potential generated by nerve stimulation, not movement)
            - Acceleromyography (requires movement of the thumb, overinterprets recovery of response)
            - Kinemyography (requires movement of the thumb, overinterprets recovery of response)
- Site of monitoring: central vs. peripheral motor nerve unit
    - Adductor pollicis movement with ulnar nerve stimulation is primary monitoring site.
    - Central muscles (e.g., diaphragm, orbicularis oculi) are resistant to nondepolarizing NMBA.
        - Dosing based on central muscles will result in overdosing of NMBA and increased incidence of residual NMB in PACU.

ANTAGONISM OF RESIDUAL NEUROMUSCULAR BLOCK

- Residual NMB is associated with several adverse outcomes:
    - Airway obstruction
    - Inadequate ventilation
    - Hypoxia
    - Difficulty swallowing
    - Diplopia
    - Poor patient experience
- Facilitating recovery requires increasing the ACh concentration relative to the NMBA through the administration of anticholinesterases (e.g., neostigmine) or sugammadex.

Anticholinesterases

- Mechanism: inhibit acetylcholinesterase at the neuromuscular junction, allowing the ACh to overcome the competitive block of the ACh receptor
- Determinants of speed and adequacy of recovery
    - Efficacy of antagonism depends on the amount of NMBA relative to ACh available to bind to the ACh receptor.
    - Recovery occurs most reliably when neostigmine is administered only once a significant degree of spontaneous recovery of neuromuscular function has occurred (TOF ratio >0.4).
    - Once acetylcholinesterase is maximally blocked, administering additional neostigmine will not further enhance recovery.
    - Neostigmine will not facilitate recovery from deep levels of NMB.
- Adverse effects
    - Vagal effects: bradycardia, prolonged QT, asystole
    - Other muscarinic parasympathetic effects including bronchospasm, increased secretions, miosis, increased intestinal tone
    - Adverse effects due to stimulation of the muscarinic receptors can be mitigated by concomitant administration of an antimuscarinic agent, such as glycopyrrolate or atropine.
- Dosing
    - Dependent on the depth of NMB, duration of action, and timing of the last dose of the NMBA
    - Neostigmine 30 mcg/kg recommended when the TOF ratio is >0.4. Greater doses should be administered at deeper levels of NMB.
- Pharmacokinetics and pharmacodynamics
    - Bolus dose onset: 7 to 11 minutes for neostigmine
    - Elimination is through the kidney and is slowed in patients with renal disease.

Selective Relaxant Binding Agents: Sugammadex

- Mechanism: encapsulates NMBAs in the plasma so that they are no longer available to bind to the ACh receptor at the neuromuscular junction
- Will facilitate recovery from rocuronium- or vecuronium-induced block in a 1:1 ratio
    - Has greater affinity for rocuronium
    - An adequate amount of sugammadex must be administered to facilitate complete and sustained recovery.
- Pharmacokinetics and pharmacodynamics
    - Effectively antagonizes all depths of NMB – even after administration of an intubating dose of rocuronium

- Antagonizes residual NMB within 2 to 3 minutes of administration
- Doses range from 2 to 16 mg/kg, with larger doses being administered at the deeper levels of NMB.
- Inadequate reversal can produce recurrence of NMB.
- The sugammadex–rocuronium complex is eliminated through the kidneys.

- Adverse effects
  - Bradycardia (can be severe), tachycardia, nausea and vomiting, dry mouth, dizziness, myalgias, headache, and anaphylaxis (rare)
  - Dose-dependent transient prolongation of activated partial thromboplastin time and prothrombin time (without increased risk of bleeding)

QUESTIONS

THE NEUROMUSCULAR JUNCTION

1. A patient has received a nondepolarizing NMBA. What explains the phenomenon of post-tetanic potentiation when monitoring with a peripheral nerve stimulator?

STRUCTURE–ACTIVITY RELATIONSHIPS

2. In the table, assign an NMBA type for the given structure of NMBA. Choices for NMBA type include depolarizing NMBA, nondepolarizing benzylisoquinolinium NMBA, or nondepolarizing steroidal NMBA.

Structure	NMBA Type
CH_3, O, O, CH_3; $H_3C-NCH_2CH_2OCCH_2CH_2COCH_2CH_2N-CH_3$; CH_3, CH_3	
CH_3, O, O, CH_3, O, N, N^+, CH_3, HO, H_2C	
H_3CO, H_3CO, O, O, OCH$_3$, OCH$_3$; $^+N-(CH_2)_3-OC-CH_2CH_2=CHCH_2CH_2-CO-(CH_2)_3-N^+$; CH_3, H_3C, CH_2, CH_2; H_3CO, OCH_3, OCH_3, H_3CO, OCH_3, OCH_3	

DEPOLARIZING NEUROMUSCULAR BLOCKING AGENTS: SUCCINYLCHOLINE

3. What conditions are most likely to result in life-threatening hyperkalemia after succinylcholine administration?

NONDEPOLARIZING NEUROMUSCULAR BLOCKING AGENTS

4. What is the relationship between the potency of an NMBA and its onset time?
5. A patient with end-stage renal disease and a K^+ level of 6.0 mEq/L requires an emergent craniotomy because of an expanding subdural hematoma. His pulse is 60 bpm, and his blood pressure is 180/100 mm Hg. Which NMBA will you administer during induction to facilitate endotracheal intubation?

MONITORING THE EFFECTS OF NONDEPOLARIZING NEUROMUSCULAR BLOCKING AGENTS

6. When monitoring with a peripheral nerve stimulator, why is quantitative assessment of depth of neuromuscular blockade more accurate than qualitative assessment? What are the benefits of accurate assessment of the TOF ratio?
7. A patient in the PACU is hypoxic following emergence and extubation. Intraoperatively, NMB had been maintained with rocuronium, and he received sugammadex 2 mg/kg to facilitate recovery from a post-tetanic count of 2. What will you do, and why?

ANTAGONISM OF RESIDUAL NEUROMUSCULAR BLOCK

8. A patient has received sugammadex to reverse residual rocuronium-induced NMB after a laparoscopic procedure when the surgeon realizes that reexploration of the abdominal cavity is required because of bleeding. What NMBA should be administered, and why?
9. A young, otherwise healthy patient received a single dose of 0.9 mg/kg rocuronium to facilitate intubation 75 minutes earlier. Qualitative assessment of muscle strength demonstrates four equal responses to TOF stimulation at the end of surgery. Should the patient be extubated without receiving a reversal agent?

ANSWERS

THE NEUROMUSCULAR JUNCTION

1. When a normal impulse arrives at the motor nerve terminal, the rapid release of ACh indicates that only those vesicles close to the membrane participate in exocytosis. However, with repetitive stimulation, additional vesicles are moved toward the motor nerve terminal and are subsequently released, which accounts for post-tetanic potentiation observed during NMB. (161)

STRUCTURE-ACTIVITY RELATIONSHIPS

2. (164)

Structure	NMBA Type
CH_3 O O CH_3 $H_3C-NCH_2CH_2OCCH_2CH_2COCH_2CH_2N-CH_3$ CH_3 CH_3	Depolarizing NMBA
CH_3, O, O, CH_3, N^+, CH_3, CH_3, N, O, HO, H_2C	Nondepolarizing steroidal NMBA
H_3CO, H_3CO, $^+N-(CH_2)_3-OC(=O)-CH_2CH_2=CHCH_2CH_2-C(=O)O-(CH_2)_3-N^+$, CH_3, H_3C, CH_2, CH_2, OCH_3, OCH_3, H_3CO, OCH_3, OCH_3, H_3CO, OCH_3, OCH_3	Nondepolarizing benzylisoquinolinium NMBA

DEPOLARIZING NEUROMUSCULAR BLOCKING AGENTS: SUCCINYLCHOLINE

3. The best-described conditions associated with hyperkalemia after succinylcholine administration include burns, trauma, spinal cord injury, or other major neurologic damage. The risk of hyperkalemia begins approximately 24 hours after injury, the time needed for development of extrajunctional atypical ACh receptors. These extrajunctional receptors can also develop after several days of immobilization, such as in an ICU patient. (167)

NONDEPOLARIZING NEUROMUSCULAR BLOCKING AGENTS

4. Rocuronium, with an ED_{95} of 0.3 mg/kg, is the least potent of the available NMBAs and, because of this, would have the quickest onset of effect. The lower potency requires a greater quantity of the NMBA to be administered for the desired effect, creating a greater diffusion gradient to move the NMBA into the neuromuscular junction where it can bind to the ACh receptor. Additionally, doses of 3 to 4 times the ED_{95} of rocuronium can be administered to further shorten its onset of effect without adverse hemodynamic effects. The onset of doses of this magnitude mimics that of succinylcholine.

However, administration of these large doses of rocuronium, or any intermediate-acting NMBA, will increase its duration of action (the time to recovery to 25% baseline T1 strength). While administration of 0.6 mg/kg rocuronium has a clinical duration of action just under 40 minutes, administrations of 0.9 and 1.2 mg/kg have clinical durations of action of more than 50 and 70 minutes, respectively. (168–169)

5. While this patient would not be expected to have an exaggerated hyperkalemic response to the administration of succinylcholine, his serum K^+ is elevated, and even the expected and normal increase in serum K^+ of 0.5 mEq/L could be sufficient to cause an arrhythmia. Therefore avoiding the use of succinylcholine would be prudent. While any NMBA could be used, in a situation such as the one described here, use of an NMBA with a rapid onset of effect may be preferred. (167)

MONITORING THE EFFECTS OF NONDEPOLARIZING NEUROMUSCULAR BLOCKING AGENTS

6. While qualitative assessment of TOF monitoring is better than clinical tests of muscle strength such as head lift, neither visual nor tactile evaluation of the response to TOF stimulation allows accurate assessment of the strength of the fourth response to the strength of the first response. This is presumably because the middle two responses increase the difficulty in comparing the fourth response to the first response. Clinicians, regardless of years of practice or clinical expertise, cannot reliably detect the presence of fade in the TOF unless there is > 60% fade (i.e., when TOF ratio ≤ 0.4). Use of a double-burst stimulation pattern with qualitative monitors improves the sensitivity of monitoring such that fade can be appreciated as long as it is > 40%, or the second response is 60% or less than the first response. Neither of these stimulus modalities detects more subtle degrees of block (TOF ratio > 0.4–0.6 but TOF ratio < 0.9) that can compromise patient respiratory function, length of stay, satisfaction, or likelihood of developing postoperative pulmonary complications. Accurate determination of TOF ratio requires quantitative assessment.
Accurate quantitative monitoring is necessary for several reasons. The choice and dose of reversal agent are based in part on the quantitative TOF ratio. For example, if TOF ratio is >0.9, no reversal is required. If TOF ratio indicates a shallow level of block (TOF ratio ≥0.6), the dose of neostigmine can be < 0.03 mg/kg. Prior to tracheal extubation, confirmation of full recovery from NMB will provide assurance that residual NMB should not be present in the PACU. (173–174, 178–180)

7. The patient's hypoxia is likely related to residual NMB. Sugammadex, 2 mg/kg, is an inadequate dose to reverse recovery from a profound depth of NMB (a post-tetanic count of 2) regardless of how long ago the last dose of NMBA was administered. Dosing of sugammadex is based on the response to neuromuscular stimulation and is guided as follows:

Response to Neuromuscular Stimulation	Sugammadex Dose (mg/kg)
PTC = 0	16
PTC = 2 to TOF count = 1	4
TOF count = 2–4 (if TOF ratio <0.9)	2

PTC, post-tetanic count; TOF, train-of-four.

Therefore this patient should receive an additional 2 mg/kg of sugammadex. (176, 180)

ANTAGONISM OF RESIDUAL NEUROMUSCULAR BLOCK

8. When NMB has to be reintroduced after reversal with sugammadex, it is likely that there will still be sugammadex available to bind additional steroidal NMBA. Because of this, the depth of block obtained through administration of a steroidal NMBA is difficult to predict. Because sugammadex will not bind the benzylisoquinolinium NMBAs, either cisatracurium or atracurium can be administered to reestablish NMB after administration of sugammadex. (182)

9. When determined with qualitative monitoring, four apparently equal responses to TOF stimulation may be observed when the patient has recovered to a TOF ratio ≥ 0.4, but <0.9, which is inadequate recovery for safe extubation. Therefore a reversal agent should be administered – either sugammadex 2 mg/kg or neostigmine 0.03 mg/kg. There is significant interpatient variability in spontaneous recovery of neuromuscular function after NMB, and no period of time will guarantee complete spontaneous recovery. With the passage of 75 minutes since administration of that single dose of rocuronium, the average time of recovery of the first response in the TOF can vary between roughly 30 and 90 minutes. Variability in the time required for complete recovery of neuromuscular function, a TOF ratio ≥ 0.9, is even greater. (168, 173–174)

Chapter

12 ANESTHETIC NEUROTOXICITY

Mary Ellen McCann and Sulpicio G. Soriano

INTRODUCTION

- General anesthesia unequivocally results in neuronal cell death and neurocognitive impairments in laboratory animals.
- The US Food and Drug Administration (FDA) requires warnings be added to the labels of general anesthetic and sedation drugs.

FDA Issued Drug and Safety Communication

The FDA has warned that "repeated or lengthy use of general anesthetic and sedation drugs during surgeries or procedures in children younger than 3 years or in pregnant women during their third trimester may affect the development of children's brains."

- Reports from the 1950s first described abnormal behavior after general anesthesia in both children and older persons.
- Most anesthetics and sedative drugs are classified as γ-aminobutyric acid (GABA) receptor agonists, *N*-methyl-D-aspartate (NMDA) glutamate receptor antagonists, or a combination of the two.
  - Both have been implicated in causing anesthetic-induced developmental neurotoxicity (AIDN).

ANESTHETIC DRUGS AS A CAUSE FOR NEURODEGENERATION AND LONG-TERM NEUROCOGNITIVE DEFICITS

Basic Science of Anesthetic-Induced Developmental Neurotoxicity

- A neurotoxic effect of anesthetic drugs at all stages of neurodevelopment, from the fetus to the aged, has been clearly demonstrated in preclinical reports.
- AIDN was first described in fetal and postnatal rats exposed to halothane.
- Subsequently, several commonly used anesthetic agents were found to induce neuroapoptosis and behavior changes in the developing rat brain.

Age-Dependent Vulnerability of Anesthetic

- Neurodevelopment progresses through several steps that include neurogenesis, neuronal morphogenesis, migration, synaptogenesis, and remodeling.

Steps of Neurogenesis

- Progenitor cells proliferate and differentiate into neurons or glial cells.
- Neurons undergo terminal differentiation and can no longer replicate.
- Dendrites and axons extend from the cell bodies to form synapses with other neurons.
- Central nervous system (CNS) neural development (up to 70%) is regulated by:
  - Early elimination during embryonal stage
  - Programmed cell death (apoptosis) modification of the CNS after birth
- Redundant progenitor cells and neurons that do not migrate properly or make synapses are physiologically pruned by apoptosis.
- Neurogenesis is ongoing throughout life, from the fetus to older persons.

- Anesthetic drugs are powerful modulators of neuronal circuits, affecting neurogenesis from the fetus to older persons.
  - Isoflurane produces neuronal cell death in brain regions where neural progenitor cells reside.
- Maximal susceptibility to AIDN is likely during the time of brain growth spurt, which occurs from the last trimester until 3 to 4 years old in humans.
- Exposure to anesthetic drugs in laboratory models during their respective times of brain growth spurt results in anesthetic-induced neuroapoptosis.

Characterization of Anesthetic-Induced Developmental Neurotoxicity

Key Features of AIDN

Pathologic Apoptosis
- AIDN hallmark is accelerated apoptosis.
- Can be activated by stressors, including glucocorticoids, heat, radiation, starvation, infection, hypoxia, pain, and anesthetics

Impeded Neurogenesis
- Neurogenesis in animals is affected by anesthetics in an age-dependent manner.
- Neural stem cells are variably affected from neonates to adults.

Altered Dendritic Development
- Anesthetics variably affect dendritic spine formation and density in an age-dependent manner.

Aberrant Glial Development
- Migration and synaptogenesis of neurons during development are guided by glial cells.
- Isoflurane interferes with the release of brain-derived neurotrophic factor (BDNF), depriving developing neurons of trophic support.

Anesthetic Effects on Spinal Cord

- Isoflurane and nitrous oxide exposure in very young rat pups increased apoptosis in the spinal cord, but no motor functional disabilities were detected.
- In neonatal rats, intrathecal ketamine acutely increased apoptosis and decreased spinal function at postnatal day 35.
- In the same animal model, intrathecal bupivacaine did not increase spinal cord apoptosis.

Neuroinflammation and Alzheimer-Related Neuropathology

- Sevoflurane increases markers of neuroinflammation in young (but not adult) mice, as does surgical trauma.
- Preclinical reports demonstrate that anesthesia and surgery may increase expression of β-amyloid, a biologic precursor of Alzheimer disease.
- Neuroinflammation and Alzheimer disease neuropathology may be a potent combination for this population that could diminish neurocognitive function.

Neurocognitive Function

- Neurocognitive function decrements occur after fetal and neonatal exposure to anesthetic drugs in rodents.
- Ketamine or sevoflurane exposure in neonatal rhesus monkeys has resulted in subsequent decreased recognition memory and emotional reactivity at an older age.

Relevant Anesthetic Durations and Concentrations

- Anesthetic duration may be more relevant than concentration.
- Anesthetics with <1 hour duration did not cause increased neuroapoptosis in animal models.
- The neurotoxicity potential of individual anesthetics and/or combined anesthetics is unclear.

Anesthetic and Sedative Drugs

- Although GABA is inhibitory in the mature brain, GABA agonists (volatile anesthetics, benzodiazepines, barbiturates, and propofol) have been found in preclinical studies to be an excitatory and apoptotic agent during early stages of brain development.
- NMDA receptor antagonists (ketamine) also are excitatory and lead to excitatory and apoptotic neuronal and glial cell death.

Alleviation of AIDN

- Anesthetic-induced cell death and neurobehavioral deficits in neonatal pups exposed to volatile anesthetics can be mitigated by concurrent exposure to an enriched environment, exercise, lithium, estrogen, erythropoietin, melatonin, and dexmedetomidine.

CLINICAL EVIDENCE FOR NEUROTOXICITY

- The combination of high doses, prolonged or repeated exposure to anesthetic drugs, and vulnerable age is directly related to neuronal cell death in laboratory models.
- Published reports implicating that general anesthesia is harmful to children are limited to retrospective epidemiologic analyses.
- This evidence may be confounded by the effects of surgery and the effects of the underlying comorbid conditions.
  - Most of the studies have attempted to control for obvious confounders, but the retrospective nature of these investigations makes it impossible to control for all the known and unknown confounders.
- The epidemiologic data are nondefinitive, with some studies demonstrating an effect but other studies showing no effect.
- Two clinical reports that prospectively examined children receiving surgery and anesthesia (GAS and PANDA studies) did not demonstrate a decrement in cognitive function.

INTRAOPERATIVE COURSE AND NEUROCOGNITIVE OUTCOMES

- The developing central nervous system is a critical period of plasticity and is exquisitely sensitive to its internal milieu.
- The environmental milieu, anesthesia, surgery, coexisting medical conditions, and the perioperative setting all have the potential to influence brain development.

Intraoperative Factors Influencing Neurocognitive Outcome

Arterial Blood Pressure
- Optimize cerebral protection by maintaining cerebral autoregulation.
- Target value for the individual neonate may not be precisely known.
- Prolonged induction and protracted hypotension are best avoided in neonates.

Carbon Dioxide Tension
- Hypocapnia leads to alkalosis, cerebral vasoconstriction, and decreased cerebral perfusion.
- Hypocapnia decreases the ability of hemoglobin to release oxygen.
- Maintain end-tidal CO_2 >35 mm Hg in infants and children undergoing general anesthesia when possible.

Oxygen Management
- Antioxidant defenses are not well developed at birth.
- Hypoxia in premature infants increases production of reactive oxygen species.
  - Reactive oxygen species cause cell stress and apoptosis.
- Hypoxia and anoxia can lead to early cell death.

Temperature
- In neonates who have experienced prior hypoxic-ischemic injury:
  - Mild hypothermia is neuroprotective.
  - Hyperthermia is associated with neurocognitive disabilities.

Serum Glucose
- Extremes of hyperglycemia and hypoglycemia are associated with adverse outcomes.

CONCLUSIONS

- Laboratory investigations definitively demonstrate that anesthetic and sedative drugs are potent modulators of CNS development and function throughout the life span.
- These can lead to neuroapoptosis, altered dendritic formation, synaptogenesis, and subsequent neurocognitive deficits.
- Retrospective clinical reports in pediatric and elderly surgical populations are inconclusive.
- Because anesthetic and sedative drugs are essential in the management of surgical patients, anesthesia providers should be sensitive to the possibility that brain development in younger years and its decline in older patients can be an issue for perioperative care and focus on potential contributory factors.

QUESTIONS

INTRODUCTION

1. Is anesthetic neurotoxicity limited to pediatric patients?
2. Is the issue of anesthetic neurotoxicity a recent finding?
3. Has any regulatory agency commented on the issue of anesthetic neurotoxicity?

ANESTHETIC DRUGS AS A CAUSE FOR NEURODEGENERATION AND LONG-TERM NEUROCOGNITIVE DEFICITS

4. What are the primary receptors that are the targets of anesthetic drugs and the purported cellular intermediaries for the reported toxicity in preclinical reports?
5. What are the neurodevelopmental processes that are impaired with exposure to anesthetic drugs?
6. How does the developmental stage of the GABAergic neuron affect its excitatory state?
7. Does neuronal apoptosis always impair neurodevelopment?
8. Is there an age-dependent impact on dendritic development after exposure to anesthetic drugs?
9. What is the preclinical link between anesthesia and Alzheimer disease in older animal models?
10. Neonatal rat pups exposed to volatile anesthetics have been shown to develop learning deficits. Which interventions mitigate this adverse outcome?
11. What are the three factors that increase the development of neuronal cell death in neonatal laboratory animals exposed to anesthetic drugs?

CLINICAL EVIDENCE FOR NEUROTOXICITY

12. Recent retrospective reports detected neurocognitive deficits after exposure to surgery and anesthesia. What are the drawbacks of these investigations?
13. Are there any prospective reports that examine the impact of surgery and anesthetic at an early age on subsequent neurocognitive function?

INTRAOPERATIVE COURSE AND NEUROCOGNITIVE OUTCOMES

14. Are there any other perioperative factors that can impair subsequent neurocognitive function?
15. Parents are in your office for surgery and want to know the long-term risks of general anesthesia for their 6-month-old infant. They have concerns about the possible neurocognitive effects of general anesthesia and are contemplating a regional anesthetic rather than a general anesthetic. What is your advice to them?

ANSWERS

INTRODUCTION

1. Preclinical reports clearly demonstrate a neurotoxic effect of anesthetic drugs at all stages of neurodevelopment. This effect spans from the fetus to the aged. (185)
2. Abnormal behavior has been reported in the 1950s in both children and the elderly after general anesthesia. Halothane was initially reported to be toxic to rodents in the 1960s. (186)
3. The Food and Drug Administration (FDA) held several open hearings and on December 14, 2016, published a cautionary perspective on the use of anesthetic drugs in patients under 3 years of age. The FDA warned that "repeated or lengthy use of general anesthetic and sedation drugs during surgeries or procedures in children younger than 3 years or in pregnant women during their third trimester may affect the development of children's brains." In 2017 the FDA approved label changes warning of possible neurotoxicity to the labels of general anesthetic and sedation drugs, and in 2018 the FDA issued another drug safety communication and review about anesthetic and sedation drugs. (185)

ANESTHETIC DRUGS AS A CAUSE FOR NEURODEGENERATION AND LONG-TERM NEUROCOGNITIVE DEFICITS

4. Anesthetic and sedative drugs that are classified as γ-aminobutyric acid (GABA) receptor agonists, *N*-methyl-D-aspartate (NMDA) glutamate receptor antagonists, or a combination of the two have been implicated in causing developmental neurotoxicity. General anesthesia and sedation can be achieved by inhalation or intravenous administration of specific drugs. There is less evidence that α_2-adrenergic receptor agonists such as dexmedetomidine cause neurodevelopmental neurotoxicity. (185–186)
5. Neurodevelopment progresses through several steps that include neurogenesis, neuronal morphogenesis, migration, synaptogenesis, and remodeling. Exposure to anesthetic drugs impaired these processes and has been implicated in the subsequent neurobehavioral deficits observed in laboratory animals. (186–187)
6. GABAergic general anesthetics act on the GABA receptor. Although GABA is inhibitory in the mature brain, it has been found in many preclinical studies to be an excitatory agent during early stages of brain development. The immature $Na^+/K^+/2Cl^-$ transporter protein NKCC1 produces a chloride influx leading to neuron depolarization. Therefore GABA remains excitatory until the GABA neurons switch to the normal inhibitory mode when the mature chloride transporter, KCC2, is expressed, which actively transports chloride out of the neural cell. This switch begins around 15th postnatal week in term human infants but is not complete until about 1 year of age. (186)
7. The proliferative stage of neurogenesis produces an overabundance of progenitor cells that develop into neural and glial cells. Neural development is regulated by early elimination during embryonal and programmed cell death during postnatal modification of the central nervous system. Redundant neural progenitor cells and neurons that do not migrate properly or make synapses are physiologically pruned by apoptosis. (186–187)
8. Dendrites and axons extend from the cell body to form functional synapses with other neurons. Exposure to ketamine and isoflurane decreases synapse and spine density in very young infant rats. However, in slightly older rats, exposure to anesthetic drugs leads to an increase in dendritic spine formation. The implications of both the decrease in dendritic spine formation at a very young age and an increase in slightly older animals are unclear, but these different effects highlight the impact of specific developmental stages. (187)
9. Preclinical reports demonstrate expression of biological precursors of Alzheimer disease after surgery and general anesthesia. Experimental surgery on mice increased β-amyloid accumulation in the hippocampus. Furthermore, exposure to isoflurane leads to increased τ and β-amyloid levels in cell culture and rodent brains. (187)
10. Anesthetic-induced cell death and neurobehavioral deficits in neonatal pups exposed to volatile anesthetics can be mitigated by concurrent exposure to an enriched environment, exercise, lithium, estrogen, erythropoietin, melatonin, and dexmedetomidine. (188)
11. The combination of large doses of anesthetic, prolonged or repeated exposure to anesthetic drugs, and vulnerable age is directly related to neuronal cell death. (188)

CLINICAL EVIDENCE FOR NEUROTOXICITY

12. Most published reports implicating that general anesthesia is harmful to children are limited to retrospective epidemiologic analyses. This evidence may be confounded by the effects of surgery and the effects of the underlying comorbid conditions. Most of the studies have attempted to control for obvious confounders, but the retrospective nature of these investigations makes it impossible to control for all the known and unknown confounders. Large database clinical investigations from Canada and Sweden reveal that exposure to surgery and anesthesia at age >2 to 4 years of age increased the odds ratio of cognitive deficits but not to the extent of previously published retrospective reports from smaller populations. Scrutiny of these large data sets reveals a lower percentage in academic achievement scores for toddlers undergoing ear, nose, and throat surgery. This finding suggests that early derangements in hearing and speech may have an impact on subsequent cognitive domains assessed by school performance. (189)
13. Two clinical reports that prospectively examined children receiving surgery and anesthesia (GAS and PANDA studies) did not demonstrate a decrement in cognitive function. The GAS study randomized infants requiring inguinal herniorrhaphy surgery to receive either sevoflurane general anesthesia or nonsedated regional anesthesia. When these children reached both 2 years and 5 years of age, there were no differences in cognition between the sevoflurane or regional anesthesia groups. A report on a smaller group of children exposed to anesthetic before 1 year showed deficits in measures of long-term recognition memory but no differences in familiarity, intelligence quotient, and Child Behavior Checklist scores. (188–189)

INTRAOPERATIVE COURSE AND NEUROCOGNITIVE OUTCOMES

14. The developing central nervous system is exquisitely sensitive to its internal milieu. Because critical periods of plasticity during brain development are modulated by the environmental milieu, perioperative conditions have the potential to influence brain development. Maternal deprivation, hypoglycemia, hypoxia, and hypotension and hypocarbia leading to cerebral ischemia during these critical periods of development may lead to neuronal injury and altered neurodevelopment. There also could be a synergistic or additive effect of stressful physiologic environment and anesthetic neurotoxicity. (188)
15. You advise them that they are correct to be concerned based on the animal data. The epidemiologic data are nondefinitive with some studies demonstrating an effect but other studies showing no effect. The only published prospective randomized trial (GAS study) in children thus far did not show a neurocognitive difference between general and regional anesthesia. (189)

Chapter

13 PREOPERATIVE EVALUATION

Lorraine M. Sdrales and Manuel C. Pardo, Jr.

INTRODUCTION

- Goals of preoperative evaluation include
  - Understanding nature and extent of proposed surgery
  - Assessing risk of coexisting medical conditions
  - Deciding whether to order preoperative tests
  - Discussing options for anesthesia care
  - Understanding and addressing patient concerns

HISTORY AND PHYSICAL EXAMINATION

- Preoperative history and physical have same structure as a general medical evaluation, with focus on perioperative implications.
- History of present illness includes age, sex/gender, surgical diagnosis and proposed procedure, surgeon, and health care facility.
- Past medical history
  - Current medical conditions
  - Hospitalizations
  - Medications: prescription, over the counter, herbals
  - Allergies: date and nature of reaction
- Past surgical and anesthesia history
  - Prior anesthesia records including details of airway management
  - Patient's prior experience and anesthetic complications
- Social history
  - Tobacco, alcohol, and substance use
  - Social determinants: e.g., housing, transportation, employment, access to care
- Family history of reactions to anesthesia
- Review of systems
  - Assessments of nutrition, frailty, functional status, OSA screening, cognitive function (in older patients)
- Physical examination
  - Vital signs
  - Exam: airway, pulmonary auscultation and cardiovascular at minimum

PREOPERATIVE EVALUATION OF COMMON COEXISTING DISEASES

- Management may be based on evidence-based practice guidelines, clinical guidelines based on expert opinion, or clinical judgment.

Neurologic

- Parkinson disease
  - Increased perioperative risk
    - Cardiovascular: autonomic dysfunction
    - Pulmonary: dysphagia, impaired cough, aspiration pneumonia
    - Neurologic: bradykinesia, insufficient strength, fall risk
    - Infectious: risk of urinary tract infections, bacterial infections
  - Evaluate comorbidities and medication/treatment regimen
    - Continue home regimen closely
    - Monoamine oxidase-B inhibitors stopped 1 to 2 weeks prior to surgery

Cardiovascular

- Several specialty societies have published guidelines for evaluation and management of patients with cardiovascular disease undergoing noncardiac surgery.
  - American College of Cardiology/American Heart Association (ACC/AHA) guideline is commonly used.
- Coronary artery disease
  - Risk factors: hypertension, dyslipidemia, diabetes mellitus, obesity, chronic kidney disease
  - 2014 ACC/AHA preoperative clinical guideline for stepwise approach to evaluating patients for noncardiac surgery

2014 ACC/AHA Guideline Steps
Step 1: Emergent? Yes, risk stratify and proceed with surgery.
Step 2: Acute coronary syndrome? Yes, evaluate and treat with goal-directed medical therapy (GDMT).
Step 3: Estimate risk of major adverse cardiovascular events (MACE).
Step 4: Low risk for MACE, proceed with surgery.
Step 5: If elevated risk for MACE, assess functional capacity. Moderate or excellent functional capacity, proceed with surgery.
Step 6: If poor or unknown functional capacity, might testing change management? If yes, cardiac stress testing. Negative result – GDMT and proceed with surgery. Positive result – percutaneous coronary intervention, coronary artery bypass grafting, GDMT, and/or surgery alternative as indicated
Step 7: If no, GDMT and proceed with surgery or surgery alternative

    - Risk calculators to estimate risk of major adverse cardiac event include:
        - Revised Cardiac Risk Index (RCRI)
        - American College of Surgeons National Surgical Quality Improvement Program (NSQIP)
        - Cardiovascular Risk Index (CVRI)
    - Functional capacity assessment guides need for cardiac testing
        - Use of metabolic equivalents (METs) is subjective and may be less accurate than Duke Activity Status Index (DASI)
- Hypertension
    - Risk factor for cardiovascular disease, stroke, and end-stage renal disease (ESRD)
    - Angiotensin-converting enzyme inhibitors (ACEIs) and angiotensin receptor blockers (ARBs) have been associated with intraoperative hypotension.
        - A 2018 metaanalysis showed no difference in mortality, major cardiac events, stroke, or acute kidney injury in patients who withheld ACEIs or ARBs compared to patients who continued them,
    - 2017 – ACC published Recommendations for Treatment of Hypertension in Patients Undergoing Surgical Procedures for the patients as follows:
        - If on chronic β-blockers, continuing is recommended for major surgery.
        - Continuing antihypertensives is reasonable for elective surgery.
        - ACEI or ARB discontinuation can be considered for major surgery.
        - If systolic blood pressure >180 or diastolic blood pressure >110, deferring elective surgery may be considered.
        - Abrupt discontinuation of β-blockers or clonidine can be harmful.
        - If β-blocker naïve, a β-blocker should not be started on the day of surgery.
- The patient receiving anticoagulant therapy
    - Disease states may include mechanical heart valve, atrial fibrillation, and venous thromboembolism (VTE).
    - The American College of Chest Physicians published guidelines in 2022 for the perioperative management of antithrombotic therapy per evidence-based data.
    - Must balance risk of discontinuation (venous or arterial thromboembolism) with the risk of surgical bleeding or an anesthetic intervention (e.g., neuraxial block)
    - If discontinuation of vitamin K antagonist (VKA) anticoagulation is needed, the decision of whether to bridge with heparin is guided by the risk of VTE or arterial thromboembolism (ATE) and patient history.
        - High risk: bridging therapy is suggested.
        - Moderate risk: bridging therapy is a clinical decision based on the patient and the surgery (bleeding, hemostasis potential).
        - Low risk: bridging therapy is not suggested.
    - Direct oral anticoagulant (DOAC) advantages over heparin include
        - More predictable pharmacokinetics
        - Fewer drug interactions
        - Lower risk of intracranial bleeding
        - Shorter half-lives and less need for bridging anticoagulation
    - DOAC dose adjustment is necessary in patients with chronic kidney disease.
        - DOAC discontinuation date before surgery depends on bleeding risk and patient's creatinine clearance.
    - The American College of Cardiology in 2017 published a suggested algorithm to decide if bridging is necessary in patients with nonvalvular atrial fibrillation.
- The patient receiving antiplatelet therapy
    - For primary or secondary prevention of coronary or cerebral artery thrombosis, as either monotherapy or dual antiplatelet therapy (DAPT)
    - Periprocedural management of monotherapy or DAPT is a complex clinical decision considering multiple factors, including risk of thrombosis and bleeding.
    - In some cases, one or both antiplatelet agents may be continued perioperatively.
    - DAPT management after PCI is guided by the type of stent and the individual circumstance.
        - 2016 guidelines recommend delaying elective surgery for 30 days after bare metal stent and 180 days after drug-eluding stent.

Pulmonary

- Postoperative pulmonary complications (PPCs) are associated with increased patient mortality.

Possible Postoperative Pulmonary Complications
▪ Respiratory infection
▪ Respiratory failure
▪ Pleural effusion
▪ Atelectasis
▪ Pneumothorax
▪ Bronchospasm
▪ Aspiration pneumonitis

- The estimated incidence after major surgery is <1% to 23%.
- No evidence-based, high-quality studies of perioperative interventions to reduce the risk of PPCs
- Lack of agreement of useful preoperative predictive models

Major Predictors of Postoperative Respiratory Failure

Patient Related	Procedure Related
Preoperative hypoxemia	Emergency surgery
Preoperative respiratory symptoms	Upper abdominal surgery
History of congestive heart failure	Thoracic surgery
History of liver failure	Duration of surgery >3 hours

Endocrine

- Diabetes mellitus
  - Major risk factor for postoperative complications
  - Hyperglycemia is associated with cardiovascular events, wound infection, pneumonia, and sepsis
  - Preoperative evaluation of diabetes
    - Type of diabetes
    - Current pharmacologic therapy
    - Current glycemic control including hypoglycemic and hyperglycemic episodes (HbA_{1c} can be a guide)
      - If patient has poorly controlled diabetes, consideration of postponing the procedure must include a risk/benefit assessment.
    - Long-term sequelae (gastroparesis, neuropathy, cardiovascular disease, peripheral vascular disease)
    - Perioperative medication management plan
      - Based on patient's baseline status
      - Avoid hypoglycemia during time of NPO.

Perioperative Medication Management of Diabetes

Patient's Baseline Status	Medication Strategy
On oral hypoglycemic	Hold oral agents on morning of surgery
On SGLT2 inhibitors	Discontinue 3–4 days prior surgery (risk of "euglycemic DKA")
Type 2 diabetes Oral hypoglycemic and insulin therapy	Hold oral agents on morning of surgery Reduce long-acting insulin by 25% on night prior to surgery Hold short-acting insulin on morning of surgery
Type 1 diabetes Intermittent insulin therapy	Reduce long-acting insulin by 25% on night prior to surgery Correctional short-acting insulin every 2–4 hours morning of surgery Basal insulin at all times (risk of DKA, metabolic abnormalities)
Type 1 diabetes Insulin pump therapy	Determine if insulin pump can be used perioperatively based on duration, location, and stress of surgery
Degludec (Tresiba)	Very long-acting insulin with duration of action of 42 hours May require dose reduction 1 additional day prior to surgery

Hematologic

- Thrombocytopenia (platelets $<150 \times 10^9$/L)
  - Proceeding with surgery is based on patient factors, quality of platelet function, and type of surgery.
    - For nonneuraxial surgery, common goal is platelets $>50 \times 10^9$/L.
    - For neurosurgery or posterior eye surgery, common goal is platelets $>100 \times 10^9$/L.

Infectious Disease

- Surgical site infection
  - Associated with morbidity and mortality
  - Glycemic control
    - CDC recommends perioperative glucose target of 200 mg/dL.
    - Other institutions recommend 180 mg/dL.
    - No consensus on target HbA_{1c}
  - Antiseptic prophylaxis
    - Antimicrobial prophylaxis per published clinical guidelines
    - CDC recommends preoperative antiseptic soap shower, normothermia, and adequate perioperative oxygenation.
- Infective endocarditis
  - AHA published guidelines in 2007, reconfirmed in 2021, for the prevention of infective endocarditis (IE).

- IE prophylaxis is only recommended for patients with cardiac conditions associated with the highest risk of adverse outcome.
- For these patients, antibiotic prophylaxis is reasonable when undergoing the following procedures:
  - All dental procedures involving manipulation of periapical gingival tissues or with perforation of oral mucosa
  - Procedures on the respiratory tract
  - Procedures on infected skin, skin structures, or musculoskeletal tissue

Cardiac Conditions Associated With the Highest Risk of Adverse Outcome From Endocarditis

Prosthetic cardiac valve or cardiac valve repair using prosthetic material
Previous infective endocarditis
Congenital heart disease (CHD)
Unrepaired cyanotic CHD, including palliative shunts and conduits
Completely repaired CHD with prosthetic material or device within 6 months
Repaired CHD with residual defects at the site or adjacent to prosthetic patch or device
Cardiac transplant recipients who develop cardiac valvulopathy

Geriatrics

- Advanced age is associated with an increased likelihood of coexisting diseases and associated physiologic changes.
- Frailty
  - Defined as a syndrome of a decrease in physiologic reserve and function resulting in vulnerability to stressors
  - Vulnerable to adverse outcomes due to cumulative declines across multiple physiologic systems
  - Severe frailty is associated with increased perioperative morbidity and mortality.
  - No high-quality randomized studies to evaluate for interventions that will provide for improved long-term postoperative outcomes

PREOPERATIVE TESTING

- The ASA Practice Advisory for Preanesthesia Evaluation advises against routine preoperative tests.
- Selective preoperative tests can be used to guide or optimize perioperative decision making and management.
- Testing should be evidence-based, necessary, and not duplicative or harmful.
- The American Board of Internal Medicine (ABIM) Foundation has "Choosing Wisely" recommendations from specialty societies.

ABIM Choosing Wisely Recommendations

American Society of Anesthesiologists advises 1) no baseline laboratory studies for patients without significant disease undergoing low risk surgery and 2) no baseline diagnostic cardiac testing (i.e., TEE/stress testing) in patients with asymptomatic stable cardiac disease.
Society of General Internal Medicine advises no routine preoperative testing before low-risk surgical procedures.
American College of Surgeons advises against routine chest radiographs in ambulatory patients with unremarkable history or physical exam.
American Academy of Ophthalmology advises against preoperative medical tests for eye surgery unless specifically medically indicated.
American College of Cardiology advises against cardiac stress tests, advanced cardiac imaging, or coronary calcium scoring for preoperative cardiac risk assessment in patients undergoing low-risk noncardiac surgery.

Rationale for Selective Testing

- In general, tests should be ordered if the diagnosis or assessment of a medical condition will affect the anesthetic management or perioperative care plan.

Recommendations for Ordering Selective Preoperative Tests

Test	Recommendation	Reference
Electrocardiogram	Reasonable in patients with known cardiovascular or cerebral vascular disease for moderate or high-risk surgery	ACC/AHA
Electrocardiogram	May be indicated for patients with known cardiovascular risk factors	ASA
Chest radiograph	1) To evaluate clinical suspicion for acute unstable chronic cardiopulmonary disease that could influence patient care 2) Selectively in patients with advanced age or other increased risk	American College of Radiology
Hemoglobin or hematocrit	Consider the procedure and the patient's age and history (e.g., liver disease, anemia, coagulopathies, bleeding, hematologic disorders)	ASA
Coagulation studies	Consider the procedure and patient's history (e.g., bleeding disorders, renal or liver dysfunction)	ASA

Test	Recommendation	Reference
Serum chemistries	Consider patient's use of medications or alternative therapies, perioperative therapies, and patient's history (e.g., endocrine disorders, risk of or known renal or liver dysfunction)	ASA
Urinalysis	Indicated when urinary tract symptoms are present or for specific procedures (e.g., prosthesis implantation, urologic procedures)	ASA

Pregnancy Testing

- The ASA Practice Advisory for Preanesthesia Evaluation recommendations include
  - Pregnancy testing may be offered to female patients of childbearing age for whom the result would alter the patient's management.
  - Pregnancy testing should not be mandatory.
  - Preanesthetic education materials should be given to patients to allow informed decision-making.

Preoperative Transfusion Testing

- Transfusion testing includes blood type and antibody screening, crossmatch for packed red blood cells (PRBCs), or the preparation of blood products such as plasma or platelets.

Potential Negative Implications of Preoperative Transfusion Testing

Transfusion Testing Not Ordered	Transfusion Testing Ordered
If urgent intraoperative transfusion needed or patient's antibody screen is positive: ▪ PRBCs not available ▪ Emergency-release blood may be needed ▪ Increased risk of transfusion reaction	Type and cross ordered in low bleeding risk situation: ▪ PRBCs are "reserved" for patient ▪ Those PRBCs are not available to other patients during that time Type and screen ordered in minimal bleeding risk situation: ▪ Low-value and wasteful use of resources, time, and equipment

- Maximum surgical blood order schedule (MSBOS) is created by analyzing perioperative transfusion history data.
  - Advises either 1) no testing, 2) type and screen only, or 3) type and cross for a specific number of PRBC units
  - Surgery specific
  - Institution specific
  - Does not reflect patient conditions such as anemia or coagulopathy or other patient-specific surgical bleeding risk

RISK ASSESSMENT

- Tools for perioperative risk include risk scores (e.g., ASA Physical Status and Revised Cardiac Risk Index) and risk prediction models (e.g., NSQIP calculator).
- Practical considerations of individual risk assessment
  - Is the perioperative risk elevated relative to that of a healthy patient?
  - Is additional testing necessary to further evaluate the risk?
  - Can additional therapy reduce the risk?
  - Based on the above, should there be changes to surgery date, location (outpatient vs. inpatient), anesthesiologist assignment (e.g., subspecialty trained), or the anesthetic plan?

ASA Physical Status

- Brief descriptions of each class make it simple to use.

ASA Physical Status Classification

Class	Description
I	Normal healthy patient
II	Patient with mild systemic disease
III	Patient with severe systemic disease
IV	Patient with severe systemic disease that is a constant threat to life
V	Moribund patient who is not expected to survive without the operation
VI	Declared brain-dead patient whose organs are being removed for donor purposes
"E"	Added to denote condition in which a delay (not well defined) in treatment will lead to a significant increase in the threat to life or body part

- Has been used to make decisions about the patient's perioperative plan
- ASA has added case descriptions to improve interrater reliability.
- Final decision of the classification is made on the day of surgery by the anesthesiologist.

MEDICATION MANAGEMENT

- Evaluation of perioperative risks of continuing or discontinuing medications
- Use evidence-based guidelines if available

NPO GUIDELINES

- Reduce the risk of the pulmonary aspiration of gastric contents
- Risk factors include gastroesophageal reflux, dysphagia, and poor motility disorders.
- ASA minimum preoperative fasting recommendations are based on ingested material
  - Clear liquids – 2 hours
  - Breast milk – 4 hours
  - Infant formula or nonhuman milk – 6 hours
  - Light meal (e.g., toast and clear liquids) – 6 hours
  - Fried foods, fatty foods, meat – additional time may be needed (≥8 hours)
- Additional instructions may include medications (e.g., proton pump inhibitors) or participation in enhanced recovery after surgery protocols (e.g., carbohydrate drinks).

INFORMED CONSENT FOR ANESTHESIA

- Providing a patient with information that allows them to make an informed choice about their care
  - The *reasonable person* standard most commonly applies: the disclosure of information that a hypothetical reasonable person would want.
  - Includes patient's condition, procedures, risks, and postoperative pain plan
  - Risk-benefit discussion of anesthetic options
  - Perioperative risks of coexisting diseases
- Often on day of surgery and may include decisions for type of anesthesia
- Analgesics and anxiolytics may impair the patient's capacity for consent.
- The US Joint Commission does not require a separate written consent form for anesthesia.

PREOPERATIVE EVALUATION CLINICS

- Increases anesthesiologist-guided preoperative counseling, communication with patients, protocol development, and postoperative care coordination.
- Can reduce surgical cancelations and possibly in-hospital mortality

Enhanced Recovery Pathways

- Multidisciplinary and often include a preoperative component

Preoperative Optimization

- Preoperative clinics with sufficient lead time prior to surgery can identify if optimization is necessary for certain issues, such as anemia, malnutrition, complex pain, smoking, frailty, or coagulation.
- Prehabilitation refers to interventions to enhance functional capacity to improve tolerance to the physiologic stress of surgery.
  - Improved physical fitness
  - Dietary interventions
  - Antistress interventions
  - Cessation of adverse health habits

Inpatient Preoperative Evaluation

- Often urgent or emergent surgery
- Geriatric acute hip fracture patients have lower mortality if surgery is within 24 to 48 hours of admission.
  - Early evaluation for correctable factors such as hypovolemia, anemia, hypoxemia, electrolyte abnormalities, and correction of anticoagulant effects
  - Additional testing that delays surgery should be selective (e.g., acute coronary syndrome).
  - ERAS pathways (e.g., multimodal analgesia) for these patients can decrease time to surgery and length of stay and decrease the complication rate.

QUESTIONS

HISTORY AND PHYSICAL EXAMINATION

1. What elements of the preanesthesia assessment differ from the routine history and physical done in an outpatient medicine setting?

PREOPERATIVE EVALUATION OF COMMON COEXISTING DISEASES

2. Complete the following table of organ system manifestations of Parkinson disease and perioperative implications.

	Physiologic Change	Potential Perioperative Consequence
Cardiovascular		
Pulmonary		
Neurologic		
Immune system		

3. How should medications be managed perioperatively for patients with Parkinson disease?
4. For a patient with known coronary artery disease undergoing noncardiac surgery, how does their risk for a major adverse cardiac event influence the preoperative plan?
5. Compared to clinical practice 10 years ago, which types of active cancer are now considered to place patients at high risk for periprocedural thromboembolism?
6. Is heparin bridging necessary for patients on direct oral anticoagulants (DOACs) at high risk for periprocedural thromboembolism?
7. When should antiplatelet therapy be continued in the perioperative period?
8. For patients with type 2 diabetes receiving oral hypoglycemic and insulin therapy, how should these medications be managed preoperatively?
9. Is antibiotic prophylaxis for infective endocarditis required in a patient with a history of aortic valve replacement undergoing laparoscopic cholecystectomy?

PREOPERATIVE TESTING

10. In the table, indicate whether preoperative testing is indicated for the condition described. (209–211)

	Yes	No
Should baseline laboratory studies be ordered for a patient having surgery for the first time?		
Should a 32-year-old sexually active woman undergoing general anesthesia receive a mandatory pregnancy test prior to surgery?		
Should an ECG should be ordered for a 72-year-old patient undergoing open inguinal hernia repair?		
Should a urinalysis be ordered for a patient scheduled for a total hip replacement?		
Should a chest radiograph should be ordered for a patient with asthma scheduled for bilateral mastectomy with DIEP flap reconstruction?		

NPO GUIDELINES

11. For the following items, indicate if they can be consumed 2, 4, 6, or 8 hours prior to surgery:
    a. Orange juice with pulp
    b. Apple juice
    c. Coffee with milk
    d. Black coffee
    e. Breast milk
    f. Nonhuman milk
    g. Toast with peanut butter

INFORMED CONSENT FOR ANESTHESIA

12. What are the components of informed consent? Is the anesthesia provider required to mention the possibility of death?

PREOPERATIVE EVALUATION CLINICS

13. What are some potential benefits of a preoperative clinic?

ANSWERS

HISTORY AND PHYSICAL EXAMINATION

1. In addition to the routine elements of a history and physical, the preanesthesia assessment includes the patient's history of prior anesthetics, family history of problems with anesthesia, an OSA screening, and an airway exam. (196)

PREOPERATIVE EVALUATION OF COMMON COEXISTING DISEASES

2. This table highlights the organ system manifestations of Parkinson disease and their perioperative implications. (198)

	Physiologic Change	Potential Perioperative Consequence
Cardiovascular	Autonomic dysfunction	Hemodynamic instability
Pulmonary	Dysphagia, impaired cough	Aspiration pneumonia
Neurologic	Decreased muscle strength	Bradykinesia, fall risk
Immune system	Increased risk of infection	Risk of UTIs, bacterial infections

3. Patients with Parkinson disease should continue their home medication schedule as closely as possible throughout the perioperative period to avoid exacerbation of symptoms. (198)
4. A patient's risk of major adverse cardiac events (MACE) can be calculated using a risk score calculator, such as the Revised Cardiac Risk Index (RCRI). In accordance with the ACC/AHA guidelines, patients with a history of coronary artery disease undergoing noncardiac surgery with a low risk of MACE can proceed with surgery. If the risk of MACE is moderate or high, the next step is to objectively measure the patient's functional capacity, which can be done by assessing their highest metabolic equivalents (METs) or using the Duke Activity Status Index (DASI). If the patient has moderate, good, or excellent functional capacity (e.g., METs ≥4, the patient can proceed with surgery without further testing. If the patient has poor (<4 METs) or unknown functional capacity, a discussion with the patient and the perioperative team should determine whether further testing would affect the treatment plan. For example, one deciding factor may be whether surgery would be delayed for revascularization (PCI or CABG) if a cardiac stress test results positive for inducible ischemia. (198–201)
5. Compared to 10 years ago, active cancers now considered to place patients at high risk of periprocedural thromboembolism include pancreatic cancer, myeloproliferative disorders, primary brain cancer, gastric cancer, and esophageal cancer. (202–204)
6. Heparin bridging is suggested for patients who are at high risk for venous or arterial thromboembolism and who must discontinue their VKA prior to surgery. Similar patients on DOACs are less likely to need bridging given the shorter-half lives of DOACs compared to VKAs. (201)
7. The periprocedural management of antiplatelets is a multifactorial decision. One or both (in cases of DAPT) may be continued if the perceived benefit outweighs the risk. For patients on DAPT after percutaneous coronary intervention (PCI), those who will be undergoing surgery within 6 months after placement of a drug-eluting stent and within 1 month of placement of a bare metal stent may be advised to continue antiplatelet therapy during the perioperative period, depending on the type of surgery. (205)
8. Patients with type 2 diabetes receiving an oral hypoglycemic agent should hold this medication on the morning of surgery. For those who are also on insulin therapy, long-acting insulin should be reduced by 25% on the night prior to surgery; short-acting insulin should be held on the morning of surgery. (209)
9. Regardless of the type of prosthetic aortic valve, antibiotic prophylaxis solely to prevent infective endocarditis is not recommended for patients undergoing gastrointestinal tract procedures such as laparoscopic cholecystectomy. (210)

PREOPERATIVE TESTING

10. In the table, indicate whether preoperative testing is indicated for the condition described. (209–211)

	Yes	No
Should baseline laboratory studies be ordered for a patient having surgery for the first time?		X
Should a 32-year-old sexually active woman undergoing general anesthesia receive a mandatory pregnancy test prior to surgery?		X
Should an ECG should be ordered for a 72-year-old patient undergoing open inguinal hernia repair?		X
Should a urinalysis be ordered for a patient scheduled for a total hip replacement?	X	
Should a chest radiograph should be ordered for a patient with asthma scheduled for bilateral mastectomy with DIEP flap reconstruction?		X

NPO GUIDELINES

11. The food or drink listed must be held for the corresponding interval prior to surgery. (216)
    a. Orange juice with pulp – 8 hours
    b. Apple juice – 2 hours
    c. Coffee with milk – 8 hours
    d. Black coffee – 2 hours
    e. Breast milk – 4 hours
    f. Nonhuman milk – 8 hours
    g. Toast with peanut butter – 8 hours

INFORMED CONSENT FOR ANESTHESIA

12. The informed consent should include information about the procedure, choices for anesthesia and postoperative pain management, and the potential risks and benefits of each considering the patient's medical condition and co-existing diseases. The risks of anesthesia discussed with the patient are typically what would be reasonable given the circumstance and must not always include all potential morbidities and death. (215)

PREOPERATIVE EVALUATION CLINICS

13. A preoperative clinic has the potential to reduce surgical cancelations and postoperative length of stay, which also reduces hospital costs. Patient outcomes may be improved with reduced morbidity and in-hospital mortality if there is sufficient time prior to surgery to medically optimize the patient for issues such as anemia, malnutrition, smoking, and others. Finally, the patient may be informed, have questions answered, and anxiety allayed through preoperative contact with a clinician (216).

Chapter

14 CHOICE OF ANESTHETIC TECHNIQUE

Manuel C. Pardo, Jr.

INTRODUCTION

- Choosing an anesthetic technique begins with the proposed surgical procedure and incorporates the patient's preferences for care and their coexisting diseases.

TYPES OF ANESTHESIA

- General anesthesia
  - A drug-induced, reversible state characterized by
    - Unconsciousness
    - Amnesia
    - Immobility
    - Control of autonomic nervous system (ANS) responses to noxious stimulation
- Regional anesthesia
  - Neuraxial (spinal, epidural, caudal) anesthesia
  - Peripheral nerve blocks
- Monitored anesthesia care (MAC)
  - Originally referred to the anesthesiologist providing anesthesia services to a patient receiving local anesthesia or no anesthesia at all
  - MAC may include varying levels of sedation, analgesia, and anxiolysis

CHOOSING AN APPROPRIATE ANESTHETIC TECHNIQUE

- If regional anesthesia is being considered
  - Major factor is the location of the surgical incision and operative field.
  - If regional block will not provide adequate coverage, general anesthesia is required.
- Procedures for which MAC may be an appropriate choice
  - No surgical incision (e.g., endoscopy)
  - Surgical procedure is not associated with pain, or analgesia can be completely provided with local anesthesia (e.g., many catheter-based procedures by cardiologists or interventional radiologists).
- Anesthetic techniques can be combined to meet patient or surgical goals. Examples:
  - A procedure started with MAC during which the patient's pain is greater than expected may require conversion to general anesthesia.
  - General anesthesia for the surgical procedure plus neuraxial or peripheral nerve blockade for postoperative analgesia (e.g., patient undergoing thoracotomy who receives general anesthesia plus epidural catheter)
- Multidisciplinary enhanced recovery pathways have been used for patients undergoing a variety of surgeries including
  - Colorectal
  - Orthopedic
  - Hepatic
  - Pancreatic
  - Gynecologic
- Potential outcome benefits of enhanced recovery pathway
  - Decreased hospital length of stay
  - Decreased morbidity
  - Faster return to work

PRACTICAL ASPECTS OF ANESTHESIA CHOICE

General Anesthesia

- Preoxygenation
  - Defined as deliberate replacement of nitrogen in the patient's functional residual capacity (FRC) with oxygen
  - Provides a margin of safety if apnea or airway obstruction develops during induction of general anesthesia
- Inhaled induction
  - Commonly chosen for pediatric patients who do not have an intravenous (IV) catheter in place
- IV induction
  - Most common technique in the adult patient
  - Steps in induction sequence
    - Preoxygenation
    - IV anesthetic administered
    - Patient loses consciousness

- Anesthesia provider begins mask ventilation
- Neuromuscular blocking drug administered to obtain intubating conditions
- Tracheal intubation
- Mechanical ventilation
- Maintenance anesthetic started

  - Rapid sequence induction (RSI)
    - An alternate approach designed to minimize risk of gastric contents regurgitation and pulmonary aspiration
    - Goal is to minimize time between onset of unconsciousness and tracheal intubation.
    - RSI steps
      - Preoxygenation
      - IV anesthetic administered
      - Immediate administration of rapid-onset neuromuscular blocking drug
      - Patient loses consciousness
      - Cricoid pressure application
      - Avoidance of mask ventilation
      - Tracheal intubation
      - Release of cricoid pressure after confirmation of endotracheal tube placement
- Airway management
  - Mask ventilation after IV or inhaled induction
  - Direct laryngoscopy or supraglottic airway placement
  - Alternate approach if airway management is anticipated to be particularly challenging
    - Awake tracheal intubation
    - Awake tracheotomy
    - IV induction of anesthesia after airway is secured
- Maintenance of anesthesia
  - Anesthesia is typically maintained with a combination of drugs, each titrated to a desired anesthetic goal.

Regional Anesthesia

- Surgery on the extremities may be amenable to peripheral nerve blockade as the primary anesthetic.
  - Peripheral nerve blockade rarely results in significant sympathectomy or hypotension.
- Neuraxial anesthesia (e.g., spinal or epidural anesthesia) can provide excellent operating conditions for surgery on the lower abdomen or lower extremities.
  - Higher levels of neuraxial blockade (mid-thoracic or higher) can result in profound sympathectomy and hypotension.

MAC

- During MAC, pharmacologic sedation is often provided by administering opioids or a hypnotic medication.
- Analgesia for the procedure can be provided by topical or local anesthetic administration.
- The most dangerous risk during MAC is respiratory depression from excessive sedation.

Strategies for Multimodal General Anesthesia

- Like multimodal analgesia for postoperative pain, the concept of multimodal general anesthesia involves targeting multiple components and pathways of anesthesia.
- Antinociceptive drugs include opioids, ketamine, dexmedetomidine, lidocaine, and nonsteroidal antiinflammatory drugs; use of multiple drugs creates an opioid-sparing effect.
- Unconsciousness and amnesia can be maintained with propofol or an inhaled anesthetic (e.g., sevoflurane).
- Immobility can be provided centrally by inhaled anesthetic or propofol, as well as by a neuromuscular blocking drug.

QUESTIONS

TYPES OF ANESTHESIA

1. What are the three major choices of anesthetic technique?
2. What are the main characteristics of general anesthesia?
3. For a patient receiving monitored anesthesia care (MAC), what are the definitions of minimal sedation, moderate sedation, and deep sedation?

CHOOSING AN APPROPRIATE ANESTHETIC TECHNIQUE

4. What patient or procedural factors suggest that general anesthesia is the most appropriate anesthetic technique?
5. Is MAC a safer anesthetic technique than general anesthesia or regional anesthesia?

PRACTICAL ASPECTS OF ANESTHESIA CHOICE

6. Which patients may benefit from rapid-sequence induction of anesthesia compared to a standard intravenous induction?
7. What is the approach to anesthetic medication administration during a procedure with MAC?
8. What are the most common reasons to convert from MAC to general anesthesia?

ANSWERS

TYPES OF ANESTHESIA

1. The three main anesthesia types include general anesthesia, regional anesthesia (which includes peripheral nerve blockade and neuraxial blockade), and monitored anesthesia care. A given procedure may be appropriately managed by more than one type of anesthesia. (221)
2. General anesthesia is a drug-induced, reversible state characterized by unconsciousness, amnesia, immobility, and control of the autonomic nervous system responses to noxious stimulation. (221)
3. The American Society of Anesthesiologists (ASA) has defined a continuum of depth of sedation, as well as a definition of general anesthesia. The major differences involve patient response to increasing degrees of stimulation, as noted in the table. Other aspects of the level of sedation include the impact on airway patency, spontaneous ventilation, and cardiovascular function. (222)

Continuum of Depth of Sedation: Definition of General Anesthesia and Levels of Sedation/Analgesia

	Minimal Sedation (Anxiolysis)	***Moderate Sedation/ Analgesia ("Conscious Sedation")***	***Deep Sedation/ Analgesia***	***General Anesthesia***
Responsiveness	Normal response to verbal stimulation	Purposeful* response to verbal or tactile stimulation	Purposeful* response following repeated or painful stimulation	Unarousable even with painful stimulus
Airway	Unaffected	No intervention required	Intervention may be required	Intervention often required
Spontaneous ventilation	Unaffected	Adequate	May be inadequate	Frequently inadequate
Cardiovascular function	Unaffected	Usually maintained	Usually maintained	May be impaired

*Reflex withdrawal from a painful stimulus is NOT considered a purposeful response.
Table from American Society of Anesthesiologists. Continuum of Depth of Sedation: Definition of General Anesthesia and Levels of Sedation/Analgesia. Last amended October 23, 2019.

CHOOSING AN APPROPRIATE ANESTHETIC TECHNIQUE

4. First, the location of the surgical incision and operative field may not be suitable for topical, local, or regional anesthesia. Certain surgical procedures compromise airway integrity or respiratory function to a degree that requires an endotracheal airway and mechanical ventilation, thus requiring general anesthesia. Patient characteristics that make regional anesthesia an inappropriate choice include inability to cooperate with the regional anesthesia technique, certain neurologic diseases, coagulopathy, or infection at the planned regional anesthesia cutaneous puncture site. (222)
5. While MAC may be considered less invasive due to the lack of an artificial airway or regional block, the risks are not necessarily reduced. For example, an ASA analysis of closed malpractice claims documented a comparable incidence of injury severity when comparing MAC to general anesthesia. Respiratory depression from sedative medication is an important mechanism of injury in these patients. (223)

PRACTICAL ASPECTS OF ANESTHESIA CHOICE

6. Patients with increased risk of gastric aspiration may benefit from a rapid-sequence induction of anesthesia, including those with clinically significant gastroesophageal reflux disease (e.g., still symptomatic despite medical therapy), delayed gastric emptying, known full stomach, or unknown fasting state. (225)

7. For procedures without nociception (e.g., radiologic imaging) or minimal nociception (e.g., small cutaneous incision amenable to local anesthetic infiltration), the anesthesia provider can administer pharmacologic sedation to achieve minimal, moderate, or deep sedation. Commonly administered sedatives include benzodiazepines, opioids, propofol, or dexmedetomidine. Respiratory depression from sedation is an ever-present concern during MAC. (227)
8. Common reasons to convert from MAC to general anesthesia include patient intolerance, patient-related complications (e.g., hemodynamic instability, hypoxemia), or procedural factors (e.g., change in procedure, extended surgical time, bleeding, or surgical request). (227)

Chapter

15 ANESTHESIA DELIVERY SYSTEMS

Stephen D. Weston

THE ANESTHESIA WORKSTATION

- Anesthesia delivery systems evolved from portable devices to the modern anesthesia workstation with multiple functions and safety features.
- Inhaled anesthetic delivery
  - Precise delivery of volatile anesthetics
  - Rebreathing of anesthetic gases after removal of carbon dioxide
  - Safety features
    - Display of inspired and exhaled anesthetic concentrations
- Oxygen delivery
  - Precise metering of oxygen and other breathing gases
  - Safety features
    - Display inspired oxygen concentration and gas pipeline and backup tank supply pressures
    - Prevent hypoxic gas mixtures caused by operator error or gas supply failure
    - Provide a breathing circuit manual oxygen flush feature
    - Possess a backup supply of oxygen
- Ventilation of the patient's lungs
  - Manual ventilation with adjustable breathing circuit pressure
  - Mechanical ventilation with ICU-like ventilator capability
  - Safety feature
    - Measure and display ventilatory parameters
    - Display of inspired and exhaled carbon dioxide concentrations
- Remove excess anesthetic gases
  - Scavenge excess gas from the breathing circuit and remove from the room
- Information display
  - Integrated platform for displaying anesthetic, hemodynamic, and respiratory parameters
  - Integration with the electronic medical record

The Anesthesia Workstation

- A full E-cylinder and a self-inflating manual resuscitation bag must be present at every anesthetizing location prior to commencing any anesthetic.
- "When in doubt, bag!" (i.e., manually ventilate the patient's lungs if there is any concern about machine function).

FUNCTIONAL ANATOMY OF THE ANESTHESIA WORKSTATION

Gas Supply System

High-Pressure Section: Auxiliary E-Cylinder Inlet

- Backup oxygen E-cylinder a required feature of the anesthesia machine
  - Hanger yoke assembly with pin index safety system (PISS)
- Oxygen (O_2)
  - Full tank 2200 psig (pounds per square inch gauge)
  - 650 L oxygen
  - Linear relationship between tank pressure and remaining oxygen
- Nitrous oxide (N_2O)
  - Full tank 750 psig
  - Full tank 1600 L of N_2O, mostly in liquid form
  - Tank remains at 750 psig until all liquid N_2O vaporized; tank is 75% depleted at this time.
- Pressure in the oxygen E-cylinder is *never* checked as part of the automatic machine check.
- Oxygen tank must be closed during normal operation.
  - Prevents unnoticed emptying of the tank in case of pipeline failure
- Gas delivered preferentially from the pipeline gas
  - If suspected oxygen pipeline contamination, must disconnect workstation from pipeline
  - Merely opening E-cylinder will not suffice.

Intermediate-Pressure Section

- Gas pipeline inlet: central gas supply source
  - Pipeline gases at 50-55 psig
  - Oxygen, air, and nitrous oxide typically used
- Connector systems
  - Diameter index safety system (DISS) connector
  - Quick coupler system
- Oxygen flush valve
  - 100% oxygen at high flow delivered to the breathing circuit
  - Used to overcome circuit leaks
  - Rapidly increases inhaled oxygen concentration

- Risk of barotrauma or awareness under anesthesia (dilution of inhaled anesthetic) if used inappropriately
- Pneumatic safety systems
  - Oxygen supply failure alarm sounds if oxygen supply pressure drops.
  - "Fail-safe valve" reduces or shuts off flow of other gases if oxygen supply pressure drops.
- Auxiliary oxygen flowmeter
  - Convenience for low-flow oxygen devices
  - Safety feature in case of power failure

Low-Pressure Section

- Flow control assemblies
  - Operator-selected total fresh gas flow
  - Electronic flow control assemblies increasingly common
  - Mechanical flow control devices (flowmeters) common either as primary or backup systems
  - Glass flow tubes in mechanical assemblies historically a source of leaks
- Proportioning systems
  - Device on machines with mechanical flow control assemblies; prevents user from selecting a hypoxic fresh gas flow
    - Links flow of oxygen and nitrous oxide
  - Electronically controlled systems programmed to prevent users from selecting hypoxic mixture
- Vaporizer mount and interlock system
  - Vaporizer mount allows detachment and replacement of vaporizers and introduces additional point for leaks or flow obstruction.
  - Interlock system prevents flow to more than one vaporizer at a time.

Anesthetic Vaporizers

Physics

- Ideal gas law
  - For gas within a container, the pressure (force per unit area) exerted by the gas on the walls of the container is directly proportional to the number of molecules of gas present and to the temperature, and inversely proportional to the volume of the container.
- Dalton's law of partial pressures
  - In a mixture of gases, each gas exerts its own pressure.
  - The total pressure of the mixture can be calculated by adding together the pressure of each gas.
- Volume percent
  - The percentage of volume occupied by a gas relative to the sum of all gases present
- Partial pressure
  - The pressure exerted by an individual gas
- Vaporization
  - The movement of molecules of a volatile liquid (such as liquid anesthetic) from the liquid phase to gas phase at a gas/liquid interface, such as the interface between anesthetic liquid and the carrier gas in the vaporizer
- Condensation
  - The movement of molecules from gas phase to liquid phase at a gas/liquid interface
- Saturated vapor pressure of a volatile anesthetic
  - When the equilibrium between rates of vaporization and condensation is reached, the gas is said to be *saturated* with anesthetic.
  - The anesthetic molecules in the gas exert a partial pressure, known as the saturated vapor pressure.
  - The saturated vapor pressure is a physical property of a volatile liquid.
    - Saturated vapor pressure rises with temperature.
    - Saturated vapor pressure is not affected by change in atmospheric pressure.
- Latent heat of vaporization
  - Energy is required for vaporization to occur.
  - Latent heat of vaporization is the energy required to change 1 gram of a particular liquid into vapor at a constant temperature.
  - In practice, the energy needed for the vaporization of anesthetic molecules is extracted from the surrounding liquid, resulting in cooling of the remaining liquid.
  - Vaporization therefore retards further vaporization.
- Boiling point
  - The temperature at which saturated vapor pressure equals atmospheric pressure
  - Most volatile anesthetics' boiling point is higher than encountered clinically.
  - Desflurane's boiling point of 22.8°C (73°F) at sea level mandates special vaporizer design to control agent delivery.

The Physics of Volatile Anesthetics

- The characteristic *saturated vapor pressure* of each volatile anesthetic liquid is unique to that anesthetic agent.
- This requires that anesthetic vaporizers be *agent-specific.*
- Saturated vapor pressure rises with temperature.
- Saturated vapor pressure is independent of atmospheric pressure.
- The process of vaporization results in cooling of the remaining liquid.
- The boiling point of the volatile anesthetics is higher than commonly encountered clinical conditions, except for desflurane.

Modern Vaporizer Types

- Variable bypass vaporizers
    - Regulate the concentration of vaporizer output by diluting gas saturated with anesthetic with a larger flow of gas that *bypasses* the vaporizing chamber.
    - The concentration dial controls (varies) the ratio of the fresh gas flow that bypasses the vaporizing chamber to the flow that enters the vaporizing chamber.
    - The diverting ratio to achieve a specific concentration depends on the physical characteristics of the volatile anesthetic liquid, and therefore the vaporizers are *agent-specific.*
    - Temperature compensation is achieved mechanically within the vaporizer, reducing vaporizing chamber flow as temperature increases.
    - Safety considerations
        - Agent-specific filling devices help prevent mis-filling.
        - Overfilling or tipping can allow liquid agent into the bypass chamber, resulting in high anesthetic output.
        - Vaporizers are common source of leaks in the anesthesia system and can be hard to detect.
- Desflurane dual-gas blender
    - Desflurane is unsuited for variable bypass vaporizer.
        - High saturated vapor pressure would require very high bypass flows.
        - Moderate potency requires a greater number of molecules being vaporized, leading to much greater cooling.
        - It would be difficult to compensate for this cooling effect through vaporizer design.
        - Boiling point can be encountered in normal operation, leading to uncontrolled vaporizer output.
    - Electrically heated desflurane sump provides source of pressurized desflurane vapor.
    - Concentration dial controls the blending of this vapor with the fresh gas flow.
    - Although the dialed concentration is stable as barometric pressure drops, the delivered partial pressure of desflurane is lower.
        - At high altitudes, the anesthesia provider must compensate by increasing the dialed concentration of desflurane relative to the decrease in barometric pressure.
- Cassette vaporizers
    - Control unit internal to the anesthesia workstation, with programming to integrate agent, temperature, carrier gas, and fresh gas flow rate
    - Changeable agent-specific cassettes magnetically coded to allow the anesthesia machine to identify the agent
    - Bypass ratio computer-controlled for all agents other than desflurane
    - With desflurane, function can switch between carefully metered bypass flow and, at higher temperatures, injection of desflurane vapor.
- Injection-type vaporizers
    - Under microprocessor control, liquid anesthetic can be injected into heated vaporizing chambers.

ANESTHETIC BREATHING CIRCUITS

Circle Breathing Systems

- Seven essential components
- Fresh gas inlet
    - Fresh gas flows into the circle system from the common gas outlet.
- Unidirectional valves
    - Inspiratory and expiratory valves
    - Permit positive-pressure breathing
    - Ensure no rebreathing of gas until carbon dioxide (CO_2) absorption has occurred
- Corrugated breathing circuit tubing
    - Large-bore tubing minimizes resistance.
    - Tubing constitutes most of the volume of the system.
    - The tubing is compliant, such that significant volume is "lost" in distending the tubing.
- Y-piece
    - Y-piece is the point at which the inspiratory and expiratory limbs of the circuit merge.
    - Dead space of the circle system begins at Y-piece.
    - Gas sampling line located at Y-piece, allows measurement of inspiratory and expiratory gases.
- Adjustable pressure-limiting valve
    - Operator-adjustable relief valve, also called "pop-off" valve
    - Above set pressure, gas vented to the scavenge system
    - Allows spontaneous breathing at atmospheric pressure, continuous positive airway pressure (CPAP), or positive-pressure manual ventilation
    - Switching from bag to mechanical ventilation via selector switch excludes the valve from the breathing circuit.
- Anesthesia reservoir bag or "breathing bag"
    - Functions
        - Reservoir for exhaled gas and excess fresh gas
        - Means of delivering manual ventilation or assisted spontaneous breathing
        - Visual/tactile means of monitoring spontaneous breathing
        - Partial protection against excessive positive pressure
    - Designed to be the most compliant part of the breathing circuit
        - Distends to several times its nominal volume at a plateau pressure <60 cm H_2O

- Carbon dioxide absorbent
  - Allows exhaled anesthetic vapor to be rebreathed, increasing the efficiency of the anesthetic
  - Most absorbents use calcium hydroxide [$Ca(OH)_2$] to react with the exhaled CO_2
    - $CO_2 + Ca(OH)_2 \rightarrow CaCO_3 + H_2O$ + heat
  - Small amounts of strong bases are typically added to catalyze the reaction.
  - Reaction of the anesthetic agent with strong base
    - Sevoflurane can degrade to compound A, nephrotoxic in rats, but not shown to be clinically significant in humans.
    - Desiccated absorbents can degrade anesthetics and lead to clinically significant carbon monoxide levels.
    - Modern CO_2 absorbents reduce the amount of strong base.
  - Indicator dye changes color when absorptive capacity exhausted.

Additional Components of the Circle Breathing Systems

- Filters and heat moisture exchangers (HMEs)
  - HMEs placed at the Y-connector conserve the patient's warmth and humidity.
  - Bacterial/viral filters prevent transmission of microbes from the patient to the machine, and vice versa.
- Heated humidifiers
  - Circle circuits with active humidification system can help prevent hypothermia.
  - Added cost and complexity
- Inspired oxygen concentration monitor
  - Required to be in the inspiratory limb or sampling from the patient Y-connector
  - Must alarm within 30 seconds if the inspired oxygen concentration drops below a set limit
  - Patient's last line of defense from receiving a hypoxic gas mixture
- Flow sensors
  - Exhaled gas flow sensor is required for display of patient tidal volume.
- Breathing circuit pressure sensors
  - Breathing circuit pressure required to be displayed continuously
  - Required alarms
    - High pressure
    - Continuous positive pressure
    - Negative pressure
    - Threshold pressure (to alert to potential disconnect during mechanical ventilation)

Circle System Function

- Amount of rebreathing depends on fresh gas flow and thus is up to the anesthesia provider.
- Semi-open operation
  - High gas flow at or above patient minute ventilation
  - High venting of waste gas to the scavenge system
- Semi-closed operation
  - Significant rebreathing with some waste flow to the scavenge
  - Low-flow anesthesia is semi-closed operation with fresh gas flow <1 to 2 L/min
  - Advantages
    - Decreased use of volatile agents
    - Improved temperature and humidity control
    - Reduced environmental contamination
  - Disadvantages
    - Difficulty in rapidly changing anesthetic depth
    - Theoretical possibility of accumulating unwanted exhaled gases or anesthetic degradation products
- Closed operation
  - Oxygen inflow set to exactly match metabolic demand
  - Complete rebreathing with no gas vented to scavenge
  - Measured quantity of liquid anesthetic added to the circuit
  - Technically challenging, not routinely used
- Patient inspired gas versus fresh gas composition
  - Gas in the circle system circuit is a mixture of fresh gas flow and patient's expired gas (after CO_2 removal).
  - At low fresh gas flow rates, the contribution of exhaled gas is more pronounced.
  - Exhaled oxygen concentration is lower than inhaled.
    - Potential for hypoxic inhaled oxygen concentration even when fresh gas flow is not hypoxic, particularly at low flows
- Set anesthetic concentration versus end-tidal anesthetic concentration
  - The set anesthetic concentration is the concentration in the fresh gas flow.
  - Exhaled anesthetic concentration may be lower, higher, or the same as the fresh gas concentration.
  - Early in anesthetic course, exhaled anesthetic concentration lower than inhaled due to anesthetic uptake
    - With low flow particularly, the set concentration may need to be significantly higher than the desired end-tidal concentration.
- Circle system disadvantages
  - Complex design with potential for disconnection, misconnection, obstruction, and leak
  - High spontaneous work of breathing
  - Large tubing compressible volume potentially compromises tidal volume delivery.

Mapleson Breathing Systems

- Breathing circuits with fresh gas flow and a reservoir to meet inspiratory flow requirements

- Unlike circle system, bidirectional flow without a CO_2 absorber
  - Higher fresh gas flow required to prevent rebreathing
- Different arrangements of the components lead to different efficiencies (flow required to prevent significant rebreathing).
- Efficiency can differ depending on whether spontaneous or controlled breathing.
- Generally not efficient for providing inhaled anesthetics
  - High gas flows required to prevent rebreathing
  - Difficult to connect to scavenge system

Mapleson Breathing Systems

- Mapleson breathing circuits lack one-way valves and CO_2 absorber.
- All Mapleson breathing circuits are compatible with spontaneous ventilation.
  - Flow rate needed to avoid rebreathing depends on particular circuit.
- Any Mapleson circuit with a reservoir bag can be used to assist spontaneous breathing or provide controlled breaths.
  - Mapelson E (Ayre's T-piece) has no reservoir bag.
- Mapleson F (Jackson-Rees system) often used for anesthesia transport
- Bain breathing system has fresh gas tubing coaxial within the corrugated expiratory limb.

Self-Inflating Manual Resuscitators

- Compressible reservoir that automatically expands on release
- Does not require gas flow for use, unlike anesthesia machine or Mapleson circuits
- Two one-way valves
  - Nonrebreathing valve between bag and patient directs expiratory flow to expiratory port
  - Bag inlet valve opens as bag refills to allow fresh gas and/or room air to be entrained
- Optional features
  - Oxygen reservoir
  - Pop-off valve
  - Positive end-expiratory pressure (PEEP) valve

ANESTHESIA VENTILATORS

Bellows Ventilators

- Bellows serves as volume reservoir for breathing gas.
- Bellows encased in rigid, airtight housing
- Pressurized gas flows into the housing to compress the bellows, thereby delivering a tidal volume.
  - Can be described as "bag in a bottle"
- Standing bellows
  - Also called "ascending bellows," rise on exhalation
  - In event of circuit leak or disconnection, bellows will fall, alerting provider.
- Hanging bellows
  - Also called "descending bellows," fall on exhalation
  - Bellows activity appears normal in event of circuit disconnection.
- Drive gas typically oxygen
  - In event of pipeline failure, gas is conserved by switching to manual ventilation.

Mechanically Driven Piston Ventilators

- Computer-controlled stepper motor controls piston activity to compress gas and deliver tidal volume.
  - Conceptually similar to "syringe plunger"
- Breathing bag serves as the reservoir for rebreathing.
  - Not excluded from the circuit, as with bellows ventilators
- Fresh gas decoupling
  - During inspiration, fresh gas is excluded from being added to the tidal volume.
  - Added instead to the breathing bag
  - On piston return stroke, the piston chamber draws from the breathing bag plus fresh gas flow.

Other Anesthesia Ventilator Systems

- Volume reflector
  - Compact rigid coil interposed between the patient and the breathing bag, or ventilator serves as gas reservoir while preventing mixing between the two ends of the tube.
- Turbine or blower technology
  - Mechanical energy is used to spin a small fan at very high speeds to create pressure and flow.

Target-Controlled Inhalational Anesthesia

- In traditional anesthesia practice, the provider selects the composition and rate of the fresh gas flow.
  - Composition of the inspired gas can differ markedly from the fresh gas composition.
- In target-controlled inhalational anesthesia, the provider selects the desired end-tidal anesthetic agent level and end-tidal oxygen concentration.
  - These goals are achieved by the machine, under electronic control.
  - Proprietary algorithms are used to achieve the targets.
- Advantages include reduced anesthetic consumption.

Fresh Gas Flow Compensation and Fresh Gas Decoupling

- Traditionally, the amount of fresh gas flow that occurred during the inspiratory cycle was added to the tidal volume, such that changes in fresh gas flow could change tidal volume.

- Modern anesthesia workstations have engineering features to prevent this tidal volume variability.
  - Fresh gas flow compensation uses electronic control to adjust bellows movement, for example, as the fresh gas rate changes.
  - Fresh gas decoupling excludes the fresh gas from the inspiratory limb during inspiration.

Scavenge Systems

- A malfunctioning or improperly adjusted scavenge system can cause sustained high pressure or negative pressure in the patient's breathing circuit.
- Pollution of the operating room with waste anesthetic gases can result from problems with the scavenge system.
- Automated machine checks cannot assess the function of the scavenge system.

SCAVENGING SYSTEMS

- Collection and removal of waste anesthetic gas
  - Reduces exposure of operating room (OR) personnel to anesthetic gases
  - Reduces fire risk associated with oxygen-rich environment
- Active versus passive scavenging systems
  - Active systems are connected to a vacuum source.
    - Most hospital systems are active.
  - Passive systems vent the waste gas into the hospital's ventilation system or via a hose directly to the building's exterior.
- Open versus closed scavenging systems
  - Open systems allow room air to be entrained into the waste gas flow.
  - Closed systems do not entrain room air.
- Open, active scavenging interface
  - Reservoir canister open to OR atmosphere
  - Waste anesthetic gas discharged into bottom of canister intermittently
  - Vacuum used to create continuous flow from canister into hospital central vacuum system
  - Continuous flow higher than overall rate of discharge from the anesthesia machine, but intermittent discharges that exceed that rate can be tolerated
  - Entrains room air when vacuum rate exceeds waste gas flow rate
- Closed, active scavenging interface
  - Waste anesthetic gas discharged into a reservoir bag
  - Reservoir bag connected to continuous suction
  - At peak waste gas discharge, bag will fill and empty during inspiratory phase.
  - Safety valves required for positive- and negative-pressure relief
- Disadvantages
  - Added complexity
  - Excessive vacuum can create negative pressure in the breathing circuit.
  - Obstruction of the scavenging system can lead to excess positive pressure and potential barotrauma.
  - Can contribute to distracting alarm conditions
  - Inappropriately set or malfunctioning system can lead to venting of waste gas into the OR.

CHECKING YOUR ANESTHESIA WORKSTATION

- ASA's Recommendations for Preanesthesia Checkout Procedures (2008)
  - 15-item daily checkout
  - 8-item checkout prior to any subsequent anesthetic
  - Focus on *availability* of key equipment and assessing the *function* of that equipment.
- **No automated checkout ensures that the basic safety requirements for safe anesthesia care have been met.**

Item 1: Verify Auxiliary Oxygen Cylinder and Self-Inflating Manual Ventilation Device Are Available and Functioning (Daily)

- Tank must be present and full, with attached regulator, flowmeter, and cylinder wrench as needed.
- A flow-inflating bag (Mapleson-type circuit) is not adequate.

Item 2: Verify Patient Suction Is Adequate to Clear the Airway (Every Case)

- Often set up by an anesthesia technician, but the anesthesia provider must verify this item prior to commencing the anesthetic.

Item 3: Turn On Anesthesia Delivery System and Confirm That AC Power Is Available (Daily)

Item 4: Verify Availability of Required Monitors and Check Alarms (Every Case)

- ASA *Recommendations* include presence of monitoring supplies, functional tests of monitoring equipment, and functional tests of alarm conditions.
- In practice, many anesthesia providers test the function of monitoring equipment by placing them on the patient and do not necessarily test alarm function before each case.

Item 5: Verify That Pressure Is Adequate on the Spare Oxygen Cylinder Mounted on the Anesthesia Machine (Daily)

- Accomplished by opening the tank on the back of the machine and assessing the tank gauge pressure
- Tank should otherwise remain closed to prevent inadvertent emptying.

Item 6: Verify That Piped Gas Pressures Are 50 psig or Higher (Daily)

- Daily check of pipeline pressures
- More detailed inspection and/or test of low-oxygen pressure alarm may be specified in local protocols.

Item 7: Verify That Vaporizers Are Adequately Filled and, if Applicable, That the Filler Ports Are Tightly Closed (Every Case)

- The provider is responsible for ensuring an adequate supply of anesthetic agent if an inhaled anesthetic is planned.

Item 8: Verify That No Leaks Are Present in the Gas Supply Lines Between the Flowmeters and the Common Gas Outlet (Daily)

- Investigate the anesthesia machine for low-pressure leaks in the low-pressure section of the anesthesia machine including the vaporizers.
- Method for carrying this out depends on the model of anesthesia workstation.
- Importance of local protocols and machine familiarity

Item 9: Test Scavenging System Function (Daily)

- Not part of any automated procedure

Item 10: Calibrate, or Verify Calibration of, the Oxygen Monitor, and Check the Low Oxygen Alarm (Daily)

- The oxygen analyzer is the only monitor that detects actual oxygen concentration delivered to the patient.

Item 11: Verify Carbon Dioxide Absorbent Is Not Exhausted (Every Case)

- Color indicator change should be assessed before each case.
- Presence of inspired CO_2 on capnography during the case is evidence of exhausted absorbent.

Item 12: Perform Breathing System Pressure and Leak Testing (Every Case)

- Ability to sustain positive pressure in the breathing circuit must be assessed prior to commencing any anesthetic.
- May be performed manually or as part of an automated machine check

Item 13: Verify That Gas Flows Properly Through the Breathing Circuit During Both Inspiration and Exhalation (Every Case)

- Automated machine checks ineffective at detecting valve obstruction
- "To-and-fro" breathing test, hand-ventilating a test lung, is recommended.

Item 14: Document Completion of Checkout Procedures (Every Case)

- Documentation by the provider in the patient's anesthesia record

Item 15: Confirm Ventilator Settings and Evaluate Readiness to Deliver Anesthesia Care (Anesthesia Timeout) (Every Case)

- Six-item checklist immediately prior to induction of anesthesia
  - Monitors are functional.
  - Capnogram tracing is present.
  - Oxygen saturation by pulse oximetry is being measured.
  - Flowmeter and ventilator settings are properly working.
  - Manual/ventilator switch is set to manual.
  - Vaporizer is adequately filled.

QUESTIONS

FUNCTIONAL ANATOMY OF THE ANESTHESIA WORKSTATION

1. What are the components of the high-pressure section of the anesthesia workstation?
2. Describe the safety system that minimizes the chance of seating the wrong gas cylinder on the anesthesia machine.
3. Explain why auxiliary E-cylinders should be closed during normal operation.
4. In case of a pipeline contamination or crossover (e.g., nitrous oxide in the oxygen pipeline), what will happen if the oxygen E-cylinder is opened?
5. Explain how to calculate the contents remaining in an oxygen E-cylinder and a nitrous oxide E-cylinder.
6. Describe the diameter index safety system (DISS) and quick coupler system.
7. What are some possible complications of the oxygen flush valve?
8. What is the oxygen source for the auxiliary oxygen flowmeter?
9. What is the purpose of a mechanical proportioning system, and how does a proportioning system achieve this goal?
10. What is the purpose of the vaporizer interlock device?
11. What does the ideal gas law state?
12. Explain the concept of partial pressures in a mixture of gases.
13. How are volume percent and partial pressures of a gas in a mixture related?
14. Moving from sea level to elevation, what happens to the volume percent of oxygen in room air? What happens to the partial pressure?
15. Explain the concept of *saturated vapor pressure.*
16. Compare three temperature–versus–saturated vapor pressure curves: (1) water; (2) the volatile anesthetics, such as sevoflurane or isoflurane; and (3) desflurane.
17. Compare the *saturated vapor pressure* of the potent inhaled anesthetics sevoflurane and desflurane with their *clinically useful concentrations* at room temperature (20°C).
18. Describe the operating principles of a variable bypass vaporizer.
19. How does a variable bypass vaporizer compensate for the reduction in temperature that results from vaporization of the liquid anesthetic?

ANESTHETIC BREATHING CIRCUITS

20. Draw a rough schematic of the essential components of a circle anesthesia breathing system.
21. Describe the potential negative effects of unidirectional valves stuck in the open or closed position.
22. What properties of the circle system corrugated breathing tubing should be assessed during the preanesthesia checkout?
23. What are the characteristics of an ideal CO_2 absorbent?
24. What is the net reaction within the CO_2 absorbent? Why have strong bases traditionally been added to the calcium hydroxide?
25. What is a heat moisture exchanger (HME)? Where in the breathing circuit should it be placed?
26. What are bacterial/viral filters? Where should they be placed?
27. What is the difference between using the circle breathing system in a semi-open, semi-closed, and closed fashion?
28. Explain why the inspired oxygen concentration (F_iO_2) can be different from the oxygen concentration in the fresh gas selected by the operator.
29. Why does the set anesthetic concentration in the fresh gas flow need to be higher than the desired alveolar anesthetic concentration early in the course of a low-flow inhaled anesthetic?
30. Given the complexity of the circle breathing system, how should problems with the anesthesia workstation be approached?
31. How is CO_2 rebreathing avoided with the Mapleson breathing systems?

ANESTHESIA VENTILATORS

32. What is the major engineering challenge to anesthesia ventilators compared to ICU ventilators?
33. Describe the function of a bellows ventilator on an anesthesia machine.
34. In case of oxygen pipeline failure, why should the bellows ventilator be switched to manual mode?
35. Describe the function of a piston ventilator on an anesthesia machine.
36. How is target-controlled inhalational anesthesia different from traditional control of the inhaled anesthetic parameters? What are some potential advantages of target-controlled inhalational anesthesia?

SCAVENGING SYSTEMS

37. Why is scavenging of waste anesthetic gases important?
38. What is a passive scavenging system?
39. What is an active scavenging system?
40. Describe an open, active scavenging system.
41. Describe a closed, active scavenging system.

CHECKING YOUR ANESTHESIA WORKSTATION

42. What are the recommendations regarding a preanesthesia checkout procedure?
43. What is the role of an automated anesthesia machine checkout procedure?
44. The first step in the preanesthesia checkout (PAC) has nothing to do with the anesthesia machine, yet it may be the most important. What is it?
45. Does the presence of a non–self-inflating breathing circuit (such as a Jackson-Rees circuit) comply with the PAC recommendations?
46. What risk is incurred if Item 3 (*Turn on Anesthesia Delivery System and Confirm That AC Power Is Available*) is omitted?
47. Describe the elements of the anesthesia workstation that are investigated in Item 8 (*Verify That No Leaks Are Present in the Gas Supply Lines Between the Flowmeters and the Common Gas Outlet*) and the importance of this check.
48. Describe the "flow test" that fulfills preanesthesia checkout Item 13 (*Verify That Gas Flows Properly Through the Breathing Circuit During Both Inspiration and Exhalation*).
49. If the flow test is omitted, what should the anesthesia provider be aware of?
50. What are the six elements of the preanesthesia workstation "Anesthesia Time Out"?

ANSWERS

FUNCTIONAL ANATOMY OF THE ANESTHESIA WORKSTATION

1. The high-pressure section of the anesthesia workstation consists of the gas cylinders and high-pressure regulators. During normal operation, this section is not active because the hospital's central gas supply serves as the primary gas source for the machine. At least one attachment for an oxygen *E-cylinder* serves as a backup source of oxygen in case of failure of the hospital supply source. A *high-pressure regulator* reduces the variable high pressure in the E-cylinder to a lower, nearly constant pressure output to the intermediate-pressure section of the anesthesia machine. (231)
2. Gas cylinders are mounted to the anesthesia machine by a hanger yoke assembly. Each hanger yoke is equipped with the pin index safety system (PISS), which is a safeguard to reduce the risk of the incorrect medical gas cylinder being attached to the yoke. Two metal pins on the yoke assembly are arranged to project precisely into corresponding holes on the cylinder head–valve assembly of the tank. Each gas or combination of gases has a specific pin arrangement. (231–232, Fig. 15.2)
3. During normal conditions (i.e., central oxygen pipeline at appropriate pressure of 50 to 55 psig), an open oxygen E-cylinder does not become depleted because the system preferentially draws from the central pipeline. However, an open oxygen cylinder may allow the anesthesia provider to not be aware of catastrophic pipeline failure. If the oxygen tank is *already open* when pipeline failure occurs, the "low oxygen pressure" alarm, a high-intensity alarm, will not sound until the auxiliary E-cylinder is already depleted. (232)
4. Backup oxygen from the E-cylinder will not flow unless the anesthesia machine is disconnected from the pipeline, since the system is designed to preferentially draw from the pipeline as long as it is adequately pressured. (232)
5. A full oxygen E-cylinder contains 650 L of oxygen at 2200 psig. Since oxygen is a compressed gas, the gauge pressure is directly proportional to the amount of oxygen in the tank. For example, at 1100 psig, there is half a tank left (325 L of oxygen) remaining. By contrast, nitrous oxide is a compressed liquid, so the relationship between its pressure and volume is different from oxygen. A full nitrous oxide E-cylinder contains about 1600 L of gas at 750 psig. As the nitrous oxide gas flows out of the cylinder, further liquid is vaporized, and the pressure in the tank remains unchanged. Therefore the pressure of a nitrous oxide tank remains 750 psig until there is no more liquid in the tank, at which point the pressure begins to fall. By this time, at least 75% of the tank has been depleted. (232)
6. DISS connectors rely on matching diameters in the male and female connections to properly seat and thread the connection. The oxygen, air, and nitrous oxide connections are mutually incompatible. Quick couplers use pins and corresponding slots on the male and female ends, respectively, in order to ensure correct connections. These connectors can be plugged together or released with a simple twisting motion. They are especially appealing for equipment that needs to be moved between locations. (233)
7. Oxygen flushing during the inspiratory phase of positive-pressure ventilation can produce barotrauma if the anesthesia machine does not incorporate a fresh gas decoupling feature or an appropriately adjusted inspiratory pressure limiter. A defective or damaged valve can stick in the fully open position and result in barotrauma. Oxygen flow from a valve sticking in a partially open position can dilute the inhaled anesthetic agent concentration, potentially resulting in awareness under anesthesia. (233)
8. The source of oxygen for the auxiliary flowmeter is the same as for the other oxygen flow control valves—the hospital pipeline or the auxiliary E-cylinder. In cases of suspected hospital oxygen pipeline contamination or crossover, switching to an E-cylinder that is not part of the anesthesia machine, or disconnecting the machine from the pipeline, is imperative. (233)
9. The concern is that a user could mistakenly select oxygen and nitrous oxide flows that result in a hypoxic mixture. The proportioning system prevents this either by interfacing the oxygen and nitrous oxide *flows* (pneumatic–mechanical interface) or by interfacing the oxygen and nitrous oxide valves (mechanical link). Proportioning systems can override flows set by the anesthesia provider, either decreasing nitrous oxide flow or increasing oxygen flow in order to maintain a nonhypoxic fresh gas flow. (234)
10. The vaporizer interlock device ensures that fresh gas cannot flow through more than one vaporizer at a time. The design of vaporizer interlock devices varies significantly. These devices are not immune from failure, with anesthetic overdose as a potential consequence. (234)
11. The pressure within a gas-filled container is the force per unit area exerted on the walls by the gas molecules. According to the ideal gas law, that pressure is directly proportional to the *number* of molecules of gas present

within the space, directly proportional to the *temperature*, and inversely proportional to the *volume* of the container that confines a gas. (234)

12. When a mixture of ideal gases exists in a container, each gas creates its own pressure, which is the same pressure as if the individual gas occupied the container alone. The total pressure may be calculated by simply adding together the pressures of each gas. This is Dalton's law of partial pressures. (234)
13. Volume percent is the percentage of volume occupied by a gas relative to the sum of all gases present. This is the same as the individual gas's contribution to the total pressure (i.e., sum of the partial pressures of each gas present), expressed as a percentage. (234–235)
14. The volume percent of oxygen in room air remains constant at 21% at sea level and elevation. Since the total atmospheric pressure decreases as the elevation increases, the partial pressure of oxygen in room air falls as elevation increases. For example, the partial pressure of oxygen in room air is 160 mm Hg at sea level and 129 mm Hg in Denver, Colorado. (235)
15. In a closed container, anesthetic molecules will continue to escape into the vapor phase until the rate at which molecules evaporate is equal to the rate of return to the liquid phase. When this equilibrium is reached, the composition of the vapor remains constant, and the gas is said to be "saturated" with the volatile liquid. The partial pressure of the anesthetic at equilibrium is known as *saturated vapor pressure* (SVP), or simply *vapor pressure.* Vapor pressure is a physical property of a substance, with each substance having its own unique SVP at any given temperature. (235)
16. At sea level, water boils at 100°C, implying that the SVP of water is 760 mm Hg at that temperature. The SVP of water at body temperature (37°C) is 47 mm Hg. Water at room temperature (20°C) has SVP of ~18 mm Hg. Desflurane is the most volatile of the anesthetics in common clinical use. It boils at 23°C (73°F). At room temperature, its SVP is 669 mm Hg. By comparison, the SVP curves of anesthetics such as sevoflurane and isoflurane are between water and desflurane. At room temperature, sevoflurane's SVP is 157 mm Hg, and isoflurane's is 238 mm Hg. (It is not necessary to memorize these values, but rather to understand the general shape of the curves presented in the figure below. (235)

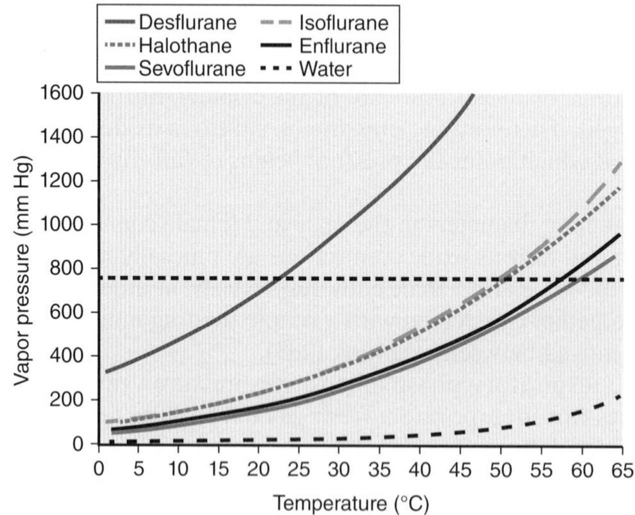

Vapor Pressure–Versus–Temperature Curves for Desflurane, Isoflurane, Halothane, Enflurane, Sevoflurane, and Water. Note that the curve for desflurane differs dramatically from that of the other contemporary inhaled anesthetic agents. Also note that all inhaled agents are more volatile than water. Dashed line indicates 1 atm (760 mm Hg) of pressure, which illustrates the boiling point at sea level (normal boiling point). (From inhaled anesthetic package insert equations and Susay SR, Smith MA, Lockwood GG. The saturated vapor pressure of desflurane at various temperatures. *Anesth Analg*. 1996;83:864–866.)

17. The SVP of the inhaled anesthetics at room temperature (20°C, 68°F) is ≥ 10-fold higher than the clinically useful dose for the inhaled volatile anesthetics. The room temperature SVP of sevoflurane is 157 mm Hg, which at 1 atmosphere would be 21% sevoflurane, whereas the MAC value for sevoflurane is 1.9%. The room temperature SVP of desflurane is 669 mm Hg, which at 1 atmosphere is 88% desflurane, compared to a MAC value of 6% (236).
18. Variable bypass refers to the method of carefully regulating the concentration of vaporizer output by diluting gas fully saturated with anesthetic agent with a larger flow of gas. The concentration control dial determines

the *diverting ratio*, the ratio of the fresh gas flow that continues through the bypass chamber to the flow diverted into the vaporizing chamber. In the vaporizing chamber, the gas flow is exposed to the liquid volatile anesthetic, exiting the chamber nearly saturated with anesthetic vapor. The anesthetic-enriched flow then mixes with the flow that bypassed the vaporizing chamber, with final concentration matching the control dial setting. (236)

19. A temperature-compensating device adjusts the diverting ratio in response to changes in the liquid anesthetic's temperature. As temperature falls, more of the fresh gas flow enters the vaporizing chamber to maintain the output concentration selected on the control dial. This is accomplished by an expansion element or temperature-sensitive bimetallic strip that changes the size of the orifice into the bypass chamber. (236, Fig. 15.4)

ANESTHETIC BREATHING CIRCUITS

20. The essential components of the circle anesthesia breathing system are fresh gas inlet, unidirectional valves (inspiratory and expiratory), corrugated breathing circuit tubing (inspiratory limb and expiratory limb), Y-piece, breathing bag, adjustable pressure-limiting valve, and CO_2 absorbent. In the figure, a bellows ventilator is shown as well. The ventilator "squeezes" the bellows, acting like the anesthesia provider's hands. (239)

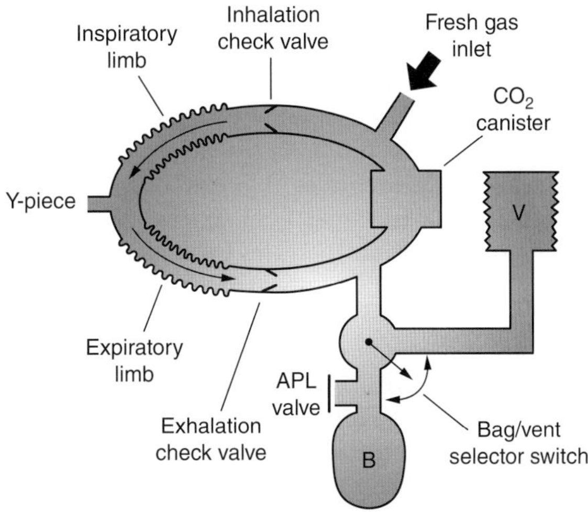

Schematic Diagram of the Components of a Circle Anesthesia Breathing System. Rotation of the bag/vent selector switch permits substitution of an anesthesia machine ventilator (V) for the reservoir bag (B). The volume of the reservoir bag is determined by the fresh gas inflow and adjustment of the adjustable press-limiting (APL) valve. (From Brockwell RC, Andrews JJ. Delivery systems for inhaled anesthetics. In: Barash PG, Cullen BF, Stoelting RK, eds. *Clinical Anesthesia*. Philadelphia, PA: Lippincott Williams & Wilkins; 2006:557–594.)

21. The unidirectional valves in the circle system permit positive-pressure breathing and prevent rebreathing of CO_2. If stuck in the open position, rebreathing of CO_2 may occur. Unidirectional valves stuck in the closed position can cause total occlusion of the circuit, leading to breath stacking and barotrauma. (239)
22. The circle system utilizes large-bore tubing designed to provide minimal resistance and resist kinking. Due to the tubing compliance, some of the tidal volume intended for the patient is lost to distention of the tubing. Many modern workstations perform a compliance test to compensate for this effect. This compliance testing should be performed with the actual circuit that will be used for anesthesia delivery. If circuit length will be increased using an extension, the compliance, leak, and flow tests should be performed with the extension in place. (239)
23. Characteristics of an ideal CO_2 absorbent include a lack of reactivity with common anesthetics, an absence of toxicity, low resistance to airflow, minimal dust production, low cost, ease of handling, and high efficiency. It should also be easy to assess for absorbent depletion (i.e., a diminished ability to remove CO_2). Finally, the container that houses the absorbent should be easy to remove and replace, should maintain breathing circuit integrity if quickly replaced during use, and should impose minimal risk of causing breathing system leaks or obstruction. (240)

24. Carbon dioxide reacts with calcium hydroxide to yield calcium carbonate, water, and heat:

$$CO_2 + Ca(OH)_2 \rightarrow CaCO_3 + H_2O + \text{heat}$$

The reaction above is slow. Carbon dioxide reacts quickly with strong bases such as sodium hydroxide or potassium hydroxide. Because the strong bases are regenerated in the subsequent step, they are catalysts for the net reaction.

25. HMEs function by absorbing warmth and moisture as exhaled gas moves through in one direction, and then returning that warmth and humidity to the next breath as the inspired gas moves through in the other direction. HMEs therefore function only when placed between the Y-connector and the patient. (241)
26. Bacterial/viral filters are used to prevent the transmission of microbes from the patient to the machine and hence potentially to other patients. Such filters are often placed on the expiratory limb of the anesthesia circuit where it connects to the anesthesia machine, and many circuit manufacturers ship their circuits with this filter already in place. During the COVID-19 pandemic, the addition of a second filter at the Y-connector was recommended for COVID-positive patients. HME filters (HMEFs) are available to serve both functions at the patient Y-connector. (241)
27. The extent of rebreathing of exhaled gas depends on the fresh gas flow rate. A circle system operated in a *semi-open* manner connotes a high fresh gas flow rate with minimal rebreathing and high venting of waste gas through the APL valve or the waste gas valve of the ventilator. In *semi-closed* operation, significant rebreathing occurs, but some waste flow is vented to scavenge. A *closed* system is one in which the rate of oxygen inflow exactly matches metabolic demand, rebreathing is complete, and no waste gas is vented (APL valve remains closed). A volatile anesthetic agent is added to the breathing circuit in liquid form in precise amounts or is initially introduced through the vaporizer. (242)
28. The gas within the circle system is filled with a combination of the patient's exhaled gases (after removal of CO_2) plus the fresh gas flow that is added. As the fresh gas flow rate decreases, the proportion of the circuit that is made up of the patient's exhaled gas increases. The patient's exhaled gas will have a lower oxygen concentration than the inhaled, and at low fresh gas flow, this exhaled oxygen concentration will have a greater contribution to the circuit concentration than the fresh gas concentration. Therefore the inspired oxygen concentration reaching the patient will be lower than the fresh gas oxygen concentration that is first entering the circuit. (242)
29. Early in an inhaled anesthetic, a larger proportion of the volatile agent in the inspired breath will be taken up by the patient, with less exhaled back into the circuit. The concentration of anesthetic in the circuit will therefore be significantly lower than the concentration in the fresh gas flow. As the patient's tissues become saturated with anesthetic, the uptake of anesthetic agent decreases, and the exhaled concentration of agent is similar to the fresh gas concentration of agent. (242)
30. *Ventilate first and troubleshoot once the patient is safe.* No anesthetic should commence without a self-inflating resuscitation bag and oxygen E-cylinder present. (243)
31. Unlike the circle system, there is bidirectional flow in the Mapleson systems, and they lack a CO_2 absorber. To eliminate CO_2 and prevent rebreathing, they depend on an appropriate fresh gas inflow rate. If fresh gas flow rates are inadequate, the dead space and alveolar gas are not cleared during the expiratory phase, and there will be rebreathing. The amount of CO_2 rebreathing with each system is affected by multiple factors, including the fresh gas inflow rate, minute ventilation, and ventilation mode (spontaneous or controlled). In spontaneous ventilation, the Mapleson A is most efficient (requires the least fresh gas flow to prevent rebreathing), while it is the least efficient in controlled ventilation. The other Mapleson systems do not exhibit such a marked difference between spontaneous and controlled ventilation. (243, Fig 15.7)

ANESTHESIA VENTILATORS

32. ICU ventilators are open circuit, using entirely fresh gas for each breath, and venting all exhaled gas into the patient's room. The anesthesia workstation must collect and redeliver the patient's exhaled gas. (245)
33. The flexible, collapsible bellows are housed in a rigid airtight housing. Pressurized gas flows into the housing, thereby compressing the bellows. As the bellows is compressed, the breathing gas is delivered to the patient. On exhalation, a mixture of the patient's exhaled gas and fresh gas flowing into the breathing circuit refills the bellows. Excess circuit gas is vented to the scavenging system during the expiratory pause. The bellows serves as a volume reservoir for breathing gas, and the overall function is similar to a "bag in a bottle." (245–246, Figs 15.10 and 15.11)
34. Many bellows anesthesia machines use oxygen as the drive gas. The amount of oxygen consumed by the anesthesia machine will equal the amount of oxygen selected for fresh gas flow *plus* an amount approximately

equal to the delivered minute ventilation. An E-cylinder will last much longer supplying oxygen fresh gas flow to the circle system with manual ventilation than with mechanical ventilation. (245–246)

35. Piston ventilators control the movement of a piston, much like the plunger of a syringe in a cylinder of essentially zero compliance. The ventilator has primary control over the volume displaced in the circuit and uses the data from pressure sensors to create pressure control breaths; the computerized controls can support a variety of ventilator modes. (246)
36. On anesthesia machines where the flow control valves and the anesthetic vaporizers are under electronic control, it is possible to design a system of target-controlled inhalational anesthesia. The user can select end-tidal anesthetic agent and end-tidal oxygen concentrations. The programmed algorithm adjusts the fresh gas composition and flow rate to achieve those targets. The major advantage of the target control is reduced consumption of anesthetic agent. The computer control is better able to achieve low fresh gas flow rates and the targeted parameters than anesthesia providers. A vigilant anesthesia provider could achieve similar results but at the expense of significant manipulation of the anesthesia machine's settings. (247)

SCAVENGING SYSTEMS

37. The fresh gas flow rates used during most anesthetic regimens deliver more volatile anesthetic agent and nitrous oxide than necessary, as well as more oxygen than is being consumed. Without scavenging, operating room personnel would be exposed to anesthetic gases, and there could be an increased risk of an oxygen-rich environment supporting combustion. (247)
38. Passive scavenging systems simply vent the waste gas into a heating, ventilation, and air conditioning (HVAC) system or through a hose to the building's exterior. Passive systems are not common in contemporary operating rooms. (247)
39. In active scavenging systems, the scavenge is connected to a vacuum source, such as the hospital's suction system. (247)
40. An open, active scavenge interface uses a reservoir, typically a canister, that is open to the operating room atmosphere. Vacuum is used to create a high continuous flow from the canister into the hospital central vacuum system. Waste gas is intermittently discharged into the bottom of the canister, but because of the canister's reservoir function, as long as the total evacuation rate is higher than the average waste gas flow, the system can tolerate intermittent discharges that briefly exceed that rate. The excess vacuum flow is obtained from entrained room air. The open system does not require positive- or negative-pressure relief valves because the canister is open to the atmosphere. (247–248, Fig. 15.12)
41. In a closed, active scavenging system, waste gas is discharged from the anesthesia machine into a reservoir bag that is connected to continuous suction. With peak discharge of waste gas (as at patient exhalation), the bag will expand, subsequently emptying during the inspiratory phase. The vacuum control valve must be adjusted so that the reservoir bag remains properly inflated, neither overdistended nor completely deflated. This type of scavenging system requires at least two valves. If the scavenge system pressure exceeds a preset pressure, gas is vented to the operating room through the positive-pressure relief valve. If the scavenge system pressure is too negative, then room air is entrained through the negative-pressure relief valve. (248)

CHECKING YOUR ANESTHESIA WORKSTATION

42. A complete preanesthesia checkout procedure (PAC) consisting of 15 items is recommended by the American Society of Anesthesiologists (ASA) each day before the anesthesia workstation is first used or whenever the anesthesia workstation is moved to a new location. An abbreviated version consisting of eight items should be performed before each subsequent case. (248, Table 15.3)
43. None of the automated checkout procedures included on contemporary anesthesia machines can ensure that the basic safety requirements for safe delivery of anesthesia care have been met. Furthermore, many anesthesia providers are not fully aware of what elements are checked by the automated procedures. Even review of user's manuals does not always make it obvious. (248)
44. Item 1 in the PAC list is *Verify Auxiliary Oxygen Cylinder and Self-Inflating Manual Ventilation Device Are Available and Functioning*. The anesthesia provider must always be prepared to keep the patient alive without the assistance of the anesthesia machine. The most important safety check in any anesthesia location prior to commencing the day's procedures is the presence of a self-inflating manual ventilation device and a source of oxygen that is separate from the anesthesia workstation and hospital pipeline oxygen supply. These items must be present at every anesthetizing location. (249)

45. A non–self-inflating Mapleson-type breathing circuit is *not* adequate to meet this item. The presence of a self-inflating resuscitation bag is required. (249)
46. If a case is inadvertently started on battery backup power, the first obvious sign of power failure can be catastrophic system shutdown when the backup batteries are exhausted. Prior to commencing the day's anesthetic procedures, functioning AC power should be verified. (250)
47. The daily check for leaks in the low-pressure system, from the flow control valves, through the vaporizers, and to the common gas outlet, tests for occult leaks that might contribute to problems with ventilation, a hypoxic gas mixture, or inadequate depth of anesthesia. Some anesthesia workstations include an outlet check valve, mandating a negative pressure leak check, covered in users' manuals. Additionally, most vaporizer leaks are not detected unless the vaporizer is set to *on*. Therefore a thorough low-pressure leak test can require testing multiple vaporizers, depending on machine configuration. Some automated machine checks may have the ability to test for leaks in the vaporizer, but many do not, emphasizing the need for machine familiarity. (250–251)
48. In the "flow test," a test lung is placed at the Y-piece, and the anesthesia provider assesses inspiratory and expiratory flow by alternately compressing the breathing bag and the test lung. The unidirectional valves can be visually inspected; obstructed valves can also be felt during the to-and-fro breathing. (251)
49. Although the flow test is recommended prior to every anesthetic, in practice it is often omitted. If omitted, providers must be cognizant of the fact that unidirectional valve malfunction and breathing circuit obstruction have not been ruled out before starting the case. Automated machine checks typically do not assess for (or detect) obstruction to flow within the breathing circuit. (251)
50. The final item in the 15-item checklist is *Confirm Ventilator Settings and Evaluate Readiness to Deliver Anesthesia Care*, also called Anesthesia Time Out. The anesthesia provider confirms the following six items prior to the induction of anesthesia: (1) monitors are functional; (2) capnogram tracing is present; (3) oxygen saturation by pulse oximetry is being measured; (4) flowmeter and ventilator settings are properly working; (5) manual/ventilator switch is set to manual; (6) vaporizer is adequately filled. (252)

Chapter

16 AIRWAY MANAGEMENT

Maytinee Lilaonitkul and Andrew Infosino

ANATOMY AND PHYSIOLOGY OF THE UPPER AIRWAY

Nasal Cavity

- Function – warms and humidifies inspired air
- Accounts for 50% to 75% of total airway resistance
- Sensory innervation
  - Ethmoidal branch of ophthalmic nerve (cranial nerve [CN] II)
  - Maxillary division of trigeminal nerve (CN V)

Oral Cavity and Pharynx

- Borders of oral cavity – hard and soft palates (superior), faucial arches (posterior), buccal mucosa (lateral), and tongue (floor)
- Pharynx composed of nasopharynx, oropharynx, and hypopharynx
- Airway resistance mainly caused by the tongue, controlled by genioglossus muscle
- Sensory innervation
  - Oral cavity and anterior two-thirds tongue: maxillary division of trigeminal nerve
  - Posterior one-third tongue, soft palate, and oropharynx: glossopharyngeal nerve
  - Hypopharynx: superior laryngeal nerve, a branch of the vagus nerve

Larynx

- Located at level of 3rd to 6th cervical vertebrae
- Function – protects lower airways and prevents aspiration
- Cartilages
  - Three unpaired – epiglottis, thyroid, cricoid
  - Three paired – arytenoids, corniculates, cuneiforms
- Cricoid cartilage is the only cartilage with full ring structure.
- Vocal cords are the narrowest part of adult airway.
- Motor and sensory innervation: superior laryngeal nerve (CN X) and recurrent laryngeal nerve (CN X)

Trachea

- 10 to 15 cm long and connects the larynx to the carina
- Sensory innervation: recurrent laryngeal nerve (CN X)

AIRWAY ASSESSMENT

History and Anatomic Examination

- Worsening airway symptoms (e.g., hoarseness or stridor)
- Medical history of obstructive sleep apnea (OSA), radiation therapy to the neck, or risk of pulmonary aspiration
- Congenital or acquired conditions affecting the airway (e.g., trauma, neoplasia, infection)
- Previous surgery to airway
- A review of previous anesthesia records, including any difficulty encountered with airway management

Physical Examination Findings

Oropharyngeal Space

- Predictors of difficult direct laryngoscopy
  - Mallampati score of III or IV
  - An interincisor gap <4.5 cm and/or a receding mandible, micrognathia
  - Upper lip bite test (ULBT) class III (lower incisors cannot bite upper lip)

Thyromental/Sternomental Distance

- Measurements correlating with poor laryngoscopic view
  - Thyromental distance <6 cm or 3 fingerbreadths
  - Sternomental distance <12.5 to 13.5 cm.

Atlanto-occipital Extension/Cervical Spine Mobility

- Limitations in neck extension/flexion can lead to difficulty aligning oral, pharyngeal, and laryngeal axes during direct laryngoscopy.

Body Habitus/Other Examination Findings

- Findings predicting difficulty in both mask ventilation and direct laryngoscopy include male sex, age ≥46 years, BMI ≥30 kg/m^2, presence of a thick neck, teeth, and/or beard.

Cricothyroid Membrane

- Important to identify before airway instrumentation in patients with difficult airways
- Located at superior border of cricoid cartilage

Additional Airway Investigations

- Imaging (CT/MRI) for detailed evaluation of complex airway pathologies
- Nasal endoscopy for pathologic airway swelling, distortion, or periglottic lesions

Principles of Preoperative Airway Assessment

- Always look at previous anesthetic records for any previous airway management difficulties.
- Using multiple airway evaluation tests offers greater predictive value of a difficult airway than any single test.
- Predicting for difficulty in ventilating and oxygenating is more important than predicting for difficulty in laryngoscopy.
- Aspiration is the most common cause of death among major anesthesia airway complications – ALWAYS assess for risk of aspiration.
- Assess and prepare for patients at risk of rapid desaturation postinduction as this will affect the time available to secure the airway.

AIRWAY MANAGEMENT TECHNIQUES

Face Mask Ventilation

- Difficulties are caused by inadequate seal, excessive gas leak, or resistance.
- Factors associated with difficult mask ventilation: age >55 years, BMI >30 kg/m^2, a beard, lack of teeth, OSA, Mallampati class III or IV, history of neck radiation, male sex, limited ability to protrude the mandible, and history of an airway mass or tumor

Preoxygenation

- Breathing 100% oxygen via well-sealed facemask to achieve an end-tidal oxygen level >90%
  - 3 minutes of tidal volume breathing or 8 deep breaths in 60 seconds
- Allows for approximately 9 minutes of apnea without desaturation in a healthy, nonobese adult
  - Decreased functional residual capacity will decrease time to oxygen desaturation with apnea (e.g., obesity, pregnancy).
  - For obese patients, 25-degree head-up position or noninvasive positive-pressure ventilation can improve preoxygenation.
- Facemask ventilation technique
  - Left hand: jaw thrust, chin lift, and facemask counterpressure to achieve adequate seal
  - Right hand: positive-pressure ventilation via reservoir bag at insufflation pressure <20 cm H_2O to minimize insufflation of the stomach

Managing Inadequate Facemask Ventilation

Signs
- Absent or minimal chest rise/breath sounds
- Absent or inadequate exhaled carbon dioxide
- Stomach insufflation

Late signs
- Cyanosis
- Low oxygen saturation
- Hemodynamic changes due to hypoxemia or hypercarbia

Management
- Airway adjuncts
  - Oral airways (require deep anesthesia to prevent gag reflex)
  - Nasal airways (relatively contraindicated in patients with coagulopathy or basilar skull fractures)
- Shaving or trimming a beard prior to induction
- Use two-handed facemask technique; a second person can assist with positive-pressure ventilation.
- Ensure adequate depth of anesthesia.
- If all measures fail, proceed to supraglottic airway insertion or intubation.

Supraglottic Airways

- Sized according to the patient's weight
- Uses
  - Primary mode of airway management in ambulatory surgery
  - Conduit for endotracheal intubation
  - Rescue oxygenation and ventilation
- Contraindicated in patients with high risk of aspiration
- Assess risk/benefit if patient is nonsupine or surgery is abdominal or of long duration.
- Advantages over ETT: easier to place, less hemodynamic changes with insertion and removal, less coughing and bucking with removal, and no need for neuromuscular blockade to facilitate placement
- Adequate tidal volume should be achieved with minimal oropharyngeal leak at positive pressure breaths <20 cm H_2O.

Managing Unsuccessful Supraglottic Airway Placement
Predictors of difficult SGA placement or failure ▪ Small mouth opening ▪ Supraglottic or epiglottic disease ▪ Fixed cervical spine ▪ Poor dentition/edentulous or large incisors ▪ Male sex ▪ Surgical table rotation ▪ Increased BMI (>30kg/m^2) **Common causes** ▪ Inadequate depth of anesthesia ▪ Downfolding of epiglottis ▪ Inadequate seal **Management** ▪ Increasing depth of anesthesia ▪ Repositioning the patient's head or SGA ▪ Adjusting the amount of air in the cuff ▪ Upsizing or downsizing the SGA ▪ Convert to an ETT if problems persist despite these maneuvers

Laryngeal Mask Airways (LMAs)

- LMA Unique: single-use version of LMA classic
- LMA Fastrach: used with special ETT that aligns better to airway
- LMA ProSeal/Supreme: improved oropharyngeal seal allows higher airway pressures with second lumen for esophageal vent or orogastric tube placement
- LMA Flexible: wire-reinforced, flexible airway tube

Air-Q Intubating Laryngeal Airways

- Shorter shaft, larger internal diameter, shape, and detachable connector facilitate endotracheal intubation.

i-gel Supraglottic Airways

- Single use with soft, preshaped, gel-like, noninflatable cuff with a gastric port and a wide-bore airway channel to facilitate endotracheal intubation

Endotracheal Intubation

- Direct laryngoscopy is the most common way to secure an airway.
- Proper positioning to align the oral, pharyngeal, and laryngeal axes achieves direct view of the glottic opening.
- Laryngoscopic view is described according to the Cormack–Lehane classification system.
  - Grade III or IV views are associated with difficult intubation.

Rapid-Sequence Induction of Anesthesia with Cricoid Pressure

- Definition: rapid induction of anesthesia and neuromuscular blockade followed immediately by laryngoscopy and intubation
- Cricoid pressure – external downward compression of the cricoid cartilage to occlude the esophagus – is used to prevent aspiration of gastric contents although its use remains controversial.
- Cricoid pressure can be released if it impedes oxygenation, ventilation, or visualization of the glottis.

Difficult Airway Management

- A difficult airway includes difficult mask or SGA ventilation, laryngoscopy, or endotracheal intubation.
- Difficult endotracheal intubation is defined as the inability to intubate despite multiple attempts; occurs in up to 7% of patients.
- Inadequate airway planning and inappropriate management are the main factors leading to patient harm in a difficult airway.
- The most common failures include perseverance on failed techniques, failure to use an SGA for rescue oxygenation, delay in calling for help, and delay in attempting a surgical airway.
- Cognitive aids such as difficult airway algorithms should be used (See algorithm on next page).
- Consider these management principles in patients with anticipated difficult airway:
  - Awake intubation vs. intubation after the induction of general anesthesia
  - Initial intubation method via noninvasive vs. invasive techniques
  - Video laryngoscopy as an initial approach to intubation
  - Maintaining vs. ablating spontaneous ventilation
- Perform awake intubation, when appropriate, in patients with one or more of the following risk factors in addition to a suspected difficult intubation.
  - Expected difficult ventilation with facemask or SGA
  - Increased risk of aspiration
  - Poor tolerance of brief apneic episodes
  - Expected difficulty with emergency invasive airway rescue technique
- A difficult airway cart should be immediately available.
- Apneic oxygenation techniques after induction of anesthesia can delay the onset of hypoxia and allow more time for safe airway manipulation.
  - Application of nasal cannula oxygen with flow rates up to 15 L/min
  - Application of high-flow nasal cannula with flow rates of 30 to 70 L/min in high-risk patients

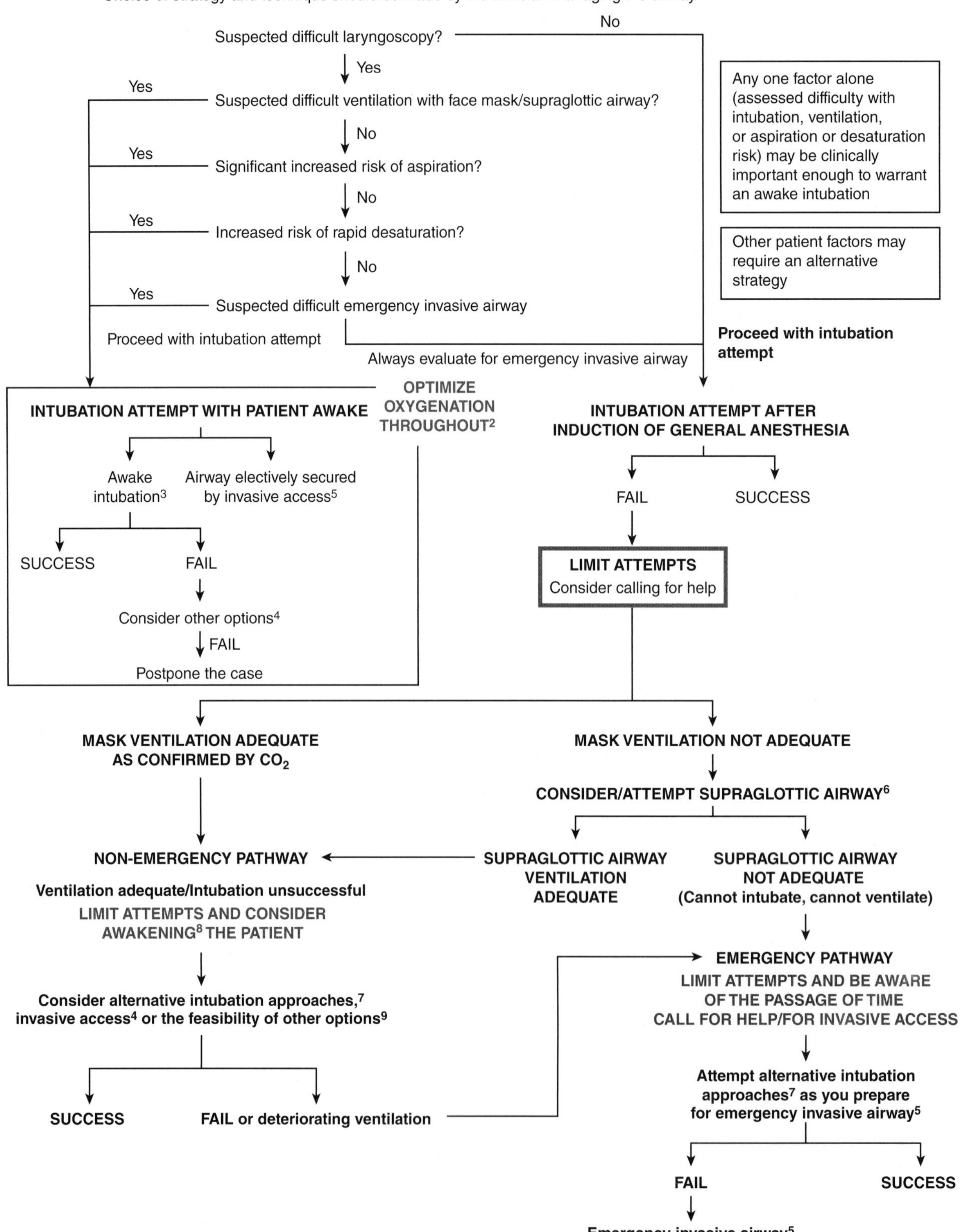

Figure from Apfelbaum JL, Hagberg CA, Connis RT, et al. 2022 American Society of Anesthesiologists practice guidelines for management of the difficult airway. Anesthesiology. 2021. doi: 10.1097/ ALN.0000000000004002. Epub ahead of print. PMID: 34762729.

Principles of Difficult Airway Management

- Have the "difficult airway equipment cart" and algorithm available in the room.
- Ensure that a skilled individual is present or immediately available to assist.
- Remember that patients do not die from failure to intubate but from failure to oxygenate.
- Consider awake intubation in patients with suspected difficult laryngoscopy and suspected 1) difficult face-mask/SGA ventilation, 2) difficult invasive airway, 3) increased risk of aspiration, and 4) increased risk of rapid desaturation.
- In an asleep patient with a difficult airway, always consider an alternative device and ways to optimize the technique (e.g., repositioning) with each new attempt.
- Limit the number of attempts at tracheal intubation or supraglottic airway placement to avoid potential injury and complications.
- Make the decision to perform cricothyroidotomy early in a "can't intubate, can't ventilate" situation. This should be performed by trained personnel whenever possible.

Direct Laryngoscopy

Technique for Direct Laryngoscopy

- Hold the laryngoscope in the left hand.
- Insert the blade on the right side of the mouth and move it to midline, shifting the tongue to the left. Then advance forward and centrally toward the epiglottis.
- Hold the wrist rigid as the laryngoscope is lifted along the axis of the handle to cause anterior displacement of the soft tissues. Rotating or tilting of the handle can damage the patient's upper teeth or gums and must be avoided.
- Manipulation of the patient's thyroid cartilage externally on the neck, using backward upward rightward pressure (BURP), may improve laryngoscopy view.
- Hold the endotracheal tube (ETT) in the right hand and advance it toward the glottis from the right side of the mouth until the proximal end of the cuff is 1 to 2 cm past the vocal cords. Some ETTs will have a black line to guide the optimal position of the vocal cords.
- Carefully remove the laryngoscope blade and inflate the endotracheal cuff with air to create a seal. This seal facilitates positive-pressure ventilation of the lungs and decreases aspiration risk.
- Cuff pressure should be <30 cm H_2O to minimize mucosal ischemia of the trachea.
- Correct placement in the trachea can be confirmed by:
  - Detection of end-tidal CO_2 with capnography (gold standard)
  - Symmetric chest rise and bilateral breath sounds with manual ventilation, cuff palpation at sternal notch
- The ETT can be secured in position with tape, commonly at 21- to 23-cm ETT marking at the lips in adults.

Choice of Direct Laryngoscope Blade

- Curved laryngoscope blade (e.g., Macintosh 3 – standard size for adults)
  - Larger flange more easily displaces tongue to the left.
  - Tip is advanced into the vallecula to elevate epiglottis.
- Straight blade (e.g., Miller 2 – standard size for adults)
  - Smaller profile is beneficial for patients with a small mouth opening.
  - Tip is passed beneath the laryngeal surface to directly elevate the epiglottis.

Video Laryngoscopy

- A video laryngoscope has a video camera at the distal end of the blade, enabling the glottis to be visualized indirectly on a video monitor without alignment of the oral, pharyngeal, and tracheal axes (e.g., GlideScope, C-MAC, McGrath Scope).
- It has higher first-pass intubation success rates than direct laryngoscopy.
- Uses
  - Initial approach for patients with anticipated difficult airway (e.g., micrognathia, inability to flex or extend neck)
  - Initial approach for high-acuity patients in the emergency department or critical care setting
  - Rescue technique for failed direct laryngoscopy
  - Teaching tool for novice trainees
  - Patients with transmissible respiratory infection (e.g., tuberculosis, COVID-19)
- Video laryngoscope blades include the curved Macintosh-style blades, straight Miller-style blades, and angulated blades.
- Angulated blades – fixed angle (60 degrees for GlideScope)
  - Visualization of the glottis achieved with minimal flexion or extension of the patient's head and neck
  - Useful in patients with anterior larynxes
  - Blade is inserted midline in the mouth, and the ETT requires a preshaped stylet that matches the curvature of the blade

ETT Stylets, Introducers, and Airway Exchange Catheters

Stylets

- Curve and stiffen the ETT, facilitating initial passage through the glottis
- The distal tip of the stylet should not protrude past the end of the ETT to minimize the potential for airway trauma.

Introducers (Gum Elastic Bougie, Frova Intubating Introducer)

- Used to facilitate intubation in patients with a poor laryngoscopic view
- Distal angulated tip that, when passed into the glottis, results in feeling characteristic clicking against the tracheal cartilages. This will not be felt in esophageal placements.
- An ETT (≥6.0 mm) is advanced over the introducer into the airway, and the introducer is then removed.
- The gum elastic bougie is solid, whereas the Frova intubating introducer has an internal channel to accommodate a stiffening rod or allow jet ventilation.

Aintree Intubation Catheter (AIC)

- Has a 19 Fr catheter with a 4.7-mm lumen that can accommodate a standard adult flexible fiberoptic bronchoscope
- Primarily used for intubating (ETT size ≥7.0 mm) through an SGA with fiberoptic guidance
- Rapi-Fit adapters allow for connection to a jet ventilator, anesthesia circuit, or Ambu bag

Cook Airway Exchange Catheter (AEC)

- Designed for ETT exchange in 11, 14, and 19 Fr sizes, all 83 cm in length
- Hollow lumen allows for jet ventilation or oxygenation through a connection to an anesthesia circuit or Ambu bag.
- Insertion to 20- to 22-cm depth is usually sufficient for orotracheal tube exchange.
- Laryngoscopy can help displace soft tissue and facilitate replacement of an ETT over the AEC.
- The Cook extra-firm soft tip AEC is 100 cm long, available in 11 or 14 Fr sizes, designed for double-lumen tube exchange.

Flexible Fiberoptic Endotracheal Intubation

- Can be useful for difficult airway management
- Performed through the nose or mouth in awake, sedated, or anesthetized patients
- The approach is dependent on the risk of a difficult airway and the cooperation of the patient.
- The nasal route is relatively contraindicated in patients with platelet abnormalities or coagulopathy.
- May be challenging in patients with masses in the upper airway (e.g., infection, neoplasm, edema) and those with copious secretions or bleeding
- Equipment, medication setup, and patient preparation are paramount to the success of fiberoptic endotracheal intubation.

Awake Fiberoptic Endotracheal Intubation

- Usually indicated in patients with a history of a difficult airway or an unstable cervical spine as it allows for continuation of spontaneous breathing and assessment of neurologic function after intubation
- Patient cooperation is critical to this technique.
- The nasal route is usually easier because the angle of curvature of the ETT naturally approximates that of the patient's upper airway.

Patient Preparation

- Administer an antisialagogue (glycopyrrolate 0.2–0.4 mg IV) preprocedure
- Sedation can be carefully administered.

Airway Anesthesia

- Airway anesthesia is achieved by topical application of local anesthetic and/or by specific nerve blocks.
  - Total maximum dose of lidocaine should not exceed 7 mg/kg to minimize risk of local anesthesia toxicity.
- Topical anesthesia for the airway
  - Spray (upper airway) or nebulize (smaller particles to lower airway)
    - 4% lidocaine is used due to the broad therapeutic window.
    - Avoid local anesthetics with specific risks, including benzocaine (methemoglobinemia) and tetracaine (narrow therapeutic window).

Nose and Nasopharynx

- Vasoconstriction of nasal vessels with 0.05% oxymetazoline hydrochloride (HCl) spray intranasally to minimize bleeding risk
  - Phenylephrine is systemically absorbed and should be avoided.
- Topical anesthesia: lidocaine solution applied directly via soaked cotton-tipped swabs or pledgets, or by nasal airways externally covered in lidocaine ointment

Tongue and Oropharynx

- Atomized or nebulized 4% lidocaine solution
- Gargle 2% viscous lidocaine for tongue and oropharynx
- Glossopharyngeal nerve block
  - Inject 2 mL of 2% lidocaine 0.5 cm deep at the base of each anterior tonsillar pillar.

Larynx and Trachea

- Atomized or nebulized 4% lidocaine solution
- Superior laryngeal nerve block
  - 22- to 25-G needle is "walked" off the cephalad edge of the thyroid cartilage or caudal edge of the hyoid bone. Inject 2 to 3 mL 2% lidocaine on each side.
- Transtracheal block
  - Advance a 20-G IV catheter through the cricothyroid membrane with an attached syringe filled with 4 mL 2% lidocaine.
  - Once air is aspirated, remove the needle, and advance the catheter. Inject the lidocaine at end-expiration to enhance spread during inspiration.

Fiberoptic Intubation Techniques

Technique for Fiberoptic Intubation

- Soften the ETT in warm water and lubricate before use.
- Suction must be immediately available throughout the procedure.
- For nasal intubation, advance the lubricated ETT into the pharynx aiming posteriorly, and use as a conduit for the fiberoptic scope.
- For oral intubation, use a channeled oral airway or have an assistant extend the patient's tongue to create pharyngeal space.
- Identify the tracheal rings and carina as the fiberoptic bronchoscope passes through the vocal cords.
- Place the bronchoscope 4 to 5 cm above the carina, and advance the ETT over it.
- Resistance to advancement often means that the ETT is affected on an arytenoid, and the ETT should be rotated and gently advanced.
- Use the fiberoptic bronchoscope to confirm depth of ETT placement before withdrawing it.

Fiberoptic Endotracheal Intubation After Induction of General Anesthesia

- This technique is used when the patient is not cooperative or when mask ventilation is not anticipated to be difficult.
- It can be done either through the nose or the mouth with the patient breathing spontaneously or under controlled ventilation.
- Supplemental oxygen can be delivered via nasal cannula or a nasal airway connected to the anesthesia breathing circuit during the procedure.
- Oropharyngeal space can be increased by jaw thrust, specialized oral airways, inflating the ETT cuff in the pharynx, or applying traction on the tongue.

Rigid Fiberoptic Intubating Stylets

- Incorporates fiberoptic imaging allowing visualization from the tip of the ETT
- ETT is loaded onto the rigid shaft of the stylet and advanced into the trachea
- Can be used with or without direct laryngoscopy for normal and difficult airways
- Useful for patients with limited mouth opening or cervical spine mobility
- High failure rate among novice users

INVASIVE AIRWAY ACCESS

- Part of difficult airway algorithm after unsuccessful intubation, and oxygenation or ventilation is not possible via mask or SGA.
- Relative contraindications include disease of the anterior aspect of the neck (tumors, infection, stenosis), laryngeal or tracheal disruption, or coagulopathy.

Techniques for Invasive Airway Access

Cricothyroidotomy

- Can be planned when a noninvasive technique is not possible (e.g., facial trauma, upper airway bleeding, or upper airway obstruction) or emergent to secure an airway
- Performed with patient in sniffing position
- Percutaneous cricothyrotomy
  - Uses the Seldinger technique
  - A needle is advanced at a 90-degree angle through the cricothyroid membrane while aspirating with an attached syringe.
  - Once air is aspirated, the needle should be directed *caudally* at a 30- to 45-degree angle.
  - A guidewire is then advanced through the needle, followed by removal of the needle, a small incision adjacent to the wire, and placement of a combined dilator and airway.
  - The wire and dilator are removed, leaving the airway in place.
- Surgical cricothyrotomy
  - A vertical skin incision, followed by a horizontal incision of the cricothyroid membrane through which a standard ETT or tracheostomy tube is placed
  - A tracheal hook, dilator, AEC, or bougie can assist in placement of the airway.

Transtracheal Jet Ventilation Via the Cricothyroid Membrane

- Puncture the cricothyroid membrane at a 90-degree angle with a catheter over a needle connected to a syringe.
- When air is aspirated, the catheter should be advanced off the needle into the trachea angled 30 to 45 degrees *caudally*.
- The catheter is then connected to a high-pressure oxygen source.
- Potential complications include pneumothorax, pneumomediastinum, bleeding, infection, and subcutaneous emphysema.

Retrograde Endotracheal Intubation

- Used in difficult airway cases, particularly when there is bleeding, airway trauma, decreased mouth opening, or limited neck movement
- The cricothyroid membrane is punctured with a needle attached to a syringe.
- After aspiration of air to confirm that the needle is in the trachea, the syringe is detached and a guidewire is threaded through the needle in a *cephalad* direction and then retrieved from the mouth with a forceps.
- An ETT is threaded over the wire until it stops on impact with the anterior wall of the trachea. Guidewire tension is reduced, allowing further passage of ETT before wire removal.

Endotracheal Extubation

- Can be performed awake (generally safest) or deep (before the return of protective airway reflexes)
- Endotracheal extubation during a light level of anesthesia (disconjugate gaze or breath-holding) increases the risk of laryngospasm.

- Deep extubation is associated with less coughing and hemodynamic effects on emergence.
  - May be beneficial in patients at risk for adverse effects of increased intracranial or intraocular pressure, bleeding into the surgical wound, or wound dehiscence
  - Relative contraindications include previous difficult facemask ventilation or endotracheal intubation, high risk of aspiration, restricted access to the airway, obstructive sleep apnea, or morbid obesity.
- Extubation of the trachea is always elective, and postponing extubation may be appropriate in some cases when the patient has increased risk for requiring reintubation.

Steps for Endotracheal Extubation

- Prior to extubation
  - Reverse any residual neuromuscular blockade.
  - Administer 100% oxygen.
  - Suction oropharynx.
  - Place a bite block to prevent biting and occlusion of the ETT.
- Extubation criteria include
  - Spontaneous respirations with adequate minute ventilation
  - Satisfactory oxygenation
  - Satisfactory acid-base status
  - Hemodynamic stability
  - Ability to follow commands
- Deflate the ETT cuff immediately before extubation.
- Administer 100% O_2 by facemask immediately after extubation, and confirm adequate ventilation and oxygenation.
- A plan for reintubation should be made in patients at risk of failed extubation and those with difficult airways (e.g., airway edema, morbid obesity, and respiratory insufficiency).
  - Extubation over an AEC or insertion of supraglottic airway before extubation provides a conduit to reintubation.

COMPLICATIONS

Complications During Laryngoscopy and Endotracheal Intubation

- A sore throat occurs in up to 40% of patients and is often self-limiting.
- Dental damage (1 in 4500 patients)
- Airway trauma – risk is increased in patients with difficult airways that require multiple laryngoscopies for intubation.
- A sympathetic nervous system response to laryngoscopy can have adverse effects in patients with preexisting hypertension, ischemic heart disease, or certain neurological conditions.
- Aspiration is the most common cause of death among major anesthesia airway complications.
- Accidental esophageal intubation
- Endobronchial intubation resulting in increased shunting and inadequate oxygenation

Complications After Endotracheal Extubation

- One-third of adverse airway events occur during emergence or recovery from anesthesia.
- Inadequate oxygenation and ventilation following extubation that may result from laryngeal edema, laryngospasm, or bronchospasm
- Most laryngospasm episodes can be treated with the application of positive pressure through a facemask and jaw thrust. If severe, may require the administration of propofol or muscle relaxants (e.g., rocuronium or succinylcholine)
- Excessive endotracheal cuff pressures over a prolonged period can cause tracheal mucosa damage and result in airway edema and subsequent tracheal stenosis.

AIRWAY MANAGEMENT IN INFANTS AND CHILDREN

Airway Management Differences Between Infants and Adults

- Anatomic and physiologic differences between the infant airway and the adult airway decrease as children grow and resolve by 12 to 14 years of age.

Major Differences Between the Infant Airway and the Adult Airway

- Larynx in infants is located higher in the neck at C3–C4.
- Infant's tongue is larger in proportion to the size of the mouth.
- Infant epiglottis is larger, stiffer, more omega-shaped, and oriented more posteriorly.
- Narrowest portion of infant airway is the cricoid cartilage.
- Infant's head has a more prominent occiput.
- Infant's nares are relatively smaller.
- Infants have higher oxygen consumption per kilogram.

Managing the Normal Airway in Infants and Children

History

- Problems with previous anesthetics
- Review of prior anesthetic records
- Snoring or obstructive sleep apnea

- Syndromes with mandibular hypoplasia
- Syndromes with cervical abnormalities

Physical Examination

- Exam may be challenging if child is fearful or unable to cooperate.
- Neck flexion and extension
- Mallampati classification
- Examine profile of airway for micrognathia or mandibular hypoplasia
- Presence and location of loose teeth

Preanesthetic Medication and Parental Presence During Induction of Anesthesia

- Parental presence during induction increasingly common
  - Minimizes need for preanesthetic medication in infants and children
  - Member of the perioperative team should escort parents out of operating room after the induction of anesthesia and can address any parental concerns.
- Preoperative anxiety
  - Anxious parents can transfer their anxiety to their children.
  - Preoperative anxiety is associated with posthospitalization behavioral changes: nightmares, separation anxiety, enuresis, eating disorders, and temper tantrums.
- "Unpleasant" induction experience can increase anxiety for subsequent anesthetics.
- Preoperative visits or telephone consultations should address anxiety in children and parents.
  - Child life services: age-appropriate play therapy and preoperative instruction
  - Coaching for older children and teenagers on reducing anxiety
- Preanesthetic medication in very anxious children aged >6 months
  - Intravenous midazolam if an IV catheter is present
  - Oral midazolam: 0.5 mg/kg up to 20 mg
  - Midazolam may also be given intranasally, intramuscularly, or rectally.
  - Older uncooperative children may require intramuscular ketamine: 3 mg/kg.

Induction of Anesthesia

- IV induction with propofol is safer and quicker than inhalational induction.
- Inhalational induction with oxygen, nitrous oxide, and sevoflurane, then establish IV after the infant or child loses consciousness
- Establish airway with supraglottic airway or ETT.
  - Neuromuscular blocking drugs such as rocuronium can facilitate laryngoscopy.

Direct Laryngoscopy and Endotracheal Intubation

- Optimal position with neck/shoulder roll
- Oropharynx: tongue shifted to left, laryngoscope blade midline, ETT entering from right
- External pressure at the level of the thyroid or cricoid cartilage can bring the vocal cords into view.
- Confirmation of endotracheal intubation with chest rise and end-tidal CO_2
- Determine proper depth of ETT.
  - Palpate ETT cuff in suprasternal notch.
  - Bilateral auscultation
- Reconfirm ETT placement after changing patient position.
  - Shorter tracheal length in children predisposes them to endotracheal tube malposition (endobronchial intubation, inadvertent extubation).

Airway Equipment

Nasal and Oral Airways

- Nasal and oral airways can relieve upper airway obstruction during induction/emergence.
  - Nasal airways: placed through nares after lubricating exterior
  - Oral airways: displace tongue anteriorly and should be properly sized

Supraglottic Airways

- SGAs can facilitate ventilation and oxygenation and deliver inhalational agents.
  - Routine airway and difficult airway management
  - Conduits for fiberoptic endotracheal intubation
  - Do not protect against aspiration
- Laryngeal mask airways
  - Available in eight sizes (1, 1.5, 2, 2.5, 3, 4, 5, and 6)
  - LMA supreme: additional channel to vent esophagus/stomach
  - Confirm position by auscultation and end-tidal CO_2.
  - Inflate cuff to minimize leak.
- Air-Q intubating laryngeal airways
  - Large-diameter shaft that facilitates endotracheal intubation
  - Available in six sizes (1, 1.5, 2, 2.5, 3.5, and 4.5)
  - Air-Q Blocker has an additional lumen to vent the esophagus/stomach.
- i-gel supraglottic airways
  - Thermoplastic elastomer with a soft gel-like noninflatable cuff
  - Integral bite block and channel to vent the esophagus/stomach
  - Available in seven sizes (1, 1.5, 2, 2.5, 3, 4, and 5)

Endotracheal Tubes

- Cuffed Versus Uncuffed Endotracheal Tubes
  - Cuffed ETTs advantages compared with uncuffed ETTs
    - Minimize the need for repeat laryngoscopy
    - Allow for lower fresh gas flows
    - Decrease the amount of inhalational agents used
    - Decrease the concentrations of inhalational agents in operating rooms
    - Cuffed tubes do **not** increase the incidence of postextubation croup.
    - Ideally cuff pressure should be measured and adjusted with a manometer to maintain a cuff pressure of 20 to 25 cm H_2O.
  - Uncuffed ETTs: confirm that leak pressure is <25 cm H_2O.
  - Suction catheters – should be available in appropriate size to suction the ETT

Microcuff ETTs

- Cuff is polyurethane membrane only 10-μm thick.
- Cuff is cylindrical in shape rather than round or oval.
- Cuff placed closer to the tip of the ETT
- Available in nine sizes (3, 3.5, 4, 4.5, 5, 5.5, 6, 6.5, and 7)

Stylets

- Can facilitate ETT placement during laryngoscopy
- Available in four sizes (6, 8, 10, and 14 Fr)

Laryngoscopes

- Straight blades have a smaller anterior-posterior profile and are easier to use in infants and small children.
- Curved blades have larger flanges and more effectively shift the tongue to the left.

ETTs and Laryngoscopes for Infants and Children

- ETT size: $\frac{16 + age}{4}$
- Subtract 0.5 for cuffed ETTs.
- Laryngoscope blades:
  - <1 year of age: Miller 1
  - 1–3 years of age: Miller or Wis-Hipple 1.5
  - 4–10 years of age: Miller 2
  - >10 years of age: Miller 2 or Macintosh 3

Video Laryngoscopy

- Video laryngoscopy is useful for managing both expected and unexpected difficult airways.
  - Allows for a view of the glottic opening without needing to align oral, pharyngeal, and laryngeal axes
  - Useful for patients with limited neck extension, hypoplastic mandibles, and "anterior" airways
  - Excellent tool for teaching laryngoscopy as both learner and instructor can both view the monitor simultaneously
- GlideScope video laryngoscopes
  - Reusable titanium scopes available in MAC T3, MAC T4, and angulated LoPro T2, T3, and T4 models
  - Single-use spectrum scopes available in straight blades (Miller S0, Miller S1), curved blades (DVM S3 and S4), and angulated blades (LoPro S1, S2, S3, and S4)
- C-MAC video laryngoscopes
  - Reusable C-MAC straight blades (Miller 0 and Miller 1), Macintosh style curved blades (MAC 2, 3, and 4), and angulated D blades (Pediatric D and Adult D)
  - Single use C-MAC Five S laryngoscopes Miller 0, Miller 1, Macintosh 3, Macintosh 4, and angulated adult D blades
- McGrath MAC video laryngoscopes
  - Reusable video laryngoscope inserted into a single-use plastic blade with a video screen mounted on the handle of the laryngoscope
  - Macintosh style curved blades (MAC 1, MAC 2, MAC 3, and MAC 4) and angulated D blade

Fiberoptic Bronchoscopy

- Useful for patients with limited mouth opening and/or limited neck flexion/extension
- Disadvantages: limited field of view, blood and/or secretions can obscure view
- Smallest bronchoscope is 2.2 mm for 3.0-mm ETT but has no suction channel and inferior optics.
- Fiberoptic bronchoscope should be at least 1 mm smaller than ID of ETT.
- Asleep fiberoptic intubation is more commonly performed than awake intubation in infants and children.
- Oxygenation via nasal cannula can minimize desaturation during fiberoptic intubation.
- Nasal fiberoptic intubation: oxymetazoline hydrochloride 0.05% nasal spray can minimize bleeding from the nasal mucosa
- Oral fiberoptic intubation: SGA can function as a conduit and shield bronchoscope from secretions/blood

Managing the Difficult Airway in Infants and Children

- Familiarity with pediatric difficult airway algorithm is essential.
- Asleep rather than awake airway management is typical in infants and children with difficult airways.
- Higher oxygen consumption in infants leads to faster desaturation and poses an additional time constraint.

Unexpected Difficult Airway

- Call for additional help from anesthesia colleagues.
- Call for surgeon for possible surgical airway.
- Call for pediatric difficult airway cart.
- Do not persist with multiple attempts at laryngoscopy.
- Consider SGA to oxygenate/ventilate.
- Consider video laryngoscope.

Expected Difficult Airway

- Minimize premedications that have ventilatory depressant effects.
- Additional anesthesia colleague
- Surgeon available for possible surgical airway
- Consider SGA, fiberoptic bronchoscopy, or video laryngoscopy.

Tracheal Extubation in Infants and Children

Deep Versus Awake Extubation

- Both deep and awake extubation are viable options for infants and children.
- Consider awake extubation in patients with difficult airways and/or decreased airway tone.
- Deep extubation may decrease the risk of airway complications including coughing and desaturation but may increase the risk of postoperative airway obstruction.

Postextubation Stridor

- Infants and small children are at higher risk for postextubation stridor because of the small diameter of their airways.
- Mechanism: pressure on the tracheal mucosa causes venous congestion and edema, most commonly from
  - Uncuffed tube that is too large
  - Cuffed tube that is overinflated
- Additional risk factors
  - Multiple endotracheal intubation attempts
  - Unusual position of the head during surgery
  - Increased duration of surgery
  - Surgical procedures that involve the airway
- Presentation: respiratory distress in the PACU with nasal flaring, retractions, increased respiratory rate, audible stridor, and decreased oxygen saturation
- Treatment
  - Mild symptoms with minimal respiratory distress: humidified oxygen and prolonged observation in PACU
  - Moderate symptoms with respiratory distress: aerosolized racemic epinephrine and admission to PICU for observation
  - Severe symptoms with desaturation unresponsive to racemic epinephrine may require emergent reintubation with a smaller ETT

Obstructive Sleep Apnea

- Infants and children with OSA are at increased risk for airway obstruction in the postoperative period.
- Carefully titrate opioids and other medications that depress ventilation.
- Consider awake extubation rather than deep extubation in these patients.
- Infants and children with OSA require a higher level of postoperative monitoring with continuous oxygen saturation monitoring and may require PICU admission.

Laryngospasm

- Infants and younger children are more prone to laryngospasm than adults.
- Most laryngospasm occurs during induction or emergence from anesthesia.
- Treatment
  - Initial treatment with continuous positive-pressure ventilation with facemask with 100% oxygen
  - If patient desaturates or becomes bradycardic, treat with propofol if IV is present, IM rocuronium, or IM succinylcholine if no IV is present.

Extubation After a Difficult Intubation

- Awake extubation recommended
- Full reversal of neuromuscular blockade
- Confirm that any airway edema from surgery or positioning has fully resolved (consider nasal fiberoptic airway exam).
- Difficult airway cart and equipment for reintubation should be immediately available.

QUESTIONS

ANATOMY AND PHYSIOLOGY OF THE UPPER AIRWAY

1. What is different about the cricoid cartilage compared with the other tracheal cartilages, and what is its clinical relevance in anesthesia?
2. You are asked by your patient to make sure they are comfortable during an awake oral fiberoptic intubation. What is the sensory innervation to the airway, and what are some techniques that can be used for patient comfort?

AIRWAY ASSESSMENT

3. Check the boxes in the table matching the preoperative airway physical examination findings that are associated with difficult airway management for the given technique.

Physical Examination Findings	Mask Ventilation	SGA Ventilation	Direct Laryngoscopy	Cricothyroid Membrane Access
High BMI (>30 kg/m^2) and increased neck circumference (>40 cm)				
Male sex				
Female sex				
Edentulous				
Prominent upper incisors				
Reduced interincisor gap (<3 cm)				
Mallampati class III or IV				
Limited ability to protrude lower mandible				
Limited cervical spine mobility				
Reduced neck tissue compliance secondary to previous irradiation				
Thyromental distance <6 cm				
Beard				

4. Your next patient is scheduled for an elective laparoscopic cholecystectomy. He has not had previous surgery, has had no medical illnesses, has fasted, and is not obese. After preoperative airway assessment, you suspect difficult laryngoscopy but do not anticipate difficulty with mask ventilation. According to the ASA Difficult Airway Algorithm, is proceeding with direct laryngoscopy and intubation after inducing general anesthesia an acceptable next step for airway management?

AIRWAY MANAGEMENT TECHNIQUES

5. Describe features of the newer generation supraglottic airways that make them different from LMA Classic.
6. What are some complications of the SGA? Can uncomplicated SGA placement result in nerve injuries?
7. Name some indications for endotracheal intubation.
8. Explain the difference between ETT stylets, introducers, and airway exchange catheters, and their potential complications.

9. What are some of the patient risk factors that may make awake intubation an appropriate airway management plan?
10. Why is visualization more difficult during fiberoptic endotracheal intubation in an asleep patient?

INVASIVE AIRWAY ACCESS

11. In an emergent situation, does a percutaneous or a surgical cricothyrotomy have a better success rate?

COMPLICATIONS

12. What are the benefits, indications, and contraindications to extubation before the return of protective airway reflexes (deep extubation)?

AIRWAY MANAGEMENT IN INFANTS AND CHILDREN

13. Describe the differences between the pediatric and the adult airway and the clinical significance, using the table below.

Airway Anatomy	Infant	Adult	Clinical Significance
Level of larynx			
Tongue			
Epiglottis			
Narrowest part of airway			
Head size relative to body			
Nares			

14. An 8-year-old patient presents for elective outpatient surgery. Describe some factors that influence premedication, parental presence during induction, and the choice of induction technique.
15. What are the disadvantages and advantages of cuffed ETTs in infants and children?
16. How does one determine if an uncuffed ETT is too small or too large?
17. Describe the limitations of flexible fiberoptic intubation in infants and children.
18. What are some risk factors for postextubation croup in infants and children?
19. How is postextubation croup treated in infants and children?
20. What is the postoperative risk for pediatric patients with obstructive sleep apnea, and how should they be managed?
21. When does laryngospasm typically occur in infants and children, and how is it treated?

ANSWERS

ANATOMY AND PHYSIOLOGY OF THE UPPER AIRWAY

1. The cricoid cartilage is the most cephalad tracheal cartilage and is the only one that has a full ring structure. Applying external pressure on the cricoid cartilage (Sellick maneuver) compresses the underlying upper esophagus against the cervical vertebrae with the intent to minimize spillage of gastric content into the pharynx during rapid sequence induction. The cricoid cartilage is also an important anatomical landmark for procedures such as cricothyroidotomy, tracheostomy, transtracheal jet ventilation, and transtracheal block. (255)
2. The airway can be divided into sensory "zones" of oropharynx (glossopharyngeal nerve), larynx above the vocal cords (superior laryngeal nerve, internal division), and larynx below the vocal cords (recurrent laryngeal nerve). Topical anesthesia to the tongue and oropharynx can be achieved by gargling, nebulizing, or spraying lidocaine solution. Nebulization has the advantage of wider coverage. For denser anesthesia of the larynx and trachea, superior laryngeal nerve and transtracheal blocks can also be performed prior to the fiberoptic intubation. Alternatively, a "spray-as-you-go" technique via the brochoscope can be used while advancing the fiberoptic scope. (256)

Motor and Sensory Innervation of Larynx

Nerve	Sensory	Motor
Superior laryngeal, internal division	Epiglottis Base of tongue Supraglottic mucosa Thyroepiglottic joint Cricothyroid joint	None
Superior laryngeal, external division	Anterior subglottic mucosa	Cricothyroid membrane
Recurrent laryngeal	Subglottic mucosa Muscle spindles	Thyroarytenoid membrane Lateral cricoarytenoid membrane. Interarytenoid membrane Posterior cricoarytenoid membrane

AIRWAY ASSESSMENT

3. The table below identifies which preoperative airway physical exam findings correlate with the associated difficult airway management. (259)

Physical Examination Findings	Mask Ventilation	SGA Ventilation	Intubation	Cricothyroid Membrane Access
High BMI (>30 kg/m^2) & increased neck circumference (>40 cm)	•	•	•	•
Male gender	•	•		
Female gender				•
Edentulous	•	•		
Prominent upper incisors		•	•	
Reduced interincisor gap (<3 cm)		•	•	
Mallampati class III or IV	•		•	
Limited ability to protrude lower mandible	•		•	
Limited cervical spine mobility	•		•	•

Physical Examination Findings	Mask Ventilation	SGA Ventilation	Intubation	Cricothyroid Membrane Access
Reduced neck tissue compliance secondary to previous irradiation	•		•	•
Thyromental distance <6 cm			•	
Beard	•			

4. It is reasonable to attempt to intubate under general anesthesia in this scenario. If, however, the patient had any other factor increasing airway risk (predicted difficulty with mask or SGA ventilation, aspiration risk, rapid desaturation risk, or suspected difficult emergency invasive airway), an awake intubation is advised. (255, Fig. 16.1)

AIRWAY MANAGEMENT TECHNIQUES

5. The newer-generation supraglottic airways (e.g., LMA Fastrach, LMA ProSeal or Supreme, Air-Q, and i-gel) have one or more of the following features: (1) improved airway seal to allow for ventilation with higher airway pressures, (2) a second lumen that acts as an esophageal vent to keep gases and fluid separate from the airway and facilitate placement of an orogastric tube, (3) an airway channel that can be used as a conduit for intubation, and (4) a bite block that is present in the airway shaft. SGAs can be classified as (1) first generation: simple breathing tube connected with a mask that seals the laryngeal inlet (e.g., Classic LMA, LMA-Unique) or (2) second generation: as above, with added features for gastric drainage and improved protection against aspiration with higher seal cuff pressure (e.g., Proseal LMA, LMA-Supreme, i-gel). (263–266)
6. Complications of SGA placement include sore throat, bronchospasm, postoperative swallowing difficulties, edema, and pulmonary aspiration. Known nerve injuries include laryngeal nerve injury and hypoglossal nerve paralysis. (265)
7. Indications for endotracheal intubation include the following:
   - Provide a patent airway
   - Prevent inhalation (aspiration) of gastric contents
   - Need for frequent suctioning
   - Facilitate positive-pressure ventilation of the lungs
   - Operative position other than supine
   - Operative site near or involving the upper airway
   - Airway maintenance by mask or supraglottic airway device difficult (Box 16.1, 267)
8. Malleable metal stylets are used to stiffen and provide curvature to an ETT to help facilitate laryngoscopy and tracheal intubation. Complications include bleeding, oropharyngeal trauma, tracheal trauma, and sore throat. A bougie or an introducer is used when there is a poor laryngoscopic view and difficulty passing an ETT. They are shaped with a curve near the distal tip, which facilitates placement into the airway. An ETT can be advanced over the bougie or introducer into the airway. Airway exchange catheters are designed for exchange of ETTs. When placed prior to extubation, they can also be left in the airway as a conduit for reintubation in the case of failed extubation. Tracheal laceration, bronchial laceration, and gastric perforation are all complications of tracheal tube exchangers. (272)
9. Awake intubation should be performed in patients with one or more of the following risk factors in addition to a suspected difficult intubation.
   - Expected difficult ventilation with face mask or SGA
   - Increased risk of aspiration
   - Poor tolerance of brief apneic episodes
   - Expected difficulty with emergency invasive airway rescue technique (273)
10. An important difference in performing fiberoptic laryngoscopy in an anesthetized patient is that the soft tissues of the pharynx, in contrast to the awake state, tend to relax and limit space for visualization with the fiberoptic bronchoscope. Using jaw thrust, using specialized oral airways, expanding the ETT cuff in the pharynx, or applying traction on the tongue may overcome this problem. (275)

INVASIVE AIRWAY ACCESS

11. Emergent percutaneous and surgical cricothyrotomy have similar success rates, and the choice of technique should depend on the provider's proficiency. More important is that the decision to perform cricothyroidotomy be made early in a "can't intubate, can't ventilate" situation. (275)

COMPLICATIONS

12. Tracheal extubation before the return of protective airway reflexes (deep tracheal extubation) is generally associated with less coughing and attenuated hemodynamic effects on emergence. This may be preferred in patients at risk from adverse effects of increased intracranial or intraocular pressure, bleeding into the surgical wound, or wound dehiscence. Previous difficult facemask ventilation or difficult endotracheal intubation, high risk of aspiration, restricted access to the airway, obstructive sleep apnea or obesity, and a surgical procedure that may have resulted in airway edema, bleeding or increased irritability are relative contraindications to deep tracheal extubation. (277)

AIRWAY MANAGEMENT IN INFANTS AND CHILDREN

13. Differences between the pediatric and the adult airway, and the clinical significance of each is described in the table below. (278-279)

Airway Anatomy	Infant	Adult	Clinical Significance
Level of larynx	C3–C4	C4–C5	The tongue is shifted more superiorly, closer to the palate, which can cause airway obstruction in situations such as the inhalation induction of anesthesia.
Tongue	Larger in proportion to the size of the mouth	-	Makes direct laryngoscopy more difficult and can contribute to obstruction of the upper airway during sedation, inhalation induction, or emergence from anesthesia
Epiglottis	Relatively larger, stiffer, more omega shaped, and angled in a more posterior position	-	Blocks visualization of the vocal cords during direct laryngoscopy
Narrowest part of airway	Cricoid cartilage	Vocal cords	Uncuffed ETTs that are correctly sized can protect the airway from aspiration in children.
Head size relative to body	Head and occiput are relatively larger		The proper position for direct laryngoscopy and tracheal intubation in an adult is often described as the sniffing position with the head elevated and the neck flexed at C6–C7 and extended at C1–C2. An infant, on the other hand, requires a shoulder roll or neck roll to establish an optimal position for facemask ventilation and direct laryngoscopy.
Nares	Smaller	Larger	This can offer significant resistance to airflow and increase the work of breathing, especially when secretions, edema, or bleeding narrow them.

14. Parental presence during the induction of anesthesia can minimize the need for preanesthetic medication, although anxious parents can transfer their anxiety to their children. Alternatively, a preanesthetic medication such as midazolam (oral, intranasal, IM, or rectal administration) can facilitate separation of the child from the parents and the inhalational induction of anesthesia. In a child without an intravenous catheter in place, an inhalational induction of anesthesia through a facemask is generally the best approach in a healthy, cooperative child. (280)

15. The disadvantage of a cuffed ETT compared with an uncuffed ETT is that a smaller cuffed than uncuffed tube is required, which can increase resistance through the ETT and the work of breathing. The advantages of cuffed ETTs are that they (1) minimize the need for repeated laryngoscopy, (2) allow for lower fresh gas flows, (3) decrease the amount of inhalational agent used, and (4) decrease the concentrations of anesthetic gasses detectable in operating rooms. Cuffed tubes do not increase the incidence of postextubation croup compared with uncuffed tubes. (282)
16. The leak pressure is used to determine if an uncuffed ETT is too large or too small. The leak pressure when using uncuffed ETTs in infants and children should be 20 to 25 cm H_2O. If the leak pressure is too high, a smaller ETT should be used, and if the leak pressure is too low, a larger ETT should be used. (282)
17. The limitations of the smaller flexible fiberoptic bronchoscopes used in infants and small children include (1) limited field of vision, (2) view that is easily obscured by secretions and/or bleeding, (3) inferior optics compared to larger adult bronchoscopes because of fewer fiberoptic bundles, and (4) no suction channel. It is also unlikely that infants and children will cooperate with an awake fiberoptic endotracheal intubation, so it is usually necessary to induce anesthesia and manage the airway with the patient asleep. (283–284)
18. Postextubation croup occurs most commonly when either an uncuffed ETT that is too large or an overinflated cuffed ETT is used. The resulting mechanical pressure on the tracheal mucosa causes venous congestion and edema, and in severe cases can even compromise the arterial blood supply causing mucosal ischemia. The resulting edema can narrow the tracheal lumen, especially in infants and small children. Because resistance to flow in an ETT is inversely proportional to the radius of the lumen to the fourth power, 1 mm of edema in an infant airway is much more significant than 1 mm of edema in an adult airway. Other risk factors for postextubation croup include multiple tracheal intubation attempts, unusual positioning of the head during surgery, increased duration of surgery, and procedures involving the upper airway, such as rigid bronchoscopy. (286)
19. Treatment of postextubation croup or stridor depends on the degree of respiratory distress. Mild symptoms can be managed with humidified oxygen and prolonged observation in the postanesthesia care unit. More severe cases may require aerosolized racemic epinephrine and postoperative observation in an intensive care unit. Patients whose respiratory distress is severe and not relieved with these measures may need to be reintubated with an ETT smaller than the one previously used. Steroids administered intravenously for preventing upper airway edema are more beneficial when given before the airway is instrumented and should be administered before procedures such as rigid bronchoscopy. (286)
20. Infants and children with obstructive sleep apnea are at significant risk for airway obstruction, respiratory distress, and the potential for apnea in the postoperative period. At baseline these infants and children hypoventilate, which results in hypercapnia and often arterial hypoxemia while asleep. Residual inhaled anesthetics or residual neuromuscular blockade can depress airway reflexes, skeletal muscle tone and strength, and respiratory drive and result in significant airway compromise in infants and children with obstructive sleep apnea. These patients should be extubated awake and monitored postoperatively with pulse oximetry and apnea monitoring. High-risk patients should be monitored postoperatively in an intensive care unit setting. Opioids must be carefully titrated both intraoperatively and postoperatively because they can depress the ventilatory drive and contribute to significant hypercapnia and arterial hypoxemia in these infants and children. (286)
21. Laryngospasm most commonly occurs during either inhalational induction of anesthesia or the emergence from anesthesia often after extubation or removal of a supraglottic airway device. Most laryngospasm episodes in pediatric patients can be treated successfully with continuous positive pressure ventilation via facemask with 100% oxygen, while applying a chin lift and jaw thrust. The positive pressure may have to be as high as 50 cm H_2O to successfully break the laryngospasm. If positive pressure is not successful and the infant or child is desaturating or bradycardic, further intervention is necessary. If there is IV access, laryngospasm should be treated with approximately 0.6 to 1.0 mg/kg of IV propofol and, if necessary, 0.2 to 0.3 mg/kg of IV rocuronium. If there is no IV access, laryngospasm should be treated with 0.6 to 1.0 mg/kg of IM rocuronium or 1.5 to 2.0 mg/kg of IM succinylcholine. (286)

Chapter

17 SPINAL, EPIDURAL, AND CAUDAL ANESTHESIA

David W. Hewson, Richard Brull, and Alan J.R. Macfarlane

PRINCIPLES

- Central neuraxial blocks include spinal, epidural, and caudal blocks.
- All result in some degree of sympathetic, sensory, and motor blockade.

PRACTICE

- Single-injection spinal blocks: anesthesia for lower abdominal, pelvic, obstetric, and lower limb surgery
- Continuous catheter-based epidural infusions: obstetric labor analgesia, postoperative pain relief, as a part of enhanced recovery after surgery (ERAS) protocols
- Caudal blocks: anesthesia and analgesia in children
- Indwelling long-term spinal catheters: chronic malignant and nonmalignant pain
- Informed consent, noninvasive monitoring, intravenous access, and available resuscitation equipment are essential preparation for neuraxial block placement.

EVIDENCE

- Impact of central neuraxial blocks on morbidity and mortality is challenging to demonstrate.
    - Respiratory complications are reduced compared with systemic opioid analgesia.
    - Outcome benefits appear greatest when neuraxial anesthesia is used alone rather than combined with general anesthesia.

ANATOMY

- There are 7 cervical, 12 thoracic, 5 lumbar vertebra, and a sacrum.
- Spinal cord is continuous with medulla oblongata (proximally) and terminates as filum terminale and cauda equina (distally).
- Spinal cord termination is variable: L3 in infants; L1 or L2 in adults
- Spinal cord is surrounded by pia, arachnoid, and dura mater.
    - Pia: innermost membrane, highly vascular
    - Arachnoid: delicate, nonvascular; principal barrier to drugs crossing into the cerebrospinal fluid (CSF)
    - Dura mater: tough, fibroelastic membrane
- Subarachnoid (intrathecal) space contains cerebrospinal fluid.
- Epidural space
    - Bounded by posterior longitudinal ligament (anteriorly), pedicles and intervertebral foramina (laterally), and ligamentum flavum (posteriorly)
    - Contents: nerve roots, fat, areolar tissue, lymphatics, and blood vessels
- Dural sac extends to S2 in adults and lower in children.

Spinal Nerves

- Formed by dorsal (afferent) and ventral (efferent) nerves that merge distal to the dorsal root ganglion
- Pass through the intervertebral foramen to exit spinal column

Blood Supply

- Posterior one-third of the spinal cord: two posterior spinal arteries
- Anterior two-thirds of the spinal cord: one anterior spinal artery
    - Artery of Adamkiewicz is its largest supply: arises from aorta and passes through a left intervertebral foramen between T7 and L4
    - Infarction leads to *anterior spinal artery syndrome*: motor weakness, loss of pain and temperature sensation below the affected spinal level. Proprioception and vibratory sense are spared.
    - Ischemia and infarction can be due to systemic hypotension, thrombosis, emboli, vasculopathy, trauma, or because of aortic surgery.

- Venous drainage: spinal veins and radicular veins drain into venous plexus in epidural space, which drain into azygous system.

Anatomic Variations

- Spinal nerve roots and CSF volume: affect spinal block quality, height, and regression
- Epidural space: is segmented, which may explain unpredictability in drug spread
- Epidural space contents: may influence volume of anesthetic required

MECHANISM OF ACTION

- Nerves within the subarachnoid space are more easily anesthetized compared with epidural nerves outside of the arachnoid membrane.

Differential Blockade with Neuraxial Procedures

- **Speed of neural blockade** depends on the size, surface area, and degree of myelination of nerve fibers.
- **Sensitivity to local anesthetic:** sympathetic ("B") > slow pain ("C") > pinprick pain and cold ("A-delta") > touch ("A-beta") > motor ("A-alpha.")
- Clinical onset of spinal blockade usually follows the above pattern; regression occurs in the reverse order.
- *Differential sensory blockade*: maximum block height varies by sensory modality.

Drug Uptake and Distribution

- Spinal injection: local anesthetic diffuses down its concentration gradient directly proportional to the drug mass, CSF drug concentration, contact surface area, lipid content, and local tissue area; diffusion is inversely related to nerve root cross-sectional area.
  - Diffuses along spaces of Virchow-Robin to deeper dorsal root ganglia
  - Diffuses into epidural space and taken up by blood vessels
- Epidural injection: spread is greater when there is decreased epidural space cross-sectional area, decreased epidural space compliance, decreased epidural fat, decreased local anesthetic leakage (e.g., spinal stenosis), and increased epidural venous engorgement (e.g., pregnancy).
  - Spreads through bulk flow longitudinally and circumferentially within the epidural space and taken up by epidural fat (majority)
  - Traverses dura into CSF (<20%)
  - Diffuses into the plasma compartment

Drug Elimination

- Vascular absorption accounts for drug regression in both CSF and epidural space
- Slower for drugs with higher lipid solubility that depot in epidural fat

PHYSIOLOGIC EFFECTS

Physiologic Effects of Neuraxial Blockade

Cardiovascular

- Arterial hypotension results from blockade of peripheral (T1-L2) and cardiac (T1-T4) sympathetic fibers.
  - Higher baseline sympathetic nervous system activity (e.g., in older patients) equates to greater consequent hypotension.

Systemic Vascular Resistance

- Decreases due to sympathectomy: height of sympathectomy may extend several dermatomes higher than sensory block level.

Cardiac Output

- Cardiac output: generally maintained or slightly decreased
- Severe bradycardia and even asystole: blockade of cardioaccelerator fibers (T1-T4)
- Profound bradycardia and circulatory collapse: especially in patients with hypovolemia (Bezold-Jarisch reflex)

Central Nervous System

- Cerebral blood flow: decreased secondary to arterial hypotension
- Sedation: decreased stimulation of reticular activating system (even in the absence of systemic sedatives)

Respiratory

- Decreased vital capacity: paralysis of abdominal muscles
- Overall improved respiratory function after thoracoabdominal surgery: pain relief allows improved respiratory function.

Gastrointestinal

- Increased colonic mucosal blood flow and motility: unopposed parasympathetic activity when blood pressure is maintained

Renal

- Urinary retention: questionable whether incidence truly higher than with general anesthesia

INDICATIONS

Neuraxial Anesthesia

- Spinal: favorable for surgery below abdomen, for patients with airway or respiratory disease, at an increased risk for general anesthesia, or who would benefit from remaining conscious

- Epidural: allows for more prolonged surgical anesthesia
- Spinal with indwelling catheter: when an epidural catheter is challenging or for lower-dose and/or incremental dosing (e.g., severe cardiac disease)

Neuraxial Analgesia

- Useful for labor and delivery, postoperative for hip, knee, cardiac, thoracic, or abdominal surgery, and for chronic pain management

CONTRAINDICATIONS

Contraindications to Neuraxial Blockade
Absolute ▪ Patient refusal, infection at needle insertion site, allergy to proposed drugs, inability to maintain stillness during needle puncture, or increased intracranial pressure
Relative ▪ Must be weighed against potential benefits and alternative techniques
Neurologic ▪ Myelopathy, peripheral neuropathy, spinal stenosis, previous spine surgery, multiple sclerosis, spina bifida
Cardiac ▪ Aortic stenosis or other cause of fixed cardiac output, hypovolemia
Hematologic ▪ Thromboprophylaxis and antithrombotic/thrombolytic therapy, inherited coagulopathy
Infection ▪ Fever, bacteremia, septic shock

SPINAL ANESTHESIA

Factors Affecting Block Height

Drug Factors

- Baricity – defined as ratio of density of local anesthetic solution compared to CSF at 37°C
  - Isobaric – same density as CSF
  - Hypobaric – lower density than CSF (e.g., by adding sterile water to injected local anesthetic)
    - Promotes spread to nondependent regions of intrathecal space
  - Hyperbaric – higher density than CSF (e.g., by adding dextrose to local anesthetic)
    - Promotes spread to dependent regions of intrathecal space, e.g., patient in lateral decubitus will preferentially develop blockade on the dependent side
- Dose: (volume × concentration), affects isobaric and hypobaric > hyperbaric solutions

Patient Factors

- Height, weight, age, and gender influence CSF volume and density with varying degrees of clinical importance.

Procedure Factors

- Patient positioning (up to 25 minutes after injection) and level of injection (isobaric solutions), needle type, and orientation may affect certain block characteristics.

Duration of the Block

- Dose, properties of the local anesthetic (e.g., lipid solubility), and use of additives affect block height.

Pharmacology

- pKa, lipid solubility, and protein binding affect drug uptake, distribution, and elimination (i.e., duration of clinical effect).

Short- and Intermediate-Acting Local Anesthetics

- *Procaine* – not commonly used, greater failure rate compared with lidocaine
- *Chloroprocaine* – preservative-free preferred, faster recovery than lidocaine
- *Lidocaine* – transient neurological symptoms (TNS) risk limits use
- *Prilocaine* – rarely associated with TNS, may be used in outpatient setting
- *Mepivicaine* – TNS risk similar to lidocaine, especially in hyperbaric formulation

Long-Acting Local Anesthetics

- *Tetracaine* – usually combined with vasoconstrictor for predictable duration (though avoid combination with phenylephrine due to association with TNS)
- *Bupivacaine* – often used, duration of 2.5 to 3 hours, rarely associated with TNS
- *Levobupivacaine* – less cardiotoxic than bupivacaine but risk is only theoretical for spinal anesthesia
- *Ropivacaine* – less motor block and earlier recovery than bupivacaine, but less potent

Spinal Additives

- Hydrophilic opioids: greater spread in CSF, can cause late respiratory depression
  - Preservative-free morphine can prolong analgesia for up to 24 hours.
- Lipophilic opioids: rapid vascular (systemic) and fat uptake, lesser spread in CSF
  - Fentanyl and sufentanil can prolong analgesia for 2 to 3 hours.

Vasoconstrictors

- Prolong sensory and motor blockade, but there is some concern of reducing neural blood supply (e.g., epinephrine, phenylephrine).

α_2-Agonists

- Directly act on α_2-adrenergic receptors in the dorsal horn of spinal cord to prolong sensory and motor block (e.g., clonidine, dexmedetomidine, epinephrine)
  - Clonidine can also cause hypotension and sedation lasting up to 8 hours.

Other Drugs

- Neostigmine, midazolam, ketamine, adenosine, tramadol, magnesium, and nonsteroidal antiinflammatories: not commonly used, variable or no clinical value, and unknown neurotoxic potential

Technique

Preparation

- Spinal needles either cut (Pitkin, Quincke-Babcock) or spread ("pencil point" designs Whitacre, Sprotte, Pencan) the dura.
  - Using smaller gauge and pencil point tips reduces the incidence of postdural puncture headache.
- Strict aseptic technique including wearing a facemask and skin preparation
  - Chlorhexidine with alcohol is most effective but must dry fully before skin puncture because of potential neurotoxicity and arachnoiditis.

Position

- Sitting (facilitates midline identification) or lateral decubitus position
- Position is influenced by spinal solution baricity, intravenous sedation, and risk of hypotension.

Projection and Puncture

- Needle below L1-L2 avoids risk of trauma to the spinal cord.
- The intercristal line, drawn between iliac crests, corresponds with the L4 vertebral body or L4-L5 interspace.
- Subcutaneous local anesthetic infiltration, then insertion of an introducer needle to help direct the delicate spinal needle
- Slowly advance the spinal needle until a characteristic "click" or "pop" occurs as the needle tip passes through the ligamentum flavum and dura into the intrathecal space.
  - A common reason for failure is insertion of the needle off the midline.
- Once clear CSF appears at the needle hub, the anesthetic dose should be injected at a rate of approximately 0.2 mL/sec.
- A paramedian needle approach can also be used (entry 1 cm lateral and 1 cm caudad).

Ultrasonography

- Can identify the vertebral level and optimal needle insertion location
- Reduces procedural failure rates, especially in patients with difficult anatomy (e.g., obesity), spine deformities (e.g., scoliosis), or previous spine surgery

Special Spinal Techniques

- Continuous spinal anesthesia: incremental dosing to achieve desired vertebral level for better hemodynamic stability
  - Small-gauge catheters have been associated with cauda equina syndrome.
- Unilateral (or selective) spinal anesthesia: capitalizes on baricity and positioning to select side of surgery (e.g., knee arthroscopy)

Monitoring of the Block

- Sensory: cold sensation (C fibers) and pinprick (A-delta fibers), must be two or three segments above the expected level of surgical stimulus
- Motor: modified Bromage scale scores motor block from 0 (none) to 4 (complete).

EPIDURAL ANESTHESIA

Factors Affecting Epidural Block Height

Drug Factors

- Volume and total dose of local anesthetic (1–2 mL per segment to be blocked)

Patient Factors

- Age, pregnancy, and extremes of height

Procedure Factors

- Level of injection (most important) and patient position

Pharmacology

Short- and Intermediate-Acting Local Anesthetics

- *Procaine* – unreliable and poor-quality block
- *Chloroprocaine* (2% or 3% preservative-free) – solutions with EDTA preservative associated with back pain
- *Lidocaine* (1% or 2%) – not associated with TNS, unlike spinal lidocaine
- *Prilocaine* – 2% gives mostly sensory block, 3% increased risk methemoglobinemia
- *Mepivacaine* (1%, 1.5%, and 2%) – 2% solution has onset time like lidocaine, slightly longer duration

Long-Acting Local Anesthetics

- *Tetracaine* – unreliable block height, risk of systemic toxicity

- *Bupivacaine* – cardiovascular and central nervous system toxicity risk; causes motor block with larger doses
- *Levobupivacaine* – less cardiotoxic than bupivacaine
- *Ropivacaine* – less cardiotoxic and higher seizure threshold than bupivacaine

Epidural Additives

- Vasoconstrictors: epinephrine reduces vascular absorption, prolongs blockade especially of lidocaine, mepivacaine, and chloroprocaine. May also have direct analgesic effect on α_2-receptors in dorsal horn
- Opioids: synergistically enhance local anesthetic analgesia, do not prolong motor block, and reduce dose-related side effects
  - Lipophilic (faster onset, shorter duration) are absorbed vascularly or into fat and are less likely to cross the dura.
  - Hydrophilic (longer duration, up to 24 hours for morphine) are found in higher concentrations in CSF.
- α_2-Agonists: clonidine and dexmedetomidine prolong sensory blockade, but clonidine side effects include hypotension, bradycardia, dry mouth, and sedation.
- Other drugs: ketamine, neostigmine, midazolam, tramadol, dexamethasone, and droperidol have all been studied but are not commonly used.
- Carbonation and bicarbonate: increases solution pH (nonionized proportion of local anesthetic) and increases the speed of epidural block onset

Technique

Preparation

- Surgical procedure and duration guide selection of vertebral level and local anesthetic.
- 16- or 18-G Tuohy needles are most commonly used and guide catheter cephalad.
- Flexible, radiopaque plastic catheters can be placed into the epidural space.
- Multiple-orifice catheters improve analgesia compared to single-orifice devices.

Position

- Sitting or lateral decubitus position, ideally with patients awake

Projection and Puncture

- The intercristal line (L4 to L5), the inferior angle of the scapula (T7), root of the scapular spine (T3), and vertebra prominens (C7) are important surface landmarks.
- Midline, paramedian, modified paramedian (Taylor approach), and caudal techniques may all be used to access the epidural space.
- A loss-of-resistance syringe containing air or saline is commonly used, or the "hanging drop" technique
- When the Tuohy needle passes from ligamentum flavum to epidural space, the pressure applied to the syringe plunger allows fluid to flow with minimal resistance into the epidural space.
- A catheter can be threaded and left in the space (typically to a depth of 4–6 cm).
- Before initiating a local anesthetic infusion, the epidural catheter should be aspirated (checking for blood or CSF) and a test dose administered to exclude intrathecal or intravascular placement.

Paramedian Approach

- Useful in mid- to high-thoracic region due to narrower spaces and steeper spinous processes

Use of Ultrasonography

- Preprocedural ultrasound can be useful in patients whose surface landmarks are difficult to discern or with spinal deformities.

COMBINED SPINAL-EPIDURAL ANESTHESIA (CSE)

- Allows rapid-onset spinal block and extended anesthesia and analgesia via epidural catheter
- The epidural volume extension technique also allows smaller doses of spinal local anesthetic to be used.
  - Adding local anesthetic or saline alone to the epidural space via the catheter compresses the dural sac and increases spinal block height.

Technique

- Needle-through-needle or separate spinal and epidural injections can be performed.

CAUDAL ANESTHESIA

- Deposition of medication in epidural space via the sacral hiatus
- Common in pediatric anesthesia

Pharmacology

- Similar to those described for epidural anesthesia

Technique

- Identification of the sacral hiatus where the two sacral cornua are joined by the sacrococcygeal ligament
- Advance needle at an approximatly 45-degree angle until there is a decrease or loss of resistance, and aspirate before injection.

COMPLICATIONS

Neurological

Neurologic Complications Associated with Neuraxial Anesthesia
Nerve Injury ▪ Risk factors: patients on anticoagulation, poor aseptic technique; risk greater with epidural and CSE vs. spinal anesthesia ▪ Radicular pain or paresthesia during neuraxial procedure warrants prompt needle withdrawal.
Paraplegia ▪ Direct needle trauma, vertebral canal hematoma, epidural abscess, periprocedural hypotension, adhesive arachnoiditis, misadministration of neurotoxic medications
Epidural Hematoma ▪ Presents with radicular back pain, unexpectedly prolonged blockade, bladder or bowel dysfunction ▪ Associated with traumatic needle or catheter insertion, use of larger needles (epidural > spinal) coagulopathy, female sex, and advanced age ▪ Symptoms should prompt immediate review and magnetic resonance imaging. ▪ Surgical hematoma evacuation is a time-critical intervention to prevent permanent harm.
Epidural Abscess ▪ Can present with back pain, tenderness, progressive neurological deficit, and systemic symptoms of infection ▪ Risk factors: concomitant systemic infection, diabetes, immunocompromised states, prolonged maintenance of an epidural catheter
Postdural Puncture Headache ▪ Frontal or occipital headache worse during upright posture and relieved by lying supine, associated with nausea, vomiting, neck pain, dizziness, tinnitus, diplopia, hearing loss, cortical blindness, cranial nerve palsies, seizures 2 to 3 days after procedure ▪ Loss of CSF may cause traction and compensatory intracerebral vasodilation. ▪ Associated with younger patients, female sex, larger needle size, multiple dural punctures, and when needle bevel is angled perpendicular to dural fibers during placement ▪ Management: hydration, caffeine, oral analgesics, and epidural blood patch (definitive therapy) with repeat patch if necessary
Total Spinal Anesthesia ▪ Rapidly progressive bradycardia, hypotension, loss of consciousness, apnea, and cardiac arrest ▪ Caused by inadvertent cephalad spread of local anesthetic to cervical nerve roots and brainstem

Neurologic Complications Associated with Neuraxial Anesthesia—Cont'd
Transient Neurological Symptoms ▪ Characterized by unilateral or bilateral buttock pain radiating to the legs without neurological deficits about 24 hours after resolution of spinal block ▪ Associated with lidocaine or mepivacaine spinal anesthesia, addition of dextrose or epinephrine, and lithotomy position for surgery ▪ Typically resolves spontaneously within 1 week

Cardiovascular

Hypotension

- More likely in older patients, with higher blocks, or when combined with general anesthesia
- Associated with nausea, vomiting, dizziness, and dyspnea

Bradycardia

- More likely if baseline heart rate is low, male sex, age <40 years, and prolonged duration of surgery

Respiratory

Respiratory Depression Associated with Neuraxial Procedures
▪ Caused by rostral spread of opioids to chemosensitive respiratory centers in brainstem ▪ Onset: 2 hours with lipophilic opioids, but hydrophilic opioids (e.g., morphine) can present up to 24 hours after injection ▪ More common in patients with sleep apnea, older patients, and during coadministration of systemic sedatives ▪ Monitor using respiratory rate and sedation score.

Infection

- Bacterial meningitis most commonly arises from intrathecal transmission of oral bacteria, e.g., *S. viridans*, making facemasks mandatory during all neuraxial procedures.

Wrong-Route Drug Delivery

- Inadvertent administration of a drug intended for vascular compartment into the epidural or intrathecal space, or vice versa
- International Organization for Standardization published medical small-bore connector standards, which should reduce this risk.

Backache

- Epidural analgesia is not associated with new-onset postpartum back pain for up to 6 months.

Nausea and Vomiting

- Secondary to direct emetogenic effect of opioids, hypotension, or gastrointestinal hyperperistalsis due to unopposed parasympathetic activity
- More likely in patients with a history of motion sickness, block height >T5, the development of hypotension, and morphine (vs. fentanyl or sufentanil)

Urinary Retention

- S2-S4 nerve roots blockade weakens detrusor muscle, neuraxial opioids suppress contractility and reduce the urge sensation.
- Spontaneous return of bladder function expected once sensory level regresses to less than S2-S3
- Urinary retention is associated with male sex, age (and age-specific pathologies, e.g., benign prostatic hypertrophy), long-acting local anesthetics, and intrathecal morphine.

Pruritus

- Associated with all intrathecal opioids, can be treated with naloxone or naltrexone

Shivering

- Risk higher with epidural over spinal anesthesia, and less with the addition of neuraxial opioids

Complications Unique to Epidural Anesthesia

Intravascular Injection

- Risk higher in obstetrical patients, can cause local anesthetic systemic toxicity (LAST)
- Decreased risk when placed in lateral position, administering fluid in epidural space before inserting catheter, advancing the catheter less than 6 cm, and aspirating the catheter before every dose

Subdural Injection

- Higher than expected sensory relative to motor blockade 15 to 30 minutes after injection

QUESTIONS

ANATOMY

1. What is the clinical significance of the curvatures of the spinal canal with respect to spinal and epidural anesthesia?
2. During spinal anesthesia placement, what are the tissue planes that will be traversed as the needle is advanced toward the subarachnoid space in the midline?
3. Describe the blood supply of the spinal cord. Which area of the cord is most vulnerable to ischemic insult?

MECHANISM OF ACTION AND PHYSIOLOGY

4. Compare and contrast the most significant factors that affect block height in spinal and epidural anesthesia.
5. How does the degree of lipophilicity of opioids added to a local anesthetic solution affect its duration of action after neuraxial injection?
6. What are the determinants of the onset time of extradural nerve fiber blockade?
7. What is differential sensory block?
8. Complete the following table using "increased" or "decreased" to describe the physiologic effect of neuraxial anesthesia on each organ system.

Organ System	Effect of Neuraxial Anesthesia
Cardiovascular	*Systemic vascular resistance:* *Cardiac output:* *Arterial blood pressure:*
Central nervous	*Cerebral blood flow:* *Wakefulness:*
Respiratory	*Vital capacity:*
Gastrointestinal	*Colonic mucosal blood flow and motility:*
Renal	*Urinary function:*

INDICATIONS AND CONTRAINDICATIONS

9. A patient with severe asthma, severe aortic stenosis, multiple sclerosis, and von Willebrand disease has had previous spine surgery with resulting spinal stenosis and myelopathy. Prior to seeing the patient, the surgeon discussed the benefits of neuraxial anesthesia with the patient, who refused due to fear of developing back pain. Which of the above issues are an absolute contraindication to proceeding with neuraxial anesthesia?

SPINAL ANESTHESIA

10. Complete the following table by indicating the sensory dermatome level of anesthesia necessary and the corresponding anatomical location.

Surgery	Dermatome	Corresponding Anatomic Location
Cesarean section		
Upper abdominal surgery		
Lower abdominal surgery		
Hip surgery		
Transurethral resection of prostate		
Vaginal delivery		
Lower extremity surgery		
Hemorrhoidectomy		

11. What are some advantages and disadvantages of a continuous spinal technique?

EPIDURAL ANESTHESIA

12. What are the options for identifying the epidural space during epidural placement?
13. What are some potential advantages of adding epinephrine to the local anesthetic solution used for epidural anesthesia?

COMBINED SPINAL-EPIDURAL ANESTHESIA

14. What is the potential clinical benefit of combined spinal-epidural anesthesia?

CAUDAL ANESTHESIA

15. What are some indications for caudal anesthesia?

COMPLICATIONS

16. What is the differential diagnosis of neurologic deficit following neuraxial anesthesia?
17. What factors are associated with postdural puncture headache following neuraxial anesthesia?
18. What are transient neurologic symptoms (TNS), and what are the factors associated with TNS following neuraxial anesthesia?

ANSWERS

ANATOMY

1. On a lateral view in the figure below, the vertebral canal exhibits four curvatures, of which the thoracic convexity (kyphosis) and the lumbar concavity (lordosis) are of major importance to the distribution of local anesthetic solution in the subarachnoid space. In contrast, these curves have little effect on the spread of local anesthetic solutions in the epidural space. Scoliosis is of less importance to local anesthetic spread but can make needle insertion more awkward. (291, 299)

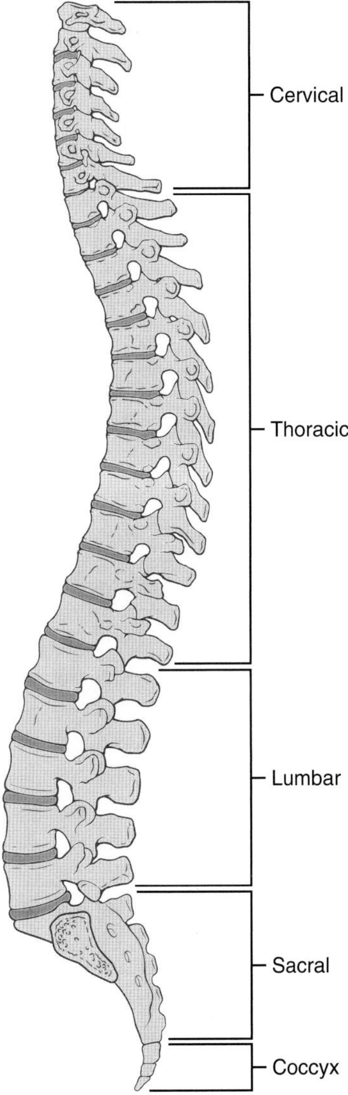

Figure from Covino BG, Scott DB, Lambert DH. Handbook of Spinal Anaesthesia and Analgesia. Philadelphia: WB Saunders; 1994:12–24.

2. As the spinal needle progresses toward the subarachnoid space, it passes through the skin, subcutaneous tissue, supraspinous ligament, interspinous ligament, ligamentum flavum, and the epidural space to reach and pierce the dura/arachnoid see figure below. The characteristic "pop" is produced by the spinal needle passing through the dura mater. (291)

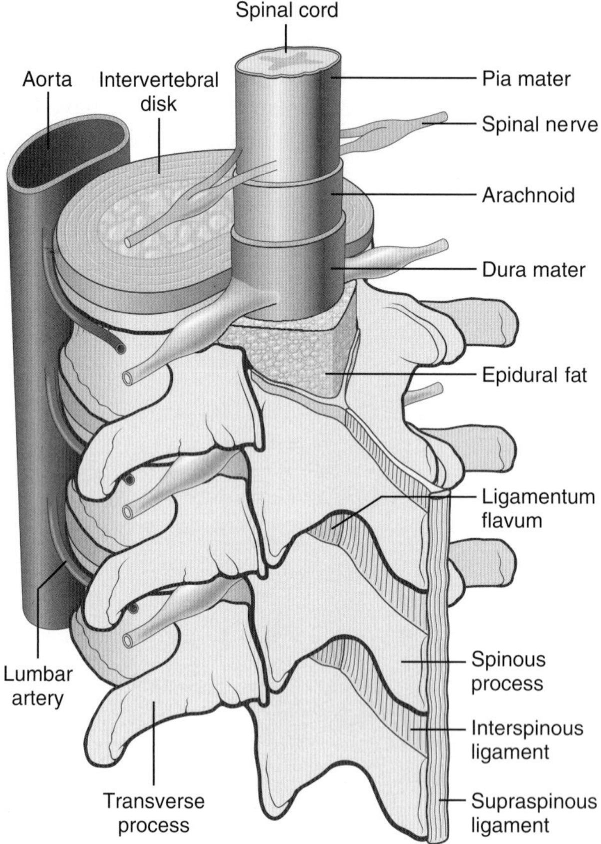

Figure from Afton-Bird G. Atlas of regional anesthesia. In Miller RD, ed. Miller's Anesthesia. Philadelphia: Elsevier; 2005.

3. The blood supply of the spinal cord arises from a single anterior and two posterior spinal arteries, as demonstrated in the figure below. The posterior spinal arteries emerge from the cranial vault and supply the dorsal (sensory) portion of the spinal cord. Because they are paired and have rich collateral anastomotic links from the subclavian and intercostal arteries, this area of the spinal cord is relatively protected from ischemic damage. This is not the case with the single anterior spinal artery that originates from the vertebral arteries and supplies the ventral (motor) portion of the spinal cord. Ischemia affecting the anterior spinal artery may result in "anterior spinal artery syndrome," characterized by motor paralysis and loss of pain and temperature sensation below the level affected. (292–294)

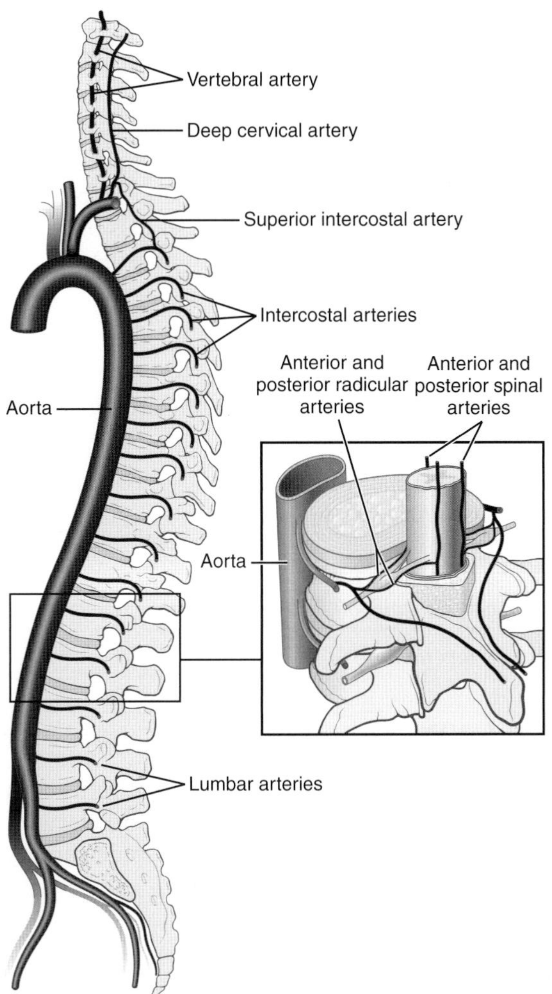

Figure modified from Covino BG, Scott DB, Lambert DH. Handbook of Spinal Anaesthesia and Analgesia. Philadelphia: WB Saunders; 1994:24.

MECHANISM OF ACTION AND PHYSIOLOGY

4. Baricity, dose, and patient positioning from time of injection to 20 to 25 minutes after are the most significant factors affecting block height for spinal anesthesia. For epidural anesthesia, the volume and total dose of local anesthetic, as well as the level of injection are most significant. (297–300, 305)
5. Lipophilic opioids, such as fentanyl and sufentanil, have a duration of action of about 2 to 3 hours after neuraxial injection due to their rapid uptake into vessels and fat. In contrast, neuraxial morphine, which is hydrophilic and poorly absorbed, has a duration of action of up to 24 hours. (301, 306–307)
6. The speed of extradural nerve fiber blockade depends on the size, surface area, and degree of myelination of the nerve fibers exposed to the local anesthetic.

After intrathecal injection of local anesthetic, loss of cold sensation (approximates sympathetic blockade) usually occurs first and can be tested by using ice or alcohol. Regression of neural blockade follows the reverse order. See table below. (293–294)

Nerve Fiber Type	Size and Myelination	Comments
B fibers	1–3 μm, minimally myelinated	Small preganglionic sympathetic fibers; most sensitive to local anesthetic blockade
C fibers	0.3–1 μm, unmyelinated	Conduct cold temperature sensation, blocked more readily than the A-delta
A-delta fibers	1–4 μm, myelinated	Mediate pinprick sensation
A-beta fibers	5–12 μm, myelinated	Conduct touch sensation, are the last sensory fibers to be affected
A-alpha fibers	12–20 μm, myelinated	Motor fibers, most resistant to local anesthetic blockade

7. Differential sensory block describes how maximum block height in neuraxial anesthesia varies according to the sensory modality. The loss of sensation to cold (and sympathetic blockade) is one to two segments higher than the loss of sensation to pinprick, which is higher still than loss of sensation to touch. (294)
8. The table below describes the physiologic effects of neuraxial anesthesia. (295)

Organ System	Effect of Neuraxial Anesthesia
Cardiovascular	*Systemic vascular resistance:* decreased *Cardiac output:* maintained or slightly decreased *Arterial blood pressure:* decreased
Central nervous	*Cerebral blood flow:* decreased *Wakefulness:* decreased
Respiratory	*Vital capacity:* decreased
Gastrointestinal	*Colonic mucosal blood flow and motility:* increased
Renal	*Urinary function:* possible retention

INDICATIONS AND CONTRAINDICATIONS

9. Absolute contraindications to neuraxial anesthesia include patient refusal, infection at the site of planned needle puncture, allergy to any of the drugs to be administered, and elevated intracranial pressure. Severe aortic stenosis, multiple sclerosis, von Willebrand disease, previous spine surgery, spinal stenosis, and myelopathy are all relative contraindications. (296–297)

SPINAL ANESTHESIA

10. The following table indicates the sensory dermatome level of anesthesia necessary, and the corresponding anatomical location for the given procedure. (297–298).

Surgery	Dermatome	Corresponding Anatomic Location
Cesarean section	T4	Nipple
Upper abdominal surgery	T4	Nipple
Lower abdominal surgery	T6-T7	Xiphoid proess
Hip surgery	T10	Umbilicus
Transurethral resection of prostate	T10	Umbilicus
Vaginal delivery	T10	Umbilicus
Lower extremity surgery	L1-L3	Inguinal ligament
Hemorrhoidectomy	S2-S5	

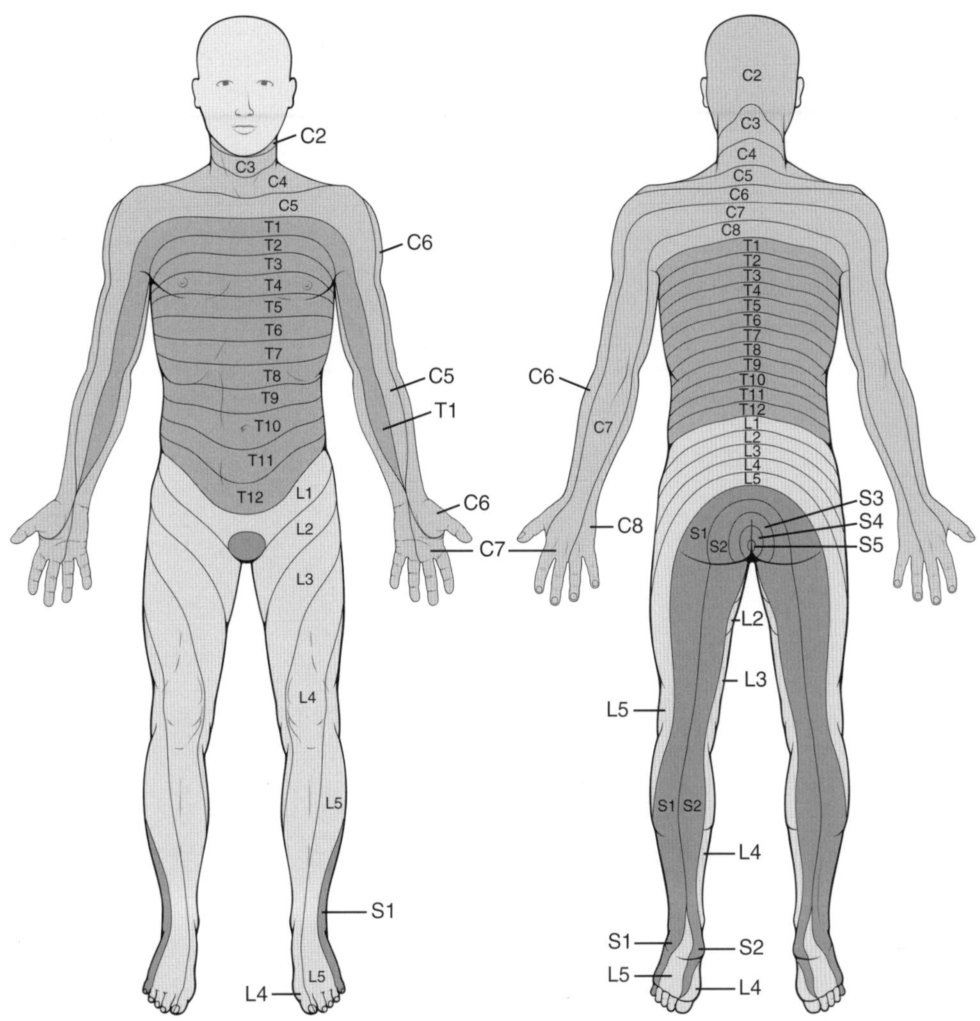

Figure modified from Veering BT, Cousins MJ. Epidural neural blockade. In Cousins MJ, Bridenbaugh PO, Carr DB, et al., eds. Neural Blockade in Clinical Anesthesia and Management of Pain. Philadelphia: Lippincott-Raven; 2009:241–295.

11. Inserting a catheter into the subarachnoid space (continuous spinal technique) permits incremental dosing and possibly greater hemodynamic stability than a higher dose, single-injection technique. A catheter also allows repeated drug administration and anesthesia for prolonged operations. The use of large-bore epidural needles and catheters for continuous spinal anesthesia poses a significant risk of postdural puncture headache. Microcatheters are available, but they may be more difficult to insert and have been associated with the development of cauda equina syndrome. It is likely that the neurotoxic injury associated with the use of high-resistance, low-flow microcatheters resulted from maldistribution of local anesthetic solution due to pooling in the dependent sacral sac. (304)

EPIDURAL ANESTHESIA

12. Identification of the epidural space during epidural placement is with the loss of resistance technique, which can be achieved many ways. With this technique, a syringe containing saline, air, or both is attached to the needle, and the needle is slowly advanced. Once the needle tip reaches and is properly seated in the ligamentum flavum, it becomes difficult to inject the saline or air, and the plunger of the syringe will "spring back" to its original position (see figure below). Upon advancing further, an abrupt loss of resistance to injection signals passage of the needle tip through the ligamentum flavum and into the epidural space. Air

is reportedly less reliable than saline in identifying the epidural space, may cause pneumocephalus, and even venous air embolism in rare cases. Saline can reduce the risk of epidural vein cannulation but may make it more difficult to detect an accidental dural puncture. The "hanging-drop" technique is an alternative method for identifying the epidural space. With this technique, a small drop of saline is placed at the hub of the epidural needle. As the needle passes through the ligamentum flavum into the epidural space, the saline drop is "sucked" into the needle by the negative pressure in the epidural space. (307–308)

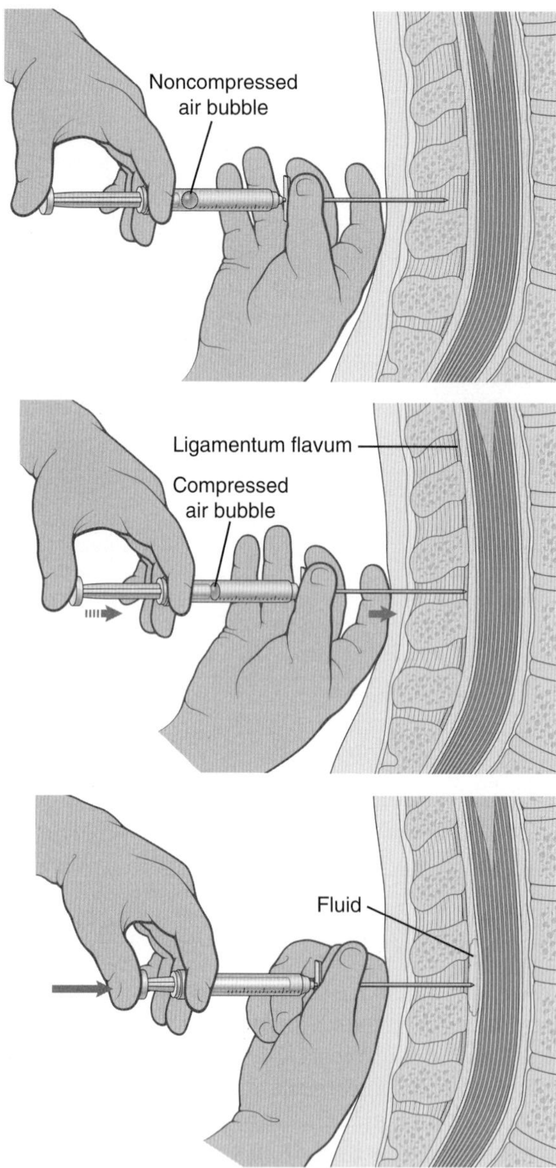

Figure from Afton-Bird G. Atlas of regional anesthesia. In Miller RD, ed. Miller's Anesthesia. Philadelphia: Elsevier; 2005.

13. Advantages of adding epinephrine to the local anesthetic solution used for epidural anesthesia include decreased vascular absorption and prolonged anesthesia and analgesia, most notably with short- and intermediate-acting local anesthetics. Epinephrine may also serve as a marker of intravascular injection that can occur with cannulation of an epidural vein. Finally, epinephrine may have some direct analgesic effects via dorsal horn α_2-receptor activation. Phenylephrine is less effective than epinephrine and is not as widely used. (306)

COMBINED SPINAL-EPIDURAL ANESTHESIA

14. Combined spinal-epidural anesthesia capitalizes on the rapid onset and intense sensory anesthesia of a spinal anesthetic and the ability to supplement and extend the duration of the block afforded by an epidural catheter. The technique is commonly used in obstetric anesthesia or in any case when the anticipated duration of surgery may last longer than an average spinal anesthetic (2–3 hours). Using a low-dose spinal anesthetic and subsequently increasing the block height gradually through incremental epidural boluses of local anesthetic or saline can offer more hemodynamic stability in high-risk patients and decrease the required dose of spinal local anesthetic. This sequential technique is termed *epidural volume extension*. (309)

CAUDAL ANESTHESIA

15. Caudal anesthesia is most used in pediatric patients undergoing surgery at or below the level of the umbilicus, such as inguinal hernia repair, circumcision, or hypospadias repair. It is less useful in adults because the spread of caudal local anesthetic in adults is unpredictable. For adults, caudal anesthesia is most used in chronic pain and cancer pain management but may also be used when the lumbar approach is not possible. (309–310)

COMPLICATIONS

16. Neurologic deficit is a rare but serious complication of neuraxial anesthesia. Direct injury may occur from needle trauma, but the injectate can also be neurotoxic. Preservatives in local anesthetics or additives have been thought to be responsible in the past for adhesive arachnoiditis and cauda equina syndrome. Profound hypotension or vascular supply disruption can cause anterior spinal artery syndrome, in which the patient will have preserved proprioception and vibratory sense. An epidural hematoma or abscess can cause ischemic compression of the spinal cord. (311–312)
17. Postdural puncture headache (PDPH) is a direct consequence of the hole made in the dura during spinal anesthesia or accidental dural puncture during epidural needle placement. Headache and other symptoms are caused by CSF leakage through the dura, which results in downward displacement of the brain with a resultant traction on pain-sensitive supporting structures. While the incidence is around 1%, patient factors that increase the risk of PDPH include younger age, female sex, and pregnancy. Procedural factors that increase the risk of PDPH include needle diameter, bevel direction during dural puncture, multiple dural punctures, and the shape of the hole created by the needle. Smaller-gauge, noncutting, pencil-point needle tips (e.g., Whitaker, Sprotte), which spread the dural fibers, reduce the risk of postdural puncture headache. (312)
18. TNS is characterized by bilateral or unilateral pain in the buttocks, commonly radiating to the legs, with no neurologic deficits. The symptoms usually occur within 24 hours of resolution of a spinal anesthetic and usually resolve spontaneously in less than a week. TNS are more common with intrathecal injection of concentrated lidocaine or mepivacaine, the addition of dextrose or phenylephrine, and solution osmolarity. The lithotomy position also increases risk. (312)

Chapter

18 PERIPHERAL NERVE BLOCKS

Andrew T. Gray and Edward Yap

INTRODUCTION

The Role of Regional Anesthesia

- Peripheral nerve blocks can provide surgical anesthesia and postoperative pain relief.
- Paresthetic-based techniques can be used alone or combined with ultrasound guidance for some regional blocks.

Preparation to Perform a Regional Nerve Block

Foundation of Knowledge

- To perform safe and effective peripheral nerve blocks, an understanding of the following is needed.
  - Peripheral neuroanatomy
  - Ultrasound technology
  - Local anesthetic pharmacology
  - Risks

Patient and Surgeon Factors

- The patient and surgeon need to consent to the nerve block.
- Surgery location is considered when deciding the type of peripheral nerve block performed.
- A thorough preoperative review to rule out any contraindications must be performed prior to a peripheral nerve block.
  - Factors to consider include medical history, allergies, prior neuropathy, concurrent anticoagulation medications

Monitors and Equipment

- Locations to perform a peripheral nerve block include a block area or operating room.
- The following monitors and equipment are needed prior to the procedure.
  - Functioning peripheral intravenous line
  - Pulse oximetry, electrocardiogram, and noninvasive blood pressure machine
  - Supplemental oxygen, emergency medications, and airway equipment must be accessible
  - Sedation may be indicated, depending on the patient's anxiety and magnitude of pain.
- For most blocks, the provider is positioned on the ipsilateral side and the ultrasound on the contralateral side of the block region.
- The choice of the ultrasound probe and needle is dependent on the location of the peripheral nerve block.
  - A catheter may be placed depending on the type of surgery, duration of hospital stay, and clinical preference.

Choice of Local Anesthetic

- Factors for the choice of local anesthesia include
  - Onset, duration, degree of block
  - Lidocaine and mepivacaine have quick onset and shorter duration.
  - Ropivacaine and bupivacaine have slower onset and longer duration.
  - Addition of epinephrine can serve as an intravascular marker and increase duration of the block.
  - Perineural steroids can also prolong peripheral nerve blocks.

Regional Block Checklist

- A standardized regional block checklist used before performing a peripheral nerve block can improve safety.
- The checklist should include surgical consent, site marking, allergies, anticoagulation status, proposed peripheral nerve block, local anesthetic dose, side of the block, monitors implemented, emergency equipment available, and sedation plan.

Risks and Prevention

- Infection
  - Infectious risk associated with a peripheral nerve block is rare.
  - An infection can cause significant morbidity and may lead to permanent neurologic injury.
  - Reduce infection rates by
    - Proper hand hygiene
    - Maximal barriers during procedure
    - Antiseptic solution at the site of insertion

- Hematoma
  - The risk of developing a hematoma depends on the proximity to vascular structures and vascular compressibility.
  - Ultrasound and proper aspiration can reduce vascular puncture.
  - A review of the patient's medical history and anticoagulation medication is important.
- Local anesthetic systemic toxicity
  - Local anesthetic systemic toxicity (LAST) symptoms can range from mild symptoms to major neurologic and cardiovascular toxicity.
  - Risk of LAST influenced by patient risk factors, concurrent medications, total local anesthetic dose, anatomic location of the peripheral nerve block
  - Decrease the risk of LAST by
    - Using the smallest effective dose
    - Incremental injection
    - Aspiration before injection
    - Intravascular marker (i.e., epinephrine)
    - Ultrasound guidance
    - Lipid emulsion resuscitation is the therapy to treat LAST.
- Nerve injury
  - Nerve injury may result from needle trauma, intraneural injection, drug neurotoxicity.
  - Serious injury is rare; transient paresthesia occurs more frequently.
  - Decrease the risk of nerve injury by
    - Ultrasound guidance
    - Limit injection pressure
    - Patient feedback
- Wrong-sided block
  - Wrong site, wrong procedure, and wrong patient peripheral nerve blocks are potentially serious medical errors.
  - This can be reduced by having a universal protocol that includes a checklist.

Preparation to Perform a Regional Nerve Block

- Thoroughly review a patient's medical history to rule out any contraindications for a peripheral nerve block.
- Understand the location of the surgery to choose the type of nerve block to be performed.
- Have a standardized checklist to use before performing a nerve block.

ULTRASOUND BASICS

Basic Ultrasound Physics

- Ultrasound waves have frequency >20 kHz.
- Piezoelectric crystals convert electrical currents into mechanical pressure waves and vice versa to generate images.
- Acoustic impedance: resistance to the propagation of ultrasound waves through tissue
  - Solid tissues: denser particles reflect waves and displayed as brighter or hyperechoic
  - Less dense tissue, less reflection of waves, displayed as darker or hypoechoic
  - Anechoic: tissues that do not reflect waves
- Improving image resolution optimizes performance of peripheral nerve blocks.
  - Increasing frequency improves resolution but decreases penetration.
  - Decreasing frequency lowers resolution but will improve the penetration.
  - Increasing receiver gain can help compensate for attenuation.

Echogenic Properties of Nerves and Tissue

- Peripheral nerves have fascicular echotexture.
- Central nerves and very small nerves are monofascicular or oligofascicular.
- Most peripheral nerves have a polyfascicular appearance.
- Nerves have a relatively constant cross-sectional area; this helps distinguish them from adjacent structures such as tendons.

Ergonomics and Transducer Manipulation

- Maintain proper posture and position to reduce fatigue.
- A comfortable grip and resting ulnar aspect of the transducer hand on the patient promote stability.
- There are five basic transducer manipulation techniques to help optimize the ultrasound image.
  - Sliding, tilting, rocking, rotation, and compression
  - Tilt to maximize the returning echoes from the peripheral nerve
  - Slide and rotate the transducer to find the needle tip
  - Rocking back—can reduce the angle of insonation, improving needle visibility
  - Compression of adjacent veins—can reduce venous puncture
- Anisotropy: reflected echoes depend on the angle of insonation

Regional Block Technique

- Most blocks can be performed with a short-axis view of the nerve.
- Needle placement techniques
  - In-plane: the entire needle shaft and tip within the plane of imaging
  - Out-of-plane: the needle tip crosses the plane of imaging as an echogenic dot

Peripheral Nerve Catheters

- Catheters placed adjacent to peripheral nerves for postoperative analgesia
- Ultrasound placement is similar to single-injection block.
- Needle system used: catheter through needle (e.g., 17-gauge Tuohy) or catheter over needle
- Peripheral nerve catheters can dislodge due to movement of skin at insertion site.

Ultrasound Basics

- Peripheral nerves have a relatively constant cross-sectional area that helps distinguish them from surrounding structures.
- Maintaining proper ergonomics while performing nerve blocks helps prevent provider fatigue.
- Practicing the five basic transducer manipulation techniques (sliding, tilting, rocking, rotation, and compression) will help optimize ultrasound images.

CERVICAL PLEXUS BLOCK

- Formed by the second, third, and fourth cervical nerves
- Superficial cervical plexus block: infiltration of local anesthetic deep to the platysma and investing fascia of the neck along the posterior lateral border of the sternocleidomastascle

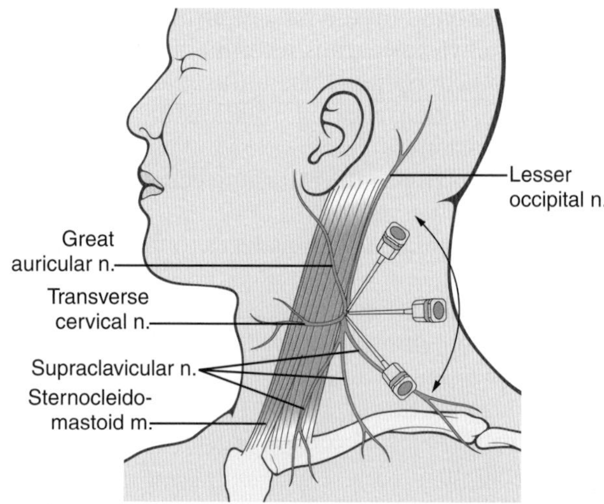

Cervical Plexus Block. (Figure modified from Brown DL, Factor DA, eds. *Regional Anesthesia and Analgesia*. Philadelphia: WB Saunders; 1996:245.)

- Anesthesia produced: area from inferior surface of the mandible to level of the clavicle
- Used to provide anesthesia in conscious patients undergoing carotid endarterectomy

UPPER EXTREMITY BLOCKS

Brachial Plexus

- Network of nerves composed of five nerve roots (C5, C6, C7, C8, and T1)
- Provides both motor control and sensory input for most of the upper extremity

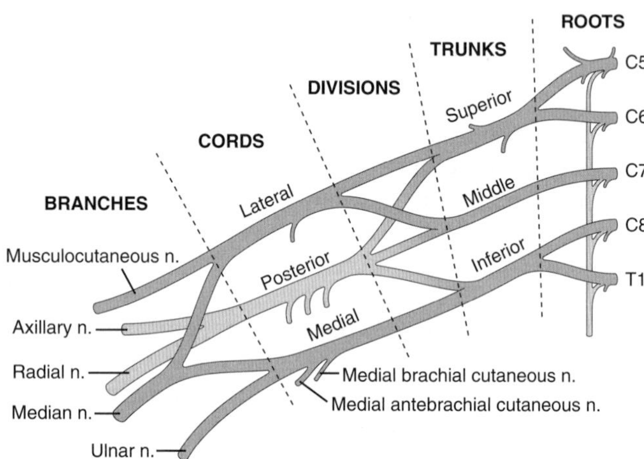

Brachial Plexus. (Figure modified from Johnson RL, Kopp SL, Kessler J, Gray AT. Peripheral nerve blocks and ultrasound guidance for regional anesthesia. In Gropper MA, ed. *Miller's Anesthesia*. 9th ed. Philadelphia: Elsevier; 2020:1459.)

- The brachial plexus does not innervate:
  - Skin over the shoulder: supraclavicular nerve of the cervical plexus
  - Medial aspect of the arm: intercostobrachial branch of the second intercostal nerve
- The C5–T1 nerve roots form ventral rami and trunks between the anterior and middle scalene muscles and then pass over the first rib and under the clavicle.
- The trunks form three anterior and three posterior divisions, which recombine to create three cords in the infraclavicular region.
- These cords divide into terminal branches in the axillary region.
- The location along the brachial plexus to block is determined by
  - Location of surgery
  - Experience
  - Patient factors (e.g., body habitus)

Interscalene Block

- Location
  - Targets the ventral rami of the brachial plexus, can spare the inferior trunk (C8, T1)
  - Suited for surgeries that involve the distal clavicle, shoulder, and upper arm

- Not always suitable for distal forearm and hand surgeries
- Performed at C6 vertebral level, where brachial plexus emerges between anterior and middle scalene muscles

- Patient position
  - Head turned to contralateral side
- Ultrasound
  - Linear probe, transverse plane
  - Nerves in short-axis view
  - Identify: middle and anterior scalene muscle, sternocleidomastoid muscle, brachial plexus ("stoplight" appearance of monofascicular C5 and bifascicular C6)
- Needle technique
  - In-plane technique, insert lateral to medial, through middle scalene
  - Local injected once in brachial plexus fascia sheath

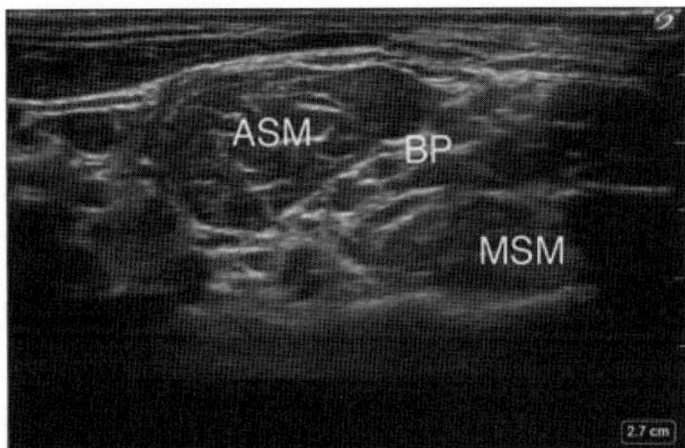

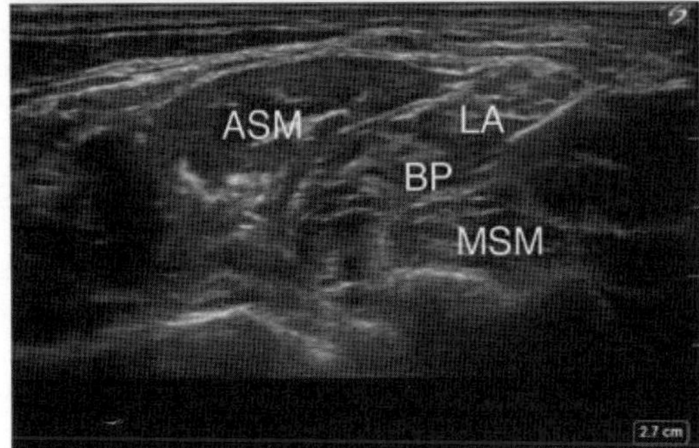

- Risks
  - Horner syndrome
  - Recurrent laryngeal nerve block
  - Epidural or subarachnoid injection
  - Vertebral artery injection
  - Pneumothorax
  - Phrenic nerve block

Supraclavicular Block

- Location
  - Injection cephalad to clavicle, adjacent to the subclavian artery where brachial plexus tightly bundled
  - Advantages: rapid onset, patient arm can remain at side
- Patient position
  - Head turned to contralateral side
- Ultrasound
  - Linear probe, transverse plane
  - Nerves in short-axis view
  - Move transducer to above the clavicle, facing caudally
  - Identify: subclavian artery over first rib, first rib, brachial plexus
- Needle technique
  - In-plane technique
  - First rib serves as backstop to needle advancement to thorax.
  - Local distributed underneath inferior trunk of brachial plexus
  - May needle multiple injections around plexus
- Risks
  - Pneumothorax most common serious complication (1% incidence)
    - Symptoms include cough, dyspnea, pleuritic chest pain
  - Phrenic nerve block (50% of procedures), usually not clinically significant

Infraclavicular Block

- Location
  - Targets medial, lateral, and posterior cords of brachial plexus
  - Suited for surgeries of the arm below the shoulder
  - Injection of the plexus underneath the clavicle
  - Advantages: close proximity of plexus to artery, consistent anatomy, stable site for catheter
- Patient position
  - Supine, arm abducted, elbow flexed, arm externally rotated if possible
- Ultrasound
  - Linear or curvilinear transducer
  - Placed medial to coracoid process in parasagittal plane
  - Nerves in short-axis view
  - Identify: pectoral major and minor muscles, axillary artery and vein, cords of the brachial plexus (may be difficult to delineate)
- Needle technique
  - In-plane technique, advanced cephalad to caudad
  - Needle directed toward space between lateral cord and axillary artery
  - Local distributed around axillary artery in U-shape

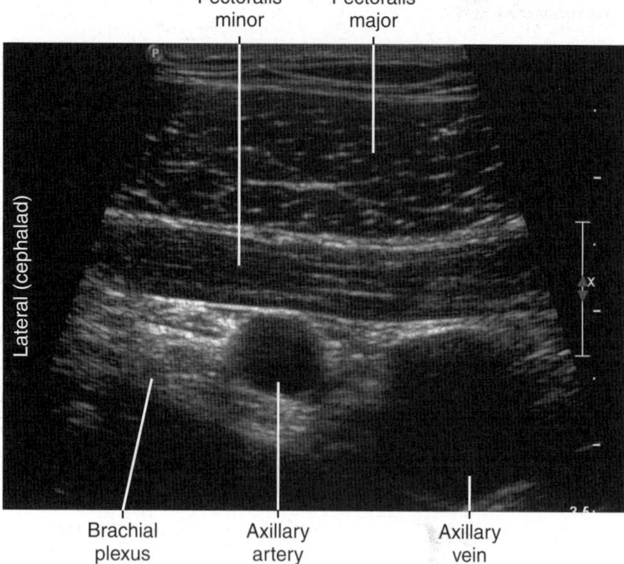

Infraclavicular Block. (From Gray AT. *Atlas of Ultrasound-Guided Regional Anesthesia*. 3rd ed. Philadephia: Elsevier; 2018:97-98.)

- Risks
  - Depth of block is a challenge.
  - Pneumothorax

Axillary Block

- Location
  - Targets terminal branches of the brachial plexus in the axilla.
    - Median, ulnar, radial, musculocutaneous nerves
  - Suited for surgeries of elbow, forearm, wrist, and hand
  - Advantages: lower risk of complications, simpler to perform
- Patient position
  - Supine, arm abducted and externally rotated
- Ultrasound
  - Linear transducer
  - Nerves and vessels in short-axis view
  - Identify: axillary artery, vein(s), terminal branches of brachial plexus, conjoint tendon, biceps, triceps, and coracobrachialis muscles
  - Nerves in relation to axillary artery: median (superficial), ulnar (medial), radial (posterior), and musculocutaneous (lateral, traversing through the coracobrachialis muscle)
- Needle technique
  - In-plane technique
  - Needle directed cephalad to caudad
  - Local injection around each terminal branch, musculocutaneous can be targeted separately

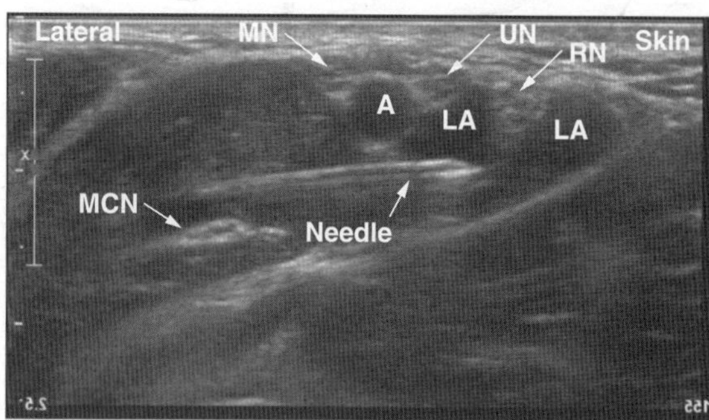

Axillary Block. (Figure from Gray AT. *Atlas of Ultrasound-Guided Regional Anesthesia*. 3rd ed. Philadelphia: Elsevier; 2018:97, 98.)

- Risks
  - Intravascular injection
  - Hematoma
  - Unsuitable for catheter
  - Lack of coverage for upper arm and shoulder

Intercostobrachial Nerve Block

- Nerve is derived from T2 and T3.
- Cutaneous innervation medial half of upper arm, supplements brachial plexus blocks
- Performed by subcutaneous infiltration in the medial half of the upper arm

Upper Extremity Blocks

- Be careful when blocking the brachial plexus at the interscalene and supraclavicular region in patients who have significant pulmonary comorbidities because it can lead to ipsilateral phrenic nerve palsy.
- The interscalene block often spares the ulnar distribution of the forearm and hand.
- The supraclavicular block provides reliable anesthesia and analgesia of upper arm, elbow, forearm, and hand; however, it has the highest risk of pneumothorax.
- The infraclavicular block provides a good location for a peripheral nerve catheter.
- The axillary block is simpler to perform and has lower risk of complications.

LOWER EXTREMITY BLOCKS

- Lower extremity nerves originate from the following plexuses.
  - Lumbar plexus: composed of the first four lumbar nerves (L1–L4)
    - Gives rise to lateral femoral cutaneous, femoral, and obturator nerves
  - Sacral plexus: composed of the first four sacral nerves (S1–S4) and receives contributions from L4 and L5
    - Gives rise to sciatic nerve

Femoral Nerve

Femoral Nerve Block

- Location
  - Largest branch of lumbar plexus, derived from L2–L4
  - Motor innervation to quadriceps
  - Sensory innervation to anterior thigh and medial leg
  - Suited for surgeries of the anterior thigh, and provides analgesia for hip, femur, knee surgeries
  - Performed distal to the point the femoral nerve passes under the inguinal ligament
  - Nerve lies lateral to femoral artery.
  - Advantages: reliable analgesia, good location for catheter, predictable and shallow anatomy
- Patient position
  - Supine
- Ultrasound
  - Linear transducer, placed transverse distal to inguinal ligament
  - Nerve in short-axis view
  - Identify: femoral artery and vein, femoral nerve (flat oval or triangular polyfascicular), sartorius and iliopsoas muscle, fascia lata/iliaca
- Needle technique
  - In-plane technique
  - Needle advanced in lateral-to-medial direction toward lateral aspect of femoral nerve
  - May feel two "pops" as the needle passes fascia lata and fascia iliaca
  - Local injected to surround nerve

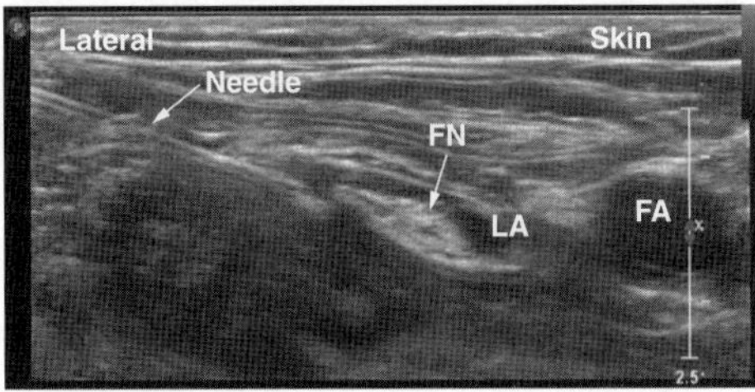

- Risks
  - Quadriceps weakness may increase risk of falls.

Adductor Canal Nerve Block

- Location
  - Adductor canal targets distal branches (mostly sensory) of femoral nerve.
  - Performed midthigh, nerve lies deep to sartorius muscle, femoral artery near the middle of sartorius muscle belly
  - Advantages: analgesia for knee surgery with minimal quadriceps weakness
- Patient position
  - Supine, leg slightly externally rotated and bent at the knee
- Ultrasound
  - Linear transducer
  - Nerve in short-axis view, may be difficult to see nerves
- Needle technique
  - In-plane technique
  - Needle advanced lateral to medial, anterior to posterior
  - Local spread under posterior fascia of sartorius muscle, lateral to femoral artery

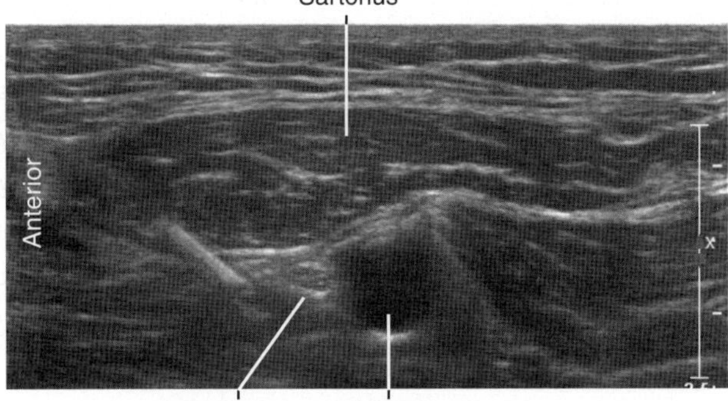

Saphenous Nerve Block Near Adductor Canal. (Figure from Gray AT. *Atlas of Ultrasound-Guided Regional Anesthesia*. 2nd ed. Philadelphia: Elsevier; 2012.)

Saphenous Nerve Block

- Terminal branch of the femoral nerve
- Sensory nerve fibers innervate medial aspect of leg, ankle, and foot.
- Can be blocked at thigh, leg, or ankle
- Adductor canal approach is often used to block the saphenous nerve in the thigh.

Sciatic Nerve

- Largest branch of the sacral plexus, consists of L4, L5, and S1–4

- Motor and sensory innervation of posterior thigh and most of leg
- Travels posterior thigh, anterior to gluteus maximus and biceps femoris
- Suited for surgeries of the posterior thigh, lower leg, foot, and ankle, and provides analgesia after knee surgery

Proximal Sciatic Nerve Block

- Location
  - Three approaches: anterior, transgluteal, and subgluteal
  - Reliably located traveling halfway between the greater trochanter of the femur and the ischial tuberosity, deep to the gluteus maximus muscle
  - Advantages: reliable posterior thigh and leg analgesia, location away from tourniquet if catheter is placed
- Patient position (transgluteal approach)
  - Lateral position with the block leg up and slightly flexed at the hip
- Ultrasound
  - Linear or curvilinear transducer
  - Nerve in short-axis view
  - Appears as a hyperechoic, polyfascicular triangular structure
- Needle technique
  - In-plane technique, longer needle may be needed
  - Directed lateral to medial, posterior to anterior, toward lateral border of nerve
  - Needle placed below fascial plane of the gluteus maximus muscle, local spread around nerve

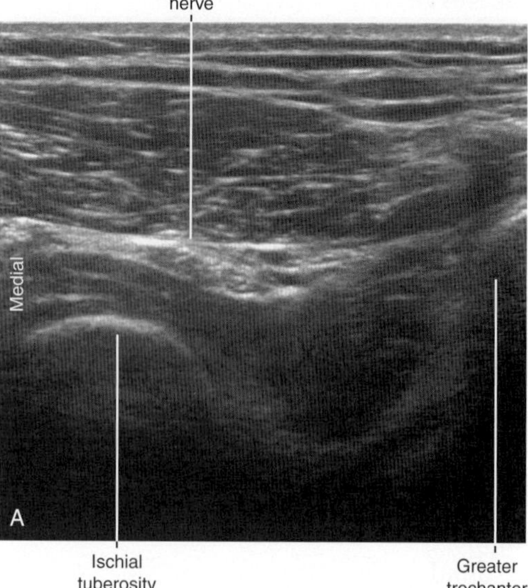

Sciatic Nerve Block Ultrasound Anatomy. (Figure from Gray AT. *Atlas of Ultrasound-Guided Regional Anesthesia*. 3rd ed. Philadelphia: Elsevier; 2018:188.)

- Risks
  - Disadvantages: hamstring weakness, foot drop, procedural discomfort

Popliteal Block of the Sciatic Nerve

- Location
  - Targets the sciatic nerve as it enters the popliteal fossa
  - Divides into common peroneal and tibial nerves
  - Suited for foot and ankle surgery
  - Combined with saphenous nerve for medial aspect of leg
- Patient position
  - Lateral position, block leg elevated, knee extended
- Ultrasound
  - Linear transducer
  - Nerve in short-axis view
  - Transducer placed in popliteal fossa
  - Identify: sciatic nerve posterior to popliteal vein and artery
- Needle technique
  - In-plane technique
  - Nerve blocked at the bifurcation of sciatic nerve (into tibial and common peroneal nerves)
  - Directed lateral to medial
  - Local spread around both components of the nerve, creating "donuts"

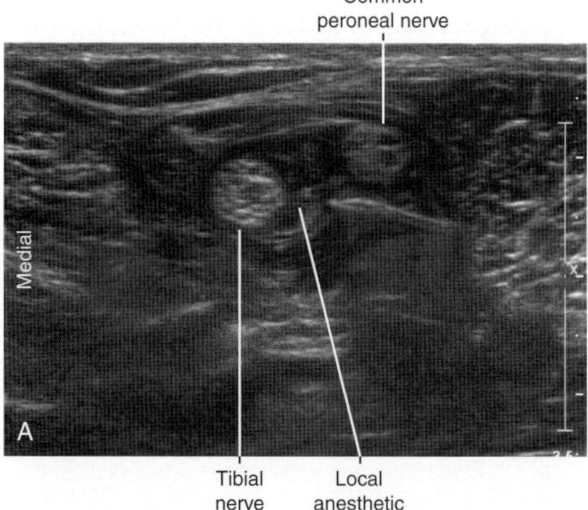

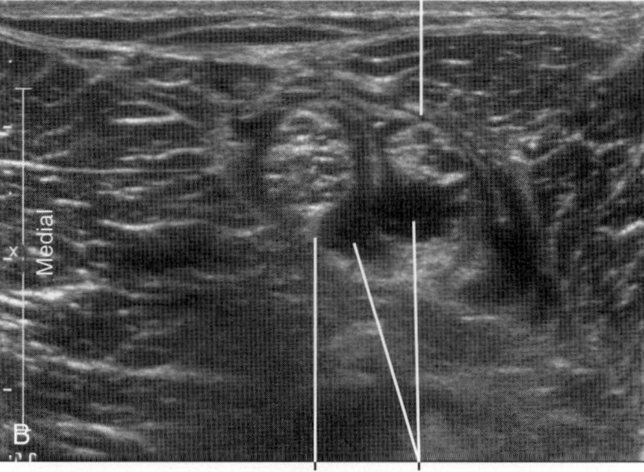

Popliteal Block of the Sciatic Nerve. From. (From Gray AT. *Atlas of Ultrasound-Guided Regional Anesthesia*. 3rd ed. Philadelphia: Elsevier; 2018:197.)

Ankle Block

- All five peripheral nerves that supply the foot can be blocked at the malleoli.

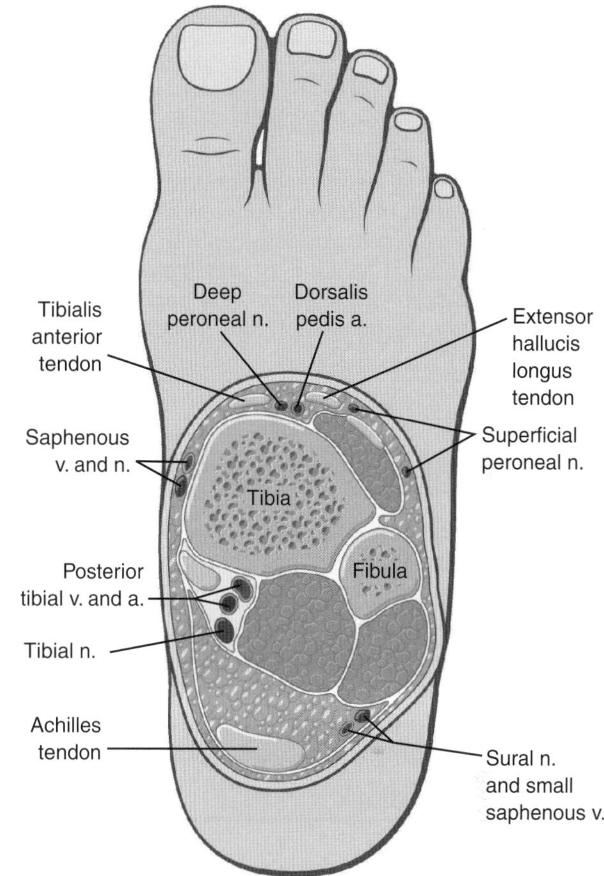

Cross-sectional Anatomy for Ankle Block. (Figure modified from Brown DL, Factor DA, eds. *Regional Anesthesia and Analgesia*. Philadelphia: WB Saunders; 1996.)

  - Tibial nerve
    - Innervates sole of the foot
    - Infiltrate 3 to 5 mL of local anesthetic in a fanning pattern around posterior tibial artery.
  - Sural nerve
    - Innervates lateral side of the foot
    - Infiltrate 5 mL local anesthetic in the groove between lateral malleolus and the calcaneus.
  - Saphenous nerve
    - Innervates medial aspect of the foot
    - Infiltrate 5 mL local anesthetic anterior to the medial malleolus near the great saphenous vein.
  - Deep peroneal nerve
    - Innervates the webbing between the first and second toes
    - Inject 5 mL local anesthetic adjacent to the anterior tibial artery.
    - Alternatively, block deep to the extensor hallucis longus tendon.

- Superficial peroneal nerve
  - Innervates the dorsum of the foot
  - Inject a subcutaneous ridge of local anesthetic between the medial and lateral malleoli over the anterior surface of the foot.

Lower Extremity Blocks

- The femoral nerve block provides analgesia to the anterior thigh and knee; however, it leads to quadriceps weakness that may be associated with higher risk of falls until block has resolved.
- The adductor canal nerve block provides analgesia for knee surgery with minimal quadriceps weakness.
- The sciatic nerve block provides anesthesia and analgesia of the posterior thigh and most of the leg, ankle, and foot. A curvilinear transducer may provide better imaging depending on patient body habitus and depth of the nerve.

CHEST AND ABDOMEN BLOCKS

- Peripheral nerve blocks for the chest and abdomen
  - Provide intraoperative and postoperative analgesia
  - Reduce systemic pain medications
  - Improve patient satisfaction
  - Improve patient discharge times from the postanesthesia care unit

Intercostal Nerve Block

- Location
  - Targets ventral rami of thoracic spinal nerves
  - Travels inferior to associated rib
    - Within subcostal groove, inferior to vein and artery
    - Between internal and innermost intercostal muscles
  - Suited for thoracic and upper abdominal surgery
- Patient position
  - Prone
- Ultrasound
  - Linear transducer
  - Short-axis view, parasagittal plane at midscapular line
  - Identify: intercostal muscles, pleura, adjacent ribs
- Needle technique
  - In-plane technique
  - Local spread in between innermost and internal intercostal muscles along inferior border of rib
  - Can be performed more centrally by injecting deep to erector spinae muscle at the lateral edge of the transverse process
- Risks
  - Pneumothorax, LAST (high-peak plasma level compared to other peripheral blocks)
  - Challenges: multiple ribs need to be blocked for dermatomal coverage

Transversus Abdominis Plane Block

- Location
  - Abdominal wall field block targeting ventral rami of T7–L1 spinal nerves
  - Nerves travel between transversus abdominis and internal oblique muscles.
  - Analgesia for lower abdominal surgery
- Patient position
  - Supine
- Ultrasound
  - Linear transducer
  - Place transverse plane, midaxillary line
  - Identify: external oblique, internal oblique, transversus abdominis muscle
- Needle technique
  - In-plane technique, longer needle may be needed
  - Needle directed in anterior to posterior direction
  - At least 20 mL local anesthetic per side
  - Local distribution between transversus abdominis and internal oblique muscles

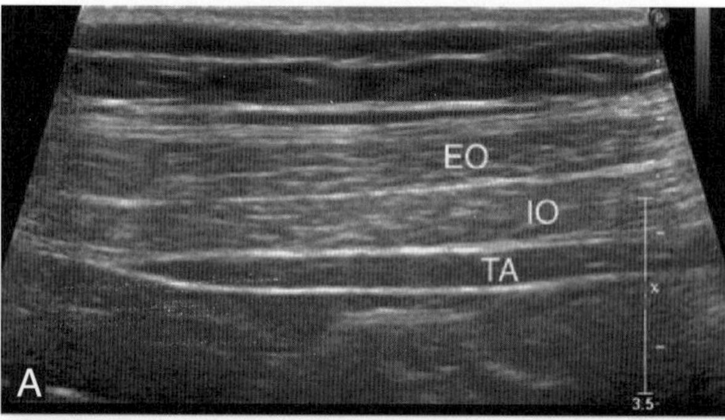

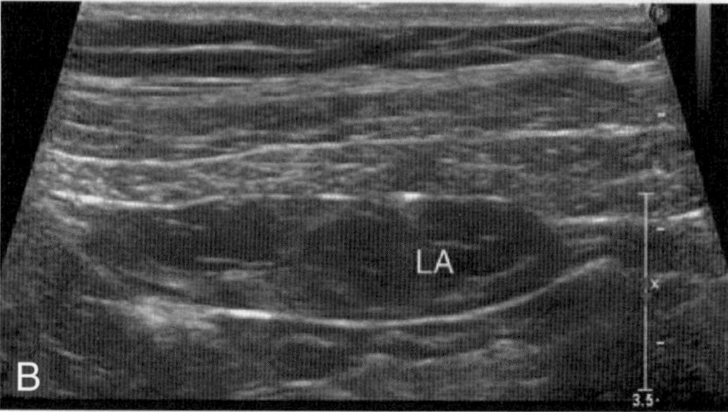

- Risks: LAST (block requires large volume of local anesthetic), intraperitoneal and intrahepatic injection

INTRAVENOUS REGIONAL ANESTHESIA (BIER BLOCK)

- A method of producing anesthesia of the arm or leg with different approach than typical peripheral nerve block
  - Exsanguination and isolation of circulation by tourniquet
  - Intravenous injection of large volume of dilute local anesthetic into isolated extremity
- Suited for procedures with minimal postoperative pain and duration 1 to 2 hours or less
- Advantages: quick onset, lasts as long as the tourniquet is inflated, may be faster than a single-shot peripheral nerve block
- Technique
  - Place small peripheral intravenous catheter in distal extremity.
  - Exsanguinate extremity with Esmarch bandage (placed distal to proximal).
  - Inflate tourniquet 250 to 275 mmHg (at least 100 mmHg above systolic blood pressure).
  - Inject plain preservative-free local anesthetic (40–50 mL for an adult arm) through intravenous catheter.
  - Remove intravenous catheter.
  - To address potential for tourniquet pain, consider using double-tourniquet technique (i.e., tourniquet with proximal and distal cuff).
    - Proximal cuff is initially inflated, allowing local anesthetic to reach extremity underneath the distal cuff.
    - When patient experiences tourniquet pain, distal cuff is inflated, then proximal cuff is deflated.
- Contraindications: any contraindication to tourniquet use (e.g., sickle cell disease)
- Challenges to use of intravenous regional anesthesia
  - Patient with extremity lacerations (escape of local anesthetic)
  - Patient with extremity fracture (may experience pain during exsanguination)
  - Development of tourniquet pain (typically after 45–60 minutes, limiting duration technique can be used)
- Risks: LAST (reduce risk by keeping tourniquet inflated for at least 20 minutes), inadequate exsanguination (leading to poor quality of block)

QUESTIONS

INTRODUCTION

1. What knowledge is needed to perform a safe and effective peripheral nerve block?
2. What are potential risks of performing a peripheral nerve block, and how can these risks be reduced?

ULTRASOUND BASICS

3. How do nerves appear on ultrasound imaging?
4. What ultrasound adjustments and techniques can be used to improve imaging?
5. Draw the appearance of a peripheral nerve in short axis with a regional block needle in-plane compared to out-of-plane.

UPPER EXTREMITY BLOCKS

6. For a given surgical site, what are the possible brachial plexus blocks that may be appropriate? How do you decide which block to perform?

Location of Surgery	Possible Brachial Plexus Block
Distal clavicle, shoulder, upper arm	
Arm below shoulder	
Elbow, forearm, hand, wrist	

LOWER EXTREMITY BLOCKS

7. What nerves and plexuses provide sensation to the lower extremity?
8. Your patient is scheduled for an open reduction, internal fixation of an ankle fracture. The patient is requesting peripheral nerve blocks and sedation, and the surgeon informs you both the medial and lateral malleoli are fractured. Which peripheral nerve block or blocks should be performed?

CHEST AND ABDOMEN BLOCKS

9. What are the benefits of peripheral nerve blocks of the chest and abdomen?

INTRAVENOUS REGIONAL ANESTHESIA

10. When is it appropriate to use intravenous regional anesthesia (Bier block) instead of a peripheral nerve block? What are the potential advantages and risks of the Bier block?

ANSWERS

INTRODUCTION

1. To perform safe and effective peripheral nerve blocks, an understanding of peripheral neuroanatomy, ultrasound technology, local anesthetic pharmacology, and risks associated with peripheral nerve blocks is needed. A thorough preoperative review of the patient's medical history, including any comorbid diseases, allergies, prior neuropathy, and concurrent anticoagulation medications, must be performed to rule out any contraindications in providing a peripheral nerve block. A standardized regional block checklist used before performing a peripheral nerve block can improve patient safety. (318–319)
2. The following table summarizes potential risks of performing peripheral nerve blockade and approaches to reducing these risks. (319–320)

Risk	Approach to Reducing Risk
Infection	Performing proper hand hygiene, using maximal barriers during procedures, and cleaning the area of the site insertion with antiseptic solution
Hematoma	Following proper hold parameters for patients who are receiving anticoagulants, using an intravascular marker (e.g., epinephrine 1:200,000), ultrasound guidance, and applying pressure to the site of insertion
Local anesthetic systemic toxicity (LAST)	Using the lowest effective local anesthetic dose, incremental injection, aspiration prior to injection, using an intravascular marker, and ultrasound guidance
Nerve injury	Use of ultrasound to identify nerves, limiting injection pressure, and patient feedback during block
Wrong-sided block	Having a universal protocol utilizing a checklist to ensure the correct patient, proper surgical site/laterality, and confirming the proposed peripheral nerve block

ULTRASOUND BASICS

3. Peripheral nerves can be recognized by their fascicular echotexture. Nerves that are closer to the spine have fewer fascicles and can be recognized by their monofascicular or oligofascicular appearance on ultrasound scans. More peripheral nerves have a polyfascicular appearance and look like a collection of small round hypoechoic dots surrounded by hyperechoic connective tissue, a pattern referred to as "honeycomb" or "bunch of grapes". See image below. (320–321)

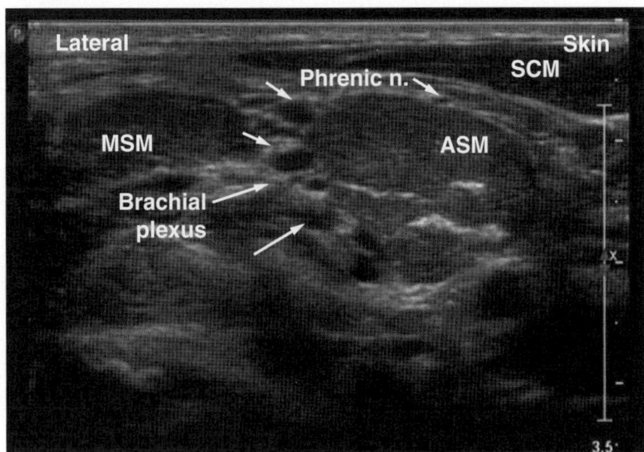

4. Increasing frequency of the ultrasound can improve the resolution of an image; however, it will decrease the penetration of the ultrasound waves. Decreasing the frequency will lower the resolution but will improve the penetration of the ultrasound. Increasing receiver gain can help compensate for attenuation. Transducer

manipulation techniques can help improve ultrasound imaging and include sliding, tilting, rocking, rotation, and compression. (320)

5. Short-axis view of the nerve is shown in both images. On the left, the needle is out-of-plane, and on the right the needle is in-plane. (321)

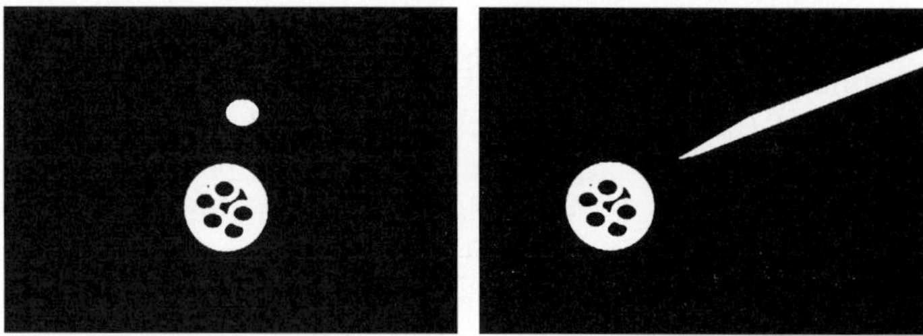

Approaches to Regional Block with Ultrasound. (From Gray AT. *Atlas of Ultrasound-Guided Regional Anesthesia.* 3rd ed. Philadephia: Elsevier; 2018:30.)

UPPER EXTREMITY BLOCKS

6. The location of the surgery, experience of the provider, and patient factors help determine where along the brachial plexus a peripheral nerve block should be performed. (322–325)

Location of Surgery	Possible Brachial Plexus Block
Distal clavicle, shoulder, upper arm	Interscalene block (spares ulnar nerve, may not be suitable for distal forearm and hand surgeries); supraclavicular block
Arm below shoulder	Infraclavicular block, supraclavicular block
Elbow, forearm, hand, wrist	Axillary block, supraclavicular block, infraclavicular block

LOWER EXTREMITY BLOCKS

7. The lower extremity innervation originates from the lumbar (L1–L4) and sacral (S1–S4, with contribution from L4–5) plexuses. The nerves that branch from these plexuses are the lateral femoral cutaneous, femoral, obturator, and sciatic nerves. The femoral nerve (L2–L4) is the largest branch of the lumbar plexus and provides motor function to the quadriceps and sensation of the anterior thigh and medial leg. The sciatic nerve (L4, L5, S1–S4) is the largest branch of the sacral plexus and provides motor function to the posterior thigh and lower leg and sensation of the posterior thigh and most of the lower leg, ankle, and foot. (327–328)
8. A sciatic block at the popliteal fossa covers sensation below the knee, except for the medial leg and ankle. A saphenous nerve block (or femoral nerve block) would need to be performed as well for surgery involving the medial leg or ankle. (327–330)

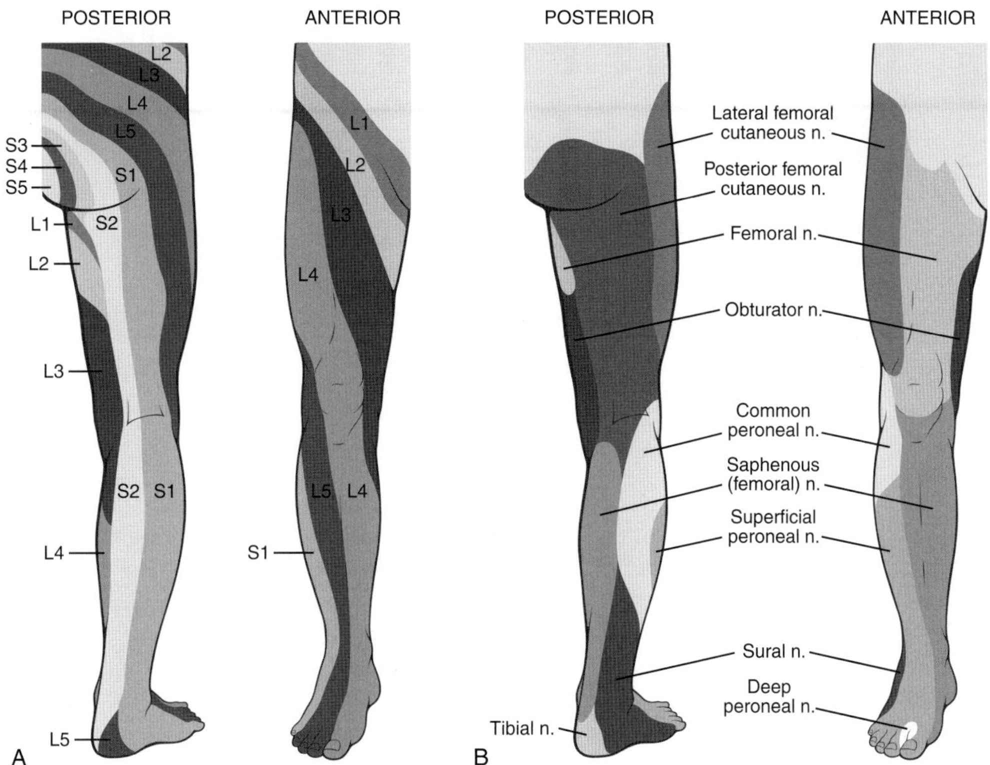

Cutaneous Distribution of Lumbosacral Nerves. (Figure modified from Horlocker TT, Kopp SL, Wedel DJ. Nerve blocks. In Miller RD, ed. *Miller's Anesthesia*. 8th ed. Philadelphia: Elsevier; 2015:1738.)

CHEST AND ABDOMEN BLOCKS

9. Peripheral nerve blocks of the chest and abdomen can provide intraoperative and postoperative analgesia, reduce systemic pain medications, improve patient satisfaction, and improve patient discharge times. (330)

INTRAVENOUS REGIONAL ANESTHESIA

10. Intravenous regional anesthesia (Bier block) is a method to provide anesthesia to the arm or leg for surgeries that have minimal postoperative pain and a duration of two hours or less. Advantages of a Bier block include its rapid onset of anesthesia, its duration and speed to perform, and its applicability to all age groups, including pediatric patients. The greatest risk of a Bier block is LAST, which is most likely to occur when the tourniquet is deflated, and large amounts of local anesthetic solution enter the systemic circulation. For this reason, bupivacaine is avoided for this type of block; the most commonly used local anesthetics include 0.5% lidocaine or chloroprocaine. Other complications of the Bier block include hematoma, engorgement of the extremity, thrombophlebitis, and subcutaneous hemorrhage. (333–334)

Chapter

19 PATIENT POSITIONING AND ASSOCIATED RISKS

Kristine Breyer and Dylan E. Masters

INTRODUCTION

- Patient positioning in the operating room
  - Facilitates planned procedures
  - Can be a source of patient injury
  - Can alter intraoperative physiology
  - Remains a significant source of perioperative morbidity
  - Is a shared responsibility between surgeons, nurses, and anesthesia providers

PHYSIOLOGIC ASPECTS OF POSITIONING

- Nonanesthetized state
  - Central, regional, and local physiologic responses maintain hemodynamics during changes in positioning.

Example of Normal Physiologic Response to Positional Changes: Reclining From Upright to Supine in the Nonanesthetized State

- Venous return increases.
- Preload, stroke volume, and cardiac output increase.
  - Arterial blood pressure briefly increases.
- Afferent baroreceptors are activated.
  - From the aorta (via the vagus nerve)
  - From the carotid sinus (via the glossopharyngeal nerve)
- Sympathetic outflow is decreased.
- Parasympathetic impulses to the sinoatrial node and myocardium increase.
  - Systemic arterial blood pressure is maintained within a narrow range.

- Anesthetized state
  - Physiologic responses that maintain hemodynamics during changes in positioning can be blunted.
  - Positional alterations in pulmonary physiology can be exaggerated.

Pulmonary Changes in Supine Position in the Anesthetized State

- Functional residual capacity (FRC) decreases when a standing patient is positioned supine; FRC is further decreased during general anesthesia.
  - Can lead to increased ventilation–perfusion mismatching
  - Increased risk of hypoxia

GENERAL POSITIONING PRINCIPLES

- During normal sleep, patients change positions.
  - Prevents prolonged compression and excessive stretch
- During anesthesia, patients lose the ability to sense injury and change position.
  - Immobility increases patients' risk for positioning injuries during surgery and anesthesia.
- Documentation
  - Preexisting physical limitations and neuropathies
  - Intraoperative positioning checks and postoperative assessments

General Principles for Patient Positioning Under Anesthesia

- Maintain spine and extremity neutrality.
- Limit the duration of extreme positions.
- Use strategic padding, especially for tissue overlying bony prominences.
- Be mindful of pressure created by all equipment.
  - Examples include surgical instruments and retractors, probes, tubes, and fluoroscopy equipment.

Supine

- Most common position for surgery
- Also called the *dorsal decubitus position*
- In classic supine: head, neck, and spine retain neutrality.
- Arm positions can vary.

- One or both arms may be abducted or adducted alongside the patient.
  - Limit arm abduction to less than 90 degrees to protect the brachial plexus from excessive stretch.
  - Limit elbow flexion to prevent ulnar nerve injury.
  - Limit elbow extension to protect against stretching of median nerve.
  - When arms are adducted, they should be held alongside body with a drawsheet.
- On arm board: hands and forearms should be supinated or in a neutral position with palms toward body.
  - Reduces external pressure on ulnar nerve

Variations of the Supine Position

- Lawn-chair position
  - Flexes hips and knees slightly
  - Legs slightly above heart level
  - Back of bed is raised, legs lowered, and slight Trendelenburg tilt
    - Reduces stress on the back, hips, and knees
    - Facilitates venous return from lower extremities
    - Reduces abdominal muscle tension
    - Often better tolerated by patients awake or under monitored anesthesia care
- Frog-leg position
  - Hips and knees are flexed.
  - Hips are externally rotated with knees supported.
    - Facilitates procedures to perineum, genitalia, and rectum
- Trendelenburg position
  - Tilted head-down in supine with the pubic symphysis as the highest part of trunk
  - Uses
    - Increase venous return during hypotension
    - Improve exposure during abdominal or laparoscopic surgery
    - Prevent air emboli during central line placement
  - Hemodynamic, respiratory, and physiologic changes
    - Autotransfusion from the legs with 9% increase in cardiac output in 1 minute, and returning to baseline within 10 minutes
    - Decreased FRC and pulmonary compliance due to shifted abdominal contents
    - Increases in intracranial pressure (ICP) and intraocular pressure (IOP)
    - Increased risk of pulmonary aspiration of gastric contents
    - Swelling of head, neck, and airway when prolonged
  - Risk of sliding and shifting when in steep Trendelenburg
    - Prevention includes use of nonsliding mattresses beneath the patient.
    - Shoulder braces can cause compression or stretch injury to brachial plexus.
- Reverse Trendelenburg position
  - Tilted so the supine patient's head is higher than any other part of body
  - Used to facilitate upper abdominal surgery
  - Decreases venous return risking hypotension, especially if hypovolemic
  - Risk of cerebral hypoperfusion
    - Invasive arterial monitoring should be zeroed at external auditory meatus.

Complications

- Backache
  - Normal spine lordosis is lost with general or neuraxial anesthesia.
  - Risk factors include patients with kyphosis, scoliosis, or history of back pain.
  - Decrease risk with extra padding at spine or slight flexion at hip and knee.
- Operating table tilt and tip over
  - Can occur when patient is positioned in reverse orientation to allow surgical access or permit passage of equipment under the table
    - Torso is opposite the pedestal of the table.
    - Risk is increased in patients with large body mass, Trendelenburg position, when bed-lengthening extensions are used, or if the bed is unlocked to move.
  - Operating table weight limits differ with reverse orientation.

Lithotomy

- Legs held by supports and abducted 30–45 degrees with knees flexed
  - Hip flexion varies with need for surgical exposure (standard, low, or high lithotomy).
  - Must raise and lower legs simultaneously to prevent spine torsion
- Used for gynecologic, rectal, and urologic procedures
- Risks
  - Neuropraxia, especially common peroneal nerve injury
    - Most common complication
    - To prevent, pad the lateral leg where nerve wraps around fibular head.
  - Crush injury to the patient's fingers
    - Confirm hand position when lower section of operating table is raised.
    - Position arms on armrests away from operating table.
  - Lower extremity compartment syndrome
    - Rare but devastating
    - Inadequate blood flow from hypoperfusion (leg elevation) or venous obstruction (limb compression or hip flexion)

        - Ischemia, edema, and rhabdomyolysis
        - Risk is highest with high lithotomy and/or prolonged surgical time.
        - Lower legs periodically for surgery beyond several hours.
- Physiologic changes
    - Cardiac output transiently increases with leg raise.
    - Lung compliance and tidal volume decrease from cephalad abdominal displacement.
    - Loss of spine lordosis can aggravate low back pain.

Lateral Decubitus

- Patient lies on nonoperative side.
- Used for surgery in thorax, retroperitoneum, hip
- Risks
    - Falling or tilting forward or backward
        - Secure well with beanbag, bedding roll and/or kidney rest.
    - Extremity injury or nerve stretch
        - Dependent leg flexed with padding between the knees
        - Arms both abducted less than 90 degrees to protect brachial plexus
        - Dependent arm on padded arm board
        - Nondependent arm supported over a padded armrest or folded bedding
    - Axillary contents compression
        - Axillary roll is placed caudal to the axilla or inflated bean bag.
        - Invasive arterial monitoring in dependent arm can detect compression of artery.
    - Excessive stretch of neck and brachial plexus
        - Maintain head in neutral position with additional head support.
    - Compression of eyes and ears
        - Tape eyes and check for compression of dependent eye.
        - Confirm dependent ear is not folded.
- Physiologic changes
    - Decreased compliance of dependent lung, favoring ventilation to nondependent lung
    - Pulmonary blood flow increases to dependent lung due to gravity.
    - Ventilation/perfusion mismatch can affect alveolar ventilation and gas exchange.

Prone

- Used for surgery in the posterior fossa, spine, buttocks, perineum and lower extremities
- Positioning is a coordinated effort including all operating room providers.
    - Endotracheal intubation, intravenous and invasive lines, and Foley catheter should all be placed with patient supine.
    - All lines and tubes should be secured prior to moving the patient.
    - Head positioning and stabilization
        - Specifically designed head rests, pillows, and mirror systems can be used.
        - Mayfield rigid head pins or Gardner-Wells tongs used in some brain and spine surgeries
    - Thorax support
        - Commercial rolls and bolsters are available (Wilson frame, Jackson table).
        - Bolsters should extend from clavicle to iliac crest.
    - Abdomen
        - Should hang relatively free without external pressure
    - Extremities
        - All extremities padded, especially at elbow to protect ulnar nerve
        - Legs padded and slightly flexed at knees and hips
        - Arms tucked in neutral position or placed next to patient's head on arm boards with less than 90 degree abduction
- Risks
    - Dislodgement or migration of lines and tubes
        - Consider disconnecting lines or monitors to facilitate the turn, and then reconnect when the patient is in the new position.
    - Neurovascular or spine injury when turning
        - Maintain head, neck, and spine neutral during turn.
        - Unstable spines are especially vulnerable.
        - Reports of cerebrovascular events
        - Consider "pre-flip" baseline recordings when neuromonitoring is available.
    - Facial pressure wounds
        - Regular checks and document that the eyes and nose are free from pressure
    - Postoperative visual loss
        - Prolonged prone positioning is one of several factors associated with ischemic optic neuropathy.
    - Head movement or slipping
        - Scalp lacerations, skull fractures, and cervical spine injury
        - Maintain an adequate depth of anesthesia to prevent movement.
        - Secure table and attachments.
        - Confirm turn lock mechanisms on Jackson table are engaged.
    - Tissue injury
        - Pendulous structures (e.g., breasts, genitalia) should be free from compression.
    - Abdominal compression
        - Problems with ventilation
        - Hypotension from inferior vena cava compression and decreased venous return

- Femoral nerve and vasculature compression
  - Can occur from lower portion of bolster
- Physiologic effects
  - Hemodynamics are well maintained.
  - Superior pulmonary function than in supine position
    - FRC and oxygenation are improved.
    - Pulmonary compliance improved in obese patients when abdomen hangs free

Sitting

- Patient's head and operative field are above the level of the heart.
- Uses
  - Some cervical spine and neurosurgical procedures, e.g., posterior fossa
  - A variation is the "beach chair" position, which is used for shoulder surgery.
  - Decreased venous pressure may reduce surgical blood loss.
- Positioning
  - Head must be adequately fixed with head strap, tape, or other rigid fixation.
  - Arms and feet are supported and padded.
  - Shoulders even or very mildly elevated
  - Knees slightly flexed
- Risks
  - Venous air embolism (VAE) is most significant complication.
    - Can lead to arrhythmias, acute pulmonary hypertension, and circulatory collapse
    - Low venous pressure and open dural venous sinuses can lead to the entrainment of air.
    - The incidence of VAE in neurosurgery in sitting position may be as high as 100%.
    - Clinically significant VAE incidence is 0.5%–3%.
    - Intraoperative detection of entrained air by transesophageal echocardiography (TEE) or precordial Doppler ultrasound
    - Multiorifice central venous catheter can be used to aspirate air in the event of a VAE.
  - Paradoxical air embolism
    - VAE leading to myocardial infarction and stroke
    - Preoperative diagnosis of an intracardiac shunt contraindicates surgery in the sitting position.
    - Transesophageal echocardiography is the gold standard for detection of intracardiac shunt.
  - Pneumocephalus
    - Occurs frequently but rarely significant
    - Symptoms include headache, confusion, seizures, and even temporary hemiparesis.
    - Must rule out intracranial bleeding or stroke
  - Head and neck swelling and macroglossia
    - Excessive neck flexion impeding cerebral venous outflow
  - Compression of laryngeal structures and tongue
    - Can be caused by excessive neck flexion combined with TEE monitoring
    - Minimum of two fingerbreadths between mandible and sternum are recommended.
- Physiologic effects
  - Hypotension from venous pooling in lower extremities
    - Compression stockings should be placed.
    - IV fluid and vasopressors may help raise mean arterial pressure.
  - Cerebral hypoperfusion
    - Can be due to excessive head and neck flexion
    - Invasive arterial pressure monitor should be placed at level of external auditory meatus.

POSITIONING FOR ROBOTIC-ASSISTED SURGERY

- Robotic-assisted surgery is increasing in prevalence in a variety of surgeries.
- Unique safety and positioning challenges
  - Table cannot be repositioned after the robot is docked.
    - Risks robot dislodgement and patient injury
  - Access to patient is limited.
    - All required lines and monitors should be placed prior to docking the robot.
  - Steep Trendelenburg causing slipping or neck stretch and brachial plexus injury
  - Endotracheal tube migration
    - Metal tray or table above the patient's face provides protection.
  - Laryngeal edema and optic neuropathy
- Physiologic effects
  - Abdominal carbon dioxide insufflation and steep Trendelenburg
    - Decrease in FRC and pulmonary compliance
    - Can be challenging with the increased ventilation requirement

PRESSURE INJURIES

- Caused by prolonged pressure inhibiting capillary blood flow over a bony prominence
- Stage 1 (intact, nonblanchable erythema) to stage 4 (full-thickness tissue loss)
- Muscle damage occurs before skin or subcutaneous tissue.
  - Likely from increased oxygen demand
- Intraoperative pressure injuries
  - Most are discovered within 72 hours of surgery.
  - Prolonged surgical time, hypotension, and hypothermia increase the risk.
    - Most are in operations lasting longer than 3 hours.

- Position influences affected area.
  - Supine: sacrum, heels, occiput
  - Prone: chest, knees
  - Sitting: ischial tuberosities
- Face, lips, tongue, and nose pressure injuries
  - Endotracheal tubes, supraglottic airways, nasogastric tubes, and other devices

BITE INJURIES

- Transcranial motor-evoked potentials used for neuromonitoring
  - Causes contraction of the temporalis and masseter muscles resulting in biting
  - Implicated in tongue (most common), lip, and tooth injuries
  - Severity can be minor bruising to laceration requiring repair.
  - Bite blocks between the molars reduces the risk.

PERIPHERAL NERVE INJURIES

- Incidence is highest in cardiac, neurosurgery, and some orthopedic procedures.
  - Upper extremity injuries are more common than lower extremity injuries.
  - Brachial plexus is most common, followed by ulnar nerve.
- Causes
  - Complex and multifactorial
  - Due to compression, stretch, ischemia, metabolic derangement, and direct trauma/laceration during surgery
- Types of injuries
  - Stretch injuries
    - Compromise of vascular plexus supplying the nerve
    - Can be obstruction in venous outflow or arterial inflow
  - Compression injuries
    - Neurapraxia: short ischemic time, focal demyelination, and usually transient dysfunction
    - Axonotmesis: anatomical disruption of the axon (without disruption of perineurium or epineurium)
    - Neurotmesis: severed or disrupted nerve and usually permanent dysfunction
- Under anesthesia
  - Early warning symptoms of pain sensation are blocked.
  - Normal spontaneous repositioning is absent.
- Positioning and padding alone cannot prevent neuropathies.

Preventing Peripheral Nerve Injuries During Surgery

- Maintain neutral position.
- Avoid stretch, overflexion, and overextension.
- Superficial nerves should be padded and weight evenly distributed.
- Ensure equipment is never resting directly on the patient.

- Retrospective study of upper-extremity position-related changes in somatosensory evoked potential recordings in 1,000 spine surgeries
  - Modification of arm position reversed 92% of upper extremity changes.
  - Incidence was significantly higher in prone "superman" and lateral decubitus positions.
  - Reversible changes were not associated with postoperative deficits.

Ulnar Nerve

- Presentation
  - Decreased sensation in the fourth and fifth fingers
  - Inability to abduct the fifth finger
  - "Claw" hand appearance (fourth and fifth digits unable to fully extend)
- Risk factors
  - Large retrospective review of risk factors for ulnar neuropathy lasting longer than 3 months
    - Very thin or very obese
    - Prolonged postoperative bedrest
    - No association with anesthetic technique or intraoperative patient positioning
  - ASA Closed Claims Project database
    - Risk factors included diabetes, alcohol use disorder, cigarette smoking, and cancer.
    - Only 9% of cases had an explicit mechanism.
    - In 27% of claims, elbow padding was explicitly stated.

Brachial Plexus

- Susceptible to stretch and compression due to superficial course in axilla and proximity to humeral head
- Presentation
  - Motor and sensory deficits are wide-ranging.
  - Sensory deficits in the ulnar distribution are common.
- Risk factors
  - Arm abduction more than 90 degrees
  - Lateral rotation of the patient's head
  - Asymmetric retraction of the sternum for internal mammary dissection
  - Direct trauma
- Injury after median sternotomy
  - Associated with the C8–T1 nerve roots
  - Position with head midline, arms at sides, elbows mildly flexed, and forearms supinated

Other Upper Extremity Nerves

- Radial nerve
  - Presentation: wrist drop, inability to abduct the thumb or extend the fingers
  - Most vulnerable at lower third of the upper arm
    - Superficial where nerve crosses in the spiral groove of the humerus
- Median nerve
  - Most vulnerable in the antecubital fossa adjacent to veins used for intravenous access
  - Risk factors
    - Use of automated blood pressure cuff below the antecubital fossa
    - Extension of the elbow beyond the comfortable range

Lower Extremity Nerves

- Sciatic nerve
  - Risk factor is from stretch in lithotomy position.
    - External rotation of the leg
    - Hyperflexion at the hip
- Common peroneal nerve
  - Risk factor is compression at head of fibula in lithotomy position.
  - Presentation: foot drop, inversion of the foot, sensory deficit
- Femoral nerve
  - Presentations
    - Decreased flexion of the hip
    - Decreased extension of the knee
    - Loss of sensation over the superior aspect of the thigh and medial/anteromedial side of the leg.
- Obturator nerve
  - Risk factors
    - Difficult forceps delivery
    - Lithotomy position
    - Excessive flexion of the thigh to the groin
  - Presentation
    - Inability to adduct the leg
    - Decreased sensation over the medial thigh
  - Cadaveric study
    - Abduction of the hips of greater than 30 degrees causes significant strain.
    - This strain is significantly reduced or eliminated by adding at least 45 degrees of hip flexion.

Lithotomy Surgical Position and Peripheral Nerve Injuries

- Lithotomy position prospective study
  - Overall incidence of nerve injury was 1.5%.
  - Most common: obturator > lateral femoral cutaneous > sciatic > peroneal nerves
  - Neuropathy evident within 4 hours of surgical end time
  - Symptoms: paresthesias and pain (no motor weakness in this study)
  - Risk factor: length of surgery greater than 2 hours
  - 14/15 patients had symptom resolution within 4 months of surgery
- Lithotomy position retrospective study
  - Lower extremity motor neuropathy > 3 months' duration
    - Incidence was 1/3608
    - Common peroneal nerve was most affected.

EVALUATION AND TREATMENT OF PERIOPERATIVE NEUROPATHIES

- ASA recommends a simple postoperative assessment of extremity nerve function in the recovery room.
- Postoperative nerve injury
  - Focused physical examination to correlate and document the sensory or motor deficits
  - Document any intraoperative events
- Neurologic consultation
  - Define neurogenic basis.
  - Localize site of the lesion.
  - Determine severity of injury to guide prognosis and management.
- Sensory neuropathies
  - Typically more transient, requiring only reassurance and follow-up
- Motor neuropathies
  - Usually includes demyelination of peripheral fibers of a nerve trunk (neurapraxia)
    - Generally requires 4–6 weeks for recovery
  - If injury to axon and intact nerve sheath (axonotmesis) or complete nerve disruption (neurotmesis)
    - Severe pain and disability
    - Recovery takes 3–12 months when reversible
    - Interim physical therapy to prevent contracture and muscle atrophy
- Electrophysiologic evaluation
  - Within 1 week, informs on characteristic and temporal pattern of injury
  - After 4 weeks, result is more definitive for site, nature, and severity of nerve injury.

PERIOPERATIVE EYE INJURY AND VISUAL LOSS

- ASA Closed Claims Project database
  - Incidence is 0.5% and accounts for 3% of claims.
  - Greater monetary settlements than nonocular injuries
- Corneal abrasions
  - By far the most common perioperative eye injury

- Natural lid reflex is abolished and tear production decreased under general anesthesia.
- Symptoms
  - Sensation of foreign body in the eye, photophobia, blurry vision, erythema
- Risk factors
  - Increased age, length of surgery, prone or Trendelenburg position, and supplemental oxygen delivery in the postanesthesia care unit
- Precautionary measures
  - Early and careful taping of the eyelids, avoiding dangling objects, and close observation as patients awaken
  - Ophthalmic ointments
  - Avoid patient rubbing eyes, especially with pulse oximeter probes, arm boards, or IV lines

- Postoperative visual loss (POVL)
  - Devastating complication
  - Multifactorial causes
  - Highest incidence in spine surgery in prone position
  - Types
    - Ischemic optic neuropathy (ION) (most common)
    - Central retinal arterial occlusion (CRAO) from direct retinal pressure
- Ischemic optic neuropathy
  - Perioperative risk factors
    - Prolonged hypotension, long duration of surgery, large blood loss, large-volume crystalloid use, anemia or hemodilution, and increased intraocular or venous pressure from the prone position
  - Patient risk factors
    - Hypertension, diabetes, atherosclerosis, morbid obesity, and tobacco use

ASA Postoperative Visual Loss Registry

- POVL after prone spine surgery was 89% ION and 11% CRAO.
- 66% of patients with ION had documented bilateral involvement.
- Patients with ION (vs. CRAO) had greater anesthetic duration, estimated blood loss, and crystalloid infusion.
- 66% of ION perioperative injury to the eye remains a rare yet devastating injury.

- Precautions
  - Perform and document frequent eye checks in the prone or lateral position.
  - Limit time in prone position whenever possible.

ANESTHESIA OUTSIDE THE OPERATING ROOM

- Maintaining patient safety is more challenging.
  - Unfamiliar environment
  - Relative lack of positioning equipment
  - Variability in staff and nursing training in patient positioning.
- Anesthesia provider responsibilities
  - Verifying the safety of each patient's position
  - Implementing guidelines for patients receiving anesthesia

QUESTIONS

PHYSIOLOGIC ASPECTS OF POSITIONING

1. How can anesthesia affect the normal physiologic responses to changes in position?

GENERAL POSITIONING PRINCIPLES

2. Who is responsible for checking patient positioning in the operating room?
3. Why is patient positioning under anesthesia so important?
4. Which upper extremity nerves are at risk for injury in the supine position, and how can this risk be mitigated?
5. What are some advantages of the lawn-chair position over the supine position?
6. How can hip dislocation occur secondary to improper frog-leg positioning?
7. How does the Trendelenburg position alter a patient's hemodynamics, pulmonary compliance, and intraocular and intracranial pressure?
8. How can brachial plexus injury occur secondary to improper Trendelenburg positioning?
9. How does the reverse Trendelenburg position affect a patient's hemodynamics?
10. At what patient level should invasive arterial blood pressure transducers be placed when a patient is in the reverse Trendelenburg position?
11. What is the concern for positioning an obese patient supine in the reverse axis on the operating table?
12. What are some potential injuries associated with the lithotomy position?
13. What is the mechanism and risk factors for lower extremity compartment syndrome secondary to lithotomy positioning?
14. What are some risks and concerns for the patient related to the lateral decubitus position and strategies to help minimize these risks?
15. How does lateral decubitus positioning affect pulmonary function?
16. What are some concerns when turning a patient from supine to the prone position?
17. What is the ideal placement of bolsters beneath the patient in the prone position and why?
18. What are the cardiopulmonary changes that occur with prone positioning?
19. For which surgical procedures might the patient be placed in the sitting position?
20. How should the patient's extremities be positioned when in the sitting position for surgery?
21. What are some complications that can occur as a result of placing the patient in the sitting position?
22. Describe the mechanism, detection, and physiologic manifestations of an intraoperative venous air embolus.
23. What is the concern regarding the patient with an anatomic intracardiac shunt scheduled for surgery in the sitting position?
24. What are the risk and symptoms of pneumocephalus in the sitting position?
25. What complications are more likely in a patient with excessive head flexion in the sitting position?

POSITIONING FOR ROBOTIC-ASSISTED SURGERY

26. What unique positioning challenges does robotic surgery pose?
27. What are some anesthetic implications of docking the robot?

PRESSURE INJURIES

28. What is the typical time course of a developing pressure injury? Which surgical procedures present the greatest risk of this complication?
29. What tissue type is at risk for pressure injuries?
30. Which body areas are at risk of pressure injuries in each of the supine, prone, and sitting positions?

BITE INJURIES

31. In what surgical scenarios are patients most likely to incur a bite injury?

PERIPHERAL NERVE INJURIES

32. What is the most common neuropathy represented by claims to the American Society of Anesthesiologists (ASA) Closed Claims Project database?
33. What are the possible mechanisms and preventive strategies for intraoperative peripheral nerve injuries?
34. What have retrospective studies of ASA closed claims shown to be patient risk factors for ulnar nerve injuries?
35. What are some positioning and surgical risk factors for injury to the brachial plexus, common peroneal, sciatic, and obturator nerves?
36. How common are injuries to the radial or median nerves?

EVALUATION AND TREATMENT OF PERIOPERATIVE NEUROPATHIES

37. How should a postoperative nerve deficit be evaluated?
38. What is the treatment and typical time course to recovery from sensory and motor neuropathies?
39. What is the value of electrophysiologic evaluation of an intraoperative nerve injury?

PERIOPERATIVE EYE INJURY AND VISUAL LOSS

40. Describe the risk factors, symptoms, and precautions to minimize risk for corneal abrasion under general anesthesia.
41. What is the mechanism for postoperative vision loss due to central retinal artery occlusion?
42. What are the surgical and patient risk factors for postoperative vision loss due to ischemic optic neuropathy (ION)?

ANSWERS

PHYSIOLOGIC ASPECTS OF POSITIONING

1. Positional changes can lead to physiologic effects, such as changes in blood pressure or pulmonary compliance. Under anesthesia, these physiologic effects can be exaggerated, and/or the physiologic responses to ameliorate these effects can be blunted. (336–337)

GENERAL POSITIONING PRINCIPLES

2. Anesthesia providers, operating room nurses, and surgeons all share responsibility for checking patient positioning for safety. Anesthesia providers should document positioning checks throughout the procedure and particularly following positioning changes. (337)
3. Even while asleep, people normally change positions to protect themselves from pressure injury and excessive stretch. Under general anesthesia patients lose the ability to change position, and sometimes patients remain in one position for long periods of time. This puts skin, soft tissue, and nerves at risk of compression, stretch, and potential injury. Sterile surgical draping often precludes the ability to easily monitor patients under anesthesia, meaning initial positioning is essential to avoid positioning-related injuries. (337)
4. The brachial plexus and ulnar nerves are at greatest risk of injury when the patient is positioned supine; proper positioning can mitigate these risks. Brachial plexus injury can occur if the arm is abducted at an angle greater than 90 degrees and the head of the humerus pushes into the axilla. Ulnar nerve injury can occur from external pressure, typically at the postcondylar groove of the humerus. The hands and forearms should be well padded in a neutral position, either supinated or with the palms toward the body, to limit external pressure on the ulnar nerve. Median and radial nerve injury can also occur, but this risk is much less. Prolonged pressure in the spiral groove of the humerus (radial nerve) and overstretching at the elbow (median nerve) should be avoided. (337–338)
5. Advantages of the lawn-chair position over the supine position include facilitated venous drainage from the elevated position of the legs; reduced stress on the back, hips, and knees; and reduced tension on the abdominal musculature. A patient may wake up with a backache after supine positioning for surgery because of the loss of normal lumbar lordotic curvature during general anesthesia or neuraxial blockade. Extra padding underneath the knee, causing slight flexion of the hip and knee may be helpful to reduce back pain. Often the lawn-chair position is better tolerated in patients who are awake or undergoing monitored anesthesia care. (338)
6. Hip dislocation can occur secondary to improper frog-leg positioning if the knees are not adequately supported and there is external pressure placed on the leg. (338)
7. The Trendelenburg position causes an autotransfusion from the legs, resulting in about a 9% increase in cardiac output in 1 minute which is sustained for about 10 minutes. After about 10 minutes the cardiovascular effects of the Trendelenburg position revert to the patient's baseline. The Trendelenburg position decreases both functional residual capacity (FRC) and pulmonary compliance from the abdominal contents displacing the diaphragm cephalad. The Trendelenburg position increases both intraocular pressure and intracranial pressure. (339)
8. Brachial plexus injury can occur secondary to improper Trendelenburg positioning in two ways. If the patient slides downward, there could be stretch on the brachial plexus, or if shoulder braces are used, there could be external compression on the brachial plexus. (339)
9. The reverse Trendelenburg position causes a decrease in venous return and could cause hypotension, particularly in patients who are hypovolemic. (339)
10. When a patient is in the reverse Trendelenburg position the invasive arterial blood pressure transducer must be placed at the level of the external auditory meatus to adequately reflect cerebral perfusion. (339)
11. When positioning an obese patient supine in the reverse axis on the operating table, the torso, and thus the heaviest part of the patient's body, is at the head of the table and opposite the weighted base. If sufficient weight is placed on the head portion, particularly if in the Trendelenburg position, the operating table can tilt and tip over. Attention must be paid to the weight limits of the operating table, noting different weight limits for different orientations. (339)
12. Lithotomy positioning can lead to injuries to the spine, the common peroneal and sciatic nerves, or the fingers (crush injury). When positioning the patient, the legs must be raised and lowered simultaneously to prevent

spine torsion. The common peroneal nerve, which wraps arounds the head of the fibula on the lateral leg, is particularly at risk for injury and should be adequately padded. The sciatic nerve can also be injured through excessive stretch from external rotation or hyperflexion at the hip. Finger crush injuries can occur during lithotomy positioning when the foot portion of the bed is raised or reattached at the end of surgery if the fingers are alongside the patient and get caught in the hinge of the operating table. (339–340, 347)

13. Inadequate arterial blood flow from leg elevation or obstructed venous outflow from compression or excessive hip flexion in the lithotomy position can lead to lower extremity compartment syndrome. Based on retrospective studies, the risk factors for positioning-related compartment syndrome are lithotomy or lateral decubitus position and prolonged surgical time (greater than 5 hours) in high lithotomy position. (340)
14. Risks associated with the lateral decubitus position include falling, nerve injury or stretch, compression of the axillary contents, and head and neck malpositioning. The patient should be well secured in lateral decubitus to prevent falling or tilting. The dependent leg should be flexed and a pillow or padding placed between the knees. The dependent arm should be placed in front of the patient on a padded arm board with an axillary roll in place, and the nondependent arm supported by pillows or blankets or with a padded arm rest. The axillary roll should be placed underneath the patient caudal to the axilla (and not in the axilla) to prevent compression injury to the brachial plexus and axillary vascular structure on the dependent side. Invasive arterial monitors should ideally be placed in the dependent arm during lateral decubitus positioning to detect neurovascular compression in the axilla. Injury to the brachial plexus can occur in the lateral decubitus position if there is lateral rotation of the neck and stretch of the brachial plexus, or by direct injury from the humeral head if the arm is abducted greater than 90 degrees. After placing the head and neck in the neutral position, the eyes should be checked for external compression and the dependent ear checked for folding. (340–341)
15. In the lateral decubitus position, the lateral weight of the mediastinum and cephalad pressure on the diaphragm decrease lung compliance of the dependent lung, favoring ventilation of the nondependent lung. Meanwhile, the dependent lung has increased blood flow due to the effect of gravity. The net effect of this is ventilation-perfusion mismatching, which can affect alveolar ventilation and gas exchange. (341–342)
16. When turning a patient from the supine to prone position, care must be taken to prevent dislodgment of all intravenous and arterial lines, as well as the endotracheal tube. The turn should be coordinated such that the head, neck, and spine are maintained in a neutral position. After turning to the prone position, the face should be checked to confirm there is no pressure on the eyes, nose or mouth. The bony prominences of the face, forehead, malar regions, and chin are also at risk of compression or pressure injury during prone positioning. When in the prone position the legs should be padded and flexed slightly at the hips and knees. The arms can be positioned tucked at the patient's side or placed on arm boards next to the patient's head. The arms should be well padded at the elbow to protect the ulnar nerve and should not be abducted greater than 90 degrees to prevent stretching of the brachial plexus. (342–343)
17. The ideal placement of bolsters beneath the prone patient is from the clavicle to the iliac crest. This placement helps reduce abdominal compression and its effects on the lungs and inferior vena cava, minimizing decreases in pulmonary compliance and venous return. Bolsters should not go beyond the iliac crests in order to protect the genitalia and femoral vessels. The abdomen and breasts should be placed medial to the bolsters in order to be free of compression. (343–344)
18. Hemodynamics are well maintained and pulmonary function is improved with prone positioning of the patient. The FRC is improved, leading to improved oxygenation in the prone position compared to the supine position. (343)
19. The sitting position is most advantageous for surgical procedures involving the superior cervical spine and the posterior fossa. A modified sitting position, or beach-chair position, is often used for shoulder surgery. (344)
20. In the sitting position, the arms should rest at the patient's sides and should be well padded and supported. The shoulders should be even or slightly elevated in order to minimize stretch injury between the neck and shoulders. The knees should be supported and padded in a slightly flexed position to reduce stretching of the sciatic nerve. (344)
21. Complications that can occur as a result of placing the patient in the sitting position include venous air embolism (and paradoxical air embolism), pneumocephalus, hypotension, cerebral hypoperfusion, head and neck swelling, and macroglossia. (344)
22. When in the sitting position for surgery, the venous system in the operative field has low pressure (above the heart), which allows a gradient for air entry. This is particularly true during intracranial surgery in which there are open dural venous sinuses. An intraoperative venous air embolus can be detected through the use of an intraoperative TEE or precordial Doppler ultrasound in the patient with adequate intravascular volume. A venous air embolism can create an air-fluid lock in the right heart, and lead to physiologic manifestations such as acute hypotension and decreased end-tidal carbon dioxide. Further complications that can occur as a

result of a venous air embolus include paradoxical air embolism, arrhythmias, acute pulmonary hypertension, and circulatory collapse. (344)

23. A patient with an anatomic intracardiac shunt is at risk for a paradoxical air embolism and subsequent stroke or myocardial infarction should a venous air embolus occur. Because some studies have shown that up to 100% of patients undergoing neurosurgery in the sitting position have some degree of venous air entrainment, patients should be evaluated to rule out an intracardiac shunt prior to planned surgery in the sitting position. Preoperative diagnosis of an intracardiac shunt is a contraindication to surgery in the sitting position. (344)
24. Pneumocephalus occurs in almost all patients undergoing cervical spine or posterior fossa surgery in the sitting position, although clinically significant pneumocephalus is rare. Symptoms of clinically significant postoperative pneumocephalus include headache, confusion, seizures, and even temporary hemiparesis. Patients with these symptoms must have the diagnosis of stroke excluded. (344)
25. Excessive head flexion in the sitting position can impede cerebral venous outflow and cerebral arterial inflow and cause brain hypoperfusion. Macroglossia can also occur, especially if TEE monitoring is combined with neck flexion. A minimum of two fingerbreadths between the mandible and the sternum is recommended for normal-sized adults to prevent these complications. (344)

POSITIONING FOR ROBOTIC-ASSISTED SURGERY

26. Robotic surgery usually requires steep Trendelenburg positioning; thus the patient must be well secured to the operating room table to avoid slipping or shifting positions due to gravity. Often a bean bag or nonslip mattress is used in addition to strapping. Caution must be exercised if shoulder braces are used in order to minimize stretch between the neck and shoulders. Laryngeal edema and optic neuropathy can result from the steep Trendelenburg positioning that may be required for many types of robotic surgery. (345)
27. Docking the robot limits direct access to the patient. Often the patient's head is located farther away from the anesthesia provider than normal, and the patient's arms are tucked bilaterally. A metal tray or table may be placed above the patient's face to provide protection from laparoscopic equipment. Specialized robot operating tables are electronically linked to the surgical robotic system. However, standard operating tables do not have this capability. For standard operating tables, moving the table for a patient docked to the surgical robotic system should not be performed. In this circumstance, moving the table risks unintended movement of surgical instrumentation inside the patient, which could lead to catastrophic outcomes. (345)

PRESSURE INJURIES

28. Pressure injuries are due to prolonged pressure that inhibits capillary flow over a bony prominence. Animal studies reveal that pressure injuries can develop in as little as 2 hours with 70 mmHg force. Pressure injuries are typically noted within 72 hours after surgery. Surgeries in which patients are most likely to incur pressure injuries include cardiac, thoracic, orthopedic, and vascular surgeries. The longer the surgery, the greater is the risk. (345)
29. Pressure injuries can vary from nonblanchable erythema to full-thickness tissue loss. Skin, soft tissue, and muscle are all at risk of injury from pressure. Interestingly, muscle damage occurs before skin and subcutaneous tissue damage, likely because of the increased oxygen requirement of muscle. (345)
30. In the supine position the sacrum, heels, and occiput are areas at risk of pressure injury. In the prone position the chest and knees are most at risk of pressure injuries, while in the sitting position the ischial tuberosities are most at risk. (345)

BITE INJURIES

31. Patients undergoing surgery that involves monitoring with transcranial motor evoked potentials are known to be at risk of a bite injury from the contraction of the temporalis and masseter muscles caused by the transcranial electrical stimulation. The tongue is most frequently injured, but lip and even tooth injuries have occurred. (346)

PERIPHERAL NERVE INJURIES

32. Claims to the ASA database reveal that ulnar neuropathy (28%) is the most common peripheral nerve injury, followed by brachial plexus (20%), lumbosacral nerve root (16%), and spinal cord (12%). Spinal cord injury and lumbosacral nerve root neuropathy were predominantly associated with regional anesthesia. (346)
33. Causes for peripheral nerve injuries are complex and multifactorial. Possible mechanisms for peripheral nerve injuries include stretch, compression, ischemia, metabolic derangement, and direct trauma or laceration during surgery. There is no clear evidence for prevention of perioperative neuropathies. Most neuropathies occur in the presence of good positioning and padding. However, maintaining neutral position, avoiding excessive extension or flexion, and adequate padding are all essential. (346–347)
34. In ASA closed claims studies, patient risk factors for ulnar nerve injuries include diabetes, alcohol use disorder, cigarette smoking, and cancer. (346)
35. Positions and surgeries associated with brachial plexus injury include arm abduction greater than 90 degrees, lateral rotation of the head, asymmetric resection of the sternum for internal mammary dissection during cardiac surgery, and direct trauma. The lithotomy position is most likely to lead to common peroneal or sciatic nerve injury. The sciatic nerve can be injured with stretch and external rotation of the leg, as well as from hyperflexion at the hip. Obturator nerve injury can occur during difficult forceps delivery, by excessive flexion of the thigh to the groin, or by lithotomy position. (347–348)
36. Fortunately, injuries to the radial or median nerves are rare. (347)

EVALUATION AND TREATMENT OF PERIOPERATIVE NEUROPATHIES

37. Evaluation and documentation of a postoperative nerve deficit should include the extent of sensory and motor deficits. A neurologic consultation can help to localize the lesion and determine severity. (348)
38. Sensory neuropathies are generally transient and resolve spontaneously over time, requiring only patient reassurance and follow-up. Most motor neuropathies are from demyelination of peripheral nerves (neurapraxia) and can take 4–6 weeks for recovery. Motor neuropathies resulting from injury to an axon or nerve disruption can cause severe pain and disability, requiring physical therapy to prevent contractures and muscle atrophy. When these injuries are reversible, recovery can take 2–12 months. (348)
39. Electrophysiologic evaluation of an intraoperative nerve injury by a neurologist in the first week may provide information regarding the characteristic and temporal pattern of the injury. Electrophysiologic evaluation after 4 weeks provides more useful information about the site, nature, and severity of the nerve injury. (348)

PERIOPERATIVE EYE INJURY AND VISUAL LOSS

40. Risk factors for corneal abrasion under general anesthesia include increased age, length of surgery, prone position, Trendelenburg position, and supplemental oxygen delivery in the postanesthesia care unit. Symptoms include the sensation of a foreign body in the eye, photophobia, blurry vision, and erythema. Precautions that can be taken to minimize the risk of corneal abrasion include careful taping of the eyelids soon after the induction of anesthesia, care regarding dangling objects when leaning over patients, ophthalmic ointments, and close observation as patients awaken. Patients may try to rub their eyes with the pulse oximeter on their finger or other equipment before they are fully awake. (348)
41. Central retinal artery occlusion is caused by direct retinal pressure or by embolism. (348)
42. Ischemic optic neuropathy (ION) accounts for the majority of postoperative visual loss complications. Risk factors for postoperative vision loss due to ION include prolonged hypotension, long duration of surgery, large-volume blood loss, large-volume crystalloid use, anemia or hemodilution, and increased intraocular or venous pressure from the prone position. It is most frequently associated with spine surgery. Patient risk factors for ION include hypertension, diabetes, atherosclerosis, morbid obesity, and tobacco use. (348)

Chapter

20 ANESTHETIC MONITORING

Ryan Paul Davis, Kevin K. Tremper, and James Szocik

INTRODUCTION

Overview

- Purpose of monitoring is to continuously assess the patient's physiologic status and the effects of surgery and anesthetic agents.
- The American Society of Anesthesiologists (ASA) established a set of basic monitoring standards, stating that the patient's oxygenation, ventilation, circulation, and temperature shall be continually evaluated.
- All monitors require calibration: some require manual calibration, some are autocalibrating, and some are empirically calibrated.

RESPIRATORY SYSTEM

Oxygenation

Inspired Oxygen

- Anesthesia machines measure inspired and expired oxygen content using amperometric and paramagnetic oxygen sensors.
  - Amperometric oxygen sensors require calibration and are slow to respond to changes.
  - Paramagnetic oxygen sensors are autocalibrating and have a rapid response to changes, allowing them to be used to measure both inspired and expired oxygen content.
    - Expired O_2 (Feo_2) concentration measurements allow for determination of complete preoxygenation/denitrogenation during induction (goal Feo_2 >85%), as well as a rough estimate of O_2 consumption.

Pulse Oximetry

- Provides a continuous noninvasive estimate of arterial hemoglobin saturation (Sao_2) by analyzing red and infrared light transmitted through living tissue, (e.g., finger, ear)
- Beer's law:
  - Basic principle of pulse oximetry
  - States that the attenuation of light is related to the properties of the material through which the light is traveling
- Oxyhemoglobin and deoxyhemoglobin absorb red and infrared light differently.
- Two wavelengths are used for conventional pulse oximetry.
  - Red at 660 nm and infrared at 940 nm
- To obtain a signal that is associated with the arterial blood, the device analyzes two components of light absorption (AC and DC), at two wavelengths (red and infrared).
  - AC – the pulsatile component of the absorbers (the expanding arterials)
  - DC – the nonpulsatile component of light absorption
  - The ratio (R) is defined as $\frac{AC_{Red}/DC_{Red}}{AC_{IR}/DC_{IR}}$
  - R ranges from 0.4 at 100% to 3.4 at 0%
    - When R is 1.0—that is, equal in both the red and infrared—the pulse oximeter will read an O_2 saturation of 85%.

Dyes and Dyshemoglobins

- Carboxyhemoglobin absorbs light like oxyhemoglobin, which artificially elevates the oxygen saturation (reading closer to sum of oxyhemoglobin and carboxyhemoglobin).
- Methemoglobin absorbs both red and infrared light to a high degree, thus driving the ratio toward 1, and the oxygen saturation toward 85%.
- Dyes also absorb both red and infrared light, with oxygen saturation decreasing toward 85%; however, dyes are cleared rapidly, so changes are transient.
- Motion artifact or low perfusion causes a low signal-to-noise ratio (noise in numerator and denominator), with resulting trend in oxygen saturation toward 85%.
- Dark skin color can produce artificially high Spo_2 values by ≥2% at Sao_2 values <90% (more pronounced with darker skin and lower saturation values).

Ventilation

- Depth, pattern, and frequency can be assessed by:
  - Observation: patient's chest rise or the rebreathing bag on the anesthesia machine
  - Auscultation: rate and depth, and can help clinician make diagnoses
    - Bronchospasm: wheezing or decreased breath sounds
    - Endobronchial intubation or pneumothorax (PTX): unilateral breath sounds
    - Pulmonary edema: auscultatory rales

Airway Pressures

- Increased peak airway pressures are caused by increased airway resistance or decreased chest wall compliance.
  - Causes include bronchospasm, endobronchial intubation, pneumothorax, pulmonary edema, kinked ETT or circuit, malfunctioning valve.
- Decreased airway pressures may result from multiple causes.
  - Circuit leak or disconnection, inadvertent tracheal extubation, failure of fresh gas delivery, ventilator setting error, excessive scavenging suction, or other issues with the anesthesia machine
- Plateau pressure is an airway pressure measured during volume-controlled ventilation, after an end inspiratory pause, i.e., when respiratory gases have stopped moving.
  - Plateau pressure is a reflection of lung/chest wall compliance.
  - The difference between peak inspiratory pressure and plateau pressure is a reflection of airway resistance only.
  - When airway pressures increase, evaluating the change in plateau pressure relative to peak airway pressure can determine if cause is due to lung/chest wall compliance or to airway resistance.

Tidal Volume

- Usually set at 6 to 8 mL/kg based on ideal body weight
- Once set, the respiratory rate (RR) should be adjusted to maintain end-tidal CO_2 ($ETCO_2$) in the normal range of 35 to 40 mmHg.
  - Most ventilators have pressure limits set to alarm if peak pressures are exceeded.
- All anesthesia ventilators require a "disconnect" alarm usually tied to airway pressure readings.
  - Normal pressure (no alarm) does not ensure adequate ventilation, for example esophageal intubation.

Capnography/End-Tidal CO_2

- Capnography is the analysis of continuous waveform of expired CO_2.
  - A reliable waveform is only achieved with intubated patients or secure supraglottic airway.
  - Important for monitoring adequacy of ventilation (i.e., removal of CO_2).
- Exchange of CO_2 into the alveolar space from the venous blood is efficient because CO_2 has 20 times the solubility in water that oxygen has.
  - Well-perfused alveoli achieve equilibrium with CO_2 in blood.
- Expired gas is sampled by the capnometer, producing a peak expired CO_2 close to the arterial carbon dioxide tension ($Paco_2$) if there is little or no alveolar dead space.
  - In healthy patients, $ETCO_2$ is usually 3 to 5 mmHg less than $Paco_2$ during general anesthesia.
- Tidal volume (TV) is composed of the alveolar gas volume and dead space volume.
  - Dead space is that portion of the tidal volume (TV) that does not participate in gas exchange (about one-third in healthy patients).
  - Dead space consists of alveolar, anatomical, and apparatus dead space.
  - These dead spaces contain inspired gas only and therefore no CO_2.
- Expiration has three phases on capnography.
  - Phase 0: inspiratory period
  - Phase 1: apparatus and anatomic dead space empty (no CO_2 = 0 mmHg)
  - Phase 2: increasing CO_2 from progressive emptying of alveoli
  - Phase 3: plateau phase alveolar gas (both alveolar gas and alveolar dead space)
- The $ETCO_2$ will always be lower than $Paco_2$ in large part due to alveolar dead space (the greater the alveolar dead space, the greater the difference between $ETCO_2$ and Pco_2).
- Changes in the $Paco_2$-toET-CO_2 difference can reflect changes in alveolar dead space and ventilation/perfusion (V/Q) matching.
  - Causes of increased $Paco_2$-to-$ETCO_2$ difference include any cause of decreased lung perfusion (e.g., pulmonary emboli, decreased cardiac output [CO]), which increase alveolar dead space.
- During cardiopulmonary resuscitation (CPR) for cardiac arrest, capnography is the most useful monitor for adequacy of chest compressions.
  - Goal of $ETCO_2$ >20 mmHg should be achieved.

CIRCULATORY SYSTEM

- Goal of circulatory system: maintain a constant supply of blood flow to all organs to allow them to maintain aerobic metabolism and function.

- No single characteristic determines adequacy of perfusion
- Many important variables cannot be measured, such as venous capacitance, organ blood flow/perfusion, and circulating blood volume.

Measurement of the Electrocardiogram (ECG)

- One of the ASA standard monitors is continuous monitoring of heart rate (HR) and rhythm.
- Measures electrical activity of the heart at the body surface
  - Net dipole of moment of the heart displayed on vertical axis in millivolts vs. time on horizontal axis
- Diagnostic mode on ECG in operating room removes all filtering and artifacts and helps to evaluate whether perceived intraoperative ECG changes are real.
- Preferred intraoperative method is a five-lead system using leads I, II, and III plus a single precordial lead at V_5.
  - Leads II and V_5 allow for most dysrhythmias and ischemia to be detected and evaluated.

Blood Pressure (BP) and Flow

- The circulatory system is an Ohm's law system, V = IR where
  - V is perfusion pressure
  - I is blood flow (e.g., cardiac output)
  - R is resistance
  - Systemic circulation: mean arterial pressure (MAP) – central venous pressure (CVP) = CO × systemic vascular resistance (SVR)
  - Pulmonary circulation: mean pulmonary artery pressure (MPAP) – left ventricular end-diastolic pressure (LVEDP; estimated by pulmonary capillary wedge pressure [PCWP]) = CO × pulmonary vascular resistance (PVR)
  - Each organ has its own perfusion pressure (PP).
    - Brain: MAP – intracranial pressure (ICP) or CVP (whichever is higher) = PP
    - Heart: DBP – right heart or coronary sinus pressure = PP
      - Heart perfuses itself during diastole.
- Mean BP can also be calculated using equation:

$$\text{mean BP} = \frac{Systolic\,BP + 2 \times Diastolic\,BP}{3}$$

- BP correlates directly with CO, assuming that resistance is constant (however, many clinical conditions affect resistance).

Blood Pressure: Hypotension

- Documentation of pulse and BP every 5 minutes is one of the ASA standards.
- Hypotension for adults can be defined as MAP between 55 and 65 mmHg depending on patient preoperative and procedural risk.
  - Multiple studies have shown the impact of hypotension on clinical outcomes, particularly myocardial and renal injury.

Noninvasive Blood Pressure

- Routine automatic intraoperative noninvasive blood pressure (NIBP) monitoring is performed using oscillometric method.
  - Cuff inflates above systolic blood pressure (SBP), deflates until pulse detected, deflates to maximal pulsation (MAP), and deflates until pulse not detected,
  - Readings include SBP, MAP, and diastolic blood pressure (DBP), but most accurate reading is MAP.
  - Proper NIBP cuff size: width of cuff is 40% of arm circumference
    - Cuff too small = measured BP too high
    - Cuff too large = measured BP too low
- Riva-Rocci technique
  - Insufflation of an occlusive cuff and noting the return of blood flow by palpation (SBP) or Doppler
    - Korotkoff sound auscultation at the antecubital fossa can determine both SBP and DBP.
    - Using a Doppler technique can measure BP in patients with nonpulsatile flow (e.g., left ventricular assist devices [LVADs]).

Invasive Arterial Blood Pressure Monitoring

- Intraarterial catheter is connected to pressure transducer, which converts mechanical energy of arterial pulse into electrical signal.
  - Increased length of tubing in the fluid-filled transducer setup will increase amplification artifact in the SBP measurement, whereas the MAP measurement remains fairly accurate.
- Useful for beat-to-beat BP measurements, arterial blood sampling, and assessment of patient's intravascular volume status.
- Catheter usually placed in radial artery (least risk and easily palpable); however, femoral, brachial, and dorsalis pedis arteries may be used.
  - Arterial waveforms differ with insertion site, with SBP increasing as the site becomes more distal from the heart.

Measures of Intravascular Volume Responsiveness

Systolic Pressure Variation

- In a mechanically ventilated patient, a transient drop in SBP with positive-pressure breaths predicts fluid responsiveness.
  - Fluid responsiveness is defined as an increased cardiac output after an IV fluid bolus.

- Decrease in SBP with positive-pressure ventilation is due in part to the positive intrathoracic pressure impeding venous return to the right heart.
  - Decrease in right heart stroke volume (SV) reduces left heart SV and arterial BP several heartbeats later.
  - Indirectly assesses venous capacitance and the potential for BP improvement with fluid administration
- Change in SBP with respiratory cycle from maximum to minimum is called systolic pressure variation (SPV).
  - If SBP drops >10 mmHg with a positive pressure breath = fluid responsive
  - If SBP drops <5 mmHg with a positive pressure breath = unlikely fluid responsive
- Limitations
  - Must be on positive-pressure ventilation
  - Must have regular heartbeat (i.e., no atrial fibrillation)
  - Must have closed thoracic cavity
  - Accuracy reduced in patients with increased lung or chest wall compliance, prone positioning, high peak end-expiratory pressure (PEEP)

Pulse Pressure Variation

- Derives similar information to SPV using changes in PP during the positive-pressure respiratory cycle
- $PPV\% = \dfrac{PP_{max} - PP_{min}}{(PP_{max} + PP_{min})/2} \times 100$
- May be more reliable over wider range of BP than absolute value of SPV

Stroke Volume Variation

- Uses arterial waveform and a pulse contour algorithm to estimate the SR from waveform and changes during positive-pressure respiratory cycle
- The percent reduction in estimated SV with positive-pressure ventilation is used to assess fluid responsiveness
- Same limitations as SPV

Central Venous Monitoring: CVP, PAP, and CO

- BPs alone are not sufficient to evaluate perfusion; information may be helpful in guiding patient therapy.
- Central venous access also used for administration of certain drugs and large-volume fluid resuscitation.

Central Venous Pressure

- Pressure transducers connected to central venous access can provide both a central venous pressure and CVP waveforms.
- CVP waveform has several elements resulting from events in the cardiac cycle.
  - A-wave: atrial contraction against closed tricuspid valve
  - C-wave: tricuspid bulging with ventricular contraction
  - X descent: atrial relaxation
  - V wave: atrial filling
  - Y descent: atrial emptying
- Despite physiologic basis, CVP does not appear to be good measure for guiding fluid therapy.
  - If vascular space compliance was unchanging, the relationship between volume and BP would be simple; however, many clinical factors impact venous compliance.
- CVP is valuable in the extremes: e.g., <5 mmHg more fluid may benefit cardiac filling vs. >16 mmHg implies more fluid may not be needed (similar to SPV but numbers reversed)

CVP Placement

- Central venous catheters can be placed in the right or left internal jugular, subclavian, or femoral veins with risks and benefits to each.

Pulmonary Artery Pressure and Cardiac Output

- Pulmonary artery catheter (PAC) is a 110 cm-long, balloon-tipped right heart access catheter that is advanced from central vein to right atrium to right ventricle to main pulmonary artery.
  - Can be advanced further in the pulmonary arterial system until pulmonary capillary wedge pressure (PCWP) waveform (flat tracing with loss of PA systolic and diastolic waves) appears if desired
    - PCWP estimates LVEDP.
- PAC can be used to diagnose a variety of conditions due to its ability to measure right and estimate left heart filling pressures and CO.
- Hemodynamic status can be grossly assessed by measuring wedge pressure and CO.
  - Hypovolemic shock (low PCWP, low CO)
  - Cardiogenic shock (high PCWP, low CO)
  - Septic shock (low PCWP, high CO, and low pressure)
  - Volume overload (high PCWP, high CO) in a normal heart
- Risk outweighs benefit of placing PAC in most situations resulting in a decrease in use during past 20 years
  - Risks
    - Line sepsis
    - Thrombosis
    - Pulmonary artery rupture
  - Remove as soon as possible to minimize risks

Methods of Measuring Cardiac Output

- PAC thermodilution
  - Most common method to measure CO

- Measured amount of cold water (usually 10 mL) injected into central circulation via proximal PA port and thermistor measures temperature in distal portion of PAC
  - Creates temperature reading as a curve over time
    - Area under curve is proportional to the CO.
    - Total change of temperature over time is greater in low CO states.
  - Primary role is diagnostic or to evaluate response to therapy.
  - Modified commercially available catheters can provide continuous CO data.
- Less invasive methods
  - Esophageal Doppler
    - Uses continuous ultrasound directed through esophagus and into aorta reflecting off moving blood back to the probe
    - Doppler effect (shift in frequency of the reflected signal vs. the original) used to estimate velocity.
    - SV derived using algorithm based on beat-to-beat maximum velocity-time integral (stroke distance), the descending aorta cross-sectional area, and a correction factor that transforms descending aortic blood flow into global CO
    - Estimates CO and detects hemodynamic changes in mechanically ventilated patients
- Devices now available that analyze the pulse contour of arterial waveform to estimate SV (HR × SV = CO).
  - Provides continuous estimate of CO
  - Requires assumptions about dynamic characteristic of arterial vasculature using internal databases or nomograms based on demographics
  - Limitations
    - Variable ability to detect changes in SVR
    - Difficult in certain clinical situations (intra-aortic balloon pump)
    - Accuracy of arterial waveform directly impacts system accuracy (e.g., with overdamped or underdamped waveforms)
- Devices using a finger cuff also appear promising.
  - Provides continuous estimate of CO
  - Limitations in patients with Raynaud's or peripheral vascular disease, hypothermia, or on vasopressor support

Transesophageal Echocardiographic (TEE) Monitoring

- Current gold standard for intraoperative assessment of cardiac function
- Ultrasound probe inserted into esophagus and various views of heart obtained
  - Information as to the heart valves, chamber size (indicating preload/filling pressure ("stretch"), contractile activity (ejection fraction, expressed as %), diastolic dysfunction, wall motion abnormalities
- Pulmonary embolism and cardiac tamponade can all be diagnosed with a TEE evaluation
- Limitations
  - Heavily dependent on expertise of the provider
  - Risk of esophageal injury
  - Requires access to patient's head (e.g., many surgeries with limited access intraoperatively)

CENTRAL NERVOUS SYSTEM

Processed Electroencephalogram (EEG) Monitoring

- Brain activity monitored by processed EEG monitors focused on the frontal area have been developed for convenience (compared with 18-channel raw EEG used by neurologists).
  - Developed through an empirical comparison of the awake and anesthetized EEG
  - EEG features are extracted, artifact is minimized, and an algorithm converts the EEG features to a numerical index, often ranging from 100 (awake) to 0 (isoelectric EEG). Modern displays allow anesthesia clinicians to assess EEG waveforms in real time.
  - Assesses anesthetic depth in an attempt to prevent intraoperative awareness with postoperative recall (subtherapeutic dosing) and unnecessary anesthetic administration (supratherapeutic dosing)
  - Processed EEG may provide extra layer of protection against recall in patients receiving total intravenous anesthesia (TIVA).

Minimum Alveolar Concentration Alert Monitoring

- A minimum alveolar concentration (MAC) >0.7 of inhaled anesthetic is recommended to minimize the risk of the intraoperative awareness and recall during general anesthesia.
- Alerts can inform providers when patients receive age-adjusted MAC values <0.7.
- Studies demonstrated MAC alerts are equivalent or superior to BIS monitor for preventing awareness.

Intracranial Pressure Monitoring

- Brain is enclosed in fixed cranial vault.
  - Cerebral perfusion pressure (CPP) = MAP – intracranial pressure (ICP) or CVP, whichever is higher
  - ICP normally <20 mmHg
  - Small changes in intracranial volume can cause a dramatic increase in ICP and impaired cerebral perfusion.

- ICP monitoring is useful to ensure brain perfusion for patients with conditions that increase ICP (e.g., cerebral edema, hemorrhage), or increased cerebrospinal fluid (CSF) volume (e.g., from hydrocephalus).
- Ventriculostomy
  - Insertion of catheter in a ventricle of the brain
  - Pressure transduced with transducer system (same as for vascular pressure measurement)
  - Zeroed at tragus
  - Advantages include ability to monitor and drain CSF with catheter to treat severe intracranial hypertension.
- Pressure transducer placed in subdural space
  - No zeroing required
  - Monitoring but no drainage capability

Cerebral Oximetry

- Oxygenation to portion of brain (cerebral cortex) can be monitored with reflectance oximeter.
- Uses near-infrared light similar to pulse oximeter but uses reflected infrared light through the scalp and skull from portion of cerebral cortex beneath
  - Light reflected predominantly from hemoglobin in red cells in vasculature of cerebral cortex
  - Measurement obtained is the *regional cerebral oxygen saturation* (rSO_2) with values from 1% to 100%.
  - rSO_2 typically around 70%
  - rSO_2 <50% or a 20% decrease from baseline may indicate decreased cerebral oxygenation.
- Primarily used in cardiac and vascular procedures with concern for poor brain perfusion
- May be useful for surgeries in the sitting position

PERIPHERAL NERVOUS SYSTEM

Neuromuscular Monitoring

Neuromuscular Blocker Management

- Neuromuscular blocking agents (NMBAs) must be appropriately monitored (train-of-four [TOF]), titrated, and reversed when appropriate.
- Too little intraoperative neuromuscular blockade can result in inappropriate patient movement and injury, such as premature extubation, extrusion of ocular contents with a cough or Valsalva maneuver, impalement of the bladder on a rigid cystoscope, or injury of abdominal organs.
- Residual postoperative neuromuscular blockade is associated with subclinical aspiration, hypoventilation, and airway obstruction.

Basic Physiology/Pharmacology

- Nondepolarizing NMBAs competitively inhibit the binding of acetylcholine with the receptor at the neuromuscular junction.
- Succinylcholine binds to the receptor and activates it, causing prolonged depolarization and blockade of transmission.

Neuromuscular Blockade Monitor

- Most common method to follow effects of nondepolarizing NMBA
- TOF count
  - Generates four supramaximal stimuli at 0.5-second intervals (2 Hz)
  - As degree of blockade deepens, twitches fade, then are lost
  - Even with four of four twitches present, 75% of receptors can still be blocked.
- Assessment of deep levels of blockade can be done using post-tetanic count
  - Tetanic stimulus at 50 Hz for 5 seconds, followed 3 seconds later by one twitch per second
    - The number of twitches causing muscle movement is the post-tetanic count.
  - Tetanus primes nerve terminal with more acetylcholine, allowing post-tetanic count to be performed.
- Double-burst stimulation
  - A nerve stimulation pattern designed to facilitate detection of fade
  - Two bursts of three electrical stimulations separated by 750 ms
  - Can be used for low levels of blockade
- Succinylcholine induces noncompetitive blockage, which can be followed by single twitch.
- Assessment by observation or palpation introduces variability in interpretation.
- Newer monitors are quantitative, allow more accurate measurement of TOF ratio. Full reversal is not acheived until there is zero fade in TOF

Evoked Potential

- Used for procedures where there may be neurologic injury due to mechanical trauma or ischemia
  - Spine surgery
  - Thoracic abdominal aneurysm surgery
  - Head and neck surgery
- Requires constant attention of trained personnel
- Signals affected differently by different anesthetic agents
- Requires a stimulating and sensing electrode to assess function
- Somatosensory evoked potentials (SSEPs)
  - Deliver small current to sensory nerve and measure response in the sensory cortex with scalp electrode

  - Response viewed as voltage vs. time.
  - Multiple responses averaged to reduce noise
  - Nerve injury or ischemia is associated with decrease in amplitude and increased latency of peaks in waveform vs. baseline.
    - Inhaled anesthetics (halogenated and nitrous oxide) also produce similar findings at higher doses.
    - Propofol is the best drug for maintenance during evoked potential monitoring.
    - Changes in medications need to be relayed to monitoring technician.
  - Limitation
    - Only evaluates sensory tracks (dorsal spinal cord) and not motor tracks (ventral spinal cord)
    - Intact SSEPs with damage to motor tracts can lead to false-negative results.
- Motor evoked potentials (MEPs)
  - Stimulate the motor cortex and detect response in muscle
  - Advantages
    - Ensure intact ventral spinal cord
    - More sensitive to neuronal injury and anesthetic drugs
  - Disadvantages
    - Require intact neuromuscular junction (no NMBAs)
    - MEPs profoundly affected by volatile and nitrous oxide compared with SSEPs.

TEMPERATURE

- Anesthesia interferes with normal temperature autoregulation.
- In first 30 minutes of general anesthesia, most temperature change is due to heat redistribution from core to periphery.
- Temperature is monitored to
  - Manage or prevent intraoperative hypothermia
  - Prevent overheating (e.g., from external warming devices)
  - Confirm or detect malignant hyperthermia
- Types of monitors
  - Liquid thermometers
    - Historically used orally or rectally to monitor body core temperature
  - Infrared scanners
    - Often directed at the tympanic membrane
    - Used preoperatively and postoperatively
    - Faster but subject to errors (e.g., cerumen or other obstruction)
  - Low mass, small thermistors
    - Often used intraoperatively (nasopharyngeal, esophageal)
    - Detects changes in temperature as changes in resistance which are converted and displayed
    - Accuracy is ±0.5°C.
  - Core temperature
    - True core measured in pulmonary artery, distal esophagus, tympanic membrane, or nasopharyngeal zones
    - Other sites that approximate core temperature include oral, axillary, and bladder.
      - Bladder: can be highly affected by urine flow and approaches true core at high urine flow
    - Rectal and skin temperatures have highly variable reliability relative to true core sites.

MAGNETIC RESONANCE IMAGING AND ADVERSE CONDITIONS

- Magnet can cause equipment malfunction and injury from projectile metallic objects.
  - Interferes with standard ECGs
  - Can induce a current in standard pulse oximeters, causing heating and burns
  - Extended length tubing for gas sampling and ventilator allows further distance from magnet.

MULTIFUNCTIONAL DISPLAYS AND DECISION SUPPORT

- Progressive implementation of electronic medical record (EMR) has allowed for development of integrated displays and decision support systems similar to those developed for aviation in 1980s.
  - Allows for live display and calculations to enhance information for providers
  - Helps reduce alarm fatigue and prioritize by urgency
  - Can allow for improved adherence to protocol measures (e.g., blood glucose, tidal volume)
  - Allow for effective monitoring of multiple patients by processing and displaying data effectively

QUESTIONS

INTRODUCTION

1. What four patient parameters have been mandated to be continually evaluated for all anesthetics by the American Society of Anesthesiologists Standards for Basic Anesthetic Monitoring? How frequently is it mandated that intraoperative blood pressure be measured?

RESPIRATORY SYSTEM

2. How do carboxyhemoglobin, methemoglobin, dyes, and motion artifact affect the pulse oximeter readings?

CIRCULATORY SYSTEM

3. Name characteristics of the circulation that can be monitored during anesthesia.
4. What is the clinical significance of the MAP, and how is it calculated?

CENTRAL NERVOUS SYSTEM

5. Why are processed electroencephalograms (e.g., bispectral index [BIS] or patient state index [PSI]) monitor used during anesthesia? What minimum alveolar concentration (MAC) of inhaled anesthetic is recommended to minimize the risk of intraoperative awareness and postoperative recall during general anesthesia?

PERIPHERAL NERVOUS SYSTEM

6. Describe the various modes of stimulation with a neuromuscular blockade monitor, or "twitch" monitor. What depth of neuromuscular blockade is appropriately monitored by each mode?

TEMPERATURE

7. Which temperature monitoring sites best reflect the core body temperature?

ANSWERS

INTRODUCTION

1. The American Society of Anesthesiologists has mandated that during all anesthetics the patient's oxygenation, ventilation, circulation, and temperature shall be continually evaluated. (351)

Parameter	Description of ASA Standards
Oxygenation	With general anesthesia, the oxygen (O_2) concentration of the gases administered shall be monitored. With all anesthetics, a quantitative measure of blood oxygenation (pulse oximetry) shall be used.
Ventilation	Ventilation during a general anesthetic shall be evaluated qualitatively and, if possible, quantitatively. Breathing device placement must be verified by carbon dioxide (CO_2) identification in the expired gases. Continual, quantitative measurement of CO_2 shall be used until removal of the device. With regional anesthesia, clinical signs of ventilation shall be monitored.
Circulation	For all patients, the arterial blood pressure and heart rate shall be evaluated minimally every 5 minutes.
Temperature	Temperature shall be monitored whenever clinically significant changes are intended, anticipated, or suspected.

RESPIRATORY SYSTEM

2. Carboxyhemoglobin, methemoglobin, dyes, and motion artifact all affect the pulse oximeter readings. Because carboxyhemoglobin absorbs light similarly to oxyhemoglobin, the reading will be approximately the sum of oxyhemoglobin and carboxyhemoglobin, therefore being artificially high. Because methemoglobin absorbs at a ratio of 1, it will trend to 85% saturation. This results in a lower observed value if the patient is well oxygenated and a higher observed value in hypoxic patients. Dyes produce an error like that seen for methemoglobin (trend to 85%), but because dyes are cleared rapidly from the circulation this error is only transient. Motion artifact will produce noise in the numerator and denominator and force the ratio value to 1.0, also trending the pulse oximeter readings to 85%. (353–355)

CIRCULATORY SYSTEM

3. During anesthesia, noninvasive monitors can be used to monitor heart rate and rhythm, systolic blood pressure, diastolic blood pressure, and mean blood pressure. By using invasive monitors, central venous pressure, pulmonary artery pressure, cardiac output, and systolic pressure variation (SPV) can be measured. Circulating blood volume, organ perfusion/blood flow, and venous capacitance are aspects of the circulatory system that cannot be directly measured. (362)
4. MAP is the upstream pressure for the perfusion of most vital organs. MAP is calculated as two-thirds diastolic blood pressure plus one-third systolic blood pressure: MAP = ($\frac{2}{3}$ DBP) + ($\frac{1}{3}$ SBP). (363)

CENTRAL NERVOUS SYSTEM

5. A processed EEG, such as the bispectral index (BIS) or patient state index (PSI) monitor, can be used during anesthesia to assess anesthetic depth. The purpose of these monitors is to reduce the risk of intraoperative awareness and recall during general anesthesia. A minimum alveolar concentration (MAC) >0.7 of inhaled anesthetic is recommended to minimize the risk of intraoperative awareness and recall during general anesthesia. Processed EEG may provide an extra layer of protection against recall in patients receiving total intravenous anesthesia (TIVA). (374–375)

PERIPHERAL NERVOUS SYSTEM

6. The neuromuscular blockade monitor has various settings. A post-tetanic count (PTC) is used to assess the deeper levels of block; 5 seconds of 50-Hz tetanic stimulus is given followed three seconds later by a series of twitches at 1 Hz. Slightly less deep blockade can be followed by a train-of-four (TOF). TOF uses 4 supramaximal stimuli at 2 Hz, and the number of responses (twitches) are counted. Deep blockade is zero to one of four counts present. Even with four of four present, 75% of the receptors can still be blocked. To attempt to show this residual blockade, one can use a double-burst stimulation (DBS) of two bursts of 50-Hz tetany separated by 750 ms. Alternatively, a TOF ratio can be measured quantitatively. This requires a device to compare the strength of the first and the fourth twitches. The TOF ratio and DBS have overlap in the degree of blockade monitored. Finally, sustained (5 seconds) 50- to 100-Hz tetany can be observed. This is quite painful in an awake patient. (375–376)

TEMPERATURE

7. True core body temperature is measured by probes in the PA catheter, distal esophagus, nasopharyngeal area, or tympanic membrane area. Sites that can approximate core body temperature include oral, axillary, and bladder. (377)

Chapter

21 POINT-OF-CARE ULTRASOUND

Lindsey Huddleston and Kristine Breyer

INTRODUCTION

- The uses and applications of point-of-care ultrasound (POCUS) are rapidly expanding.
  - This is likely due to increasing portability, ease of use, ability for rapid assessments, and repeat examinations.
- Ultrasound image acquisition and interpretation are essential skills for anesthesia providers.
- POCUS is now a required competency of anesthesia training.

REVIEW OF ULTRASOUND PHYSICS

- Sound waves are characterized by frequency, amplitude, and wavelength.
  - Sound waves with frequencies above 20,000 Hertz (Hz) (or 20 kHz) are termed *ultrasound.*
- *Piezoelectric effect*: the ability of certain materials to generate an electric charge in response to applied mechanical stress
  - This is how ultrasound transducers *receive* sound waves.
- *Inverse piezoelectric effect*: the conversion of electrical energy to mechanical energy, leading to a change in length in this type of material when an electrical voltage is applied
  - This is how ultrasound transducers *produce* sound waves.
- *Attenuation:* decreased amplitude of the ultrasound wave as it propagates through tissue
- *Acoustic impedance:* amount of resistance an ultrasound beam encounters as it passes through a specific tissue
  - Fluids have low acoustic impedance and produce a black (anechoic) image.
  - Solid substances (e.g., bone) have high acoustic impedance and produce a white (hyperechoic) image.
- Two-dimensional (2D) ultrasound, also called *B-mode* (for "brightness"), is the most commonly used ultrasound mode in POCUS.
  - The quality of a 2D image is determined by spatial resolution, temporal resolution, and field of view (FOV).
- *M-mode* (for "motion") is another ultrasound mode commonly used in POCUS.
  - M-mode uses a single piezoelectric crystal along a single line within the transducer beam to transmit waves.
    - The resulting image is displayed over time.

ULTRASOUND TRANSDUCERS

- High-frequency transducers
  - Shorter wavelength = superior image resolution but decreased depth of penetration
  - Example: linear transducer
  - Uses in POCUS: vascular access, nerve blocks, assessing for pneumothorax
- Low-frequency transducers
  - Longer wavelength = superior depth of penetration but decreased image resolutions
  - Examples: phased array and curvilinear transducers
  - Uses in POCUS: cardiac, abdominal (gastric and eFAST), pleural space

POCUS Transducers: Mode of Crystal Excitation

Linear

- Depth: 6 cm
- Parallel and perpendicular

Phased array

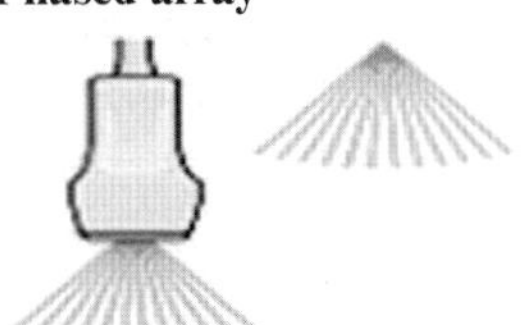

- Depth: 35 cm
- Large number of multi-directional, overlapping beams
- Evaluation of motion and flow

Curvilinear

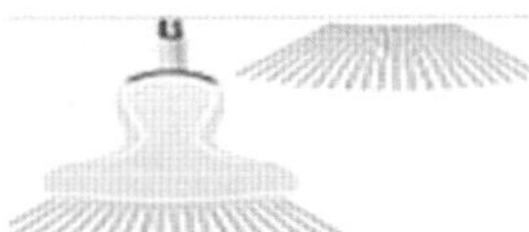

- Depth: 30 cm
- Divergent beams for wider field of view

PREPARING FOR THE EXAMINATION

- Equipment: ultrasound machine with proper probes attached, ultrasound gel, towels, blankets for covering the patient, and (potentially) an assistant
- Machine setup
  - Proper probe for exam
  - Set "examination type" or "examination mode."
  - Set the appropriate depth.
- Optimal patient positioning is key for high-quality images.

BASIC CARDIAC ULTRASOUND

Four basic views: parasternal long-axis view (PLAX), parasternal short-axis view (PSAX), apical four-chamber view, and subcostal view (see figure below)

- Probes: phased array (favored) and curvilinear

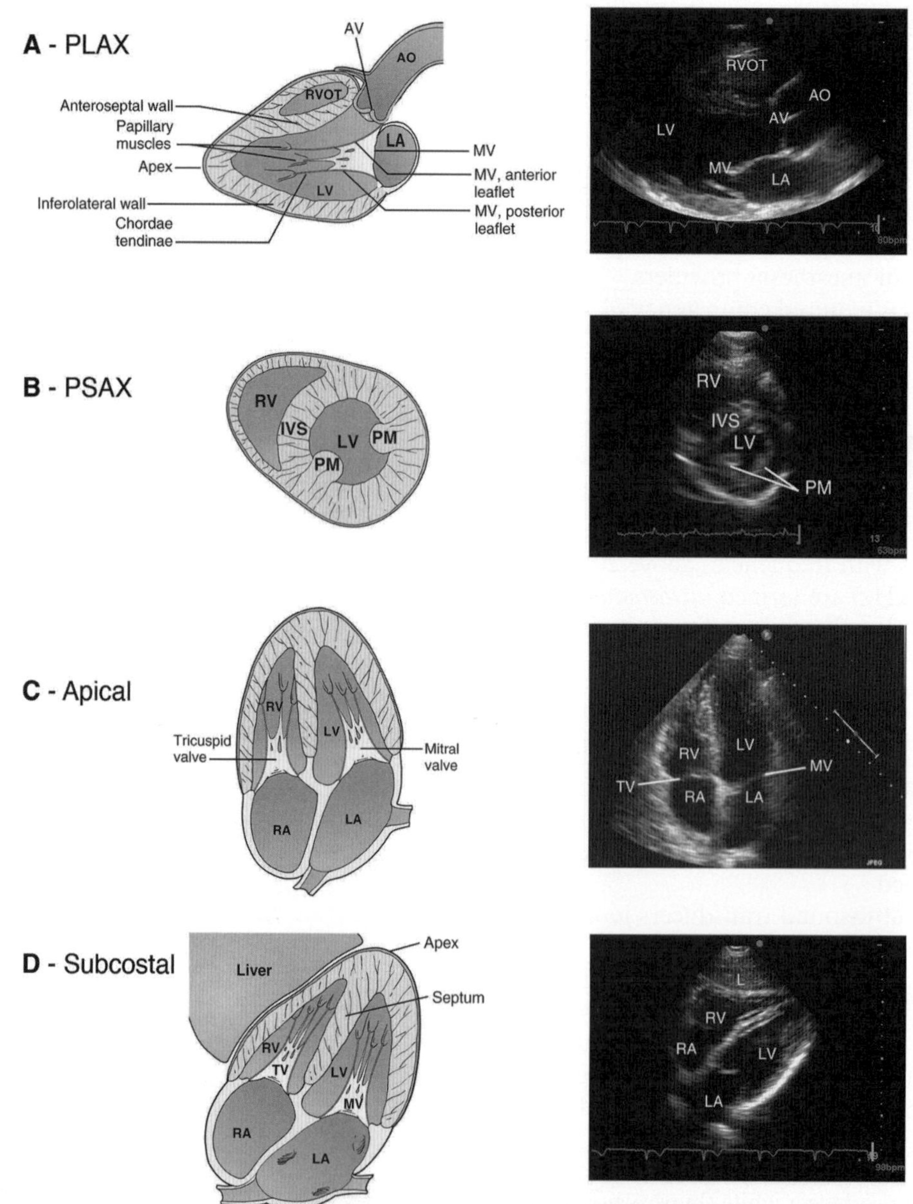

Cross-sectional anatomy and ultrasound images for the four basic cardiac ultrasound views. (A) Parasternal long axis (PLAX). Note that on an optimal PLAX view, apex is not fully visualized on the ultrasound image. (B) Parasternal short axis (PSAX) taken at the level of the papillary muscles. (C) Apical 4-chamber view. (D) Subcostal 4-Chamber view. *AO,* Aorta; *AV,* aortic valve; *IVS,* intraventricular septum; *LA,* left atrium; *LV,* left ventricle; *MV,* mitral valve; *PM,* papillary muscle; *RA,* right atrium; *RV,* right ventricle; *RVOT,* right ventricular outflow tract; *TV,* tricuspid valve. (Figure modified from Soni NJ, Arntfield R, Kory P: *Point of Care Ultrasound.* 2nd Edition, Philadelphia, PA, Elsevier, Inc., 2020: 115-122, Figures 14.4, 14.5, 14.8 and 14.10).

Parasternal Long-Axis View

- Patient position: left side down
- Initial probe position: 3rd to 5th intercostal space just to the left of the sternum
- Indicator notch: toward patient's right shoulder
- Structures to identify:
  - Left ventricle (LV); the apex of the LV should *not* be seen
  - Left atrium (LA)
  - Mitral valve (both the anterior and posterior leaflets and the annulus)
  - Left ventricular outflow tract (LVOT)
  - Aortic valve (at least two of the three leaflets)
  - Right ventricular (RV) outflow tract (RVOT)
  - Descending aorta
- Image interpretation:
  - Evaluation of LV systolic function
  - Assess for presence of pericardial effusion.
    - Distinguish pericardial from pleural fluid using descending aorta as landmark.
    - Pericardial fluid: fluid anterior to the descending aorta (or above on the ultrasound screen)
    - Pleural fluid: fluid behind the descending aorta (or below on the ultrasound screen)
  - Comparison of LVOT, RVOT, and LA chamber size
    - These chambers should have similar anterior to posterior dimensions.
    - One chamber appearing noticeably larger may be suggestive of pathology.

Parasternal Short-Axis View

- Patient position: left side down
- Initial probe position: rotate clockwise 90 degrees from PLAX
- Indicator notch: toward patient's left shoulder
- Structures to identify:
  - LV in cross section (should appear round)
  - Septum
  - Papillary muscles (approximately 3 and 7 o'clock)
- Image interpretation:
  - Evaluation of LV systolic function
  - Presence of flattening of intraventricular septum (suggests RV pressure or volume overload)
  - Presence of pericardial effusion
  - Wall motion abnormalities
  - "Kissing" papillary muscles (suggests underfilled LV)

Apical Four-Chamber View

- Patient position: left side down
- Initial probe position: anterior to the midaxillary line, usually one or two rib spaces below the nipple line
- Indicator notch: to the patient's left
- Structures to identify:
  - LA and LV
  - Apex of LV (should appear thin)
  - Interventricular septum (center of the ultrasound screen, oriented vertically)
  - RA and RV
  - Mitral valve
  - Tricuspid valve
- Image interpretation:
  - LV size and systolic function
  - RV size and systolic function
    - Use caution interpreting RV if image is foreshortened.
  - Gross function of mitral and tricuspid valve
  - Presence of pericardial effusion

Subcostal and Inferior Vena Cava Views

- Patient position: supine (knees bent to help relax abdominal muscles in awake patient)
- Initial probe position:
  - Subcostal: 2 to 3 inches below the xyphoid process, just to the right of midline
  - IVC: rotate counterclockwise approximately 90 degrees from subcostal view
- Indicator notch
  - Subcostal: to the patient's left
  - IVC: toward the patient's head
- Structures to identify
  - Subcostal
    - RA and RV
    - LA and LV
    - Mitral valve
    - Tricuspid valve
  - IVC
    - Hepatic vein draining into IVC
    - IVC draining into RA
    - Compare with/identify aorta
- Image interpretation:
  - Subcostal
    - LV size and systolic function
    - RV size and systolic function
    - Gross function of mitral and tricuspid valve
    - Presence of pericardial effusion
  - IVC
    - Absolute diameter
    - Change in diameter with respirations

Perioperative Cardiac Ultrasound

- Ultrasound can help determine (or rule out) the cause of undifferentiated shock.
- Most evidence for use with the following focused questions:
  - Is the LV systolic function normal?
  - Is there a pericardial effusion?
  - Is there a problem with the RV?
- As many views as possible should be obtained to answer questions reliably and avoid misinterpretation.

- Remember that a normal basic cardiac ultrasound does not rule out *all* cardiac etiologies of shock (e.g., severe valvular disease).
- Don't forget to use lung and abdominal ultrasound when applicable to look for other causes of shock (pneumothorax, bleeding).
- Transesophageal echocardiogram will often provide superior images in the operating room given limitations with positioning and access to the chest wall.

PULMONARY ULTRASOUND

Normal Lung Examination

- *Presence of pleural sliding:* visceral and parietal pleura slide against each other during respiration creating the appearance of movement—"shimmering"
  - In M-mode, sliding looks like a "sandy beach."
- *A-lines:* reverberation artifacts that appear as horizontal hyperechoic lines at equidistant depths from the pleura
- *B-lines:* laser-like, hyperechoic vertical lines that arise from the pleural line and extend to the bottom of the ultrasound screen

Evaluation for Pneumothorax

- Patient position: supine (or near supine)
- Initial probe position: can use any probe (just make sure to decrease depth)
  - Start on either right or left anterior chest wall in the second intercostal space.
  - Systematically examine multiple rib spaces on both sides of the chest wall.
- Indicator notch: toward patient's head
- Structures to identify:
  - Two rib shadows with bright pleural line in-between
- Image interpretation—sonographic signs of pneumothorax
  - Absence of pleural sliding (barcode appearance on M-mode)
  - Absence of B-lines
  - Absence of lung pulse
    - Pleural motion with each heartbeat; easy to recognize on M-mode
  - Presence of lung point
    - Interface where healthy lung starts and a pneumothorax ends
    - 100% specific for pneumothorax.
    - The only sign that is 100% diagnostic for a pneumothorax.
    - Other sonographic signs suggestive of a pneumothorax are also seen in other clinical scenarios (e.g., mainstem intubation, severe ARDS).

Evaluation of Interstitial and Alveolar Patterns

- Patient position: supine (or near supine)
- Initial probe position: can use any probe (just make sure to decrease depth)
  - Start on either right or left anterior chest wall in the second intercostal space.
  - Systematically examine multiple rib spaces on both sides of the chest wall.
- Indicator notch: toward patient's head
- Structures to identify
  - Two rib shadows with bright pleural line in-between
- Image interpretation:
  - Presence of more than three B-lines per intercostal space is indicative of interstitial pathology.
  - Differential diagnosis: pulmonary edema (noncardiogenic or cardiogenic), interstitial pneumonia, pulmonary fibrosis, contusion, tumor, and pneumonitis
  - The pattern of B-lines (spacing, diffuse versus focal) and clinical context will help narrow differential.

Evaluation of the Pleural Space

- Patient position: upright (if able), supine, or semirecumbent
- Initial probe position
  - Need curvilinear or phased array probe given depth of structures
  - Seated patient: footprint of ultrasound probe perpendicular to the skin on the lateral chest wall just below the clavicle
  - Supine or semirecumbent patient: probe in the midaxillary line, scan cranio to caudal until diaphragm visualized
- Indicator notch: toward patient's head
- Structures to identify
  - Diaphragm
  - Pleural space
  - Liver or spleen
  - Kidney (if posterior)
- Image interpretation
  - Pleural fluid = anechoic space between the visceral or parietal pleura
  - "Spine sign" (visualization of the vertebral bodies in the thoracic cavity above the diaphragm) = presence of fluid
  - Quality of fluid: simple versus complex, free-flowing versus loculated
  - Quantity of fluid
    - Lung ultrasound can detect effusions as small as 20 mL.
  - Consolidated lung will show air bronchograms (hyperechoic lines and dots within the area of consolidated lung).
    - Immobile air bronchograms are more likely atelectasis.

- Mobile/dynamic air bronchograms are more specific for pneumonia.

Intraoperative Pulmonary Ultrasound: Diagnosis of Acute Hypoxemia

- Acute hypoxemia is a common intraoperative event that requires prompt diagnosis and management.
- Ultrasound is readily available for use in the operating room and can aid in diagnosis of hypoxemia.
- Lung hypoxemia findings and possible diagnoses include:
  - Absence of sliding—pneumothorax or endobronchial intubation
  - Multiple B-lines—acute pulmonary edema
  - Normal lung ultrasound—bronchospasm, pulmonary embolus
- Remember to perform a systematic exam interrogating multiple rib spaces and both lung fields.

ABDOMINAL ULTRASOUND

FAST Exam

- Focused assessment with sonography in trauma (FAST)
  - Originally developed and most specific in blunt trauma patients to identify:
    - Hemothorax (fluid in the chest cavity)
    - Hemoperitoneum (free peritoneal fluid)
    - Hemopericardium (fluid in the pericardial sac)
  - Also useful in hypotensive patients at risk for intraperitoneal hemorrhage
  - Four views—right upper quadrant (RUQ); left upper quadrant (LUQ); pelvic; subcostal (or subxiphoid)
  - eFAST (extended) adds views to evaluate for pneumothorax.
- Patient position: supine, arms slightly abducted from the patient's side
- Initial probe position
  - RUQ view: right midaxillary line approximately at the level of the subxiphoid
  - LUQ view: just posterior to midaxillary line approximately at the level of the subxiphoid
  - Pelvic view: midline just above the pubic bone
  - Subcostal view: 2–3 inches below the xyphoid process, just to the right of midline
- Indicator notch: by convention, toward patient's right or head in each view
- Structures to identify
  - RUQ view: liver, diaphragm, kidney
  - LUQ view: spleen, diaphragm, kidney
  - Pelvic view: bladder (fluid filled, hypoechoic structure)
  - Subcostal: see above in cardiac ultrasound
- Image interpretation: in each view, try to identify the following structures/locations assessing for free fluid
  - RUQ view
    - Above the diaphragm (supradiaphragmatic)
    - Below the diaphragm (subphrenic)
    - Hepatorenal (Morrison pouch)
    - Inferior tip of the liver
    - Inferior tip of the kidney
  - LUQ view
    - Above the diaphragm (supradiaphragmatic)
    - Below the diaphragm (subphrenic)
    - Splenorenal
    - Inferior tip of the liver
    - Inferior tip of the kidney
  - Pelvic view
    - Hypoechoic pockets to the side of the bladder
    - Fluid behind the bladder or uterus

Gastric Ultrasound

- Patient position: first supine (or near supine); then right lateral decubitus (RLD)
- Initial probe position: perpendicular to the skin in the epigastric region just below the subxiphoid margin
- Indicator notch: toward patient's head
- Structures to identify:
  - Liver, aorta (longitudinal), pancreas, and the superior mesenteric artery
  - Gastric antrum short axis (can be differentiated from bowel by the thick, hypoechoic muscularis layer surrounding the hyperechoic serosa and mucosal layers)
- Image interpretation
  - Qualitative assessment
    - *Empty:* gastric antrum will either appear collapsed and flat or round to ovoid shape with thick walls, often described as a "bull's eye"
    - *Fluids present*: clear liquids will appear anechoic or hypoechoic, and the antrum will distend and become thin-walled
    - *Solids present*: initially after eating-air ingested prevents visualization of the structures deep to the antrum, appearance is of "frosted glass". Later-antrum distends and appears to be full of contents with heterogenous echogenicity.
  - Quantitative assessment
    - Cross-sectional area in RLD position
    - Volumes <1.5 mL/kg = normal/low risk for aspiration
    - Volumes ≥ 1.5 mL/kg = higher than normal aspiration risk

Gastric Ultrasound

Consider gastric ultrasound in the following clinical scenarios:
- Unknown fasting state
- Concern for delayed gastric emptying (obesity; severe diabetes; medication use such as GLP-1 agonists, opioids, etc.)

Potential interventions if high gastric volume identified:
- Delay elective surgery.
- Administer antacids.
- Use endotracheal tube and rapid sequence intubation.
- Decompress stomach with nasogastric tube prior to intubation.

CONCLUSION AND FUTURE DIRECTIONS

- Perioperative POCUS is a core training competency in anesthesiology.
- Other applications for perioperative POCUS include evaluation for deep venous thrombosis and ocular pathologies.
- As anesthesia providers become more skilled in POCUS, the applications are likely to expand further.

QUESTIONS

REVIEW OF ULTRASOUND PHYSICS

1. Describe the piezoelectric effect and inverse piezoelectric effect. How do they relate to medical ultrasound imaging?
2. What is acoustic impedance? How does it apply to the structures commonly viewed in medical ultrasound?

BASIC CARDIAC ULTRASOUND

3. What are the four questions to answer when assessing LV systolic function in the parasternal long axis view?
4. What is foreshortening? How does it affect image acquisition and interpretation in the apical four-chamber view?

PULMONARY ULTRASOUND

5. Describe the four sonographic signs to evaluate for a pneumothorax. Which of these signs is 100% specific for a pneumothorax?
6. What is the "spine sign"? What information does it provide about the pleural space?

ABDOMINAL ULTRASOUND

7. Where is the most common place for fluid to collect in the RUQ view of the FAST exam? Where is the most common place for fluid to collect in the LUQ view?
8. How can volume of gastric contents be calculated using ultrasound? What volume is considered higher than normal risk for aspiration?

ANSWERS

ULTRASOUND PHYSICS

1. Ultrasound transducers are composed of numerous piezoelectric crystals. These piezoelectric crystals have unique electromechanical properties that allow them to convert electrical charge into mechanical energy (the piezoelectric effect). They can also do the opposite—convert mechanical energy into electrical energy (the inverse piezoelectric effect). When an electric current is applied to the piezoelectric crystals of an ultrasound transducer, the crystals start to vibrate and produce sound waves (or ultrasound waves). This is an example of the inverse piezoelectric effect. Alternatively, when the piezoelectric crystals on the transducer are hit by a reflected ultrasound wave, they begin to vibrate (mechanical energy). These mechanical vibrations are converted to electrical energy and sent to the ultrasound machine, which interprets the electrical charges to create an image. This is an example of the piezoelectric effect. (383–384)
2. Acoustic impedance is a physical property of a tissue. It a measure of the resistance an ultrasound beam encounters as it passes through a tissue, which depends on the physical density of the tissue and the velocity of the soundwave transmitted through the tissue medium. In medical ultrasound, when an ultrasound wave is transmitted, the angle of transmission changes once a new tissue or medium is encountered, based upon the acoustic impedance of the two opposing substances. The difference in acoustic impedance between the two substances changes the reflection angles. Fluids generally have a low acoustic impedance, and therefore most sound waves are transmitted through the fluid and not reflected back to the transducer, producing a black or anechoic image. More solid substances (e.g., bone) generally have a higher acoustic impedance, causing more waves to be reflected back and producing a very bright white or hyperechoic signal. (384)

BASIC CARDIAC ULTRASOUND

3. The four questions to answer when assessing LV systolic function in the parasternal long axis view are (1) Is the LV chamber (cavity) size changing between systole and diastole? (2) Are the walls of the LV (myocardium) getting thicker? (3) Is the anterior leaflet of the mitral valve hitting the septum? (4) Is the annulus of the mitral valve moving toward the apex? (385–386)
4. Foreshortening occurs when the ultrasound beam does not cut through the true apex of the left ventricle. This causes the apex of the LV to appear rounded and thick rather than thin and bullet shaped. Foreshortened images can lead to three important data misinterpretations: (1) any abnormalities of the LV apex will not be seen (e.g., LV thrombus); (2) LV function may appear better than it actually is; and (3) a normal, healthy RV may artifactually appear larger in size with reduced function. (387)

PULMONARY ULTRASOUND

5. The four sonographic signs to evaluate for a pneumothorax are (1) absence of pleural sliding; (2) absence of B-lines; (3) absence of lung pulse; (4) presence of lung point, which is 100% specific for pneumothorax. The figure below depicts an algorithm for diagnosis of pneumothorax with ultrasound. (391, 394)

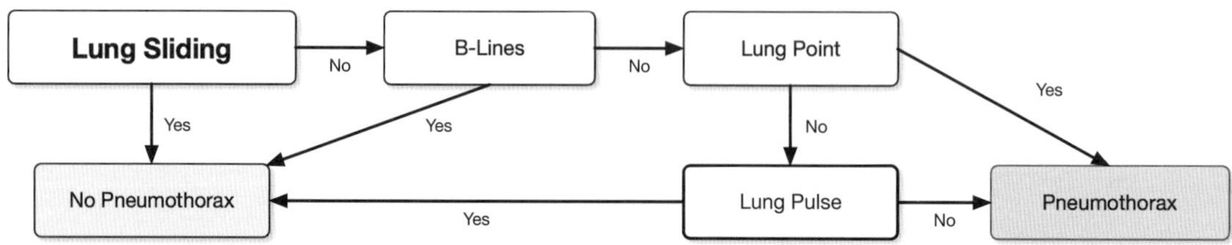

Sample diagonostic algorithm for pneumothorax.

6. The "spine sign" is visualization of the vertebral bodies in the thoracic cavity above the diaphragm (see figure below). These are not usually seen in this location and indicate the presence of fluid in the pleural space. (393, 395)

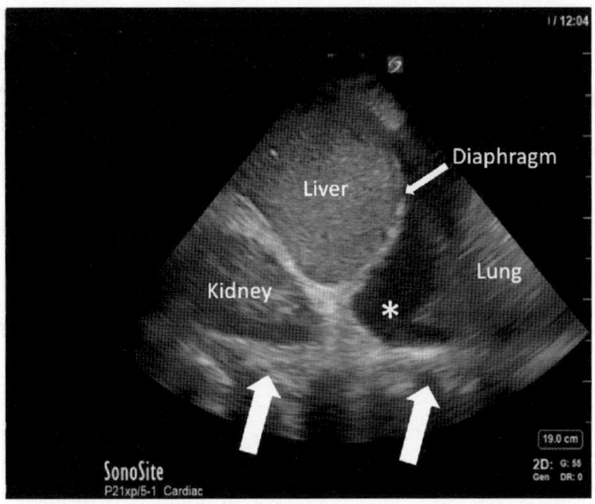

Right sided pleural effusion with anechoic pleural fluid (*asterisk*) and consolidated lung adjacent to the pleural fluid. Note that the spine shadow is seen both below and above the diaphragm (*arrows*). When the spine shadow is seen above the diaphragm, this is termed "spine sign" and is an indirect indicator of the presence of pleural fluid.

ABDOMINAL ULTRASOUND

7. The most common place for fluid to collect in the RUQ FAST view is the potential space between the liver and kidney, also known as the Morrison pouch. In the LUQ view, the most common place for fluid to collect is between the spleen and the diaphragm. (394–395)
8. The volume of gastric contents can be calculated in two ways. The first is to measure the antral cross-sectional area (CSA) in the right lateral decubitus position. This can be done by measuring the craniocaudal and anterior-posterior diameters of the antrum from serosa to serosa and then calculating the area using the formula for the area of an eclipse ($CSA = (AP \times CC \times \pi)/4$). Alternatively, some ultrasound machines allow the operator to trace the circumference of the antrum at the level of the serosa and then automatically calculate the CSA. Once the CSA is calculated, the volume can be estimated using mathematical models that stratify by patient age. Volumes $\geq$1.5 mL/kg may indicate delayed emptying or a nonfasted state and are associated with a higher-than-baseline risk of aspiration. (399)

Chapter

22 ACID-BASE BALANCE AND BLOOD GAS ANALYSIS

Amreen Savanna Rahman and Linda L. Liu

DEFINITIONS

Acids and Bases

- Bronsted and Lowry definition: acids are proton (H^+) donors, and bases are proton acceptors.
- Biologic molecules are weak acids or bases that reversibly donate or bind H^+.

Acidemia and Acidosis

- pH < 7.35 is *acidemia.*
  - The process of lowering the pH is *acidosis.*
- pH > 7.45 is *alkalemia.*
  - The process of raising the pH is *alkalosis.*
- A patient can have a mixed disorder but can only be acidemic or alkalemic.

Base Excess (BE)

- BE is a calculated value based on plasma pH, pCO_2, and hemoglobin.
- BE > 0 is a base excess.
  - The amount of strong acid to return 1 L of whole blood to pH 7.4
  - Base excess suggests a metabolic alkalosis.
- BE < 0 is a base deficit.
  - The amount of strong base to return 1 L of whole blood to pH 7.4
  - Base deficit suggests a metabolic acidosis.
- BE is often used as a surrogate measure for lactic acidosis in clinical practice.

REGULATION OF THE HYDROGEN ION CONCENTRATION

Acid-Base Status Overview: Normal Values and Physiologic Adaptations to Changes

Normal values at 37°C
- Arterial hydrogen ion **concentration** is 35 to 45 mmol/L.
- Arterial pH is 7.45 to 7.35, respectively.
- Plasma bicarbonate ion concentration is 24 ± 2 mEq/L.

Physiologic systems to buffer acid-base disturbances:
- Buffer systems
  - Immediate chemical response
- Ventilatory response
  - In minutes, whenever possible
- Renal response
  - Days, but can nearly completely restore pH

Buffer Systems

- Buffer systems consist of a base molecule and weak conjugate acid that respond to acid-base disturbances.

Bicarbonate Buffer System

- Bicarbonate is a base molecule, and carbonic acid is the weak conjugate acid.
  - CO_2 combines with water, catalyzed by carbonic anhydrase.
  - Carbonic acid is formed, which deprotonates to form bicarbonate.

Hemoglobin Buffer System

- Histidine residues with multiple protonatable imidazole side chains
  - CO_2 will diffuse into the red blood cells (RBCs) and combine with water.
  - Carbonic acid is formed, which deprotonates.
  - The H^+ binds Hb, while the bicarbonate ion will exchange with Cl^- back into plasma.

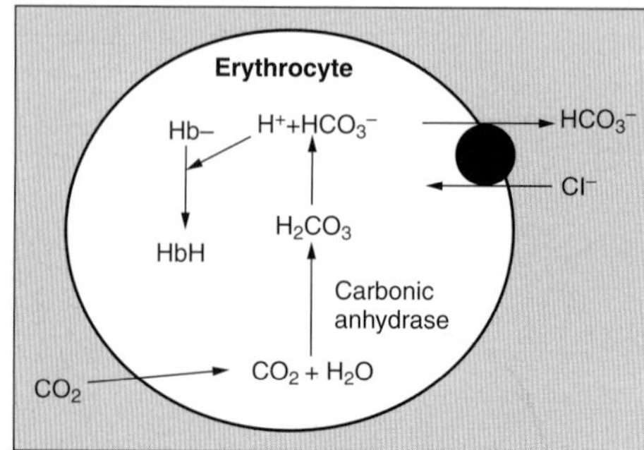

Hemoglobin buffering system. Carbon dioxide freely diffuses into erythrocytes, where it combines with water to form carbonic acid, which rapidly deprotonates. The protons generated are bound up by hemoglobin. The bicarbonate anions are exchanged back into plasma with chloride.

Ventilatory Response

- Central chemoreceptors at medulla respond to changes in CSF pH.
  - CO_2 crosses blood-brain barrier and increases CSF $[H^+]$.
  - Minute ventilation increases 1–4 L/min per 1mm Hg increase in $PaCO_2$.
  - Response is linear except at extreme values.
    - High $PaCO_2$ can lead to CO_2 narcosis.
    - Low $PaCO_2$ can lead to the apneic threshold.
- Peripheral chemoreceptors are located at the bifurcation of the common carotid and along the aortic arch.
  - Receptors respond to PaO_2, $PaCO_2$, pH, and arterial perfusion pressure.
  - Respiratory centers are stimulated via the glossopharyngeal nerve.
  - Most sensitive to PaO_2
    - Patients after bilateral carotid endarterectomies mostly lack hypoxic ventilatory drive.
- Ventilatory response does not fully correct an acid-base disturbance.
  - Overcorrection of a metabolic alkalosis will cause hypoventilation leading to hypoxemia.
  - This would trigger the hypoxic ventilatory drive to breathe.

Renal Response

- Slower than the ventilatory response
- Proximal tubule reabsorbs bicarbonate catalyzed by carbonic anhydrase.
- Ammonia diffuses into the tubular fluid, combines with H^+ to form NH_4^+
  - Remains in the tubule to be excreted

ANALYSIS OF ARTERIAL BLOOD GASES

Sampling

- Sampling sites are readily cannulated arteries (radial, brachial, femoral).
- Venous blood gases can be used to approximate $PaCO_2$ in most clinical situations.
  - Venous pH usually 0.03–0.04 less than arterial
- ABG should be drawn in a heparinized syringe without air bubbles.
  - Air bubbles can equilibrate with the blood and influence results.
  - Expedient analysis and placement on ice avoid oxygen consumption and CO_2 generation (by white blood cell metabolism).

Temperature Correction

- Hypothermia will lower the partial pressure of gases in solution.
  - The pCO_2 and pO_2 will decrease, and bicarbonate will not change.
  - ABG with pH 7.4, pCO_2 43 mm Hg taken at 37°C will have a pH of 7.5 and pCO_2 of 31 mm Hg at 30°C.
- Methods to managing ABGs in hypothermic patients

Alpha-Stat

- Measures all blood gases at 37°C and allows for pH drift with temperature changes
- Strive to keep the ABG measured pH at 7.4 during hypothermia.
  - The true pH is higher.

pH-Stat

- Maintain the pH static at 7.4 based on the core temperature.
- Add CO_2 to compensate for the hypothermia to maintain a corrected pH of 7.4.
  - In the ICU, compensation can be achieved by lowering the ventilatory rate.
  - Some suggest this can improve cerebrovascular perfusion during hypothermia.

Oxygenation

- Hypothermia left-shifts the oxygen-hemoglobin dissociation curve.
  - Oxygen readily binds to hemoglobin but more difficult to unload at tissues

DIFFERENTIAL DIAGNOSIS OF ACID-BASE DISTURBANCES

Adverse Responses to Acidemia and Alkalemia

- The consequences of severe acidosis or alkalosis are more rapid and profound with respiratory than with metabolic causes.

Effects of Severe Acidemia and Alkalemia

- Acidemia can lead to decreased myocardial contractility and catecholamine release.
  - Severe acidemia ($pH < 7.2$) decreases myocardial responsiveness to catecholamines, so myocardial depression is revealed.
- Severe alkalemia ($pH > 7.6$) leads to decreased cerebral and coronary blood flow due to arteriolar vasoconstriction.

Respiratory Acidosis

- Results when minute ventilation is inadequate relative to CO_2 production.
  - Causes can be increased CO_2 production or decreased CO_2 elimination or increased rebreathing or absorption of CO_2.

Compensatory Responses and Treatment

- Kidneys increase H^+ secretion and bicarbonate reabsorption.
  - Compensatory response from kidneys takes hours to days.
- For severe acidosis, the patient may need interim ventilatory support.

Chronic Respiratory Acidosis

- Ventilation strategies in patients with chronic respiratory acidosis should avoid hyperventilation.
  - Relative hypocapnia can lead to CNS irritability and cardiac ischemia.
  - If pCO_2 is normalized, compensatory bicarbonate excretion can complicate ventilator weaning by increasing minute ventilation requirement.

Respiratory Alkalosis

- Results when minute ventilation is increased relative to carbon dioxide production
  - $PaCO_2$ is diminished relative to bicarbonate levels.
- Decreased pCO_2 and increased pH trigger central and peripheral chemoreceptors to decrease the drive to breathe.

Compensatory Responses and Treatment

- Kidneys compensate by decreasing reabsorption and increasing excretion of bicarbonate.
- Treatment is directed at correcting the underlying disorder.

Metabolic Acidosis

- Due to an increase in acids other than carbon dioxide
- Compensatory increase in ventilation begins within minutes.
  - Some patients may require ventilatory support.
- Can be categorized into anion gap and nonanion gap acidosis

Causes of Metabolic Acidosis

Anion gap
- Lactic acidosis, ketoacidosis, uremia, toxins (methanol, ethylene glycol, ethanol, aspirin, paraldehyde, INH)

Nongap
- Excess of chloride, GI losses, renal losses, drugs (acetazolamide)

Anion Gap

- Anion gap (AG) is the difference between measured cations and anions.
- $AG = [Na^+] - ([Cl^-] + [HCO_3^-])$
  - Normal is 8–12 mEq/mL.
  - Need to correct for albumin greater or less than 4.4 g/dL
    - Decrease AG by 2.5 mEq/L per 1 g/dL decrease in albumin, and vice versa.
- If there is an anion gap, determine the Δgap.
  - $\Delta gap = (AG - 12) + HCO_3^-$
    - $\Delta gap < 22$ suggests concurrent nongap metabolic acidosis.
    - $\Delta gap > 26$ suggests concurrent metabolic alkalosis.
- The most common unmeasured anions are lactic acid and keto acids.

Nonanion Gap

- Nonanion gap acidosis can result from Cl^- replacing bicarbonate.
- Examples include bicarbonate wasting processes such as renal tubular acidosis and diarrhea, or excessive resuscitation with normal saline (>30 mL/kg/h).

Strong Ion Difference

- Alternative approach to categorizing metabolic acidosis
- Distinguishes six primary acid-base disturbances by incorporating albumin
- Does not appear to offer an advantage over the traditional approach

Compensatory Responses and Treatment

- Carotid body chemoreceptors trigger increased alveolar ventilation.
- Renal excretion of H^+ ions
- When chronic, bone buffers may act as a buffer leading to loss of bone mass.

Treatment of Severe Metabolic Acidosis

- Consider sodium bicarbonate in extreme anion gap metabolic acidosis with hemodynamic instability.
  - The patient must have the capacity to ventilate off the byproduct of bicarbonate, which is CO_2.
- Treat the underlying cause of the acidosis (e.g., hypoperfusion leading to lactate, DKA-forming ketones).

Metabolic Alkalosis

- Due to increased bicarbonate or decreased hydrogen ions
  - Increased bicarbonate absorption in response to hypovolemia, hypokalemia, hyperaldosteronism
  - Loss of H^+ from GI tract or kidneys

Compensatory Responses and Treatment

- Alveolar hypoventilation leading to CO_2 retention
  - Can only compensate by up to 75%
- Increased reabsorption or decreased secretion of H^+ by the kidneys
  - Depends on the presence of cations (sodium, potassium) and chloride
  - Fluid repletion with saline and potassium chloride may be necessary.
- Treat the cause of the acid loss.

Diagnosis

- Determine the direction of the disorder: pH < 7.35 or > 7.45.
- Is the process primarily metabolic or respiratory disorder?
  - Based on pCO_2 and bicarbonate
- If the process is respiratory: chronic or acute?
  - Chronic respiratory process: pH change of 0.03 for every 10 mm Hg change in pCO_2 from 40 mm Hg
  - Acute respiratory process: pH change of 0.08 for every 10 mm Hg change in pCO_2 from 40 mm Hg
- If a metabolic process: acidosis or alkalosis? Is the respiratory compensation adequate?
  - If primarily metabolic acidosis
    - Calculate anion gap.
    - If anion gap is present, calculate Δgap.
    - Use Winter's formula, $pCO_2 = (1.5 \times HCO_3^-) + 8$, to see if there is a concurrent respiratory acidosis or alkalosis.
  - If primarily metabolic alkalosis
    - Calculate expected $pCO_2 = (0.7 \times HCO_3^-) + 21$ to see if there is a concurrent respiratory acidosis or alkalosis.

OTHER INFORMATION PROVIDED BY ANALYSIS OF ABG AND PH

Ventilation

- Anatomic dead space
  - Fraction of the respiratory system not involved in gas exchange
  - Baseline amount of dead space ventilation is usually 0.25 to 0.30.
- Increased dead space ventilation decreases ventilation efficiency.
  - Causes include pulmonary embolus or decreased cardiac output.
  - Gradient between $PaCO_2$ and end-tidal CO_2 increases.

Oxygenation

- Causes of hypoxemia
  - Low inhaled FiO_2
  - Hypoventilation
  - Venous admixture

Alveolar Gas Equation

- Estimates partial pressure of alveolar O_2
  - Barometric pressure (increased altitude decreases inspired O_2)
  - Water vapor pressure
  - Inspired O_2 concentration (calculated using $PaCO_2$ and respiratory quotient)

Alveolar-Arterial (A-a) Gradient

- Estimates the percentage venous admixture
  - Deoxygenated venous blood mixing with oxygenated arterial blood (shunt)

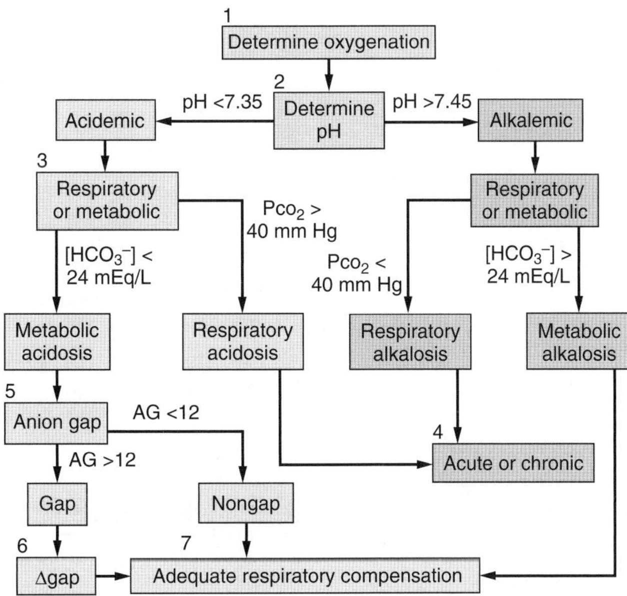

Seven Steps for Acid-Base Diagnosis. Δgap, anion gap −12 +[HCO_3^-]. If Δgap is less than 22 mEq/L, then concurrent nongap metabolic acidosis exists. If Δgap is greater than 26 mEq/L, then concurrent metabolic alkalosis exists.

- More sensitive than pulse oximetry to assess shunts
- Normal A-a gradient is <15 mm Hg breathing room air.
  - Baseline shunt exists from Thebesian and bronchial veins.
- Increased A-a gradient due to age, increased FiO_2, and vasodilators that inhibit hypoxic pulmonary vasoconstriction
  - Larger A-a gradients due to pathologic shunting
    - Right-to-left intrapulmonary shunting (atelectasis, pneumonia, and endobronchial intubation)
    - Intracardiac shunts (congenital heart disease)
  - Increasing FiO_2 in large shunts will not increase PaO_2.

PaO_2/FiO_2 Ratio

- Simple alternative to A-a gradient to assess degree of hypoxemia
- Used to determine severity of disease in ARDS patients
  - With severe disease P/F ratio is <100 mm Hg.

Cardiac Output Estimates

- Mixed PvO_2 is a balance between oxygen delivery and tissue oxygenation.
  - Sample obtained from a mixture of SVC, IVC, and cardiac venous return
    - Unwedged PA catheter
  - Can use trends from central venous PvO_2 as a proxy for mixed PvO_2
    - Central line in SVC
- Normal mixed PvO_2 value is 40 mm Hg.
- Can be used to estimate cardiac output (CO) when O_2 consumption (VO_2) is static
  - Decreased PvO_2 indicates decreased CO, leading to increased O_2 extraction.
  - Increased PvO_2 suggests higher CO.
    - Sepsis, peripheral shunting, or impaired oxygen extraction

Fick Equation

- Calculates cardiac output based on PaO_2, PvO_2, and Hb
  - Basis is that oxygen delivered to the veins equals arterial O_2 delivery minus O_2 consumption.
- CO equals O_2 consumption divided by the arterial-venous difference in O_2 content.
  - $CO = VO_2/(CaO_2 - CvO_2)$

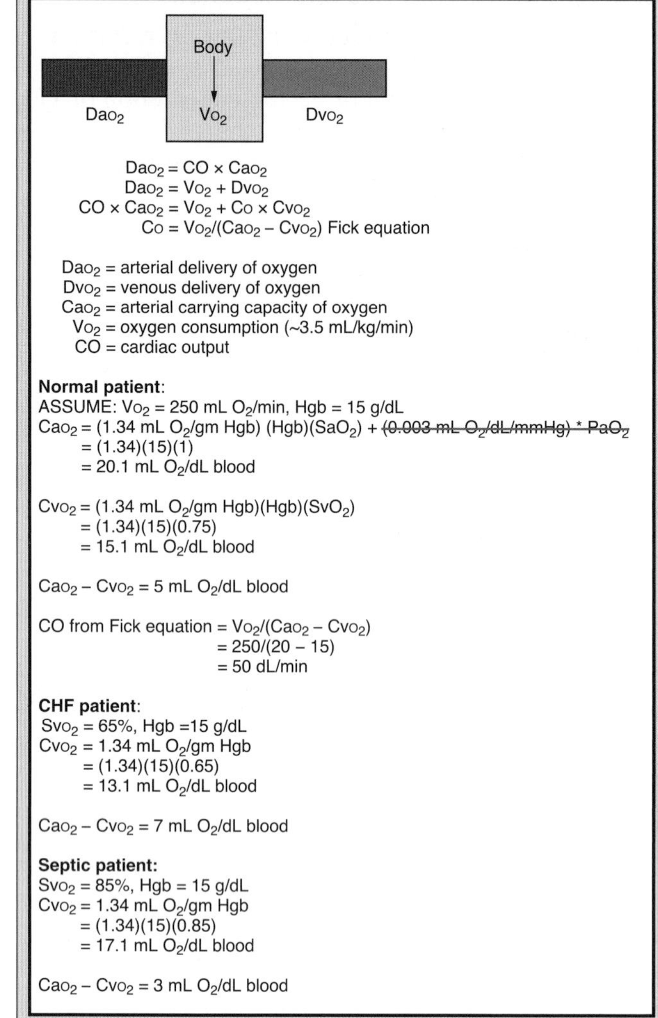

Cardiac Output Calculations. Figure depicts calculation of cardiac output via Fick equation; arterial and mixed venous oxygen content; and arteriovenous difference in normal, septic, and heart failure patients. Amount of dissolved oxygen calculated by 0.003 mLO_2 /dL/mm Hg. *PaO_2 can be ignored because of its small influence on CaO_2. CHF, Congestive heart failure.

Arteriovenous Difference

- Difference between arterial and mixed venous content
- Normal is 4–6 mL O_2/dL of blood.
- Decreased cardiac output leads to higher O_2 extraction, which increases AV difference.

Lactate Measurements

- Arterial lactate concentration is used as a marker.
  - Hypoperfusion or microcirculatory dysfunction

- Sensitive for disease severity: >2 mmol/L is considered significant
- Causes are classified into perfusion related (Type A) and nonperfusion related (Type B).

Causes of Elevated Lactate

Type A—Perfusion Related
- Distributive: sepsis, anaphylaxis
- Cardiogenic/cardiac arrest
- Hypovolemia: hemorrhagic
- Obstructive: pulmonary embolism, cardiac tamponade
- Tissue ischemia: mesenteric ischemia, burns, trauma, compartment syndrome, necrotizing soft tissue infections
- Muscle activity: tonic-clonic seizures, increased work of breathing, disorders with acute muscle rigidity (e.g., serotonin syndrome, neuroleptic malignant syndrome, malignant hyperthermia)

Type B—Nonperfusion Related
- Toxins: cyanide, carbon monoxide, cocaine, alcohol
- Medications: metformin, linezolid, HIV reverse transcriptase inhibitors, epinephrine, inhaled β_2-agonists, propofol infusion syndrome
- Malignancy
- Liver failure

QUESTIONS

INTRODUCTION

1. What is the primary derangement in the following acid-base disorders, and what is the expected compensatory response? Complete the table below with arrows indicating the direction of change.

	pH	$PaCO_2$	HCO_3^-
Metabolic Acidosis	↓		
Respiratory Acidosis	↓		
Metabolic Alkalosis	↑		
Respiratory Alkalosis	↑		

2. What are the differences between central and peripheral chemoreceptors in terms of location, triggers, response, and limitations to the response? How would these responses change in a patient with bilateral carotid endarterectomies?

ANALYSIS OF ARTERIAL BLOOD GASES

3. In a patient breathing room air, how would the presence of an air bubble in an ABG sample change the ABG results? What are the expected changes to the ABG in a patient with hypothermia?

DIFFERENTIAL DIAGNOSIS OF ACID-BASE DISTURBANCES

4. A 63-year-old woman who lives alone presents to the ED complaining of several days of watery diarrhea. An ABG shows pH 7.25, $PaCO_2$ 23 mm Hg, PaO_2 100 mm Hg; other labs include Na 134 mEq/L, Cl 119 mEq/L, HCO_3 10 mEq/L. She was given 3 L of normal saline in the ED. What acid-base abnormality is present?
5. A 32-year-old woman is found down, transported to the ED, and subsequently intubated for airway protection. Initial labs after intubation reveal an ABG with pH 7.14, $PaCO_2$ 31 mm Hg, PaO_2 386 mm Hg. Other labs include Na 142 mEq/L, K 3.4 mEq/L, Cl 100 mEq/L, HCO_3 8 mEq/L. What is the acid-base abnormality? What other lab values would be useful?

OTHER INFORMATION PROVIDED BY ANALYSIS OF ABG AND pH

6. What are the expected values for mixed PvO_2 in patients with septic shock? Cardiogenic shock?

ANSWERS

1. The main acid-base derangement is represented by two arrows, while the compensatory response is represented by one arrow. (405–407)

	pH	paCO_2	HCO_3^-
Metabolic Acidosis	↓	↓	↓↓
Respiratory Acidosis	↓	↑↑	↑
Metabolic Alkalosis	↑	↑	↑↑
Respiratory Alkalosis	↑	↓↓	↓

2. The following table highlights the differences between central and peripheral chemoreceptors. (402)

	Central Chemoreceptors	Peripheral Chemoreceptors
Location	Medulla	Common carotid, aortic arch
Triggers	CSF pH, PaCO_2	PaO_2, PaCO_2, perfusion pressure
Response	Increase minute ventilation	Hypoxic ventilatory drive
Limitations	CO_2 narcosis or apneic threshold	Attenuated by anesthesia and eliminated in patients with bilateral carotid endarterectomies

3. An air bubble in an ABG syringe can cause a falsely elevated pO_2 value from equilibration of air and blood pO_2 values. Hypothermia will lower the pCO_2 and pO_2, and thus pH will drift upward. Bicarbonate values will not change. A sample drawn at 37°C with a pH 7.4, pCO_2 43 will have a pH 7.5, pCO_2 31 at 30°C. (403)
4. When interpreting acid-base abnormalities, approach the problem in a systematic and stepwise fashion.
   Step 1: Determine oxygenation.
   Step 2: The patient has a pH of 7.25, so there is an acidosis.
   Step 3: The primary derangement is metabolic as evidenced by the $HCO_3 < 24$ mEq/L.
   Step 4: The next step is to calculate an anion gap, $[134 - (119 + 10)] = 5$. This is a nonanion gap metabolic acidosis.
   Step 5: There is no anion gap, so this step in determining Δgap is skipped.
   Step 6: To determine respiratory compensation, we can use Winter's formula, $PaCO_2 = 1.5\,(HCO_3^-) + 8$.
   Based on this formula, this patient has a nongap metabolic acidosis with appropriate respiratory compensation. The most likely etiology is due to her diarrhea, which is a bicarbonate wasting process, with chloride replacing the bicarbonate from the normal saline resuscitation. (408–409)
5. Again, take a stepwise approach to this acid-base abnormality.
   Step 1: Determine oxygenation.
   Step 2: There is an acidosis as the pH is 7.14.
   Step 3: The primary dysfunction is metabolic based on the bicarbonate of 8.
   Step 4: The AG is 34, which is elevated. A normal AG is expected to be 8–12.
   Step 5: $\Delta gap = (AG\text{-}12) + HCO_3^-$. A $\Delta gap > 26$ indicates that there is a concurrent metabolic alkalosis here.
   Step 6: Determine whether there is adequate compensation using Winter's formula, $PaCO_2 = 1.5\,(HCO_3^-) + 8$.
   The calculated or expected pCO_2 is lower than actual pCO_2, so there is a concurrent respiratory acidosis as well. Recalling the differential for anion gap metabolic acidosis, this could be a toxic ingestion, lactic acidosis, ketoacidosis, or uremia. Gathering further details and lab findings such as a lactate, BUN, serum ketones, toxicology screen, and urine studies would aid in narrowing the differential. In summary, this patient has three primary acid-base disorders: anion gap metabolic acidosis, metabolic alkalosis, and respiratory acidosis. (408–409)
6. Septic shock is typically a vasodilatory shock state with high cardiac output. Despite increased circulation, there is decreased oxygen extraction, so the expected PvO_2 will be higher than normal. In cardiogenic shock, there is decreased delivery due to decreased cardiac function, leading to increased oxygen extraction from the blood that is being circulated, especially at the coronaries, leading to a decreased mixed PvO_2. (412)

Chapter

23 HEMOSTASIS

Genevieve Manahan

INTRODUCTION

- Normal physiologic hemostasis is a constant balance between two processes:
  - Procoagulant pathways generating localized hemostatic clot
  - Counterregulatory mechanisms that inhibit uncontrolled thrombus propagation or premature thrombus degradation

NORMAL HEMOSTASIS

- Primary hemostasis—platelet deposition at a site of vascular endothelium injury
- Secondary hemostasis—stabilization of a primary clot reinforced by crosslinked fibrin

Vascular Endothelial Role in Hemostasis

- Normal vascular endothelial cells reduce unprovoked thrombosis through antiplatelet and anticoagulant activity.
  - Vascular endothelial antiplatelet mechanisms
    - Negatively charged vascular endothelium repels platelets.
    - Production of potent platelet inhibitors prevents adhesion of platelets (prostaglandin I_2, nitric oxide).
    - Expression of adenosine diphosphatase (CD39) degrades adenosine diphosphate (ADP), a potent platelet activator.
  - Vascular endothelial anticoagulant mechanisms
    - Expression of thrombomodulin (TM), a cofactor for thrombin-mediated activation of protein C (an anticoagulant)
    - Production of tissue factor pathway inhibitor (TFPI), which inhibits the procoagulant activity of factor Xa and TF/VIIa complex
    - Synthesis of tissue plasminogen activator (tPA), an activator of fibrinolysis

Platelets and Hemostasis

- Endothelial injury shifts balance to promotion of platelet adhesion, activation, and aggregation.
  - Adhesion—damage to endothelial cells expose underlying extracellular matrix containing collagen, von Willebrand factor (vWF) and other platelet-adhesive glycoproteins
    - Absence of vWF (von Willebrand disease) or glycoprotein Ib-IX-V complex receptors (Bernard-Soulier syndrome) results in a clinically significant bleeding disorder.
  - Activation—platelet interaction with collagen results in secretion of thromboxane A_2 and granular contents, resulting in recruitment and activation of additional platelets
    - Alpha granules: fibrinogen, coagulation factors V and VII, vWF
    - Dense bodies: ADP, ATP, calcium, serotonin, histamine, epinephrine
  - Aggregation—recruitment of additional platelets to the site of injury
    - Newly active glycoprotein IIb/IIIa receptors promote cross-linking with fibrinogen.
    - Deficiency of glycoprotein IIb/IIIa receptors results in Glanzmann thrombasthenia.

Plasma-Mediated Hemostasis

- A cascade involving the serial activation of proenzyme and cofactors to accelerate and amplify fibrin generation by thrombin (factor IIa)
  - Extrinsic and intrinsic pathways culminate in a common pathway in which fibrin generation occurs.
    - This model is an oversimplification of in vivo hemostasis.
    - However, the construct remains useful when interpreting in vitro coagulation tests.
  - Extrinsic pathway—initiation phase with exposure of blood plasma to tissue factor (TF), which is prevalent in subendothelial tissues

    - Factor VIIa complexes with TF, factor X, and calcium to promote factor X to Xa.
    - Factor VIIa/TF complexes also activate factor IX of the intrinsic pathway.
  - Intrinsic pathway amplifies and propagates the hemostatic response to increase overall thrombin generation.
  - Final common pathway: depicts thrombin generation and subsequent fibrin formation
    - Tenase complexes produced by intrinsic (factor IXa, factor VIIIa, Ca^{2+}) and extrinsic (TF, factor VIIa, Ca^{2+}) pathways facilitate formation of prothrombinase complex, which causes a surge in thrombin generation from prothrombin.
    - Thrombin cleaves fibrinogen to create fibrin that polymerizes into fibrin strands to form clot.
    - Factor XIII is activated by thrombin and crosslinks fibrin strands.

Regulation of Coagulation

- Fibrinolysis—conversion of plasminogen to plasmin, which degrades fibrin and fibrinogen
  - Conversion to plasmin accomplished by tissue plasminogen activator (tPA) or urokinase from vascular endothelium.
  - Plasmin also inhibits factors V and VIII, reducing platelet adhesion and aggregation.
- Protein C system—regulates coagulation through inhibition of thrombin and essential cofactors Va and VIIIa
- Antithrombin (AT, formerly antithrombin III)—inhibits thrombin and factors IXa, Xa, XIa, and XIIa
  - Heparin binds AT, causing a conformational change and accelerating AT inhibition of enzymes by 100-fold.

BLEEDING DISORDERS

Inherited Bleeding Disorders

von Willebrand Disease (vWD)

- Most common inherited bleeding disease, up to 1% of the population
- Three main types (types 1, 2, and 3), most with an autosomal dominant inheritance pattern; vWD results in quantitative or qualitative deficiencies resulting in defective platelet adhesion and aggregation
- vWF is essential for platelet adhesion to the extracellular matrix (ECM) and prevention of degradation of factor VIII.
- Clinical presentation: history of easy bruising, recurrent epistaxis, menorrhagia; severe spontaneous hemorrhage can be seen in vWD type 3
- Diagnosis
  - Normal platelet count and PT
  - aPTT may have mild to moderate prolongation depending on level of factor VIII reduction.
  - Screening tests: measurement of vWF levels and platelet binding activity in the presence of ristocetin cofactor

Hemophilias

- Hemophilia A (factor VIII deficiency) and hemophilia B (factor IX deficiency)—X-linked inherited bleeding disorders
- Frequently present in childhood as spontaneous hemorrhage involving joints/deep muscle
- Severe disease is defined as <1% of coagulation factor activity (more common with hemophilia A)
- Diagnosis: prolongation of aPTT with normal PT, bleeding time, platelet count

Acquired Bleeding Disorders

Drug Induced

- Drugs with direct anticoagulant effect: heparin, warfarin, direct oral anticoagulants (DOACs), and antiplatelet drugs
- Drugs inhibiting platelet aggregation: β-lactam antibiotics, nitroprusside, nitroglycerin, nitric oxide, and selective serotonin reuptake inhibitors (SSRIs)

Vitamin K Deficiency

- Vitamin K is an essential fat-soluble vitamin required for carboxylation of factors II, VII, IX, and X and proteins C and S.
  - Present in dietary sources and synthesized by bacteria in the GI tract
- Risk factors: fasting, poor dietary intake, TPN, fat malabsorption, newborns who have yet to develop normal gut microbiota, and patients undergoing oral antibiotic therapy

Liver Disease

- The liver is a primary site of production of procoagulant factors: fibrinogen, prothrombin (factor II), factors V, VII, IX, X, XI, and XII, anticoagulants proteins C and S, and antithrombin.
- Severe liver disease impairs synthesis of factors producing platelet dysfunction, impeded clearance of activated clotting, and fibrinolytic proteins.
- Prolonged PT and possible prolongation of the aPTT do not reflect parallel decreases in anticoagulant factors and true bleeding risk.
- Thrombocytopenia results from platelet sequestration in the spleen; however, decreased plasma metalloprotease ADAMTS13 results in high levels of vWF promoting platelet aggregation.

- Many patients with balanced procoagulant and anticoagulant processes
  - However, balance can be disrupted, resulting in increased risk of bleeding or inappropriate clotting.

Renal Disease

- Chronic renal failure and uremia are associated with decreased platelet aggregation.
- Impaired platelet adhesion due to defects of glycoprotein IIb/IIIa

Disseminated Intravascular Coagulation

- Pathologic hemostatic response to tissue factor/factor VIIa complex leading to excessive activation of the extrinsic pathway
  - Natural anticoagulant mechanisms are overwhelmed, generating intravascular thrombin.
- Numerous precipitating factors including sepsis, trauma, amniotic fluid embolus, malignancy, or incompatible blood transfusions
- Presents as diffuse bleeding disorder with consumption of coagulation factors and platelets due to widespread microvascular thrombotic activity
- Labs: decreased platelet count, prolongation of PT, aPTT, thrombin time (TT), elevated fibrin and fibrin degradation products (D-dimers)

Cardiopulmonary Bypass–Associated Coagulopathy

- Initial priming results in hemodilution and thrombocytopenia, worsened by adhesion of platelets to bypass circuit.
- Induced hypothermia results in reduced platelet aggregation, decreased clotting factor production and enzymatic activity.
- Increased plasmin generation occurs during CPB, accelerating fibrinolysis.

Trauma-Induced Coagulopathy

- Commonly due to acidosis, hypothermia, and hemodilution as well as independent trauma-induced coagulopathy (TIC)
- Hypoperfusion stimulates activated protein C, which decreases thrombin.
- Tissue damage results in shedding of the endothelial glycocalyx, resulting in "autoheparinization."
- Impaired platelet responsiveness—"platelet exhaustion" from activation related to injured tissues

Treatment of Bleeding Disorders

von Willebrand Disease

- DDAVP (0.3 mcg/kg IV) releases vWF from endothelial cells and produces a near complete response in type 1 vWD.
- DDAVP is contraindicated in type 2B vWD because it may precipitate thrombocytopenia.
- Significant surgical bleeding can require use of plasma-derived vWF: factor VIII concentrate (Humate-P), recombinant vWF (Vonvendi), or cryoprecipitate.

Hemophilia

- Hematologist consultation recommended with administration of recombinant or purified factor VIII or factor IX concentrates.
- In severe hemophilia, alloantibodies to exogenous factors may form and require substitution of porcine factor VIII, administration of activated (FEIBA) or nonactivated prothrombin complex concentrates (PCCs), or treatment with recombinant factor VIIa (rFVIIa).

Disseminated Intravascular Coagulation

- Correction of precipitating underlying condition is essential.
- Supportive treatment with selective blood component transfusions as guided by coagulation studies
- Use of anticoagulation (heparin) is controversial, limited to conditions with high thrombotic risk.
- Antifibrinolytic therapy is generally contraindicated.

Platelet Disorders

- Platelet transfusions usually withheld in nonbleeding patients until count is $<10,000/\mu L$
- Repeat platelet transfusions increase the risk of antibody formation to human leukocyte antigens (HLA) or human platelet antigens.
  - Platelet alloimmunization may cause an inadequate increase in platelet counts with transfusion, and use of HLA-matched platelets may be required.
- Treatment of platelet dysfunction due to renal disease includes
  - DDAVP (0.3 mcg/kg IV)—stimulates release of vWF from endothelial cells
  - Conjugated estrogens (0.6 mg/kg IV for 5 days)—shortens bleeding times, possibly via decreased generation of nitric oxide
  - Transfusion of cryoprecipitate (rich in vWF and fibrinogen)—limited to patients with life-threatening bleeding due to risk of allogeneic blood products

PROTHROMBOTIC STATES

- Pathogenesis of thrombosis, the Virchow triad: blood stasis, endothelial injury, hypercoagulability

Inherited Thrombotic Disorders

Factor V Leiden and Prothrombin Gene Mutation

- Inheritable thrombotic predisposition is seen in up to 50% of patients with venous thromboembolism.

- Point mutations result in factor Va that is no longer susceptible to APC-mediated degradation, resulting in a prothrombotic state (factor V Leiden).
- Point mutations in prothrombin *G20210A* gene result in increased plasma concentrations of prothrombin, resulting in a hypercoagulable state.
- Homozygous mutations result in highest risk of developing DVTs, although the absolute risk of blood clots remains low in the absence of other hypercoagulable risk factors.

Protein C and Protein S Deficiency

- Protein C deficiency: autosomal dominant, affecting 1 in 500 in the general population
  - Deficiency in protein C results in venous thromboembolism (VTE), warfarin-induced skin necrosis, neonatal purpura (homozygous neonates), and fetal loss.
  - Acquired protein C deficiency is seen in DIC, liver disease, severe infection (meningococcemia), uremia, and vitamin K antagonist anticoagulation.
- Protein S deficiency: autosomal dominant, individuals are at increased risk of VTE and pulmonary embolism (PE)
  - Acquired protein S deficiency is associated with pregnancy, oral contraceptive use, DIC, human immunodeficiency virus (HIV) infection, nephrotic syndrome, and liver disease.

Acquired Thrombotic Disorders

Antiphospholipid Syndrome

- Acquired autoimmune disorder characterized by venous and/or arterial thromboses, recurrent pregnancy loss
- Associated with autoimmune disorders such as systemic lupus erythematosus or rheumatoid arthritis
- Catastrophic antiphospholipid syndrome (APS) is a severe form that results in coagulopathy, ischemic necrosis of the extremities, and multiorgan failure and is associated with a mortality rate of 30%.
- Labs: mild prolongation of aPTT and positive testing for antiphospholipid antibodies
- Patients with APS and prior thrombotic complication are at increased risk for recurrent thrombosis.

Heparin-Induced Thrombocytopenia

- Autoimmune-mediated drug reaction occurring in as many as 5% of patients receiving heparin therapy
- Presents with a mild to moderate thrombocytopenia resulting in platelet activation and increased risk of venous and arterial thromboses
- Heparin-induced thrombocytopenia (HIT) is mediated by IgG antibodies binding to platelet factor 4 (PF4).
- Risk factors: women, patients undergoing major surgical procedures and use of unfractionated heparin compared to low-molecular-weight heparin
- Clinically manifests as thrombocytopenia occurring 5 to 14 days after heparin initiation, although can be seen within 1 day with prior heparin exposure
- Confirmation of this clinical diagnosis includes HIT antibody testing with ELISA (most sensitive) followed by a serotonin release assay (SRA), which is more specific.

Treatment of Thrombotic Disorders

Inherited Thrombophilias

- Patients with VTE and positive testing for inherited thrombophilia are anticoagulated for their initial presentation; however, continuation of anticoagulation after resolution is determined by severity of presentation, presence of more than one thrombophilia, and homozygosity or heterozygosity for thrombophilia.
- Pregnant patients with known thrombophilia often are anticoagulated in the antepartum and postpartum setting.

Antiphospholipid Syndrome

- Patients with APS who experience a thrombotic complication are managed with life-long anticoagulation.
- Treatments include vitamin K antagonists, plus aspirin for patients with a history of arterial thrombosis.
- Pregnant patients with APS are often treated with low-molecular-weight heparin (LMWH) during the antepartum period.

Heparin-Induced Thrombocytopenia

- In suspected HIT, heparin is discontinued immediately.
- Alternative nonheparin anticoagulation (often a direct thrombin inhibitor—bivalirudin, lepirudin, argatroban) is administered as testing is performed due to risk of thrombosis.
- Initiation of warfarin alone is contraindicated for HIT because an initial decrease in synthesis of proteins C and S enhances a prothrombotic state.
- Platelet transfusions are not recommended unless platelets counts are <20,000/μL with signs of bleeding.
- If possible, avoidance of future heparin exposure is recommended.
  - Subsequent limited preioperative reexposure to heparin after laboratory testing to ensure an absence of PF4/heparin immune complexes is a strategy undergoing investigation.

LABORATORY EVALUATION OF HEMOSTASIS

Perioperative Bleeding Risk

- Carefully performed bleeding history remains the single most effective predictor of perioperative bleeding as well as a careful medication review relating to consumption of aspirin, nonsteroidal anti-inflammatory drugs, and supplements such as ginkgo and vitamin E.
- Standard coagulation tests used as screening are limited in their ability to reflect the in vivo hemostatic response.
- Preoperative coagulation screening tests may be indicated when planned surgery is associated with significant bleeding or in patients who are unable to provide an adequate bleeding history.
- Patients with <20% to 30% of normal coagulation factor activity or platelet counts of <50,000/μL are more likely than patients with normal values to have uncontrolled intraoperative bleeding.
- For active bleeding or surgical intervention, platelet transfusion is recommended to a goal of 50,000/μL or, in high-risk cases such as intracranial hemorrhage or neurosurgery, 100,000/μL.

Laboratory-Based Measures of Coagulation

Prothrombin Time

- Assesses the extrinsic and common pathways of plasma-mediated hemostasis
- Measures time (seconds) for fibrin clot formation to occur after mixing with tissue factor and calcium
- Sensitive to deficiencies in fibrinogen and factors II, V, VII, or X; used to monitor anticoagulation with vitamin K antagonists
- Most PT reagents contain heparin-binding chemicals; thus PT remains normal in the setting of heparin, LMWH, and fondaparinux.
- Reagent can vary; thus the international normalized ratio (INR) was introduced by the World Health Organization to normalize PT results among different laboratories.
- Prolongation of the PT should be assessed further with mixing studies.
  - Mixing patient's plasma sample with normal donor plasma results in a corrected time to clot formation in the case of a coagulation deficiency compared with presence of an inhibitor.

Activated Partial Thromboplastin Time

- Assesses the integrity of the intrinsic and common pathways of plasma-mediated hemostasis
- Measures time (seconds) for fibrin clot formation to occur after mixing with phospholipid, calcium, and an activator of the intrinsic pathway
- Detects low levels of prekallikrein, high molecular weight kininogen, factors XII, XI, IX, and VIII, as well as low levels of factors II, V, and X and fibrinogen. Most sensitive to deficiencies in factors VIII and IX
- Used to monitor unfractionated heparin and anticoagulation with parenteral direct thrombin inhibitors
- aPTT values cannot be compared between laboratories due to the lack of a reference standard.

Anti–Factor Xa Activity

- Increasingly used to monitor heparin anticoagulation instead of aPTT
- Patient plasma is combined with reagent factor Xa and an artificial substance that releases a colorimetric signal after factor Xa cleavage, thus providing a functional assessment of heparin anticoagulation effect.
- Unlike aPTT, the anti–factor Xa assay is not affected by coagulation factor deficiencies, factor inhibitors, or the presence of lupus anticoagulant when measuring heparin-bound antithrombin inhibition of factor Xa.
- Anti–factor Xa testing can also be used to measure the effect of other anticoagulants such as low-molecular-weight heparin, fondaparinux, and factor Xa inhibitors.

Thrombin Time

- Measures final step where fibrinogen is converted to fibrin
- Measures the time (seconds) for fibrin clot formation to occur after mixing sample with calcium and thrombin
- Conditions that prolong thrombin time: anticoagulant therapy, hypofibrinogenemia, dysfibrinogenemia, DIC, liver disease, high concentrations of serum proteins (multiple myeloma, amyloidosis), and circulating bovine thrombin antibodies

Fibrinogen Level

- Diluted plasma is exposed to thrombin. Time to fibrin clot formation is compared with a standard curve, and fibrinogen concentration is extrapolated.
- Immunologic fibrinogen assays are used when hypofibrinogenemia is found without an obvious clinical explanation.

Tests of Platelet Function

Platelet Count

- Determined as part of a complete blood count, performed by automated machines
- Artificially decreased platelet counts may be caused by platelet clumping or the presence of large platelets.
- Overestimated platelet counts may occur if samples contain cellular debris.

Bleeding Time

- First in vivo assay of platelet function
- A BP cuff is inflated on the upper arm with a standard 9-mm-long, 1-mm-deep incision on the forearm. Blood is blotted every 30 seconds until bleeding stops.
- A prolonged bleeding time of >11 minutes signifies either platelet dysfunction or thrombocytopenia.
- A normal bleeding time does not predict adequate hemostasis during surgery, nor does an abnormal bleeding time predict abnormal surgical bleeding; thus it is not recommended as a preoperative screening test.

Platelet Aggregometry

- Gold standard for assessment of platelet function
- Centrifugation of a sample creates platelet-rich plasma, which is added to a number of platelet agonists.
- The addition of platelet agonists stimulates platelet aggregation, resulting in a decrease in turbidity of the solution and an increase in light transmission.
- Patterns based on the kinetics and amplitude of response are associated with specific platelet disorders. Testing can also be used for monitoring antiplatelet therapy.

Point-of-Care Measures of Coagulation

Activated Clotting Time

- Activated clotting time (ACT) measures the time in seconds for formation of a clot after a contact activation initiator is added to a sample of freshly drawn whole blood.
- Fibrin clot formation is measured by way of intrinsic and common pathways; thus heparin and other anticoagulants prolong time to clot formation.
- Popular perioperative coagulation monitor during surgical cases requiring high doses of heparin due to simplicity, low cost, and linear response at high heparin concentrations

Viscoelastic Measures of Coagulation

- Measures the entire spectrum of clot formation in whole blood from early fibrin strand generation through clot retraction and fibrinolysis
- Thromboelastograph (TEG)—Whole blood is placed into a rotating cup with a sensor pin. As a clot begins to form, the pin meets increased resistance, which is translated through an electronic recorder.
- Rotational thromboelastometry (ROTEM)—Similar mechanism, with whole blood placed into a cup. However, the cup is stationary as the pin rotates.
- Variables derived from viscoelastic tracings do not correlate directly with laboratory-based tests of coagulation but do describe information on the extrinsic pathway, levels of fibrinogen, effects or presence of heparin, and resistance to lysis.
- Incorporation of viscoelastic testing in perioperative diagnostic algorithms to guide transfusion has been found to reduce overall blood product administration.

Platelet Function Analysis

- The point-of-care platelet function analyzer (PFA-100) passes citrated whole blood within a capillary tube under high shear stress.
  - Platelets begin to adhere to the membrane and form a plug, which closes the capillary aperture and is recorded as the closure time.
  - Prolonged closure times indicate platelet dysfunction but are not specific to a particular disorder.

ANTITHROMBOTIC AND PROCOAGULANT DRUGS

Antiplatelet Agents

Cyclooxygenase (COX) Inhibitors

- COX-1 maintains the integrity of the gastric lining and renal blood flow as well as initiates formation of thromboxane A_2 (TxA_2)—important for platelet aggregation and secretion
- COX-2 synthesizes prostaglandin mediators in pain and inflammation.
- Aspirin—irreversibly inhibits COX-1
  - COX-2 is 170 times less sensitive to aspirin than COX-1; only irreversibly inhibited by high doses
  - Platelets are unable to synthesize new COX-1 once the enzyme is inhibited, resulting in an inhibitory effect lasting 7 to 10 days.
  - Recovery of platelet function after aspirin requires generation of new platelets.
  - Megakaryocytes produce 10% to 12% of circulating platelets daily; near normal hemostasis expected in 2 to 3 days after the last dose of aspirin.
- NSAIDs—nonselective, reversible COX inhibitors
  - Platelet function returns to normal 3 days after discontinuation of the use of NSAIDs.
  - Selective COX-2 antagonists (celecoxib) were developed to provide pain relief without GI bleeding complications.
    - Clinical trials with selective COX-2 antagonists reported increased risks for cardiovascular complications.
    - Increased thrombotic risk thought to be caused by inhibition of prostacyclin (PGI_2) without inhibition of TxA_2

P2Y12 Receptor Antagonists

- Includes thienopyridines (e.g., clopidogrel, ticlopidine, prasugrel) and nucleoside analogs (e.g., ticagrelor and cangrelor)
  - Thienopyridines—prodrugs requiring hepatic metabolism, irreversibly inactivates ADP binding site

- Nucleoside analogs—reversible inhibitors that change conformation of the P2Y12 receptor
- Prevents binding of ADP by the P2Y12 receptor, which impairs platelet adhesion and aggregation by preventing the expression of GPIIb/IIIa on the surface of activated platelets.
- Clopidogrel—requires metabolism by *CYP2C19* for activation, causing a wide interindividual variability in inhibiting ADP-induced platelet function
  - Genetic polymorphism of *CYP2C19* and *ABCB1* is thought to affect the intestinal permeability and oral bioavailability.
  - FDA black box warning: Patients who are *CYP2C19* poor metabolizers (up to 14% of patients) are at greater risk of treatment failure, and genotype testing may be helpful.
- Ticagrelor—lower interindividual variability
  - Binds to a separate site on the P2Y12 receptor; both parent drug and metabolite have antiplatelet effects
  - Dosed twice daily
- Cangrelor—only P2Y12 inhibitor available for IV administration
  - Rapid onset/offset, with normalized platelet function within 60 minutes of discontinuation
  - May be helpful in bridging therapy for patients with drug-eluting stents who require surgery

GPIIb/IIIa Inhibitors

- Prevents platelet aggregation by decreasing the binding of fibrinogen and vWF to GPIIb/IIIa receptors on the surface of activated platelets
- Administered IV in order to limit ongoing arterial thrombosis or prevent formation of occlusive thrombi and restenosis in diseased vessels
- Abciximab—noncompetitive, irreversible inhibitor of GPIIb/IIIa
  - Inhibition continues at various levels for several days; platelet aggregation normalizes within 24 to 48 hours.
- Eptifibatide and tirofiban—competitive, reversible GPIIb/IIIa antagonists
  - Platelet aggregation returns to normal 8 hours after discontinuation.
- All medications of this class can cause thrombocytopenia, but the strongest effect is with abciximab.

Anticoagulants

Vitamin K Antagonists

- Warfarin—inhibits synthesis of factors II, VII, IX, and X and proteins C and S
- Long half-life (36 hours); complete anticoagulant effect takes 3 to 4 days due to long half-lives of preexisting coagulation factors
- During initiation, early reductions in anticoagulant protein C relative to other factors produces a hypercoagulable state and risk for thrombosis or warfarin-induced skin necrosis.
- Monitored using INR with goal of 2 to 3
  - Patients with mechanical heart valves require a higher INR goal of 2.5 to 3.5.
- Narrow therapeutic window affected by other medications, foods, alcohol
  - Also affected by genetic variations in cytochrome P450, *CYP2C9*

Unfractionated Heparin

- Mixture of different length polysaccharides with a high molecular weight
- Indirectly inhibits thrombin (factor IIa) and factor Xa by binding to antithrombin (AT)
- Short half-life, fully reversed with protamine
- Heparin resistance occurs due to hereditary insufficiency of AT or acquired insufficiency of AT from prolonged heparin administration.
  - Treatment with recombinant or plasma-derived AT concentrates
  - Plasma transfusions may also be used with increased risk of transfusion-associated circulatory overload (TACO) or other transfusion reactions.
- Monitored with aPTT or ACT
- Full-dose heparin for cardiac surgery: IV bolus of 300 to 400 U/kg
  - 1 mg protamine to 100 units of heparin is the reversal dose used at the conclusion of cardiopulmonary bypass.

Low-Molecular-Weight Heparin and Fondaparinux

- LMWH produced by cleaving unfractionated heparin into shorter fragments, resulting in greater indirect (AT-mediated) inhibition of factor Xa compared with direct thrombin (factor IIa) inhibition.
- Fondaparinux—synthetic pentasaccharide of the AT binding region of heparin selectively inhibits factor Xa at AT
- Both cannot be monitored using aPTT but can be monitored with anti–factor Xa activity levels
- Longer half-lives than heparin; can be administered subcutaneously
- Protamine is only partially effective in reversing LMWH and not effective for fondaparinux
- LMWH is contraindicated in patients with HIT.

Direct Thrombin Inhibitors

- Directly binds to thrombin, inhibiting free and fibrin-bound states
- Clinical effects monitored with aPTT or ACT.
- Hirudin—naturally occurring direct thrombin inhibitor (DTI) found in leeches

- Lepirudin—recombinant hirudin analog
- Argatroban, bivalirudin—synthetic agents
  - Argatroban—half-life of 45 minutes, preferred DTI in patients with renal insufficiency due to hepatic elimination
  - Bivalirudin—reversible DTI metabolized by plasma proteases and renally excreted
    - Often chosen in patients with both renal and hepatic dysfunction due to its short half-life of 25 minutes, but dose adjustment is required
- No reversal agents for DTI
- All DTIs interfere with INR, with argatroban having the greatest effect.

Direct Oral Anticoagulants

- Advantages over VKAs: more predictable pharmacokinetics and pharmacodynamics, fewer drug interactions
- Available reversal agents include idarucizumab and andexanet alfa—costly with limited availability
- Approved for prevention of venous thromboembolism after hip or knee replacement, treatment and secondary prevention of venous thromboembolism, prevention of stroke in nonvalvular atrial fibrillation
- Not approved for use in patients with mechanical heart valves, contraindicated in pregnancy
- Stroke prevention in atrial fibrillation—DOAC vs. warfarin
  - Decreased rates of stroke, intracranial hemorrhage and mortality. Similar rates of major bleeding events, increased GI bleeding
- Acute symptomatic VTE
  - DOACs have similar efficacy to VKAs with significantly decreased risk of major bleeding.
- DOACs divided into two broad categories by mechanism
  - Inhibition of thrombin
    - Dabigatran (Pradaxa)—first new oral antithrombotic agent approved for the prevention of ischemic stroke in patients with nonvalvular atrial fibrillation since warfarin
    - Predominantly eliminated by the kidney, dose reduction required with CrCl <30 mL/min
  - Inhibition of factor Xa—rivaroxaban (Xarelto), apixaban (Eliquis), edoxaban (Savaysa), and betrixaban (Bevyxxa)
    - Some renal clearance; however, apixaban is approved for use in patients with end-stage renal disease requiring hemodialysis
- Routine monitoring of DOAC therapy is not required due to predictable pharmacokinetics.
  - Testing for suspected overdose or need for urgent/emergent surgery:
    - Dabigatran: aPTT assay is nonlinear until dabigatran concentrations are quite high (>200 ng/mL)
      - Thrombin time is very sensitive—useful to detect the presence of the drug but unable to quantify the amount present
      - Dilute thrombin time or ecarin clotting time, which are both linear at clinically relevant dabigatran concentrations and are the tests of choice for monitoring
    - For direct Xa inhibitors: anti–factor Xa activity assays are best for monitoring but must be specifically calibrated for each drug

Thrombolytics

- Used to break up active blood clots, commonly used during acute myocardial infarctions, strokes, massive pulmonary embolism, arterial thromboembolism, and venous thrombosis
- Can be administered IV or directly to the site of blockage
- Mechanism: thrombolytics are serine proteases that convert plasminogen to plasmin
  - Plasmin degrades fibrinogen, fibrin, as well as cross-linked fibrin, generating fibrin-degradation products.
  - Fibrin-degradation products released include fragment X and D-dimer—both inhibit platelet aggregation
- Non–fibrin-specific agents
  - Streptokinase, produced by β-hemolytic streptococci
    - Can elicit an immune response due to bacterial protein structure
- Fibrin-specific agents
  - Recombinant tPA—alteplase, reteplase, and tenecteplase
  - May confer a lower risk of hemorrhagic complications by limiting lysis to the site of thrombosis, although data are conflicting
- Surgery or puncture of noncompressible vessels is contraindicated within a 10-day period after the use of thrombolytic drugs.

Procoagulant Drugs

Antifibrinolytics

- Lysine analogs—ε-aminocaproic acid (EACA), tranexamic acid (TXA)
  - Competitively inhibits the binding site on plasminogen, leading to inhibition of plasminogen activation as well as preventing plasminogen binding of fibrin
  - Likely equivalent efficacy, shown to decrease perioperative blood loss in cardiac surgery, liver transplantation, orthopedic surgery
  - No apparent risk of thrombosis but further studies necessary
  - Risk of high-dose TXA causing seizures in patients undergoing cardiac surgery

- Serine protease inhibitor—aprotinin
  - Removed from the US market due to concerns of renal and cardiovascular toxicity; available only in Europe and Canada
- Use of TXA in trauma patients studied in the Clinical Randomisation of an Antifibrinolytic in Significant Haemorrhage 2 (CRASH-2) trial
  - Associated with reduction in all-cause mortality
  - Reduction in risk of death due to bleeding; no increase in vascular occlusive events
  - Patients who received the drug after 3 hours experienced increased risk of death from bleeding
- World Maternal Antifibrinolytic Trial (WOMAN)
  - Administration of tranexamic acid reduced death due to bleeding in women with postpartum hemorrhage.
  - Greatest benefit if given within 3 hours of birth; no increase in adverse effects

Recombinant Factor VIIa

- Increases generation of thrombin via the intrinsic and extrinsic pathways to enhance hemostasis
- Short half-life of 2 to 2.5 hours; FDA approved for patients with hemophilia
- Increased off-label use in cardiac surgery, trauma, and liver transplantation
- Limited trials have shown decreased rates of blood transfusion; however, no significant improvement in mortality rates with increased rates of venous and arterial thromboses (including coronary events)
- Guidelines recommend that recombinant factor VIIa no longer be used for the off-label indications of prevention and treatment in bleeding in patients without hemophilia.

Prothrombin Complex Concentrate

- Purified formulations of varying amounts of vitamin K–dependent coagulation factors
  - Four-factor PCC (FEIBA) contains factor VII, while three-factor PCC does not.
  - Derived from human plasma but treated with viral reduction process reducing infectious and noninfectious transfusion reactions
- First-line treatment for emergent reversal of VKAs due to improved safety profile and small volume of administration compared with plasma

Fibrinogen Concentrate

- FDA approved for correction of congenital fibrinogen deficiency, but increasing use for correction of acquired hypofibrinogenemia
- Pooled from human plasma and subsequently undergoes viral inactivation steps
- Benefits over plasma/cryoprecipitate include a standardized fibrinogen content, low infusion volume, decreased infectious risk, and faster time to administration due to rapid reconstitution.
- Cryoprecipitate and plasma, however, are less costly and provide additional procoagulant factors.

PERIOPERATIVE MANAGEMENT OF ANTITHROMBOTIC THERAPY

Vitamin K Antagonists

- Recommendation to stop VKAs 5 days prior to surgery if low risk for thromboembolism with restart 12 to 24 hours postoperatively in the setting of adequate hemostasis
- Patients at high risk of thromboembolism should be bridged with unfractionated heparin (UFH) or LMWH.

Heparins

- For patients undergoing bridging, infusion should be stopped 4 to 6 hours prior to surgery and resumed without a bolus dose no sooner than 12 hours postoperatively.
- After surgery with high postoperative bleeding risk, resumption of UFH should be delayed 48 to 72 hours until adequate hemostasis has been achieved.
- For patients bridging with LMWH, the last dose should be administered 24 hours prior to surgery; dosing should be resumed 24 hours postoperatively in low bleeding risk surgery and delayed until 48 to 72 hours postoperatively for surgeries with high bleeding risk.

Antiplatelet Agents

- Low-dose aspirin (ASA) has been shown to reduce the risk of stroke and myocardial infarction by 25% to 30%, and continuation of perioperative ASA therapy may confer a significant reduction in myocardial infarction and other major cardiovascular events.
- Current recommendations are to continue ASA for patients who are at moderate to high risk for cardiovascular events requiring noncardiac surgery and to stop ASA 7 to 10 days prior to surgery for patients at low risk for cardiovascular events.
- Patients on dual antiplatelet therapy (DAPT) should discontinue clopidogrel 5 days prior to cardiac or noncardiac surgery.
- For patients with recent percutaneous coronary procedures, surgery should be delayed for 30 days after bare-metal stent placement and ideally up to 6 months after drug-eluting stent placement.
  - DAPT should be continued in these patients if surgery is required before this timeframe unless the risk of bleeding outweighs the risk of thrombosis.

Neuraxial Anesthesia and Anticoagulation

- Data from randomized controlled trials to guide the timing and management of antithrombotic therapy for neuraxial anesthesia are lacking, although the American Society of Regional Anesthesia and Pain Medicine (ASRA) and the European Society of Anaesthesiology (ESA) have published guidelines to assist in management, as noted in the table below.

Emergent Reversal of Anticoagulants

- VKA—four-factor PCC with concomitant administration of vitamin K
- DTI—no direct reversal agents but generally short half-lives, supportive care recommended
- DOACs
  - Idarucizumab—humanized antibody fragment that binds to dabigatran
    - FDA approved in 2015, complete reversal occurs in minutes
  - Andexdanet alfa was approved in 2018 for the emergent reversal of rivaroxaban or apixaban.

	Time Before Puncture/ Catheter Manipulation or Removal	Time After Puncture/ Catheter Manipulation or Removal	Laboratory Tests
UFHs (for prophylaxis, ≤ 15,000 IU/d)	4–6 h	1 h	Platelet count for treatment >5 d
UFHs (for treatment)	IV 4–6 h SQ 24 h	1 h 1 h	aPTT, ACT, platelet count
LMWH (for prophylaxis)	12 h	4 h	Platelet count for treatment >5 d
LMWH (for treatment)	24 h	4 h	Platelet count for treatment >5 d
Fondaparinux (for prophylaxis, 2.5 mg/d)	36–42 h	6–12 h	Anti–factor Xa, standardized for specific agent
Rivaroxaban	72 h	6 h	Anti–factor Xa, standardized for specific agent
Apixaban	72 h	6 h	Anti–factor Xa, standardized for specific agent
Dabigatran	5 d	6 h	dTT (dilute thrombin time)
Warfarin	5 d and INR ≤1.4	After catheter removal	INR
Argatroban	Contraindicated		
Acetylsalicylic acid	None	None	
Clopidogrel	7 d	After catheter removal	
Ticlopidine	10 d	After catheter removal	
Prasugrel	7–10 d	After catheter removal 6 h with loading dose	
Ticagrelor	5–7 d	After catheter removal 6 h with loading dose	
NSAIDs	None	None	

QUESTIONS

NORMAL HEMOSTASIS

1. Describe the process of primary and secondary hemostasis.
2. Platelets are actively involved in primary hemostasis by three main processes. Name each process described below.
   ___________ At the vascular endothelium, this occurs due to exposed extracellular matrix containing collagen, von Willebrand factor, and other glycoproteins.
   ___________ Secretion of alpha granules and dense bodies
   ___________ Recruitment of additional platelets to the site of injury

BLEEDING DISORDERS

3. Disseminated intravascular coagulation (DIC) may be precipitated by many underlying conditions. List common conditions associated with DIC in the categories below.

Category	Conditions
Infections	
Malignancy	
Obstetric causes	
Massive inflammation	
Toxic/immunologic	
Other	

4. Describe the coagulation abnormalities that occur in patients with severe liver disease.

PROTHROMBOTIC STATES

5. What clinical signs are associated with antiphospholipid syndrome?
6. What laboratory tests are used to diagnose heparin-induced thrombocytopenia?

LABORATORY EVALUATION OF HEMOSTASIS

7. In the preoperative setting, what are the first steps in determining a patient's perioperative bleeding risk?
8. What anticoagulation effects can be monitored by an anti-Xa assay? Are there advantages to using anti-Xa assays to monitor unfractionated heparin?

ANTITHROMBOTIC AND PROCOAGULANT DRUGS

9. What is the effect of aspirin on cyclooxygenase enzymes? What are the effects of NSAIDs?
10. What were the primary conclusions of the CRASH-2 and WOMAN trials of antifibrinolytic therapy?

PERIOPERATIVE MANAGEMENT OF ANTITHROMBOTIC THERAPY

11. Patients receiving antithrombotic medications typically require discontinuation prior to surgery to balance the risk of surgical bleeding with the risk of thromboembolism. Fill in the table below with appropriate timing of preprocedural medication discontinuation.

Antithrombotic Agent	Drug Name	When to Stop Before Procedure
Antiplatelet agents	ASA P2Y12 receptor antagonists GPIIb/IIIa antagonists	
Vitamin K antagonists	Warfarin	
Heparins	UFH	
	LMWH	
Pentasaccharide	Fondaparinux	
Direct thrombin Inhibitors	Argatroban Bivalirudin	
	Dabigatran	
Factor Xa inhibitors	Rivaroxaban Apixaban Edoxaban	

ANSWERS

NORMAL HEMOSTASIS

1. Primary hemostasis results from injury to vascular endothelium and subsequent platelet deposition at the injury site that forms a "platelet plug." Secondary hemostasis involves the formation of a more stable clot, which is reinforced by crosslinked fibrin. This is a complex process mediated by plasma clotting factors. (414)
2. Platelet actions during primary hemostasis include adhesion, activation, and aggregation.
   Adhesion—at the vascular endothelium, this occurs due to exposed extracellular matrix containing collagen, von Willebrand factor, and other glycoproteins. Under normal conditions the thrombogenic matrix is separated from circulating platelets, thus initiation of the platelet plug requires endothelial injury. Intact endothelial cells also possess antiplatelet and anticoagulant activity that inhibit clot formation.
   Activation—secretion of alpha granules and dense bodies. Interaction of platelets with collagen during the initial adhesion phase results in platelet activation. Platelets secrete thromboxane A_2 as well as their storage granules, which act to recruit and activate additional platelets.
   Aggregation—recruitment of additional platelets to the site of injury. Glycoprotein IIb/IIIa receptors on the surface of activated platelets have higher affinity for fibrinogen, promoting cross-linking and aggregation. (415–416)

BLEEDING DISORDERS

3. Common conditions associated with disseminated intravascular coagulation (DIC) are listed by category in the table below. (420–421)

Category	Conditions
Infections	Bacterial (gram-negative bacilli, gram-positive cocci) Viral (CMV, EBV, HIV, VZV, hepatitis) Fungal (histoplasma) Parasites (malaria)
Malignancy	Hematologic (AML) Solid tumors (prostate cancer, pancreatic cancer) Malignant tumors (mucin-secreting adenocarcinoma)
Obstetric causes	Amniotic fluid embolism Preeclampsia/eclampsia Placental abruption Acute fatty liver of pregnancy Intrauterine fetal demise
Massive inflammation	Severe trauma Burns Traumatic brain injury Crush injury Severe pancreatitis
Toxic/immunologic	Snake envenomation Massive transfusion ABO blood type incompatibility Graft versus host disease
Other	Liver disease/fulminant hepatic failure Vascular disease (aortic aneurysms, giant hemangiomas) Ventricular assist devices

4. Severe liver disease impairs the synthesis of procoagulant factors, including fibrinogen, prothrombin (factor II), factors V, VII, IX, X, and XII, and anticoagulants protein C, S, and antithrombin. Patients with portal hypertension also have thrombocytopenia from platelet sequestration in the spleen. Fibrinolysis can also be abnormal as certain inhibitors of fibrinolysis are decreased; however, other inhibitors are increased. Overall, patients have a reduction in both procoagulant and anticoagulant factors, putting them at risk for both bleeding and inappropriate clotting. (420).

PROTHROMBOTIC STATES

5. Antiphospholipid syndrome (APS) is an acquired autoimmune disorder characterized by both venous and arterial thromboses and pregnancy loss. A severe form, catastrophic APS, results in coagulopathy, ischemic necrosis of the extremities, multiorgan failure, and a significant mortality rate of 30%. (422–423)
6. Heparin-induced thrombocytopenia (HIT) is an autoimmune-mediated drug reaction which presents with a mild to moderate thrombocytopenia and increased risk of venous and arterial thromboses. HIT is a clinical diagnosis, but HIT antibody testing is used for confirmation. The first test used is the enzyme-linked immunosorbent assay (ELISA) which is sensitive but not specific. In patients with a positive ELISA test, the more specific serotonin release assay should be sent for confirmation. (423)

LABORATORY EVALUATION OF HEMOSTASIS

7. As bleeding history remains the most effective predictor of perioperative bleeding, risk assessment should begin with a thorough history of prior excessive bleeding after surgery, trauma, or childbirth. Oral surgery and dental extractions in particular serve as good tests of hemostasis due to increased fibrinolytic activity in mucus membranes. A thorough medication review related to a history of aspirin, NSAIDs, anticoagulants, and supplements should be performed. (423–424)
8. Anti–factor Xa testing can measure the anticoagulant effect of unfractionated heparin, low molecular weight heparin, fondaparinux, and factor Xa inhibitors. Use of anti-Xa monitoring for unfractionated heparin may be useful in patients with coagulation factor deficiencies, factor inhibitors, or presence of lupus anticoagulant, which influences the accuracy of aPTT. (425)

ANTITHROMBOTIC AND PROCOAGULANT DRUGS

9. Aspirin is an irreversible COX inhibitor. As COX-2 is less sensitive to aspirin than COX-1, the primary inhibition is of COX-1 only. Recovery of platelet function requires generation of new platelets because platelets are unable to synthesize new COX-1 once the enzyme is inhibited.

   There are two types of NSAIDs; the first are nonselective, reversible COX inhibitors. The second are selective COX-2 antagonists and primarily affect prostaglandin mediators in pain and inflammation without effect on platelet hemostasis. Platelet function after nonselective NSAID use will return to normal 3 days after discontinuation. (427–428)
10. Both trials studied the use of tranexamic acid (TXA) as an adjunct to reduce bleeding through a reduction in fibrinolysis. The CRASH-2 trial, which focused on trauma patients, showed an association with reduction in all-cause mortality and reduction in risk of death due to bleeding, with no increase in vascular occlusive events when TXA was administered within 3 hours. The WOMAN trial of TXA in women with postpartum hemorrhage showed a reduction in death due to bleeding with the greatest benefit if given within 3 hours of birth. (431)

PERIOPERATIVE MANAGEMENT OF ANTITHROMBOTIC THERAPY

11. The table below summarizes appropriate timing of preprocedural medication discontinuation. (434)

Antithrombotic Agent	Drug Name	When to Stop Before Procedure
Antiplatelet agents	ASA P2Y12 receptor antagonists GPIIb/IIIa antagonists	7 d 7–14 d 24–72 h
Vitamin K antagonists	Warfarin	2–5 d
Heparins	UFH	6 h
	LMWH	12–24 h
Pentasaccharide	Fondaparinux	3 d (prophylactic dosing)
Direct thrombin Inhibitors	Argatroban Bivalirudin	4–6 h 3h
	Dabigatran	2–4 d (longer if renal impairment)
Factor Xa inhibitors	Rivaroxaban Apixaban Edoxaban	2–3 d 2–3 d 2–3 d

Chapter

24 FLUID MANAGEMENT

Nathalia Mavignier and Matthieu Legrand

INTRODUCTION

- Fluid administration in the perioperative period has two essential goals.
  - Ensure adequate intravascular volume to maintain cardiac output and tissue perfusion
  - Prevent electrolyte and acid-base disturbances
- Major decisions in perioperative fluid management
  - Choosing the appropriate fluid
  - Deciding the appropriate timing and volume of fluid to be administered

PHYSIOLOGY OF FLUID BALANCE

- Approximately 60% of body weight is attributed to total body water, which can be divided into the following components noted in the figure below:
  - Intracellular component (~55%)
  - Extracellular components (~45%)
    - Intravascular fluid (~7.5%) and plasma fluid (~5.5%) are present within the vascular system.
    - Interstitial fluid (~20%) surrounds the cells.
- The distribution of extracellular fluid between the plasma and interstitial compartments affects the choice of fluids administered.
- Transcapillary fluid shifts are driven by competing Starling forces across the endothelial membrane.
  - Hydrostatic pressure
    - Physical force of fluids against endothelial barriers
    - Strongest driver of fluid movement
    - Capillary hydrostatic pressure (P_c) decreases relative to interstitial hydrostatic pressure (P_i) as fluid traverses a capillary bed.
  - Oncotic pressure
    - Osmotic pressure generated by the presence of proteins
    - Capillary oncotic pressure increases relative to interstitial oncotic pressure as fluid traverses a capillary bed.

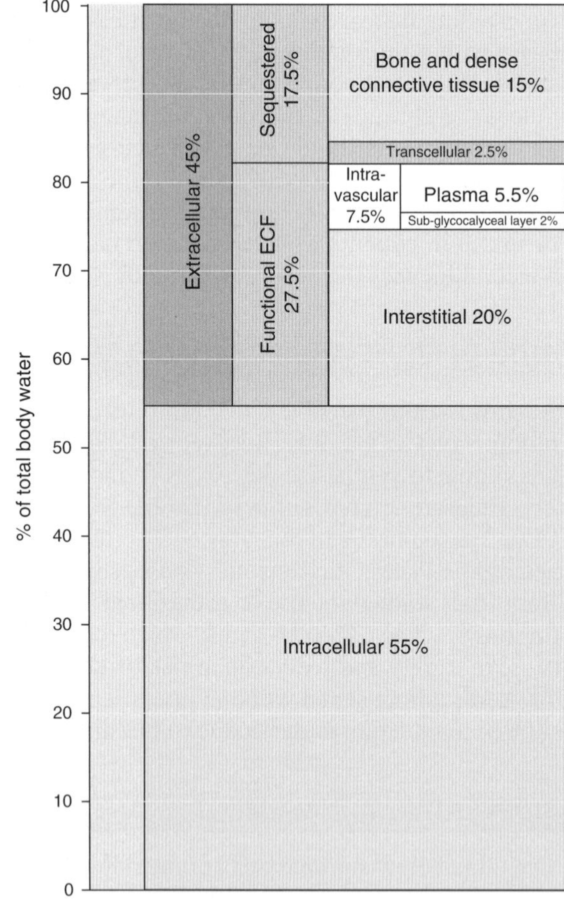

Distribution of Total Body Water. (From Edwards MR, Grocott MPW. Perioperative fluid and electrolyte therapy. In Gropper MA, et al, ed. Miller's Anesthesia. 8th ed. Philadelphia: Elsevier; 2015)

  - Endothelial permeability
    - The endothelium is coated by the glycocalyx, a thin gel-like layer that allows regulation of endothelial permeability.
    - The glycocalyx may be degraded by inflammation, trauma, and increased intravascular hydrostatic pressure.
- Electrolytes move freely across endothelial membranes.
  - Therefore electrolytes provide insignificant osmotic forces in transcapillary fluid equilibrium.

- However, electrolytes play a critical role in fluid shifts between the intracellular and extracellular compartments.
- The choice of replacement fluids can alter the relative electrolyte balances and water distribution between compartments.
- Knowledge of the normal fluid composition listed in the table below may inform fluid management decisions in an individual patient.

Electrolyte	Plasma Fluid (mEq/L)	Intracellular Fluid (mEq/L)	Extracellular Fluid (mEq/L)
Sodium	142	10	140
Potassium	4	150	4.5
Magnesium	2	40	2
Calcium	5	1	5
Chloride	103	103	117
Bicarbonate	25	7	28

FLUID REPLACEMENT SOLUTIONS

- Considering individual fluid compositions is required when choosing the appropriate replacement fluid.
- Osmolarity between the intracellular and extracellular compartment is maintained equally due to the osmotic forces.
- Tonicity of a solution will affect osmolar equilibrium via the movement of water.
  - Hypotonic fluids shift water toward the intracellular compartment.
  - Hypertonic fluids shift water toward the extracellular compartment.
  - Isotonic fluids produce no water shifts.

Crystalloids

- Crystalloid solutions are a mixture of electrolytes and water.
- Classification of crystalloids is based on two factors.
  - Composition
    - Balanced (electrolyte ratios similar to plasma), e.g., lactated Ringer's, Plasma-Lyte
    - Unbalanced, e.g., normal saline
  - Tonicity (hypo-, hyper-, or isotonic relative to plasma)
- Crystalloid solutions do not contribute to oncotic pressure because they diffuse out of the intravascular space shortly after administration.
- The distribution kinetics of crystalloids follows the balance of the extracellular compartment. Of the total crystalloid volume infused
  - 15%–20% will remain inside the vessels after 15–20 minutes.
  - 80%–85% will move to the interstitium (i.e., a ratio of 1:4, 1 part remaining intravascular to 4 parts moving intersitial).

Normal Saline

- Normal saline (0.9% NaCl) is a slightly *hypertonic* solution with supraphysiologic concentrations of sodium and chloride.
- Administration of normal saline can produce unwanted effects.
  - Hyperchloremic metabolic acidosis due to the decrease in the strong ion difference (SID) with saline administration
    - SID is the difference in charge between the strong cations (i.e., Na^+, K^+, Ca^{2+}, Mg^{2+}) and strong anions (i.e., Cl^-, lactate, ketoacids, sulfates).
    - The figure below illustrates Stewart's approach to acid-base equilibrium when a fluid such as normal saline (SID 0) is administered (normal plasma SID is 40).

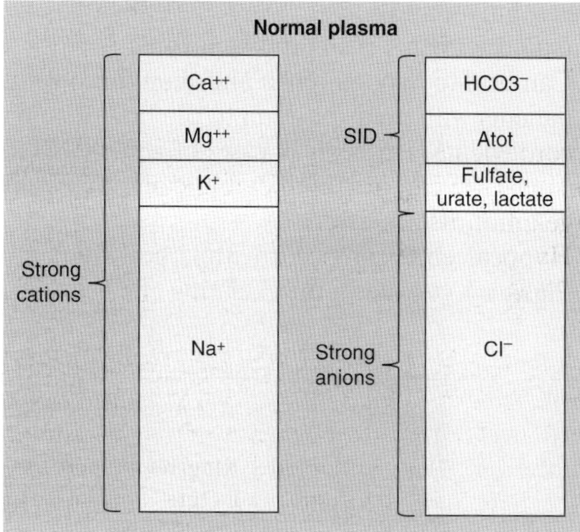

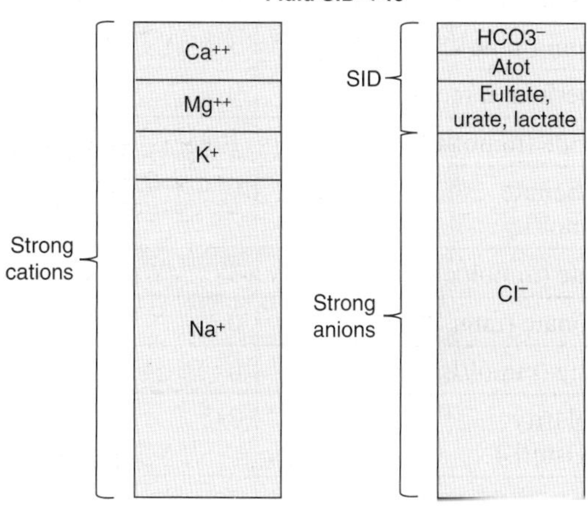

Stewart Approach to Acid-base Equilibrium. SID = strong ion difference. *Top,* normal plasma. Plasma SID is normally around 40. *Bottom,* SID <40, which can result after resuscitation with a solution that has SID <40.

- Increased plasma potassium concentration may occur with saline-induced metabolic acidosis.
- Risk of acute kidney injury (AKI) may increase.
    - Mechanism may be chloride-induced vasoconstriction of the glomerular afferent arterioles and potentially decreased renal blood flow.

Balanced Crystalloid Solutions

- Solutions (e.g., lactated Ringer's, Plasma-Lyte) whose composition tries to mimic the electrolyte balance of the plasma
- Most contain an anion buffer, such as lactate, acetate, and gluconate, to maintain the electroneutrality of the solution.
    - Metabolism of lactate, acetate, and gluconate leads to plasma release of bicarbonate, i.e., an alkalinizing effect.
    - As a result, lactated Ringer's and Plasma-Lyte have a higher SID (27 and 50, respectively).
- Balanced solutions are the fluid of choice when a large volume of fluids is required, e.g., in major surgeries, burns, and sepsis.
- Lactated Ringer's is slightly hypotonic.
    - Can lead to hyponatremia and should be avoided in patients with predisposition to cerebral or spinal cord edema, especially in cases of acute CNS injury
- Plasma-Lyte can lead to metabolic alkalosis when large amounts are given.
    - Hypocalcemia can occur with large-volume Plasma-Lyte due to the chelating effects of acetate.

Other Crystalloid Solutions

- Sodium bicarbonate administration can lead to metabolic alkalosis, hypocalcemia, and hypernatremia.
- Hypertonic saline (i.e., 3% NaCl) should be used only for intracranial hypertensive emergencies or patients with acute symptomatic hyponatremia.
    - The intravascular fluid shifts with hypertonic saline are temporary and come with risks of hypernatremia and peripheral vein thrombophlebitis.
- Dextrose 5% in water (D5W) is often used as a parenteral alternative to free water replacement.
    - The dextrose is immediately metabolized; the free water will then freely diffuse into the intracellular compartment.
    - Administration of D5W may lead to hyperglycemia and hyponatremia.
    - Clinical use of D5W includes the following conditions.
        - Correcting symptomatic hypernatremia (i.e., intracellular dehydration) in patients unable to receive enteral water
        - Prophylaxis of hypoglycemia (e.g., patients receiving insulin)
        - Prophylaxis of "ketosis fasting" in individuals who remain without enteral nutrition for a prolonged period (e.g., postoperatively)
- The following table lists the composition of commonly used replacement fluids.

	Normal saline	Ringer's lactate	Ringer's acetate-gluconate (PlasmaLyte)	Ringer's acetate-malate (Isofundine)	Hydroxyethyl starch 6% 130/0.4 (Voluven)	Gelatin (Gelofusine)	Albumin 4% (Albumex 4)
Sodium (mmol/L)	154	130	140	140	154	154	148
Potassium (mmol/L)	0	4	5	4			
Calcium (mmol/L)	0	3	0	2.5			
Magnesium (mmol/L)	0	0	3	1			
Chloride (mmol/L)	154	109	98	127	154	120	128
Bicarbonate (mmol/L)	0	0	0	0			
Lactate (mmol/L)	0	28	0	28			
Gluconate (mmol/L)	0	0	23	0			
Acetate (mmol/L)	0	0	27	24			
Osmolarity (mOsm/L)	308	275	294	304	308	274	250
SID	0	27	50	20	0	34	20

Composition of Common Replacement Fluids. Data from Heming N, Moine P, Coscas R, Annane D. Perioperative fluid management for major elective surgery. *Br J Surg*. 2020;107(2):e56-e62. doi:10.1002/bjs.11457, and Noritomi DT, Pereira AJ, Bugano DD, et al. Impact of Plasma-Lyte pH 7.4 on acid-base status and hemodynamics in a model of controlled hemorrhagic shock. *Clinics (Sao Paulo)*. 2011;66:1969–1974.

Colloids

- Colloid solutions contain water, electrolytes, and macromolecules such as albumin or synthetic starches.
- The macromolecules confer this type of solution with a high plasma oncotic pressure.
  - Colloid solutions can maintain the intravascular volume for longer than crystalloid solutions.
  - Smaller amounts of colloid solution are needed to maintain the same amount of intravascular volume compared to crystalloid solutions.
- However, the intravascular half-life of colloids may be less than expected in patients with increased vascular permeability.
- So far, use of colloids has not been shown to improve perioperative outcomes when used in surgical patients.
- Artificial colloids (e.g., hydroxyethyl starch [HES]) are associated with more complications (e.g., AKI, bleeding).

Albumin

- Albumin accounts for up to 50% of the total plasma protein content and up to 70%–80% of plasma oncotic pressure.
- Common concentrations of albumin as a resuscitation fluid include
  - 5% albumin (osmotic strength equal to that of normal plasma, around 20 mmHg), and
  - 25% albumin (often administered after large-volume paracentesis)
- The interstitial compartment contains the larger absolute amount of albumin—even though the concentration is lower than in plasma (most of albumin physiologically "leaks" into the interstitial compartment).
  - Infused albumin is able to move into the interstitial compartment.
  - Transfer is expected to be faster when the glycocalyx layer is degraded and vascular permeability increases.
- Summary of studies comparing albumin replacement to crystalloids in the patient with critical illness
  - Albumin did not demonstrate a mortality benefit compared to crystalloid in patients admitted to the intensive care unit.
  - An impact on outcome in patients with septic shock is possible but not definitive.
- In the surgical population, albumin has unknown potential benefits.
  - Unlike synthetic colloids, albumin has no effect on coagulation.
  - Since albumin is processed from human blood components, it may be unacceptable as a resuscitative fluid in some patients who are Jehovah's Witnesses.

Synthetic Colloids

- Synthetic colloids are made with synthetic large molecules built off a base of either starch, dextran, or gelatin.
- Hydroxyethyl starch
  - Can be identified by three numbers: concentration (%), molecular weight, and molar substitution (e.g., 6% HES 130/0.4)
  - Administration of HES can result in several complications.
    - Increased mortality and increased renal injury compared to use of crystalloids in critically ill patients
    - Increased risk of postoperative AKI, which makes the use of HES undesirable in the surgical population
    - Increased incidence of anaphylactoid reactions and pruritus
    - Reduction in circulating factor VIII and von Willebrand factors resulting in impaired platelet function
    - Development of coagulopathy among healthy volunteers, critically ill patients, and postsurgical patients
- Dextran
  - Water-soluble polymer of glucose synthesized by certain bacteria
  - Available in solutions with different molecular weights, e.g., 40 kDa (dextran 40) and 70 kDa (dextran 70)
  - The half-life is relatively long and varies according to molecular weight.
    - After 12 hours, about 30% of dextran 40 and 60% of dextran 70 remain intravascular.
  - Potential side effects of dextran solutions include anaphylactic and anaphylactoid reactions, increased bleeding times, and, rarely, noncardiogenic pulmonary edema.
  - There are no high-quality data on efficacy and safety.

HEMODYNAMIC MONITORING FOR FLUID RESPONSIVENESS

- Fluid responsiveness refers to the likelihood of an increase in stroke volume after an intravenous fluid bolus.
  - An increase in stroke volume or cardiac output by ≥10%–15% after a fluid challenge is indicative of fluid responsiveness.
- Surrogates of stroke volume include systolic pressure variation (SPV) and pulse pressure variation (PPV).
  - SPV and PPV can be easily measured with an intraarterial catheter during controlled mechanical ventilation.

- SPV values of >10 and PPV values of >10%–15% have been used to predict fluid responsiveness in controlled, mechanically ventilated patients in sinus rhythm who are not making spontaneous respiratory efforts.
  - Patient position and intrathoracic pressure also affect accuracy of SPV and PPV in predicting fluid responsiveness.
- The passive leg raise test has been shown to be informative in predicting fluid responsiveness in critically ill patients; however, surgical conditions may preclude its use.

- Central venous pressure (CVP) has been a consistently poor predictor of fluid responsiveness.

PERIOPERATIVE FLUID STRATEGIES FOR OPTIMAL VOLUME STATUS

- Optimal fluid management depends on the invasiveness and type of surgery as well as the individual patient's hemodynamic status.
  - Both too-restrictive and too-liberal fluid administration strategies have been associated with worse outcomes.
- Approaches to optimize intraoperative fluid therapy include the following aims.
  - Avoid fluid overload due to the risk of tissue and organ edema.
  - Avoid a restrictive fluid strategy than can lead to increased risk of AKI in major abdominal strategy.
- Goal-directed fluid therapy (GDFT) with cardiac output monitoring to titrate fluids and inotropes improves outcome after major noncardiac surgery.
  - This appears to be mostly driven by greater use of inotropes.
  - In GDFT, fluid is titrated to optimize stroke volume and cardiac output.
  - Use of GDFT algorithms have improved postoperative morbidity and decreased hospital lengths of stay, primarily in high-risk patients undergoing major abdominal surgery.
  - Inotropic agents may be added for persistently low cardiac output despite appropriate fluid challenges.

Perioperative Fluid Management Considerations

- Preference should be given to balanced crystalloid solutions over normal saline in the absence of known hyponatremia or hypochloremia.
- There are uncertainties regarding the potential benefits and risks of albumin despite a high cost.
- Hydroxyethyl starch solutions have been shown to be nephrotoxic, associated with bleeding, and should be avoided.
- While fluid overload should be avoided, restrictive fluid practices have been associated with a higher risk of AKI.
- Tailored fluid administration with hemodynamic monitoring should be considered to guide fluid responsiveness in high-risk patients undergoing major surgery.

QUESTIONS

PHYSIOLOGY OF FLUID BALANCE

1. What factors determine transcapillary fluid shifts?

FLUID REPLACEMENT SOLUTIONS

2. Do crystalloid solutions contribute to oncotic pressure? Why or why not?
3. What are the consequences of administering normal saline in large volumes?
4. Which perioperative settings are most appropriate for use of balanced crystalloid solutions?
5. What are the main indications for hypertonic saline administration? What are the risks?
6. What are the primary indications for intravenous dextrose solutions?
7. What are the clinical uses and potential side effects of hydroxyethyl starch (HES) solutions?

HEMODYNAMIC MONITORING FOR FLUID RESPONSIVENESS

8. What is the definition of "fluid responsive" after an intravenous fluid bolus?
9. What are the surrogate measurements of stroke volume most commonly used during surgery? What factors influence their accuracy?
10. What is the predictive value of central venous pressure (CVP) for fluid responsiveness?

PERIOPERATIVE FLUID STRATEGIES FOR OPTIMAL VOLUME STATUS

11. What are the risks associated with fluid overload in the perioperative period? What are the risks associated with a restrictive fluid strategy?
12. Describe in detail a liberal fluid strategy for adults undergoing major abdominal surgery.
13. What is goal-directed fluid therapy (GDFT), and how does it improve outcomes after major noncardiac surgery?

ANSWERS

PHYSIOLOGY OF FLUID BALANCE

1. Transcapillary fluid shifts are determined by competing Starling forces. Capillary hydrostatic forces (the strongest driver of fluid movement) decrease as plasma oncotic pressure increases across a capillary bed. (437)

FLUID REPLACEMENT SOLUTIONS

2. Crystalloid solutions do not contribute to oncotic pressure because they diffuse out of the intravascular space shortly after administration. (438)
3. The administration of normal saline in large volumes may lead to hyperchloremic metabolic acidosis and renal dysfunction. Furthermore, the acidosis may result in an increase of plasma potassium concentration. (438–439)
4. Balanced solutions are the fluid of choice when a large volume of fluids is required, such as occurs in major surgeries, burns, and sepsis. As described in the prior question, large-volume normal saline administration consistently produces a hyperchloremic metabolic acidosis and may cause AKI. (438–439)
5. Hypertonic saline should be used only for intracranial hypertensive emergencies or symptomatic patients with acute hyponatremia. The effects of intravascular fluid shifts may induce hypernatremia. Another potential risk is peripheral vein thrombophlebitis; hypertonic saline should be administered in a central vein if possible. (439–440)
6. Dextrose solutions are indicated to correct symptomatic hypernatremia (i.e., intracellular dehydration) in patients unable to receive enteral water. Other indications include prevention of hypoglycemia (e.g., patients with diabetes who receive insulin but who are not permitted oral carbohydrate intake) and of "ketosis fasting" in individuals who remain NPO postoperatively. (440)
7. Hydroxyethyl starch (HES) solutions are used for volume replacement and in the treatment of hypovolemia. However, administration of HES can be associated with acute kidney injury, anaphylactoid reactions, pruritus, and dilutional coagulopathies. The mechanism of coagulopathy also includes a reduction in circulating factor VIII and von Willebrand factors, and impaired platelet function. (441)

HEMODYNAMIC MONITORING FOR FLUID RESPONSIVENESS

8. Fluid responsiveness is defined as an increase in stroke volume or cardiac output by ≥10%–15% after an intravenous fluid bolus. (441)
9. Surrogate measurements of stroke volume include systolic pressure variation (SPV) and pulse pressure variation (PPV); both require an intraarterial catheter for measurement. Stroke volume can also be estimated with noninvasive devices analyzing pulse oximeter or arterial line waveforms. Conditions such as low tidal volume mechanical ventilation, right heart failure, irregular cardiac rhythm, and patient position changes can influence the accuracy of stroke volume estimation. Invasive measurement of stroke volume can be achieved using a pulmonary artery catheter. (441–442)
10. The predictive value of CVP for fluid responsiveness has been consistently poor. However, patients with very low CVP values (<5 mm Hg in mechanically ventilated patients) are more likely to be fluid responsive. (442)

PERIOPERATIVE FLUID STRATEGIES FOR OPTIMAL VOLUME STATUS

11. Fluid overload in the perioperative period can lead to tissue and organ edema, which can be detrimental to patient outcomes. On the other hand, a restrictive fluid strategy in the perioperative period can increase the risk of AKI, particularly in high-risk patients undergoing major abdominal surgery. (442)
12. A liberal fluid strategy for adults undergoing major abdominal surgery includes crystalloid administration of 10 mL/kg body weight during the induction of anesthesia, followed by a dose of 8 mL/kg/h until the end of surgery and adjusted based on hemodynamic status. (442)
13. GDFT involves using cardiac output monitoring to titrate fluids and inotropes to optimize stroke volume and cardiac output. GDFT has been shown to improve outcomes after major noncardiac surgery, largely driven by a higher use of inotropes. (442)

Chapter

25 BLOOD THERAPY

David Shimabukuro and Nicholas V. Mendez

INTRODUCTION

- Multiple transfusions can result in severe complications.
- *Lethal triad* of hypothermia, acidosis, and coagulopathy in trauma patients is a negative clinical indicator.
- High-volume transfusion (>10 units/24 hours of packed red blood cells [PRBCs]) is associated with increased mortality.
  - There is a 10% increase in mortality for every 10 units of blood given (i.e., if given 50 units of blood, the mortality rate is 50%).

BLOOD BANKING ESSENTIALS

Whole-Blood Processing

- Collected whole blood is separated into two components.
  - PRBCs
  - Platelet-rich plasma
- Platelet-rich plasma is further separated.
  - Platelets
  - Platelet-poor plasma (which is then frozen)
- Platelet-poor plasma has multiple uses.
  - Thawed for patient use
  - Further processed to cryoprecipitate
  - Further processed to factor-poor plasma
    - Used to make albumin, IVIG, etc.

Ensuring Donor-Recipient Compatibility

Blood Type

- Routine typing for presence or absence of major red blood cell (RBC) surface membrane antigen(s) (A, B, Rh)
- Anti-A, anti-B, and Rh antibodies
  - Capable of causing rapid intravascular destruction of RBCs
  - Formed by patients whose RBC membranes lack surface A, B, or Rh antigens
    - A and B antibodies occur naturally.
    - Rh antibodies are produced after exposure to the antigen.

Antibody Screen

- Identifies the presence of antibodies against common minor RBC surface antigens (e.g., Kell, Kidd, Fya, Fyb).
  - Recipient serum is added to wells containing known antigens.
  - Agglutination indicates presence of an antibody.

Crossmatch

- Donor RBCs are incubated with recipient plasma to detect incompatibility.
  - Rapid agglutination (5–10 minutes) indicates incompatibility of major blood type or MN, P, and/or Lewis antigens.
  - Slower agglutination (45–60 minutes) indicates incompatibility to minor surface antigens such as Kell and Kidd.
- *Type-specific blood* indicates that only the ABO-Rh type has been determined (takes <10 minutes).
- Electronic crossmatch (5–10 minutes) is possible in specific cases.

Patient Blood Types

- Blood type A: Patient's RBCs express the A antigen and produce anti-B antibodies.
- Blood type B: Patient's RBCs express the B antigen and produce anti-A antibodies.
- Blood type AB: Patients' RBCs express both A and B antigens.
- Blood type O: No antigens are expressed, but both anti-A and anti-B antibodies are produced.

Massive Transfusion/Emergency Release Protocols

- PRBC crossmatching before release depends on the urgency of need.
  - Prior to knowing patient's blood type (e.g., exsanguination from aortic rupture), universal donor is type O-negative.
    - O-positive blood is acceptable if the patient is not a woman of childbearing age.
    - Can switch to type-specific blood when available
  - If patient's blood type is known, transfuse type-specific, noncrossmatched blood (if available) or partially crossmatched (<10 minutes) if time allows.

- Plasma type AB-negative can be given to all individuals.
  - Transfuse type-specific plasma if available.
- Platelets blood type is irrelevant as it contains no RBCs and very little plasma.

Blood Storage

- PRBCs are stored at 1–6°C for up to 42 days.
  - Storage solutions contain phosphate, dextrose, and/or adenine.
  - Adenine allows resynthesis of adenosine triphosphate needed to fuel metabolic reactions and increases RBC survival.
  - Accepted storage time is for hemolysis <1% and 24 hours after transfusion to have 75% RBC viability.
- Fresh frozen plasma (FFP) and cryoprecipitate are stored at –20°C up to 1 year.
  - Once thawed, must be used within 24 hours (FFP) and 4 hours (cryoprecipitate)
- Platelets are stored at room temperature (20°C) for up to 5 days.
  - Continuously gently agitated to prevent clumping

BLOOD COMPONENTS

Packed Red Blood Cells

- Goal is to increase the oxygen-carrying capacity of blood to improve oxygen delivery to tissues.
- One PRBC unit is 200–250 mL with a hematocrit of 70%–80%.
  - Transfusion increases adult hemoglobin by approximately 1.0–1.5 g/dL.
- Solutions for coadministration
  - If hypotonic, may cause hemolysis
  - Containing calcium (e.g., lactated Ringer) can cause clotting in the transfusion line or blood filter.
- Decision to transfuse based on measured blood loss and oxygen-carrying capacity.
  - Acute blood loss of approximately 30% of adult patient's blood volume exceeds ability of crystalloid use alone.
  - Hypotension and tachycardia as signs can be blunted by compensatory vasoconstriction, anesthesia, and other drugs.
- PRBCs:FFP:platelet ratios are used in place of whole blood in patients with large blood loss.
  - 1.5 units PRBC to 1 unit FFP
  - 1 unit apheresis platelets (or 6 pooled platelet units) to 6 units PRBCs

Crystalloid and Colloid for Acute Blood Loss

- Does not improve oxygen-carrying capacity
- May cause coagulation defects from ongoing dilution
- Crystalloid volume given should be about 3 times the volume of blood loss
- Albumin remains in intravascular space longer than crystalloid (about 12 hours).

Fresh Frozen Plasma

- One FFP unit is 200–300 mL and contains all coagulation factors except platelets.
- Uses
  - Treatment of hemorrhage from presumed coagulation factor deficiencies
  - Intraoperatively if coagulation studies are at least 1.5 times longer than normal
  - In specific ratios with PRBCs in trauma patients
  - Urgent reversal of warfarin
  - Management of heparin resistance (FFP contains antithrombin III)

Cryoprecipitate

- The fraction of plasma that precipitates when FFP is thawed from –70°C
- Contains factor VIII, fibrinogen, fibronectin, von Willebrand factor, and factor XIII
- Uses
  - Treatment of hemophilia A (high concentration of factor VIII)
  - von Willebrand factor deficiency that is unresponsive to desmopressin
  - Hypofibrinogenemia (higher concentration than FFP)

Platelets

- Treats thrombocytopenia without infusion of unnecessary blood components
- Derived from single donors (apheresis platelets) or pooled from random-donor platelets
- Uses
  - Intraoperatively if the platelet count is less than 50,000–100,000 cells/mm^3 (depends on surgery location)
  - In specific ratios with PRBCs and FFP in trauma patients

PATIENT BLOOD MANAGEMENT AND THE DECISION TO TRANSFUSE RED BLOOD CELLS

Decision to Transfuse PRBCs

- Patient blood management and degree of preoperative anemia
- Monitoring of blood loss (e.g., suction canister, sponges)
- Assessment of ongoing or likelihood of future blood loss
- Monitoring for inadequate perfusion and oxygenation of vital organs
- Quantitation of all intravenous fluids given to patient
- Monitoring for transfusion indicators (e.g., laboratory data)

Patient Blood Management

- Based on three pillars
  - Optimization of RBC mass
  - Reduction of bleeding (e.g., controlled hypotension, antifibrinolytics)
  - Optimization of physiologic tolerance of anemia
- Preoperative preparation to reduce anemia (e.g., iron, recombinant human erythropoietin)
  - Higher presurgical hemoglobin reduces overall morbidity and mortality.
- Transfuse only at the appropriate time with the appropriate therapy.

Monitoring for Blood Loss

- Visualization and gravimetric measurements of blood in sponges, drapes, and suction canisters

Monitoring for Inadequate Perfusion and Oxygenation of Vital Organs

- Standard monitors include heart rate, noninvasive blood pressure, and oxygen saturation.
- Additional analysis includes arterial blood gases, mixed venous oxygen saturation, blood pH and lactate levels, and echocardiography.
  - Systolic pressure variation/pulse pressure variation can predict responsiveness to fluid bolus.
  - Appropriate urine output suggests adequate intravascular blood volume.
- Tachycardia is an insensitive and nonspecific indicator of hypovolemia.

Monitoring for Transfusion Indicators

- Decision to transfuse PRBCs
  - Laboratory data
  - The patient's ability to compensate for decreased oxygen-carrying capacity
    - Multiple factors are considered (e.g., history of cardiac disease, age).

Hemoglobin Values and the Decision to Transfuse

- Hemoglobin >10 g/dL—rarely requires a PRBC transfusion
- Hemoglobin <6 g/dL—almost always requires PRBC transfusion
- Hemoglobin 6 to 10 g/dL—depends on patient's risk for complications and the clinical scenario

COMPLICATIONS OF BLOOD THERAPY

Transmission of Infectious Diseases

- Infection risk is markedly low.
  - Routine donor blood testing reduces risk.
  - Low-incidence risks include hepatitis B, hepatitis C, HIV, HTLV-I/II, West Nile virus, Zika virus, malaria, Chagas disease, cytomegalovirus, and possibly Creutzfeldt-Jakob disease.
- Bacterial contamination
  - Most likely with platelet concentrates due to storage at room temperature
  - Transfusion-related sepsis can be fatal.
  - Suspect sepsis if fever develops within 6 hours of receiving platelet concentrates.

Noninfectious Hazards of Transfusion

Transfusion-Related Acute Lung Injury

- Acute lung injury that occurs within 6 hours of transfusion, particularly FFP
- Dyspnea and hypoxemia due to noncardiogenic pulmonary edema exclusive of other causes
  - Type 1: without preexisting acute respiratory distress syndrome (ARDS)
  - Type 2: preexisting ARDS within the previous 12 hours
- Treatment is to immediately stop the transfusion, provide supportive care, and notify blood bank.

Transfusion-Related Immunomodulation

- Lymphocyte function is suppressed by blood transfusions, particularly PRBCs.
  - Likely via arginase
- In the setting of surgical trauma may increase the risk of postoperative infection

Metabolic Abnormalities

Hydrogen Ions

- PRBCs have a high hydrogen ion concentration.
  - Due to preservatives and erythrocyte metabolic function
  - Stored blood pH is as low as 6.7.
- Contributes minimally to metabolic acidosis in recipients

Potassium

- Potassium concentration increases progressively during storage.
  - One unit of PRBCs contains about 5–6 mEq of potassium.
- Increased caution with large-volume transfusion in patients with compromised renal function

2,3-Diphosphoglycerate

- 2,3-diphosphoglycerate (DPG) concentration decreases progressively during storage.
  - Decreased 2,3-DPG increases the affinity of hemoglobin for oxygen, decreasing oxygen availability to tissues.
- The clinical significance is unclear.

Citrate

- Citrate is an anticoagulant that is metabolized to bicarbonate.
  - Metabolic alkalosis can occur in the hours after massive transfusion.
- Citrate binds calcium and can cause hypocalcemia.
  - Mobilization of calcium from bone and metabolism to bicarbonate limits this effect.
  - Risk is higher with rapid rate of transfusion (>50 mL/min), with hypothermia or liver disease, or in neonates.

Hypothermia

- Administration of cold blood products can decrease the patient's body temperature.
- Risks
  - May worsen coagulopathy
  - Associated with increased surgical site infections and poor wound healing
- Use of fluid warmers can mitigate risk of hypothermia.
  - Overheating of malfunctioning fluid warmers can cause hemolysis.

Coagulopathy

- Clinically represented by excessive microvascular bleeding
  - Separate from inadequate surgical control of bleeding
  - Laboratory tests can confirm the presence and type of coagulopathy.

Considerations for Transfusion in the Presence of Coagulopathy
▪ Platelets – Platelet count is less than 50,000 cells/mm³. – Qualitative platelet defect exists (e.g., antiplatelet drugs). ▪ FFP – INR is greater than 1.5. – Prothrombin time is longer than 1.5 times normal. – More than one blood volume is lost (about 70 mL/kg). ▪ Cryoprecipitate or fibrinogen concentrate – Fibrinogen level is less than 100 mg/dL. ▪ Desmopressin or topical hemostatic agent (e.g., fibrin glue) – Useful for excessive bleeding ▪ Recombinant activated factor VII or vitamin K four-factor prothrombin complex concentrate – Last-resort "rescue" when standard therapy has failed – Risks inducing thromboembolic complications

Transfusion Reactions

Febrile Reactions

- Occurs in 0.5% to 1% of transfusions
- Likely caused by recipient antibodies reacting to antigens on donor leukocytes or platelets
  - Most PRBCs are leuko-reduced at the time of separation to decrease risk.
- Usually mild with body temperature rarely rising above 38°C
  - Treat by slowing the rate of transfusion and administering antipyretics.
- Severe reactions with chills and shivering may require discontinuing the transfusion.

Allergic Reactions

- Presents with urticaria, pruritus, and increased body temperature
- Treat with intravenous antihistamines; discontinue the transfusion in severe cases.

Hemolytic Reactions

- Results from incompatible blood transfusion
- Pathophysiology
  - Complement system is activated.
  - Intravascular hemolysis and spontaneous hemorrhage occur.
  - Free hemoglobin becomes detectable in plasma and urine.
- Signs
  - Hypotension, lumbar and substernal pain, fever, chills, dyspnea, and skin flushing
    - All except hypotension can be masked by anesthesia.
  - Can progress to acute renal failure and disseminated intravascular coagulation
- Treatment
  - Immediate discontinuation of the transfusion
  - Maintenance of urine output by crystalloid resuscitation and administration of mannitol or furosemide
  - Administration of sodium bicarbonate and corticosteroids is of unproven value.

AUTOLOGOUS BLOOD TRANSFUSIONS

Predeposited Autologous Donation

- For elective surgery that may require blood transfusion
- Patient must have a minimum hemoglobin 11 g/dL to be eligible.

Predepositing Autologous Blood
▪ Donation of 10.5 mL/kg of blood approximately every 5–7 days ▪ Maximum donation is 2–3 units. ▪ Last unit is collected ≥72 hours before surgery. ▪ Oral iron supplementation is recommended. ▪ Recombinant erythropoietin increases donation volume by 25% but is very expensive.

Intraoperative Blood Salvage

- RBCs are collected during surgery, then washed and returned to the patient.
- Infection or malignancy at the operative site is considered a relative contraindication.
- Complications include dilutional coagulopathy, reinfusion of heparin anticoagulant, and hemolysis.

Normovolemic Hemodilution

- A prespecified volume of the patient's blood is removed intraoperatively before surgical blood loss.
  - Crystalloid or colloid is infused to maintain intravascular volume.
- Hemodilution of the hematocrit to 27%–33% results in fewer RBCs lost per 1 mL of surgical blood loss.
- The whole blood with higher hematocrit and greater clotting ability is reinfused after surgery.

QUESTIONS

BLOOD BANKING ESSENTIALS

1. What tests are performed during a type and screen?
2. How is a crossmatch performed, and what does it determine?
3. What blood type(s) can be used during an emergency if the patient's blood type is unknown?
4. What is type-specific blood?

BLOOD COMPONENTS

5. What is the hematocrit of a unit of PRBCs? How much will a patient's hemoglobin concentration increase after a transfusion of 1 unit?
6. What is FFP, and what are indications for FFP transfusion perioperatively?
7. What is cryoprecipitate, and what are indications for its administration?
8. What are the different platelet preparations, and what are indications for a platelet transfusion?

PATIENT BLOOD MANAGEMENT AND THE DECISION TO TRANSFUSE RED BLOOD CELLS

9. What factors should be considered when deciding whether to transfuse a patient with a unit of PRBCs?
10. Describe the methods to assess for adequate organ perfusion and tissue oxygenation.

COMPLICATIONS OF BLOOD THERAPY

11. Transfusion of which blood component carries the highest risk of infection? Why?
12. What is transfusion-related acute lung injury (TRALI), and how does it present?
13. What metabolic abnormalities should be anticipated when transfusing a large volume of PRBCs?
14. How does a febrile transfusion reaction present, and how is it treated?
15. How does an allergic transfusion reaction present, and how is it treated?
16. What causes a hemolytic transfusion reaction? How does it present, and how is it treated?
17. What are the potential implications for the changes in concentration of 2,3-diphosphoglycerate (2,3-DPG) in PRBCs during storage? How might this be mitigated?

AUTOLOGOUS BLOOD TRANSFUSIONS

18. What constraints must be considered when predepositing blood prior to elective surgery?
19. What are some relative contraindications to the use of intraoperative blood salvage?
20. What are the rationale and potential advantages of the normovolemic hemodilution technique?

ANSWERS

BLOOD BANKING ESSENTIALS

1. Blood typing refers to the laboratory process of determining the presence or absence of major surface antigen(s) on the membranes of recipient RBCs, namely A, B, and Rh. Antibody screening identifies the presence of antibodies in the recipient's serum against common minor RBC surface antigens. The antibody screen is performed by combining the recipient's serum with known RBC surface antigens, and the presence of agglutination indicates that an antibody of clinical significance is likely present. (446–447)
2. A crossmatch is performed when donor RBCs from the unit to be transfused are incubated with plasma from the intended recipient. Agglutination occurs if the crossmatch is incompatible based on either major or minor RBC surface antigens. The entire crossmatch process can take up to 60 minutes and should always be performed before the transfusion of blood, if possible. (447)
3. O-negative is the blood type of choice during emergency circumstances in which the patient's blood type is unknown. Because O-negative blood lacks the A, B, and Rh major antigens, it will not be hemolyzed by anti-A or anti-B antibodies should they be present. Alternatively, O-positive blood is considered acceptable in adult patients except for circumstances in which the recipient is a woman of childbearing age. If plasma is needed, AB-negative plasma can be given to all individuals. The blood type of platelets is irrelevant as it contains no RBCs and very little plasma. (447)
4. Type-specific blood indicates that only the major blood typing has been performed to determine the ABO-Rh compatibility, which typically takes less than 10 minutes. Type-specific blood has not been assessed for minor RBC surface antigen compatibility. (447)

BLOOD COMPONENTS

5. A single unit of PRBCs has a hematocrit of 70%–80% and a volume of about 200–250 mL. Typically, a single-unit transfusion will raise an adult patient's hemoglobin concentration by approximately 1.0 g/dL. (448)
6. FFP is the fluid portion of whole blood that is frozen within six hours of donation. It contains all coagulation factors except for platelets. FFP transfusion may be indicated perioperatively if coagulation studies (e.g., PT/INR) are at least 1.5 times longer than normal in the setting of bleeding, or in specific ratios with PRBCs in trauma patients. FFP may also be indicated for urgent reversal of warfarin or in the management of heparin resistance because FFP contains antithrombin III. (449)
7. Cryoprecipitate is the fraction of plasma that precipitates when FFP is thawed. It contains factor VIII, fibrinogen, fibronectin, von Willebrand factor, and factor XIII. Cryoprecipitate is indicated in the treatment of hemophilia A, von Willebrand factor deficiency, and hypofibrinogenemia. (449)
8. Platelets are prepared either in pooled form arising from platelet concentrates from donated whole blood (termed "random-donor platelets") or from a single donor (termed "apheresis platelets"). A platelet transfusion may be indicated perioperatively to treat thrombocytopenia if the platelet count is less than 50,000–100,000 cells/mm^3 depending on the surgery being performed. Platelets may also be indicated in specific ratios with PRBCs and FFP in trauma patients. (449)

PATIENT BLOOD MANAGEMENT AND THE DECISION TO TRANSFUSE RED BLOOD CELLS

9. The decision to transfuse a patient with a unit of PRBCs is a clinical decision based on the overall risk versus benefit analysis after weighing several patient-specific factors. The pillars of patient blood management and the degree of preoperative anemia should be evaluated. The quantity of blood lost (e.g., in suction canisters, etc.) as well as the likelihood of future loss should be considered. Signs of inadequate organ perfusion should be sought and laboratory data collected to support the decision as time permits. (449–450)
10. Adequate organ perfusion and tissue oxygenation can be evaluated using standard monitors in combination with laboratory studies such as arterial blood gases, mixed venous oxygen saturation, and lactate levels. Invasive monitors can provide systolic pressure variation or pulse pressure variation to indicate fluid

responsiveness. Monitoring of urine output may be valuable as appropriate urine output suggests adequate intravascular volume. Additional studies such as echocardiography may also prove useful when available. Tachycardia and hypotension alone are not sensitive or specific indicators of hypovolemia. (450)

COMPLICATIONS OF BLOOD THERAPY

11. Transfusion of platelets, particularly platelet concentrates, carries the highest risk of bacterial contamination because they are stored at room temperature. As such, bacterial contamination of platelets is one of the leading causes of transfusion-related mortality. Sepsis should be suspected in any patient who develops a fever within 6 hours of receiving platelet concentrates. (452)
12. Transfusion-related acute lung injury (TRALI) is the development of noncardiogenic pulmonary edema within six hours of receiving a transfusion of a blood product component, particularly FFP. It can be further divided into TRALI type 1, which occurs without a preexisting acute respiratory distress syndrome (ARDS), and type 2, which occurs in the setting of preexisting ARDS within the previous 12 hours. TRALI presents with the acute onset of dyspnea and arterial hypoxemia. (452)
13. Some of the metabolic disturbances that should be considered in the setting of a high-volume transfusion include metabolic alkalosis, hypocalcemia, and hyperkalemia. While the metabolic function of RBCs increases the hydrogen ion concentration of PRBCs, it contributes minimally to the acid-base status of the patient. On the other hand, the anticoagulant preservative citrate is metabolized to bicarbonate and could result in a metabolic alkalosis in the hours following massive transfusion. Citrate also binds calcium and could cause hypocalcemia, particularly in neonates, patients receiving rapid large-volume transfusion, and patients with hypothermia or liver disease. PRBCs also contain an increased potassium concentration with increasing storage duration, with one unit of PRBCs containing about 5–6 mEq of potassium. Thus PRBC transfusion, especially with multiple units, could contribute to development of hyperkalemia. (452–453)
14. Febrile transfusion reactions present with a mild fever, with temperatures rarely rising above 38°C. It is thought to occur as a result of recipient antibodies interacting with antigens on donor leukocytes. Currently, most donated blood is leuko-reduced, thereby decreasing the likelihood of febrile reactions. Febrile transfusion reactions are treated with antipyretics and by slowing the rate of transfusion, although the transfusion should be discontinued if the fever is severe or is accompanied by chills and/or shivering. (453–454)
15. Allergic transfusion reactions usually present with urticaria, pruritis, and fever. Treatment of allergic transfusion reactions includes administration of antihistamines and discontinuation of the transfusion if the reaction is severe. (454)
16. A hemolytic transfusion reaction occurs when blood product from a donor of an incompatible blood type is transfused into the patient, resulting in activation of the complement system, intravascular hemolysis, and the development of spontaneous hemorrhage. Hemolytic transfusion reactions present with hypotension, lumbar and substernal pain, fever, chills, dyspnea, and skin flushing and may progress to acute renal failure and disseminated intravascular coagulation. Laboratory analysis will reveal free hemoglobin in the plasma and/or urine. Treatment of a hemolytic transfusion reaction involves the immediate discontinuation of the transfusion and maintenance of urine output with use of crystalloids, mannitol, and/or furosemide. Other supportive care should be provided as indicated and the reaction should be reported to the blood bank immediately. (454)
17. Increasing storage time of PRBCs is associated with progressively decreased concentrations of 2,3-DPG. This decreased concentration results in increased affinity of hemoglobin for oxygen (decreased P_{50} values), thereby making less oxygen available for tissue oxygenation. It is suspected that donated blood with shorter storage times, and higher 2,3-DPG levels, may provide better tissue oxygenation per unit transfused. However, the clinical significance of this observation remains controversial. (452)

AUTOLOGOUS BLOOD TRANSFUSIONS

18. Predeposited blood must be donated at least 72 hours before surgery to allow sufficient time for the restoration of plasma volume. The patient must also have a minimum hemoglobin concentration of 11 g/dL prior to donation. The maximum quantity of predeposited blood is 2–3 units. To reach this amount, the patient can donate a maximum of 10.5 mL/kg every 5–7 days. (454)

19. The presence of infection or malignancy at the surgical site is considered a relative contraindication for the use of intraoperative blood cell salvage. (454)
20. The goal of normovolemic hemodilution is to remove a portion of the patient's blood volume early intraoperatively and replace it with either crystalloid or colloid such that euvolemia is maintained. The end goal is a hematocrit of 27%–33%, resulting in fewer RBCs lost per 1 mL of surgical blood loss. Following surgery, the patient's blood that was removed earlier is reinfused. In addition to the loss of fewer patient RBCs, further potential advantages include the return of the patient's own whole blood, which has a higher hematocrit and therefore greater oxygen-carrying capacity. Additionally, whole blood has a greater clotting ability because it contains the endogenous coagulation factors and platelets. (454)

Chapter

26 CARDIOVASCULAR DISEASE

Grace C. McCarthy

INTRODUCTION

- Cardiovascular disease is the leading cause of global death.
  - Leading cause of death in the United States
  - Influences the risk of perioperative mortality

CORONARY ARTERY DISEASE

- Presence of coronary artery disease (CAD) may be associated with increased morbidity and mortality after noncardiac surgery.
- Routine preoperative cardiac evaluation
  - History of angina or anginal equivalents
    - Men—most common symptom is shortness of breath with exertion
    - Women—most common symptom is fatigue
    - 70% of ischemic episodes are not associated with angina
    - Up to 15% of acute myocardial infarctions are silent
    - Other relevant history: recent myocardial infarction, heart failure, aortic stenosis, medical therapy for cardiovascular disease
  - Risk factors for CAD
    - Family history of CAD (esp. age <50)
    - Physical inactivity
    - Obesity
    - Unhealthy diet high in saturated fat, trans fat, and cholesterol
    - Tobacco use
  - Exercise tolerance/functional capacity
    - Ability to walk up one flight of stairs without chest pain or shortness of breath (approximately 4 METs)
    - Moderate exercise tolerance (>4 METS) without anginal symptoms predicts low risk of cardiac complications.
  - Physical exam with focus on cardiac and respiratory findings
  - Electrocardiogram (ECG)
    - Additional cardiac testing ordered based on acuity and risk of surgery, patient history, physical exam, and exercise tolerance

Prior Myocardial Infarction

- Incidence of myocardial reinfarction (MI) in the perioperative period is related to time elapsed since previous MI
- Elective surgery should be delayed for 2 to 6 months after an MI.
  - No fewer than 60 days should elapse before noncardiac surgery.
  - Risk of perioperative repeat MI stabilizes at 5% to 6% after 6 months.
  - Risk remains elevated for up to 1 year.
- Most perioperative repeat MIs occur in the first 48 to 72 hours postoperatively.
- Coronary revascularization by stenting (percutaneous coronary intervention [PCI]) or coronary artery bypass grafting (CABG)
  - Can reduce the risk of noncardiac surgery after a prior MI
  - Routine PCI is not recommended by American College of Cardiology (ACC)/American Heart Association (AHA) outside of current clinical practice guidelines.
- Following PCI, elective noncardiac surgery should be delayed based on the need for dual antiplatelet therapy.
  - 14 days following balloon angioplasty
  - 30 days following bare-metal stent placement
  - 6 months following drug-eluting stent placement
- Coronary angiography is not routinely recommended for preoperative evaluation.

Perioperative Risk Reduction Therapy/ Medications

- Statin and β-blocker therapies
  - Continuation has been shown to reduce adverse outcomes after surgery.
- Angiotensin-converting enzyme (ACE) inhibitors and angiotensin-receptor blockers (ARBs)
  - Holding perioperatively may reduce the incidence of intraoperative hypotension.

- Platelet inhibitors for *recently* placed intracoronary stents
  - High risk of stent thrombosis and death when discontinued for surgery
  - Antiplatelet treatment should be individualized based on the patient's risk of stent thrombosis versus surgical bleeding risk.

Monitoring

- Electrocardiogram (ECG)
  - Five-lead ECG allows noninvasive monitoring for myocardial ischemia.
    - Use in patients with known or suspected CAD
  - Myocardial ischemia (demand ischemia)
    - Can manifest as ST-segment depression of at least 1 mm from baseline
  - Precordial V_5 lead
    - Most sensitive for detecting ST-segment changes characteristic of ischemia
  - Lead II
    - Most sensitive for detection of arrhythmias
- Invasive arterial blood pressure monitoring
  - May speed identification and treatment of hemodynamic changes
  - Allows for continuous measurement of stroke volume variation (SVV) and pulse pressure (PPV) variation
    - Helps predict fluid responsiveness
- Transesophageal echocardiogram (TEE)
  - Most sensitive indicator of myocardial ischemia
  - Use is reserved for selected high-risk patients.
  - Can assess response to intravenous fluid replacement and inotropic drugs on left ventricular function and cardiac output
  - Allows assessment of regional wall motion, global ventricular function, intravascular fluid volume, and associated ventricular filling
- Pulmonary artery catheter (PAC)
  - Data do not support the routine use of PACs.
  - Use is reserved for selected high-risk patients.
  - Can monitor response to intravenous fluid replacement and inotropic drugs on cardiac output

Management of Anesthesia

- Judiciously treat preoperative anxiety.
- Consider preinduction intraarterial catheter to monitor blood pressure in high-risk patients.
- Maintain heart rate and systemic arterial blood pressure within 20% of awake values.
- Avoid tachycardia and maintain hemodynamic stability.
- Avoid hypothermia.
- Continue intensive monitoring into the postoperative period for high-risk patients.

Myocardial Ischemia Detection and Management

- Use a five-lead ECG to monitor for myocardial ischemia.
- ST-elevation MI (STEMI) results from complete and prolonged occlusion of a coronary blood vessel.
  - >1-mm ST elevation in two contiguous leads on ECG
- Non-STEMI (NSTEMI) may present as ST depressions, T-wave inversions, or transient ST elevations.
  - Type 1 NSTEMI—due to atherosclerotic plaque rupture and thrombosis
  - Type 2 NSTEMI—due to myocardial oxygen supply and demand imbalance
- Tachycardia is the most common cause of oxygen supply-demand imbalance.
  - Treat tachycardia if present at the time of ischemia.
- Ensure adequate oxygenation and ventilation.
- Evaluate and treat causes of hypotension.
- Treat anemia.
- Ensure appropriate pain control.

VALVULAR HEART DISEASE

Mitral Stenosis

- Hallmark: mechanical obstruction of left ventricular diastolic filling
- Commonly due to fusion of mitral valve leaflets from rheumatic heart disease
- Increased left atrial and pulmonary venous pressure
  - Eventually results in increased pulmonary vascular resistance
- Predisposes to atrial fibrillation

Management of Anesthesia

- Avoid tachycardia and maintain sinus rhythm.
- Maintain systemic vascular resistance to maintain diastolic coronary perfusion.
- Avoid arterial hypoxemia, hypoventilation, or hypercarbia.
  - May exacerbate pulmonary hypertension and precipitate right ventricular failure
- Increased circulatory volume may lead to flash pulmonary edema and hypoxemia.

Mitral Regurgitation

- Hallmark: left atrial volume overload and decreased left ventricular forward stroke volume
- Causes include mitral valve prolapse, chronic hypertension, ischemia leading to left ventricular dilation or papillary muscle dysfunction, rheumatic heart disease, and infective endocarditis.

Management of Anesthesia

- Maintain sinus rhythm with normal or slightly elevated heart rate (80 to 100 bpm).
- Maintain DBP.

- Systemic vascular resistance (SVR) management
  - Mild decrease in SVR will improve forward flow.
  - Sudden increases in SVR may worsen mitral regurgitation.

Aortic Stenosis

- Hallmark: increased left ventricular systolic pressure with compensatory increase in left ventricular wall thickness and myocardial oxygen demand plus reduced coronary blood flow
- Causes include progressive calcification of congenitally abnormal (bicuspid) valve or calcification of normal (tricuspid) valve with age, and rheumatic fever
- May present with angina, heart failure, or syncope
- Increased risk of sudden death

Management of Anesthesia

- Maintain sinus rhythm with normal to slightly decreased heart rate (60 to 90 bpm).
- Avoid hypotension.
  - Maintain SVR to provide adequate diastolic coronary perfusion.
- Maintain intravascular volume status.
  - Left ventricular hypertrophy, reduced intracavitary volume, and associated diastolic dysfunction contribute to challenges.

Management of Anesthesia in Patients With Aortic Stenosis

- A cardiac defibrillator should be immediately available.
  - External cardiac compressions are unlikely to generate an adequate stroke volume across a severely stenosed aortic valve.
- Continuous arterial blood pressure monitoring is highly recommended.
  - Dependent on the procedure and the severity of aortic stenosis
- Avoid hypotension and maintain afterload for coronary perfusion.
- Maintain sinus rhythm and avoid extremes of heart rate.
- Maintain intravascular fluid volume.

Aortic Regurgitation

- Hallmark: decreased forward left ventricular stroke volume with decreased coronary blood flow
- Acute regurgitation
  - Most often due to infective endocarditis, trauma, or aortic dissection
- Chronic regurgitation
  - Usually due to rheumatic fever

Management of Anesthesia

- Maintain sinus rhythm with normal or slightly elevated heart rate (80 to 100 bpm).
- Maintain diastolic blood pressure.
- SVR management
  - Mild decrease in SVR will improve forward flow.
  - Sudden increases in SVR may worsen aortic regurgitation.

DISTURBANCES OF CARDIAC CONDUCTION AND RHYTHM

- ECG
  - Primary tool for diagnosis of cardiac conduction and rhythm
- Ambulatory ECG (Holter) monitoring
  - Useful to document intermittent and/or symptomatic dysrhythmias
  - Can document efficacy of antidysrhythmic therapy

Heart Block

- Classified by site of conduction block relative to atrioventricular (AV) node
  - Block above AV node usually benign and transient
  - Block below AV node more likely to be progressive and permanent
- Need for treatment depends on multiple factors.
  - Degree of heart block
  - Site of conduction abnormality
  - Presence of symptoms

Cardiac Implantable Electronic Devices (CIEDs)

- Increasing number of patient with CIEDs
  - Permanent pacemakers (transvenous or leadless)
  - Biventricular pacemakers
  - Implantable cardioverter-defibrillators (ICDs)
- Preoperative evaluation
  - Determine type of device (pacemaker and/or ICD).
  - Reason for implantation
  - Dependency on device
  - Brand/model/magnet mode settings
  - Last interrogation and device battery life
- Electromagnetic interference (EMI) most common with monopolar electrocautery above the umbilicus
- If pacemaker dependent and at high risk of EMI, place a magnet on the device or reprogram prior to procedure.
- For ICDs likely to sense EMI as a shockable rhythm, disable tachyarrhythmia detection with magnet placement or reprogram prior to procedure, as noted in the figure below.

Perioperative management of transvenous pacemakers/ICDs

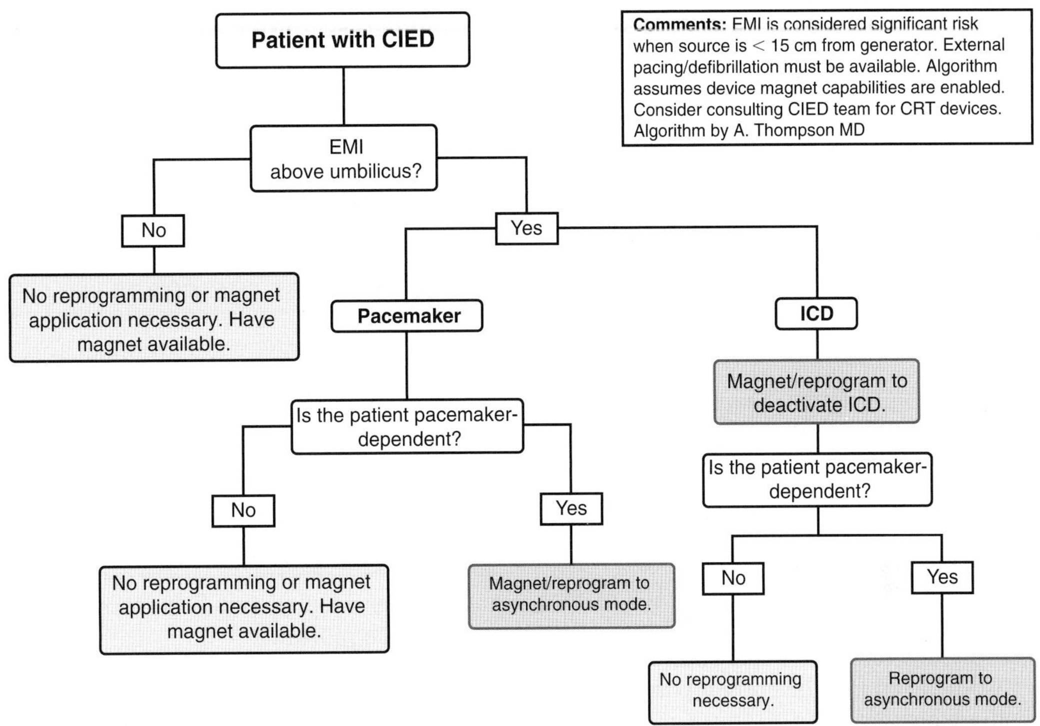

HEART FAILURE

- Hallmark: cardiac dysfunction (systolic, diastolic, or both) characterized by pulmonary and/or systemic venous congestion, and/or inadequate peripheral oxygen delivery
- Determinants of severity
  - Ejection fraction
  - Symptoms of heart failure
  - Limitations of physical activity
- Guideline-directed management and therapy (GDMT) used to evaluate and direct treatment
- Heart failure should be treated and optimized prior to elective surgery.

Management of Anesthesia

- Careful preload and afterload management to optimize cardiac output
- Consider regional anesthesia for peripheral or minor surgery.
- Minimize hemodynamic effects of general anesthesia.
  - Consider additional monitoring (arterial catheter, CVP, PA, TEE) based on patient physiology and invasiveness of surgical procedure.

HYPERTROPHIC CARDIOMYOPATHY

- Hallmark: left ventricular outflow tract obstruction (LVOTO) due to asymmetric hypertrophy of the basal interventricular septum and systolic anterior motion (SAM) of the anterior mitral leaflet
- May be inherited in an autosomal dominant fashion
- Increased risk of sudden death

Management of Anesthesia

- Goal is to decrease pressure across LV outflow tract.
  - Decrease myocardial contractility and heart rate.
    - β-Adrenergic blockade
  - Increase preload.
    - IV fluids
  - Increase afterload.
    - Phenylephrine, vasopressin
- Maintain sinus rhythm.
  - Atrial contraction needed to maintain cardiac output
  - ICD if patient has malignant arrhythmias
- Surgical procedures to treat LVOTO
  - Septal myectomy
  - Septal ablation

PULMONARY HYPERTENSION

- Hallmark: increased pulmonary artery pressure and pulmonary vascular resistance (PVR), which increases right heart afterload, resulting in right ventricular hypertrophy and dilation
- Defined as mean pulmonary arterial pressure greater than 20 mmHg

- Increased risk of perioperative morbidity and mortality
- Evaluation and optimization should occur prior to elective surgery.

Management of Anesthesia

- Goal is to avoid increases in PVR and resulting right heart failure.
  - Minimize sympathetic stimulation from anxiety, stress, pain, and inflammation.
  - Avoid hypoxemia, hypercapnia, acidosis, hypothermia, hypervolemia.
- Avoid hypotension.
  - Abrupt decreases in SVR may lead to decreased coronary perfusion and worsening right heart failure.
- For patients with severe pulmonary hypertension
  - Continuous arterial pressure monitoring helpful for hemodynamic management
  - Monitoring CVP or PA pressure, or TEE may be helpful, depending on stress of surgery.
  - Additional therapy (e.g., inotropic support, pulmonary vasodilators) may be chosen based on patient hemodynamics.

Challenges in Diagnosis of Pulmonary Hypertension

- Pulmonary hypertension is often silent and difficult to diagnose.
  - Diagnosis often delayed because symptoms can be nonspecific: dyspnea with exertion, fatigue, chest pain, and palpitations
  - Clinical symptoms often signal advanced disease.
- An elevated right ventricular systolic pressure (RVSP) >40 mmHg should prompt further evaluation for pulmonary hypertension.

CARDIAC TAMPONADE

- Hallmark: increased pericardial pressure leading to decreased diastolic filling of the ventricles, decreased stroke volume, decreased systemic arterial blood pressure
  - Compensatory tachycardia and increased systemic vascular resistance
- Pulsus paradoxus: fall of systolic blood pressure >10 mmHg during inspiration
- Risk of hemodynamic collapse and cardiogenic shock unresponsive to fluids and inotropes
- Primary therapy is pericardial drainage.

Management of Anesthesia

- Maintain myocardial contractility, arterial blood pressure, increased heart rate, and venous return.
- Avoid events/drugs that could decrease cardiac output.
- Continuous infusion of vasopressors may be necessary to maintain cardiac output and arterial blood pressure prior to pericardial drainage.
- Avoid positive pressure ventilation with significant cardiac tamponade; maintain spontaneous ventilation until drainage is imminent.

ANEURYSMS OF THE AORTA

- Most often involve the abdominal aorta
  - May involve any part of the thoracic or abdominal aorta
- Elective repair often recommended for aneurysms >5 cm to avoid spontaneous rupture.

Management of Anesthesia

- Consider prophylactic β-blocker and statin therapy to reduce mortality.
- Endovascular versus open repair of aneurysm dictates anesthetic needs.
  - Endovascular repair less invasive, may only require regional anesthesia
  - Open repair is a major procedure.
    - Requires general anesthesia
    - Invasive monitoring of arterial blood pressure
    - Consider epidural analgesia for postoperative pain.
    - Consider continuous cardiac output monitoring.

CARDIOPULMONARY BYPASS

- Cardiopulmonary bypass (CPB) provides a bloodless and motionless surgical field.
  - Allows detailed repair of the heart and great vessels
  - Supplies oxygenated blood to all organs
- CPB circuit
  - Venous reservoir
  - Arterial pump
  - Heat exchanger
  - Oxygenator
- Cannulas
  - Venous cannula
  - Arterial cannula
  - Cardiac vent cannula
  - Coronary sinus cannula
  - Cardioplegia/root vent cannula
  - Cardiotomy suckers
- Steps for initiation of CPB
  - Heparinization
  - Arterial cannulation

        - Aortic cannulation once ACT reaches appropriate duration
    - Venous cannulation
        - Right atrium or venae cavae cannulated
- Blood gas management strategies during CPB
    - Alpha stat
        - Temperature uncorrected
        - Cerebral autoregulation maintained
    - pH stat
        - Temperature corrected
        - To maintain normal pH, CO_2 is added to the CPB circuit.
        - Cerebral autoregulation uncoupled
- Steps for discontinuation of CPB
    - Rewarming
    - Deairing
        - Removal of intracardiac air via deairing cannula
    - Heart rate and rhythm
        - May require pacing if heart rate low or if heart block present
    - Drips
        - Vasopressors and/or inotropes may be necessary to separate from CPB.
    - Gas (anesthesia)
        - Restart general anesthetic.
    - Oxygen
        - Ensure appropriate oxygen flow.
    - Ventilation
        - Ensure the mechanical ventilator is on.

QUESTIONS

CORONARY ARTERY DISEASE

1. What percentage of adult patients undergoing surgery have, or are at risk for, coronary artery disease?
2. What is the most common symptom of angina in men and women?
3. What percentage of myocardial ischemic episodes are silent (not associated with angina pectoris)? What percentage of myocardial infarctions are silent?
4. What is the best indicator of a patient's cardiac reserve?
5. What determines whether a patient needs additional cardiac testing prior to surgery?
6. Is tachycardia or hypertension more likely to result in myocardial ischemia in a patient with coronary artery disease? What is the physiologic rationale?
7. How long should elective surgery be delayed after a prior myocardial infarction?
8. How long should elective noncardiac surgery be delayed following percutaneous coronary intervention (PCI)? Complete the following table:

Type of PCI	Recommended Duration of Dual Antiplatelet Therapy

9. Complete the following table, which indicates the electrocardiogram leads that are most likely to reflect myocardial ischemia in specific myocardial territories.

Electrocardigram (ECG) Leads	Coronary Artery Responsible for Myocardial Ischemia	Area of Myocardium That May Be Involved
II, III, aVF		
V_3-V_5		
I, aVL		

10. How should anesthesia be induced in patients at risk for myocardial ischemia?
11. What are some factors that influence the intensity of intraoperative monitoring by the anesthesia provider?
12. Why is hypothermia potentially dangerous for patients with coronary artery disease?

VALVULAR HEART DISEASE

13. Why are patients with mitral stenosis at an increased risk for atrial fibrillation and thrombus formation in the left atrium?
14. Why might patients with aortic stenosis have angina pectoris despite the absence of coronary artery disease?
15. Outline the hemodynamic goals and anesthetic considerations for patients with the following valvular heart diseases:

Valvular Disease	Cardiac Rhythm	Heart Rate	SVR	Volume/ Preload	Contractility
Mitral stenosis (MS)					
Mitral regurgitation (MR)					
Aortic stenosis (AS)					
Aortic regurgitation (AR)					

DISTURBANCES OF CARDIAC CONDUCTION AND RHYTHM

16. Identify the following cardiac rhythm abnormalities and list potential treatment options:

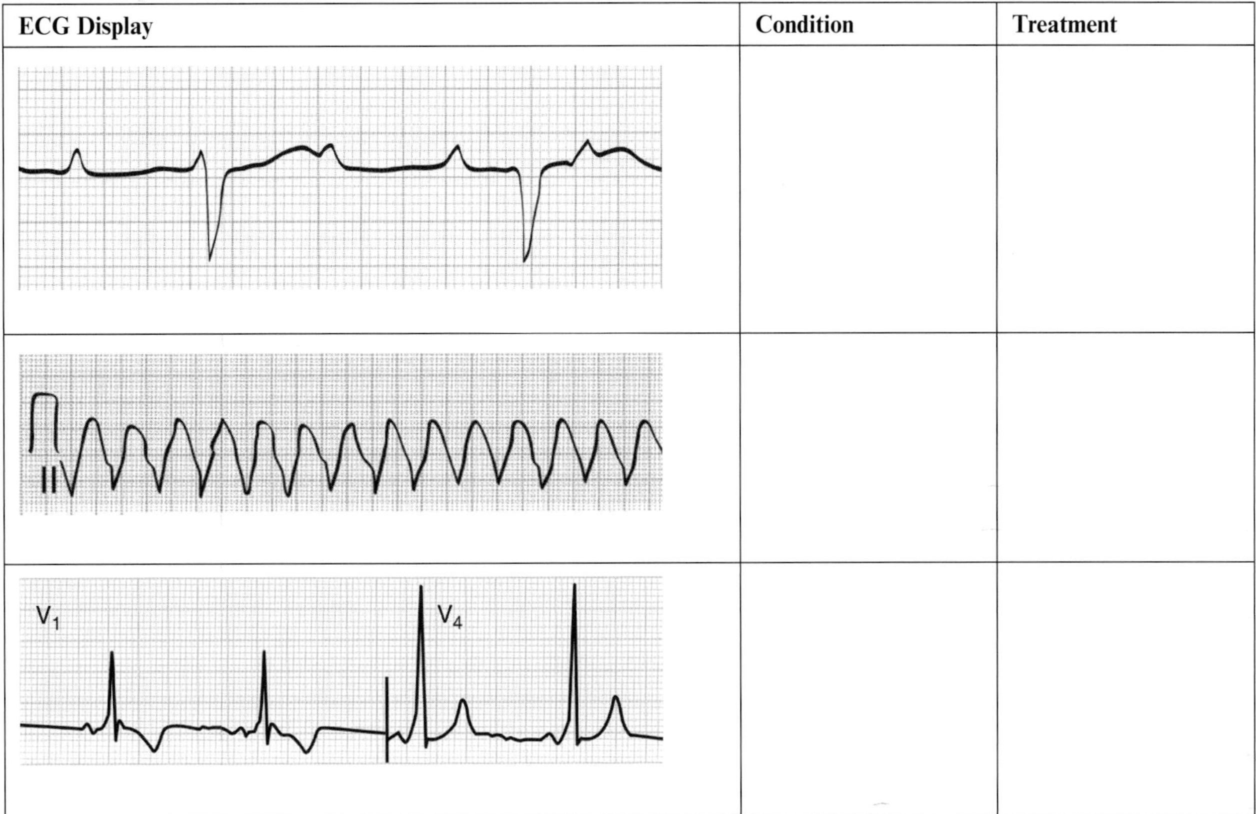

ECG Display	Condition	Treatment

17. For a patient with a known cardiac implantable electronic device (CIED), what should be determined about the device during the preoperative evaluation?
18. What is chronic resynchronization therapy (CRT), and what is the main indication?
19. How does electromagnetic interference (EMI) affect CIED function?
20. When should a CIED be reprogrammed prior to a procedure versus just placing a magnet on the device?

HEART FAILURE

21. What is the correlation between heart failure and postoperative morbidity?
22. How does positive-pressure ventilation of the lungs affect patients in heart failure?
23. Is regional anesthesia an appropriate option for patients with heart failure undergoing peripheral surgery?

HYPERTROPHIC CARDIOMYOPATHY

24. How are patients with hypertrophic cardiomyopathy (HCM) likely to present?
25. Outline the hemodynamic goals and anesthetic considerations for patients with HCM:

Cardiac Rhythm	Heart Rate	Preload	Afterload	Contractility

PULMONARY HYPERTENSION

26. What is the correlation between pulmonary hypertension and perioperative morbidity and mortality?
27. What is the goal of anesthetic management of patients with pulmonary hypertension?

28. Complete the following table by filling in each drug/agent's effect on pulmonary vascular resistance (PVR):

Drug/Agent	Effect on PVR (↑, ↓, or ↔)
Propofol	
Etomidate	
Ketamine	
Volatile anesthetics	
Nitrous oxide	
Midazolam	
Fentanyl	
Nitric oxide	
Milrinone	

CARDIAC TAMPONADE

29. Describe the physiology of cardiac tamponade.
30. What are some manifestations of cardiac tamponade?
31. What are some temporizing measures for patients with cardiac tamponade awaiting definitive treatment?

ANEURYSMS OF THE AORTA

32. What is the goal of anesthetic management of patients undergoing resection of an abdominal aortic aneurysm?
33. Which anesthetic techniques could be used for endovascular versus open repair of abdominal aortic aneurysms?

CARDIOPULMONARY BYPASS

34. How is blood drained from the vena cavae and returned to the arterial system during cardiopulmonary bypass?
35. Why is heparinization of the patient's blood necessary during cardiopulmonary bypass?
36. When is protamine administered, and what are some possible side effects of protamine administration?

ANSWERS

CORONARY ARTERY DISEASE

1. Approximately 40% of adult patients undergoing surgery have, or are at risk for, coronary artery disease. (459)
2. Angina or chest pain is not the most common anginal symptom in men and women. The most common anginal symptom in men is shortness of breath with exertion. The most common anginal symptom in women is fatigue. (459)
3. Approximately 70% of myocardial ischemic episodes are not associated with angina pectoris, and myocardial infarctions are not associated with angina pectoris approximately 15% of the time. (460)
4. The best indicator of a patient's cardiac reserve is their exercise tolerance/functional capacity. A limited exercise tolerance in the absence of significant pulmonary disease is a sign of a decrease in a patient's cardiac reserve. Alternatively, the cardiac reserve of a patient who can climb two or three flights of stairs (>4 METS) without stopping is likely adequate. Walking on level ground is a poor indicator of cardiac reserve (~2 METS). Shortness of breath with climbing one to two flights of stairs may indicate significant cardiac disease. The ability to achieve a moderate level of activity (>4 METS) without anginal symptoms predicts a low risk of perioperative complications. (460)
5. Assessment of functional capacity should help direct preoperative testing and treatment decisions, taking into account the patient's risk for CAD and the acuity and risk of surgery. For low-risk surgeries, oftentimes no additional cardiac assessment is needed prior to surgery. For patients and surgeries that carry a higher risk of perioperative major adverse cardiac events (MACE), if a patient's functional capacity is moderate or greater (≥4 METS), no additional cardiac testing is recommended. If a patient's functional capacity is poor (<4 METS) or unknown and further cardiac testing will impact decision-making or perioperative care, then pharmacologic stress testing can be considered. (460, 461)
6. Tachycardia is more likely than hypertension to result in myocardial ischemia in a patient with CAD. Tachycardia results in an increased myocardial oxygen requirement combined with a decreased myocardial perfusion time. Myocardial perfusion to the left ventricle, and thus myocardial oxygen supply, occurs during diastole. Hypertension leads to an increased myocardial oxygen requirement but also simultaneously increases myocardial perfusion. (460)
7. According to the 2014 ACC/AHA guidelines for perioperative cardiac evaluation prior to noncardiac surgery, no fewer than 60 days should elapse between recent MI and noncardiac surgery. Though significant risk reduction occurs by 60 days post-MI, the risk of reinfarction remains elevated for up to 1 year following an MI. The exact duration of the suggested delay is unclear and should be evaluated on a case-by-case basis with cardiology input as needed. (460)
8. Elective noncardiac surgery after PCI should be delayed based on the need for dual antiplatelet therapy, as noted in the table below. (460)

Type of PCI	Recommended Duration of Dual Antiplatelet Therapy
Balloon angioplasty	14 days
Bare-metal stent placement	30 days
Drug-eluting stent placement	6 months

9. The ECG leads correspond to myocardial location and can suggest the areas of myocardium that may be ischemic, as highlighted in the table below. (462)

Electrocardiogram (ECG) Leads	Coronary Artery Responsible for Myocardial Ischemia	Area of Myocardium That May Be Involved
II, III, aVF	Right coronary artery	Right atrium Sinus node Atriventricular node Right ventricle
V_3–V_5	Left anterior descending coronary artery	Anterolateral aspect of the left ventricle
I, aVL	Circumflex coronary artery	Lateral aspect of the left ventricle

10. For patients at risk of myocardial ischemia, care must be taken to achieve a smooth, hemodynamically stable induction. Patients already receiving statins and β-blockers should continue them preoperatively. A preinduction arterial line may facilitate rapid recognition of hemodynamic changes and allow immediate treatment. Careful administration of induction agents, narcotics, and inhaled agents, combined with monitoring and thoughtful vasopressor use, is essential. It is important to avoid tachycardia with associated increases in myocardial oxygen requirements. (460, 462)
11. The intensity of monitoring in the intraoperative period is influenced by the severity of the patient's cardiovascular disease, the complexity of the procedure, the choice of anesthetic technique, and a risk-benefit analysis of each type of potential monitoring. The induction of general anesthesia for even a "simple" case may result in hemodynamic collapse. Choosing a regional technique may help avoid the more profound hemodynamic changes often seen with general anesthesia. The level of monitoring should reflect the patient and surgical risk and may be escalated as needed. Intensive monitoring should continue into the postoperative period for high-risk patients. (462, 463)
12. Hypothermia predisposes patients to shivering, which leads to abrupt increases in myocardial oxygen requirements. Shivering is often accompanied by tachycardia, which can increase the risk of myocardial ischemia in patients with CAD. (463)

VALVULAR HEART DISEASE

13. Patients with mitral stenosis are at an increased risk of atrial fibrillation due to distension/stretch of the left atrium. Distension of the left atrium can predispose to stasis of blood and the formation of thrombi. Thrombi in the left atrium can lead to systemic emboli. Anticoagulation may be recommended to reduce the risk of systemic embolic events. (463)
14. Patients with aortic stenosis may present with angina pectoris, even in the absence of CAD. This is due to an imbalance in myocardial oxygen supply and demand. There is an increase in myocardial oxygen demand from left ventricular hypertrophy combined with increased left ventricular pressures and increased myocardial work. Myocardial oxygen supply is decreased due to reduced coronary blood flow as a result of the stenotic flow through the aortic valve. (464, 465)
15. Anesthetic considerations for patients with valvular heart disease must take into account the effects on cardiac rhythm, heart rate, systemic arterial blood pressure, SVR, volume status, and maintenance of cardiac output. (463–466)

Valvular Disease	Cardiac Rhythm	Heart Rate	SVR	Volume/ Preload	Contractility
Mitral stenosis (MS)	Maintain sinus rhythm	Avoid tachycardia	Maintain SVR to maintain diastolic coronary perfusion	Maintain intravascular fluid volume; increased circulatory volume may lead to flash pulmonary edema and hypoxemia	Maintain contractility
Mitral regurgitation (MR)	Maintain sinus rhythm	Normal to slightly elevated (80–100 bpm)	Mild decrease in SVR may improve forward flow; sudden increase may worsen MR	Maintain intravascular fluid volume; excessive volume expansion can worsen MR and lead to pulmonary edema	Maintain contractility
Aortic stenosis (AS)	Maintain sinus rhythm	Normal to slightly decreased (60–90 bpm)	Avoid hypotension; maintain SVR to maintain diastolic coronary perfusion	Avoid hypovolemia; maintain intravascular fluid volume	Maintain contractility
Aortic regurgitation (AR)	Maintain sinus rhythm	Normal to slightly elevated (80–100 bpm)	Mild decrease in SVR may improve forward flow; sudden increase may worsen AR	Maintain intravascular fluid volume; excessive volume expansion can worsen MR and lead to pulmonary edema	Maintain contractility

DISTURBANCES OF CARDIAC CONDUCTION AND RHYTHM

16. The anesthesia provider should rapidly recognize certain critical cardiac conduction abnormalities and be familiar with treatment options. (467)

ECG Display	Condition	Treatment
	Third-degree AV (complete) heart block	▪ Temporary: transcutaneous pacing or emergency transvenous or transesophageal pacing ▪ IV isoproterenol ▪ Permanent pacemaker placement
	Ventricular tachycardia	Stable: ▪ IV amiodarone, procainamide, lidocaine Unstable: ▪ Synchronized cardioversion
	Wolff-Parkinson-White syndrome	Stable: ▪ IV adenosine, procainamide, b-blockers Unstable: ▪ Synchronized cardioversion Catheter ablation of accessory pathways

17. If the urgency of the surgery permits, the type of device should be determined (pacemaker and/or implantable cardioverter-defibrillator [ICD])), the indication for implantation, whether the patient is dependent on the device for pacing, what brand or model device is in place, what happens when a magnet is placed on the device, when the device was last interrogated, and whether the device battery is near end of life. Most device batteries last between 5 and 10 years. (466)
18. Chronic resynchronization therapy (CRT) involves implantation of an additional pacing lead in the heart to restore the normal timing pattern of the heartbeat to allow the atria and ventricles to contract in a more organized and efficient way. CRT pacing is also termed *biventricular pacing*. CRT is indicated for symptomatic patients in sinus rhythm with moderate-to-severe heart failure with left ventricular ejection fraction ≤35% and a widened QRS interval (QRS ≥150 ms). CRT has been shown to improve ejection fraction, reverse cardiac remodeling, decrease hospitalizations, and reduce mortality. (466)
19. Cardiac implantable electronic device (CIED) function may be adversely affected by electromagnetic interference (EMI). Monopolar electrocautery is more likely to cause EMI than bipolar electrocautery. In patients who are pacemaker dependent, EMI may be sensed by the pacemaker as native cardiac electrical activity and result in inappropriate inhibition of pacing, leading to hemodynamic compromise. For patients with ICDs, EMI may be falsely interpreted as a shockable rhythm and risks intraoperative shock delivery by the device. (466)
20. For surgeries above the umbilicus, patients with CIEDs are at highest risk of EMI. For patients with true pacing dependency at high risk of EMI exposure during surgery, a magnet may be placed on a pacemaker to switch the device to asynchronous pacing, or the device may be reprogrammed to asynchronous pacing with the ability to adjust the heart rate (if the target HR is different from the magnet settings). In the case of ICDs, magnet placement will only suspend tachyarrhythmia therapies (i.e., shocks) without changing pacing settings if the device is both a pacemaker and ICD. If the patient is pacemaker dependent with an ICD/pacemaker and there is high risk of EMI exposure, the ICD/pacemaker must be reprogrammed to set the pacemaker to asynchronous pacing. Devices that are reprogrammed should be interrogated and reactivated after the surgical procedure to ensure proper function. (466, 468)

HEART FAILURE

21. The preoperative presence of heart failure is highly correlated with postoperative morbidity. Elective surgery should not be performed in patients with untreated heart failure. Optimization of heart failure therapy should be undertaken prior to surgery. Cardiology consultation is frequently helpful to ensure optimal guideline-directed management and therapy (GDMT). (469)
22. Positive-pressure ventilation of the lungs in patients with heart failure may be beneficial because of its effect of decreasing pulmonary vascular congestion, reducing volume overload through decreased venous return, and improvement in arterial oxygenation. Alternatively, positive-pressure ventilation may reduce volume loading and reduce cardiac output. The resumption of negative intrathoracic pressures with spontaneous ventilation can lead to increased filling pressure and worsening heart failure. Careful monitoring and control of hemodynamics during institution and discontinuation of positive-pressure ventilation are essential. (469)
23. Regional anesthesia for peripheral surgery in patients with heart failure should be considered since anesthetics with minimal hemodynamic effects are preferred. In patients with poorly controlled heart failure, local or regional anesthesia may be the safest option for peripheral surgery. Mild decreases in SVR produced by an epidural or spinal anesthetic may improve cardiac output in patients with heart failure; however, larger decreases in SVR should be avoided or preemptively treated if possible. (469)

HYPERTROPHIC CARDIOMYOPATHY

24. Hypertrophic cardiomyopathy (HCM) is commonly inherited in an autosomal dominant pattern and can present with sudden cardiac death, especially in young adults. Though patients can remain asymptomatic for decades, common presenting symptoms include angina, dyspnea, exercise intolerance, dizziness, syncope, or sudden death. (470)
25. The goal during management of anesthesia for patients with HCM is to decrease the pressure gradient across the left ventricular outflow tract. Increases in heart rate, rhythm disturbances, decreases in preload or afterload, and increases in contractility will worsen left ventricular outflow tract obstruction (LVOTO). The following table summarizes hemodynamic goals for patients with HCM. (470)

Cardiac Rhythm	Heart Rate	Preload	Afterload	Contractility
Maintain sinus rhythm; suppress arrhythmias with β-blockers; ICD for malignant arrhythmias	Avoid tachycardia; β-blockers for heart rate control	Increase intravascular fluid volume with fluids or head down position	Increase afterload with phenylephrine or vasopressin	Decrease contractility with β-blockers

PULMONARY HYPERTENSION

26. Patients with pulmonary hypertension have a significantly increased risk of perioperative morbidity and mortality. Patients with known or suspected pulmonary hypertension undergoing elective surgery should have proper evaluation and optimization prior to surgery. (470)
27. The goal of anesthetic management of patients with pulmonary hypertension is the avoidance of events or drugs that could result in an increase in pulmonary vascular resistance, which could then cause worsening right ventricular failure. Events that may result in an increase in pulmonary vascular resistance include arterial hypoxemia, hypercapnia, acidosis, hypothermia, hypervolemia, and insufficient anesthesia and analgesia. Abrupt decreases in SVR should be avoided as decreased coronary perfusion may worsen right heart failure. Using a regional technique offers the advantage of maintaining spontaneous ventilation. Although positive pressure ventilation may increase pulmonary vascular resistance, its potential benefit for improving arterial oxygenation likely outweighs its risk. (470)
28. All standard induction agents at normal induction doses have no influence on pulmonary vascular resistance (PVR). Fentanyl and midazolam also have no direct effect on PVR. Volatile anesthetics are useful for relaxing vascular smooth muscle and will not cause an increase in PVR. Nitrous oxide may increase PVR and should be avoided. Inhaled nitric oxide and milrinone are both pulmonary vasodilators and will decrease PVR. The table below summarizes each drug's effect on PVR. (470, 471)

Drug/Agent	Effect on PVR (↑, ↓, or ↔)
Propofol	↔
Etomidate	↔
Ketamine	↔
Volatile anesthetics	↔ or ↓
Nitrous oxide	↑
Midazolam	↔
Fentanyl	↔
Nitric oxide	↓
Milrinone	↓

CARDIAC TAMPONADE

29. Cardiac tamponade occurs as a result of increased intrapericardial pressure from the accumulation of fluid in the pericardial space. The increase in pericardial pressures causes a decrease in compliance of the right ventricle, reducing right ventricular filling, stroke volume, and cardiac output, causing hypotension. The decrease in stroke volume results in sympathetic nervous system activation in an attempt to maintain cardiac output. Cardiac output and systemic blood pressure in these patients becomes dependent on heart rate and on a central venous pressure that exceeds the right ventricular end-diastolic pressure. (471)
30. With clinical signs alone, it is difficult to make the diagnosis of cardiac tamponade. Manifestations of cardiac tamponade include hypotension, tachycardia, vasoconstriction, and elevated central venous pressure. Patients may present in cardiogenic shock unresponsive to fluid and inotropes, or in cardiac arrest. Pulsus paradoxus, which is a decrease in systolic blood pressure by more than 10 mmHg with inspiration, suggests that a pericardial effusion is causing cardiac tamponade. (471)
31. Temporizing measures include expansion of intravascular fluid volume, giving inotropes to increase myocardial contractility (e.g., epinephrine or norepinephrine), and the correction of metabolic acidosis, which may depress myocardial contractility. Definitive care requires drainage of the pericardial fluid. (471)

ANEURYSMS OF THE AORTA

32. The goal of anesthetic management of patients undergoing resection of an abdominal aortic aneurysm is to maintain cardiovascular and hemodynamic parameters at or near normal. Intraoperative monitoring with an arterial line allows for titration of hemodynamics as well as continuous noninvasive cardiac output monitoring and calculation of stroke volume variation (SVV) and pulse pressure variation (PPV) to guide volume replacement. Perioperative administration of β-blockers and statins may reduce perioperative mortality. (471)
33. For endovascular aneurysm repair, a less invasive regional anesthetic may be used; however, for prolonged cases general anesthesia may be preferred. Open procedures for aortic aneurysm surgery require general anesthesia. Epidural catheter placement may be helpful for postoperative pain following open abdominal aortic aneurysm surgery. (471, 472)

CARDIOPULMONARY BYPASS

34. Blood is drained from the venae cavae by the venous cannula that is inserted into the right atrium or both the superior and inferior venae cavae. Blood drains from the right side of the heart by gravity or by vacuum-assisted drainage to the cardiopulmonary bypass (CPB) reservoir. Oxygenated blood is returned to the arterial system by the arterial cannula, which is inserted into the ascending aorta. (472, 473)
35. Heparinization of the patient's blood is mandatory before institution of cardiopulmonary bypass to prevent catastrophic clotting of blood both in the patient and in the cardiopulmonary bypass machine. The CPB tubing and reservoir are nonendothelialized surfaces and represent a large surface area of foreign material that can activate native inflammatory responses as well as the coagulation cascade. The dose of heparin that is usually administered is 300 to 400 units/kg. An activated clotting time (ACT) of 400 to 500 seconds is required throughout the course of cardiopulmonary bypass with additional heparin administered as necessary. (474)

36. Once separation of cardiopulmonary bypass is complete and the patient is determined not to require any additional repair necessitating going back on bypass, protamine is administered to neutralize the heparin given for CPB. Protamine should be given slowly over 10 to 15 minutes to avoid hypotension related to rapid infusion, known as a type I reaction. There are also type II and type III reactions, which cause anaphylaxis and pulmonary hypertensive crisis, respectively. Once protamine is given, an ACT is performed to confirm normalization of values back to baseline, typically between 90 and 120 seconds. (474, 475)

Chapter

27 CHRONIC PULMONARY DISEASE

Andrew James Deacon and Peter Douglas Slinger

INTRODUCTION

Overview of Chronic Pulmonary Disease

- Categorized as obstructive or restrictive lung disease
  - Obstructive disease can be divided into reactive airway disorders (asthma) or chronic obstructive pulmonary disease (COPD).
- Many patients have more than one type of pulmonary disease.
- Using regional or local anesthesia is preferable for patients with chronic respiratory diseases.

History

- Common symptoms: cough, wheezing, shortness of breath, chest tightness, sputum production, and reduced exercise tolerance
- Assessment: recent exacerbations, current and previous therapies, emergency department visits, hospital admissions, and tobacco use

Physical Exam

- Signs: tachypnea, cyanosis, use of accessory muscles, clubbing of fingers
- Auscultation: unequal breath sounds, wheezing, rales

Laboratory Examination

Chest imaging

- Not required for all patients
- Consider if there was recent change in respiratory symptoms or signs.

Spirometry

- Simple spirometry (expired volume or flow vs. time), forced vital capacity (FVC), or forced expiratory volume in 1 second (FEV_1)
- Consider if there was recent change in symptoms or for patients with chronic lung disease undergoing lung surgery.
- Full pulmonary function tests including residual volume, functional residual capacity (FRC), and measurement of the lung diffusing capacity for carbon monoxide (D_{LCO}) are only indicated to clarify diagnosis or severity of disease, or if unclear after spirometry.

Gas Exchange

- Oxygen saturation: document preoperatively for all patients with respiratory disease
- Arterial blood gases (ABGs): document preoperatively for patients with moderate or severe lung disease at risk for postoperative mechanical ventilation or if symptoms severely worsen

ASTHMA

Clinical Presentation

- Hallmark: inflammation of the airways causing episodic, recurrent lower airway obstruction
- Treatment: steroids (inhaled and/or oral) are the most effective medications
- Pathophysiology: bronchospasm, small airway edema, mucus
- Irritant stimuli: allergens, dust, cold air, instrumentation of the airway, medications (e.g., nonsteroidal antiinflammatory drugs [NSAIDs], histamine-releasing drugs)
- Severity: defined by the amount of treatment required to control symptoms
  - Intermittent or mild persistent, moderate persistent, or severe persistent
  - Patients requiring endotracheal intubation or admission to ICU indicate higher risk
  - Peak expiratory flow (PEF) rates can be used to assess severity or guide therapy.
    - PEF $<50\%$ predicted indicates severe asthma.
    - PEF increase $>15\%$ after bronchodilator administration suggests inadequate treatment.
- Stepwise therapy
  - Inhaled short-acting β_2-agonists

- Inhaled low-, medium-, or high-dose corticosteroids daily
- Long-acting muscarinic antagonist
- Oral systemic steroids

- Suppression of the hypothalamic-pituitary-adrenal (HPA) axis after corticosteroid therapy
  - Can last for up to 10 days after a short course of oral prednisone
  - Can last for up to 1 year after larger doses, prolonged (>3 weeks) therapy, evening dosing, and continuous therapy
  - Unlikely to be caused by inhaled corticosteroids
  - The stress of surgery can precipitate an adrenal crisis.

Management of Anesthesia

- Elective surgery should be delayed 6 weeks after an exacerbation.
- Assess severity and adequacy of control.
- Exclude signs that are suggestive for a cause other than asthma, such as a fixed airway obstruction, pneumonia, tracheomalacia, or vocal cord dysfunction.
- Anesthetic techniques that promote bronchodilation and avoid airway irritants are preferred.

Principles of Perioperative Asthma Management

- Usual inhalers per routine on day of surgery
  - Inhaled β_2-agonists prior to anesthesia
- Avoid lower airway manipulation (e.g., endotracheal intubation) if possible.
  - Use regional anesthesia or an LMA/mask for general anesthesia if possible.
- Avoid medications that release histamine (e.g., thiopental, morphine, atracurium).
- Use anesthetic drugs that promote bronchodilation (e.g., propofol, ketamine, sevoflurane).
- If instrumentation of the lower airway is necessary, it should be performed after attaining a deep level of general anesthesia to decrease airway reflexes.

CHRONIC OBSTRUCTIVE PULMONARY DISEASE

Clinical Presentation

- Hallmark: inflammation of the small airways and destruction of lung parenchyma
- FEV_1/FVC ratio <70%, and the residual volume is increased.
- Clinical signs: dyspnea, hypoxemia, or hypercarbia
- Severity: defined by the predicted FEV_1
  - Stage I: >50% predicted (this category includes both mild and moderate COPD)
  - Stage II: 35% to 50% predicted
  - Stage III: <35% predicted

Carbon Dioxide Retention

- Defined as baseline $PaCO_2$ >45 mmHg on ABG
- Patients with stage II or III COPD, but cannot be predicted based on history or examination
- When given supplemental oxygen, their $PaCO_2$ values increase (increased ventilatory dead space and the Haldane effect)
- $PaCO_2$ increase above baseline leads to respiratory acidosis.

Right Ventricular Dysfunction

- Occurs in up to 50% of patients with severe COPD due to chronic hypoxemia
- Cor pulmonale occurs in 70% of adult COPD patients with an FEV_1 <0.6 L.
- Patients with a resting PaO_2 <55 mmHg should receive supplemental oxygen.
- Goal of oxygen treatment is to maintain PaO_2 at 60 to 65 mmHg at home.
- Supplemental oxygen decreases right heart strain and improves long-term survival.

Bullae

- Cystic air spaces in lung parenchyma caused by loss of structural support tissue
- When bullae occupy >50% of the hemithorax, patients present with mixed restrictive and obstructive lung disease
- Risks of positive-pressure ventilation include rupture, tension pneumothorax, and bronchopleural fistula.
- Manage with low airway pressures and avoidance of nitrous oxide
- Treatment of rupture may require chest drain and/or lung isolation.

Flow Limitation

- Increase in expiratory effort will not produce an increase in flow at that given lung volume.
- Can develop intrinsic positive end-expiratory pressure (auto-PEEP) during positive-pressure ventilation
- Auto-PEEP can result in hemodynamic collapse by obstructing pulmonary blood flow.

Perioperative Management

- Treatable complications of COPD must be actively sought and managed preoperatively.
  - Atelectasis
  - Bronchospasm
  - Respiratory tract infection
  - Congestive heart failure
- Intensive chest physiotherapy should be started preoperatively in patients with excessive sputum production

- Comprehensive pulmonary rehabilitation program increases functional capacity.
  - Chest physiotherapy, exercise, nutrition, and education
  - Programs may take months to complete.

INTERSTITIAL LUNG DISEASE

Clinical Presentation

- Hallmark: chronic restrictive lung disease due to inflammation and fibrosis of alveolar walls
- FEV_1 <70% predicted, FEV_1/FVC ratio normal or increased, and residual volume decreased
- Pathophysiology: alveolar wall inflammation and fibrosis of alveolar walls increases elastic recoil
- Causes: unknown (most common), autoimmune, inorganic dust, organic antigens, drugs, or radiation
- Severity
  - Increased respiratory effort and energy are required to prevent alveolar hypoventilation.
  - In severe cases, ventilation/perfusion (V/Q) mismatch can cause hypoxemia.

Perioperative Management

- Controlled ventilation with endotracheal tube is usually necessary for general anesthesia.
- Mechanical ventilation has risk of barotrauma and acute lung injury.
- Strategies to minimize airway pressure
  - Long inspiration-to-expiration ratios (e.g., 1:1 to 1:1.5)
  - Small tidal volumes (4–7 mL/kg ideal body weight)
  - Rapid respiratory rates
  - PEEP can be safely used.

CYSTIC FIBROSIS

Clinical Presentation

- Hallmark: abnormally viscous secretions, which can cause obstruction of the respiratory tracts, pancreas, biliary system, intestines, and sweat glands
- Inability to clear the thick purulent secretions enhances bacterial growth, leading to chronic inflammation and bronchiectasis (permanent dilation of the airways)
- Presents as a mixed obstructive and restrictive lung disease
- Autosomal recessive disorder
- Severity
  - Early mortality due to pulmonary complications including air-trapping, pneumothorax, massive hemoptysis, and respiratory failure
  - Effective sputum elimination is a key goal in the long-term management of cystic fibrosis.

Perioperative Management

- Optimize with preoperative chest physiotherapy to clear secretions.
- Endotracheal intubation with large-diameter endotracheal tube to allow endobronchial toileting and bronchoscopy

OBSTRUCTIVE SLEEP APNEA

Clinical Presentation

- Obesity is the most important physical characteristic.
- Risk factors: male gender, middle age, BMI >28 kg/m^2, alcohol and sedative use
- Pathophysiology: upper airway pharyngeal collapse when laryngeal muscles relax
  - Can be due to adenotonsillar hypertrophy or craniofacial abnormalities (retrognathia)
- Sequelae of apnea/hypopnea leading to hypoxemia
  - Cardiopulmonary dysfunction: systemic or pulmonary hypertension, cor pulmonale
  - Cognitive dysfunction: intellectual impairment, hypersomnolence, mood dysregulation
- Diagnosis
  - Presumptive: based on clinical impression or score, e.g., STOP-BANG score
  - Gold standard: polysomnography in a sleep laboratory

Definitions in Obstructive Sleep Apnea (OSA)

- Apnea: cessation of breathing for ≥10 seconds
- Hypopnea: >50% decrease in ventilation or decrease in SpO_2 by 3% to 4% for ≥10 seconds
- Severe OSA: >40 episodes of apnea or hypopnea per hour (in adults)

Treatment of OSA

- Correction of reversible factors such as weight reduction, avoidance of alcohol and sedatives, nasal decongestants
- Therapeutic options: continuous positive airway pressure (CPAP), dental appliances, upper airway surgery

Preoperative Evaluation of Patients With OSA

- Identify anticipated difficulties and coexisting diseases, and treat to the extent possible.

Potential Organ System Involvement in OSA
▪ Airway – Anticipated difficult mask ventilation – Difficult tracheal intubation ▪ Respiratory – Restrictive lung disease due to decreased chest wall compliance ▪ Cardiovascular – Systemic hypertension, pulmonary hypertension – Signs of biventricular dysfunction: cor pulmonale and congestive cardiac failure ▪ Gastrointestinal and endocrine – Esophageal reflux, fatty liver infiltration – Type 2 diabetes

Perioperative Management

- Airway management
  - Oral and nasopharyngeal airways should be available.
  - Advanced equipment to manage difficult ventilation and intubation
- Choice of anesthetic technique
  - Minimize sedatives, e.g., benzodiazepines
  - Short-acting anesthetic drugs, e.g., sevoflurane, propofol
  - Multimodal opioid-sparing analgesia
  - Avoid long-acting muscle relaxants
- Patient positioning
  - Extubate in the semi-upright position to facilitate spontaneous ventilation.
- Post-extubation
  - Equipment and drugs available to reintubate if necessary
  - Supplemental oxygen during transfer from the operating room to the postanesthesia care unit
  - CPAP available for patients who used it preoperatively
- Monitoring
  - Potential for inaccurate noninvasive blood pressure measurements
  - Consider arterial line for patients at increased risk of underlying cardiorespiratory disease and potential need for ABG monitoring.
- Vascular access
  - Possible difficult intravenous access, may require ultrasound-guided access or central venous catheter placement

Postoperative Management

- Disposition is influenced by the severity of OSA, invasiveness of surgical procedure or airway surgery, and predicted postoperative opioid use.
- A patient with increased perioperative risk of airway obstruction and hypoxemia should receive continuous oxygen saturation monitoring in ICU, a step-down or telemetry unit.

Obesity Hypoventilation Syndrome

- Definition: chronic daytime hypoxemia (PaO_2 <65 mmHg) and hypoventilation ($PaCO_2$ >45 mmHg) in an obese patient without COPD
- Pathophysiology: an interaction between sleep-disordered breathing, decreased respiratory drive, and obesity-related respiratory impairment
  - Patients exhibit signs of central apnea.
  - Pickwickian syndrome: obesity, daytime hypersomnolence, hypoxemia, hypercapnia
- Preoperative assessment: a patient with SpO_2 <96% warrants ABG analysis to assess $PaCO_2$
- Diagnosis allows for the following:
  - Planning for appropriate postoperative monitoring (ICU, step-down bed)
  - Treatment of coexisting conditions, e.g., systemic hypertension, cardiac dysrhythmias, congestive cardiac failure
  - Initiation of CPAP (ideally for 2 weeks to correct abnormal ventilatory drive)

PULMONARY HYPERTENSION

Pathophysiology

- Definition
  - Mean pulmonary artery pressure >25 mmHg on right heart catheterization
  - Systolic pulmonary artery pressure >50 mmHg on echocardiography
- Perioperative risk: respiratory complications and prolonged intubation after noncardiac surgery

Preoperative Evaluation

- The two commonly encountered types of pulmonary hypertension are caused by left-sided heart disease and lung disease.

Management of Anesthesia

- Increased right ventricular systolic intracavitary and transmural pressures may restrict right coronary artery perfusion during systole, unfavorably affecting oxygen supply at a time of increased demand.
- Avoid increasing pulmonary vascular resistance
  - Hypoxemia
  - Hypercarbia
  - Acidosis
  - Hypothermia
- Avoid impairment of right ventricular filling
  - Tachycardia
  - Arrhythmias
- Avoid decreasing systemic blood pressure
  - Ketamine is a useful drug for induction of anesthesia.

- Vasopressors, e.g., phenylephrine, norepinephrine, and vasopressin are commonly used to maintain systemic blood pressure.
  - Vasopressin increases systemic blood pressure without affecting pulmonary artery pressure.
- Inhaled pulmonary vasodilators including nitric oxide (10–40 ppm) or nebulized prostaglandins (prostacyclin 50 ng/kg/min) can be considered.
- Inotropes and inodilators (e.g., dobutamine, milrinone) decrease systemic vascular tone and can cause tachycardia, potentially worsening hemodynamics in patients with pulmonary hypertension from lung disease.
- Epidural analgesia and anesthesia
  - Lumbar epidural analgesia and anesthesia have been used in obstetric patients with pulmonary hypertension.
  - Thoracic epidural analgesia may require an inotrope or vasopressor due to the requirement for tonic cardiac sympathetic innervation in these patients.

Management Principles for Pulmonary Hypertension Secondary to Lung Disease

- Avoid hypotensive and vasodilating anesthetic drugs whenever possible.
- Ketamine does not exacerbate pulmonary hypertension.
- Support mean systemic blood pressure with vasopressors: norepinephrine, phenylephrine, vasopressin.
- Use inhaled pulmonary vasodilators (nitric oxide, prostacyclin) in preference to intravenous vasodilators as needed.
- Use thoracic epidural local anesthetics cautiously and with vasopressors and inotropes as needed.
- Monitor cardiac output if possible.

ANESTHESIA FOR LUNG RESECTION

Preoperative Assessment for Pulmonary Resection

- Respiratory complications are a major cause of morbidity and mortality after thoracic surgery.
- Atelectasis, pneumonia, and respiratory failure occur in 15% to 20% of patients, and mortality is 3% to 4%.

Objective Assessment of Pulmonary Function

- Determination whether the patient can tolerate the proposed resection
- Respiratory function assessment occurs via three independent but related areas: respiratory mechanics, gas exchange, and cardiopulmonary interaction.

Respiratory Mechanics

- The predicted postoperative FEV_1 ($ppoFEV_1$) is the best predictor of risk after lung resection.
- ppoFEV1% = preoperative FEV_1% × (100 – % of functional tissue removed)/100
  - Estimate percent functional lung removed by counting the number of lung segments.
- Patients with a $ppoFEV_1$ of >60% are at low risk of postoperative pulmonary complications, and patients with <30% are at high risk.

Lung Parenchymal Function

- DLCO reflects the ability of the lung to exchange oxygen and carbon dioxide at the alveolar–capillary interface.
- The predicted postoperative DLCO (ppoDLCO) is a useful indicator of parenchymal function, using the same calculation as FEV_1.
- Patients with a ppoDLCO of >60% are at low risk of postoperative pulmonary complications, and patients with <30% are at high risk.
- Analysis of ABG has traditionally been used to predict risk of respiratory failure.

Cardiopulmonary Interaction

- Gold standard is cardiopulmonary exercise testing to calculate a VO_{2max}.
- A VO_{2max} >20 mL/kg/min is associated with a low risk of postoperative pulmonary complications, with <10 mL/kg/min considered very high risk.
- Valid surrogate tests include the stair climb test, shuttle walk test, and 6-minute walk test.

Ventilation-Perfusion Scintigraphy

- Ventilation-perfusion scintigraphy (V/Q scan) can assess the contribution of the lung or lobe to be resected.
- If the tissue to be resected is minimally ventilated or perfused, this will modify the predicted postoperative lung function.

Preoperative Cardiac Assessment

- Intrathoracic surgery is considered by the American Heart Association as high risk for a major adverse cardiac event.
- Atrial fibrillation is common after thoracic surgery, typically occurring on postoperative day 2 or 3, with the risk reverting to baseline at week 6.
- The risk factors for atrial fibrillation include male gender, older age, magnitude of lung or esophagus resected, history of congestive cardiac failure, concomitant lung disease, and length of procedure.
- The risk of atrial fibrillation can be decreased by prophylactic diltiazem or amiodarone.

Smoking Cessation

- Pulmonary complications are reduced in patients undergoing lung resection who stop smoking preoperatively.
  - Benefits are proportional to the duration of cessation.
- Nicotine replacement and behavioral management increase the chance of successful cessation.

Assessment of the Patient With Lung Cancer

- Anesthetic considerations include mass effects, metabolic abnormalities, metastases, and medications.

Anesthetic Considerations in Patients with Lung Cancer – The Four Ms	
Mass effects	Obstructive pneumonia, lung abscess, superior vena cava syndrome, tracheobronchial distortion, Pancoast syndrome, recurrent laryngeal nerve or phrenic nerve paresis, chest wall or mediastinal extension
Metabolic abnormalities	Lambert-Eaton syndrome, hypercalcemia, hyponatremia, Cushing syndrome
Metastases	Particularly to brain, bone, liver, adrenal gland
Medications	Chemotherapy drugs, pulmonary toxicity (bleomycin, mitomycin), cardiac toxicity (doxorubicin), renal toxicity (cisplatin)

Indications for Lung Isolation

- Surgical exposure to the thorax, e.g., lung resection, mediastinal, cardiac, vascular, esophageal, and spinal surgery
- Control ventilation, e.g., for a patient with a bronchopleural fistula.
- Prevent contralateral lung soiling, e.g., pulmonary hemorrhage, bronchopleural fistula, whole-lung lavage.
- Allow differential patterns of ventilation in patients with unilateral lung injury.

Options for Lung Isolation

- Double-lumen endobronchial tube (DLT)
- Bronchial blocker
- Endobronchial (single-lumen tube)
- Endotracheal tube advanced into the bronchus

Airway Anatomy

- Knowledge of the airway anatomy allows for correct positioning and the ability to troubleshoot malposition of an airway device.

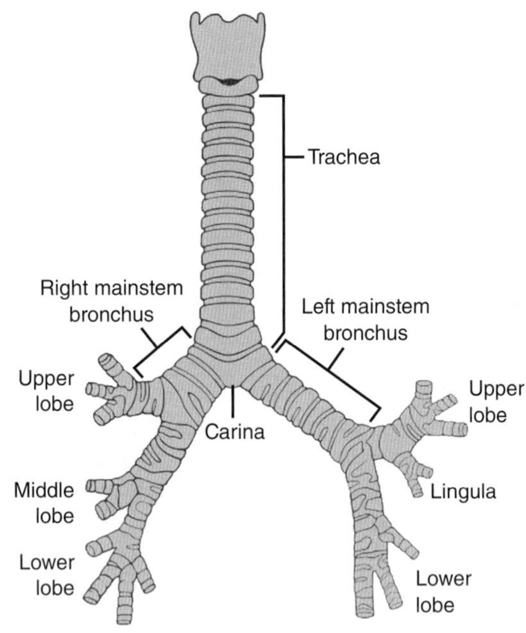

Bronchial Anatomy Relevant to Lung Isolation
▪ Carina: bifurcation is "sharp" with no further divisions seen in the left or right lumen
▪ Right main bronchus: typically 1.5–2 cm long
▪ Right upper lobe: the only trifurcation within the tracheobronchial tree, with a distinct appearance on fiberoptic bronchoscopy; aberrant takeoff at or above carina in 1 in 250 patients
▪ Left main bronchus: typically 4.5–5 cm long
▪ Lower lobes: can be identified bilaterally as the longitudinal fibers of the trachealis muscle descend into them

Sizing a Double-Lumen Endobronchial Tube

- There is no consensus for optimal sizing of a DLT.
- Ideally the bronchial tube's external diameter should be 1–2 mm smaller than the patient's bronchial diameter.
- A simplified method based on patient's sex and height can be used.
- After size selection, check a chest radiograph or computed tomography (CT) chest coronal slice to exclude aberrant anatomy such as endoluminal obstruction, significant tracheal deviation, and aberrant right upper lobe takeoff.
- A DLT should not be advanced against resistance.

Selection of Double-Lumen Tube Size Based on Adult Patient's Sex and Height

Sex	Height (cm)	Size of DLT (Fr)
Female	>160 (63 in)	37
	153–159	35
	>152 (60 in)	Consider 32
Male	>170 (67 in)	41
	160–169	39
	<159 (63 in)	Consider 37

Methods of Insertion of a Left-Sided DLT

- Blind
  - During laryngoscopy, the endobronchial lumen is advanced through the glottis; the DLT is then turned 90 degrees counterclockwise and advanced until resistance is felt.
  - This technique results in 35% malposition, so confirmation is required with auscultation and a flexible bronchoscope.
- Direct vision
  - During laryngoscopy, the endobronchial lumen is advanced through the glottis, rotated 90 degrees counterclockwise, and advanced until the tracheal cuff is just past the glottis.
  - A flexible bronchoscope is inserted into the bronchial lumen to its opening, and the DLT and bronchoscope advanced simultaneously into the correct bronchus.

Positioning a Left-Sided DLT

- Auscultation alone is unreliable to confirm correct positioning but should be used after initial placement and again after repositioning the patient.
- Bronchoscopy via tracheal lumen
  - Endobronchial portion of the DLT is confirmed to be in the left main bronchus.
  - The right upper lobe takeoff can be identified to confirm anatomic landmarks.
  - The blue endobronchial cuff is 5–10 mm distal to the tracheal carina.
- Bronchoscopy via bronchial lumen
  - Ensure the bifurcation into the left upper and lower lobe can be seen, confirming distal migration of the DLT has not led to obstruction of the left upper lobe.

Right-Sided DLT Indications

Indications for a Right-Sided DLT

- Distorted anatomy of the entrance of the left main bronchus
- External or intraluminal tumor compression
- Descending thoracic aortic aneurysm
- Site of surgery involving the left main bronchus
  - Left lung transplantation
  - Left-sided tracheobronchial disruption
  - Left-sided pneumonectomy
  - Left-sided sleeve resection

- Right-sided DLT has a modified cuff and a slot in the endobronchial lumen allowing ventilation of the right upper lobe.
- Note that a left-sided pneumonectomy can be done with a left-sided DLT, provided the DLT or bronchial blocker is withdrawn prior to stapling the left main bronchus.

Positioning a Bronchial Blocker (BB)

- A BB is inserted within a single-lumen tube via an adaptor and advanced into the left or right main bronchus, or a lobe.
  - The adaptor also allows insertion of a flexible bronchoscope and attachment to the anesthetic circuit.
- The BB cuff is inflated to obstruct the lumen, allowing lung isolation.
- A small channel within the BB allows gas to escape to provide lung deflation, application of suction, intermittent insufflation of oxygen, or application of PEEP.

Physiologic Considerations of One-Lung Ventilation in the Lateral Position

- One-lung ventilation (OLV) in the lateral position with an open chest improves V/Q matching.
  - Lung isolation: ventilation only to the dependent lung
  - Perfusion to the nonventilated, nondependent lung is decreased favoring perfusion to the dependent lung.
    - Causes of decreased perfusion include gravity and hypoxic pulmonary vasoconstriction.
- Compliance of the dependent lung decreases due to the following factors:
  - Cephalad shift of the diaphragm after induction of anesthesia and muscle relaxation
  - Mediastinal shift after creation of a pneumothorax
  - Surgical manipulation and pushing or retraction onto the mediastinum
- Application of PEEP 5–10 cm H_2O to the ventilated (dependent) lung can be beneficial.
  - Improves the decreased compliance in the ventilated lung
  - Maintains FRC, which also decreases pulmonary vascular resistance
- Changes in cardiac output can have varying effects, but typically shunt is lowest and PaO_2 greatest at a "normal" cardiac output during OLV.

Conduct of Anesthesia

- Any anesthetic technique that provides safe and stable general anesthesia can be used for thoracic surgery.
  - Volatile anesthetics impair hypoxic pulmonary vasoconstriction only at a minimum alveolar concentration (MAC) that is greater than routine use.
  - There is no clear advantage of propofol total intravenous anesthesia compared with volatile anesthesia in terms of shunt fraction and hypoxemia.
- The risk-benefit ratio for intraoperative monitoring with an intraarterial catheter and venous access favors being overly invasive from the outset.
  - A central venous catheter allows vasoactive agents to be infused for patients at increased risk of intraoperative hemorrhage (e.g., pneumonectomy, complex procedures and redo-thoracotomy).

- Devices to warm the patient and measure the temperature are useful.
  - The open hemithorax provides a large surface area for evaporative cooling.
- Continuous spirometry allows monitoring of inspiratory and expiratory volumes, pressures, and flows and can alert the anesthesia provider to problems such as bronchospasm, gas trapping, or DLT malposition.
  - A difference between inspired and expired volumes of >30 mL/breath
    - During OLV can indicate loss of lung isolation
    - During two-lung ventilation (TLV) after lung resection can indicate an air leak through lung parenchyma
  - Persistent end-expiratory flow can indicate the development of gas trapping.

Intraoperative Complications that can Occur During Thoracotomy

Complication	Cause
Hypoxemia	Intrapulmonary shunt during OLV
Sudden hypotension	Surgical compression of the heart or great vessels
Sudden changes in ventilating pressure or volume	Movement of endobronchial tube/blocker, air leak
Arrhythmia	Mechanical irritation of the heart
Bronchospasm	Direct airway stimulation Increased frequency of reactive airways disease
Hemorrhage	Surgical blood loss from great vessels or inflamed pleura
Hypothermia	Heat loss from open hemithorax

Approach to Intravenous Fluid Management

- Euvolemia is preferred: replacement of intravascular volume deficits and maintenance with a balanced salt solution
  - Restrictive fluid regimen has a higher incidence of acute kidney injury.
  - Liberal regimens risk developing interstitial and alveolar edema.

Fluid Management for Pulmonary Resection Surgery

- 2–3 mL/kg/h until the patient can drink, then discontinue intravenous fluids
- Total positive fluid balance should not exceed 20 mL/kg in the first 24-hour perioperative period.
- No fluid administration for third-space fluid losses during pulmonary resection
- Urine output >0.5 mL/kg/h is unnecessary.
- If increased tissue perfusion is required postoperatively, it is advisable to use invasive monitoring and inotropes/vasopressors rather than cause fluid overload.

Approach to One-Lung Ventilation

- The following box describes a suggested approach to OLV.

Suggested Approach to OLV

Parameter	Suggested Application	Explanation
FiO_2	Induction and early maintenance FiO_2 1.0 Decrease FiO_2 during OLV if tolerated	Aids absorption atelectasis in nondependent lung, speeding lung collapse
Tidal volume	TLV 6–8 mL/kg OLV 4–6 mL/kg	Peak airway pressure <35 cm H_2O, plateau airway pressure <25 cm H_2O
Recruitment maneuver	Before lung isolation During OLV as needed	Reverses atelectasis in ventilated lung, improving PO_2 during OLV
PEEP	Routine PEEP 5–10 cm	No PEEP in patients with obstructive disease
Respiratory rate	Respiratory rate 12–16 breaths/min	May be higher if required
PCO_2	Permissive hypercapnia during OLV	Aim to keep pH >7.2
Mode	Volume or pressure controlled	Pressure control for patients at risk of lung injury, such as bullae, preexisting lung disease, pneumonectomy, lung transplantation

Prediction of Intraoperative Hypoxia

- Higher percentage of ventilation or perfusion to the operative lung on preoperative V/Q scan
- Poor PaO_2 during TLV, particularly in the lateral position intraoperatively
- Right-sided thoracotomy
- Normal preoperative spirometry (FEV_1 or FVC) or restrictive lung disease
- Supine position during OLV

Management of Hypoxia During OLV

- Occurs in <5% of cases
- SpO_2 <94% typically indicates a problem.
- The most common cause of hypoxia is DLT malposition.

Management of Gradual Hypoxemia During OLV

Dependent/Ventilated Lung

FiO_2 1.0
Confirm position of DLT or blocker with flexible bronchoscope
Recruitment maneuver (this will transiently make hypoxemia worse)
Apply PEEP 5–10 cm (except in patients with emphysematous pathology)

Nondependent/Surgical Lung

Passive, apneic O_2 1–2 L/min via suction catheter down DLT, more effective after partial recruitment maneuver
Partial recruitment maneuver followed by CPAP 1–2 cm H_2O

Management of Gradual Hypoxemia During OLV
Nondependent/Surgical Lung
Intermittent positive-pressure ventilation
Flexible bronchoscopic lobar insufflation using O_2 connected to working channel
Selective lobar collapse using a bronchial blocker
Small tidal volume ventilation
Mechanical restriction of blood flow to the nonventilated lung (clamping pulmonary artery)
Other Measures
Cardiac output optimal
Volatile anesthetic <1.0 MAC to optimize hypoxic pulmonary vasoconstriction and V/Q matching
Venovenous ECMO

Conclusion of Surgery

- The patient should be awake, warm, and comfortable before extubation.
- Anesthetic management should be guided by the predicted postoperative FEV_1 as follows:
  - If >60%, extubate in operating room.
  - If 30% to 60%, consider extubation based on exercise tolerance, DLCO, V/Q scan, and associated diseases.
  - If <30%, staged weaning from mechanical ventilation
    - Consider extubation if >20% with thoracic epidural analgesia.

Pain Management

- Optimal analgesia consisting of both systemic and regional analgesia continues to evolve.
- The optimal choice is based on patient, surgical, and local system factors.

MEDIASTINOSCOPY

- Typically used for patients who have had an unsuccessful endobronchial ultrasound-guided transbronchial needle aspiration (EBUS)
- Surgical access is limited, and many structures may be compressed or transected.
- General anesthesia with a single-lumen tube ensures patient immobility.
- Monitor the pulse in the right hand for innominate artery (and therefore right carotid perfusion) compression by surgeon.
  - Use arterial line, pulse oximeter with plethysmograph or palpation by anesthesia provider.
  - Noninvasive blood pressure cuff on the left arm confirms innominate artery compression (i.e., normal blood pressure in left arm) with decreased perfusion in right arm (via arterial line, pulse oximetry plethysmograph, or palpation).

Anesthetic Management of Mediastinoscopy Hemorrhage

1. Stop surgery and pack the wound. There is a serious risk that the patient will approach the point of hemodynamic collapse if the surgery-anesthesia team does not realize soon enough that there is a problem.
2. Begin resuscitation and call for help, both anesthetic and surgical.
3. Obtain large-bore intravenous access in the lower limbs.
4. Place an arterial line (if not placed at induction).
5. Obtain crossmatched blood in the operating room.
6. Place a double-lumen tube or bronchial blocker if the surgeon thinks thoracotomy is a possibility.
7. Once the patient is stabilized and all preparations are made, the surgeon can reexplore the surgical incision.
8. Convert to sternotomy or thoracotomy if indicated.

MEDIASTINAL MASSES

- Patients at risk for respiratory or cardiovascular complications are those with symptoms or with significant compression of vital structures on CT scan.
  - Pulmonary arteries, atria, superior vena cava, and major airways are at risk.
- General anesthesia is potentially dangerous due to greater airway compression.
  - Lung volume decreases due to the overlying mass with cephalad shift of the diaphragm.
  - Relaxation of bronchial smooth muscle
  - Loss of normal transpleural pressure gradient and a subsequent decrease in airway caliber
- Ideally, spontaneous ventilation is maintained and paralysis avoided.
- Flow–volume loops for assessment of severity of intrathoracic airway obstruction are unreliable and not recommended for decision-making.
  - Cardiopulmonary bypass must be initiated before the induction of anesthesia in patients at high risk.
  - Rescue with cardiopulmonary bypass after cardiorespiratory arrest is unlikely to be successful and should not be relied on.

Management of Life-Threatening Complications of Mediastinal Masses

Complication	Options for Management
Airway obstruction	• Maintenance of spontaneous ventilation, avoidance of muscle relaxants • Awake fiberoptic intubation with single-lumen endotracheal or endobronchial tube placed distal to the obstruction • Patient repositioning: optimal position determined preinduction based on patient's symptoms • Rigid bronchoscopy and ventilation distal to the obstruction; experienced bronchoscopist and equipment in the room at induction
Cardiovascular collapse	• Lower limb intravenous (IV) access (large-bore IV line with or without central line) • Patient repositioning • Elective cardiopulmonary bypass preinduction in extreme cases

QUESTIONS

INTRODUCTION

1. What chronic pulmonary diseases are common in patients presenting for surgery?
2. What are some preoperative considerations when assessing patients with chronic pulmonary disease?
3. Spirometry, including flow-volume loops, have characteristic patterns in patients with restrictive and obstructive disease. In the diagram below, draw the flow-volume loop for a patient with restrictive or obstructive disease. The flow-volume loop of a patient with normal pulmonary function is provided.

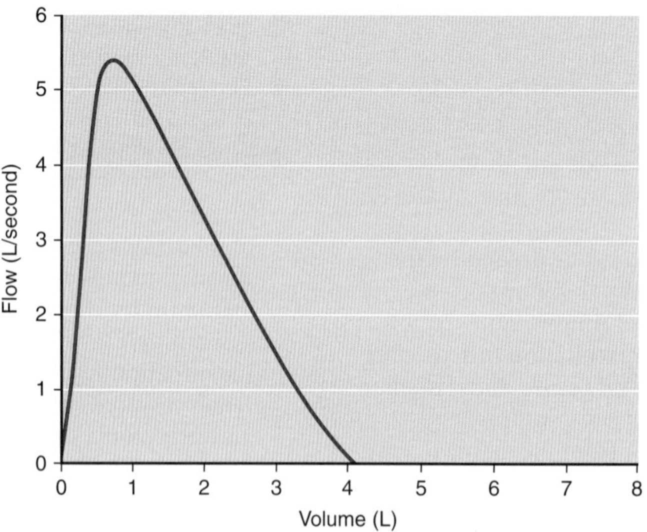

ASTHMA

4. The severity of asthma is defined by the treatment required to control symptoms. In the following table, outline the steps in asthma treatment.

	SABA	ICS	LABA	LAMA	Systemic Corticosteroids
Step 1					
Step 2					
Step 3					
Step 4					
Step 5					
Step 6					

ICS, inhaled corticosteroids; *LABA*, long-acting β_2-agonists (e.g., formoterol); *LAMA*, long-acting muscarinic antagonists (e.g., tiotropium bromide and aclidinium bromide); *SABA*, Inhaled short-acting β_2-agonists (e.g., albuterol).

5. You are scheduled to administer general anesthesia to a patient with chronic asthma undergoing a laparoscopic cholecystectomy. The patient's asthma is currently well-controlled with inhaled corticosteroids. Does the patient need preoperative chest imaging? Does the patient need perioperative stress-dose steroid supplementation?

CHRONIC OBSTRUCTIVE PULMONARY DISEASE

6. Can carbon dioxide retention be predicted from a patient's lung function test results?
7. What is the mechanism of hemodynamic collapse in a patient with severe COPD during positive-pressure ventilation?
8. Outline the cardiovascular response to severe hypercarbia.

INTERSTITIAL LUNG DISEASE

9. Outline a safe ventilation strategy for a patient with restrictive lung disease.

OBSTRUCTIVE SLEEP APNEA

10. Describe clinical symptoms and signs suggestive that a patient has obstructive sleep apnea.
11. How would you decide if a patient with obstructive sleep apnea requires postoperative monitoring in a high-dependency unit?

PULMONARY HYPERTENSION

12. For a patient with pulmonary hypertension undergoing anesthesia, what physiologic states can worsen pulmonary hypertension?
13. What are the hemodynamic goals for a patient with pulmonary hypertension undergoing anesthesia?
14. Which vasopressor increases systemic vascular resistance without increasing pulmonary vascular resistance?

ANESTHESIA FOR LUNG RESECTION

15. Calculate the predicted postoperative FEV_1 for a patient with a preoperative FEV_1 of 57% undergoing a left upper lobectomy.
16. Which objective measurements of lung function and exercise testing would indicate a patient is at low risk of postoperative pulmonary complications after thoracotomy?
17. Describe the risk factors for atrial fibrillation after thoracic surgery.

OPTIONS FOR LUNG ISOLATION

18. Describe the advantages and disadvantages of using a double-lumen endobronchial tube, a bronchial blocker, an endobronchial tube, and single lumen tube for lung isolation.
19. What size double-lumen endobronchial tube would be most appropriate for a female patient who is 165 cm tall? Or a male who is 168 cm tall? Are there any other additional factors you would consider before intubation and insertion of the DLT?
20. What is the ideal position of a left-sided double-lumen endobronchial tube?
21. How is V/Q matching improved during one lung ventilation of the dependent lung with an open thorax of the nondependent lung?
22. Describe a ventilation strategy for a patient undergoing one-lung ventilation.
23. What are the predictors of hypoxemia during one-lung ventilation?
24. What is the most common cause of desaturation during OLV with a DLT?

MEDIASTINOSCOPY

25. What structures can be compressed or transected during mediastinoscopy?
26. Describe how the placement of routine monitoring can assist with the detection of innominate artery compression during mediastinoscopy.

MEDIASTINAL MASSES

27. Outline a plan for the induction of anesthesia for a patient with a superior mediastinal mass causing 60% obstruction of their mid trachea.

ANSWERS

INTRODUCTION

1. Pulmonary diseases that are common in patients presenting for surgery include obstructive and restrictive lung disease, obstructive sleep apnea, and pulmonary hypertension. Obstructive lung diseases can be divided into reactive airway disorders (asthma) and chronic obstructive pulmonary disease (COPD). However, many patients have more than one type of lung disease. (477)
2. Preoperative considerations when assessing patients with chronic pulmonary disease include that (1) no single test of respiratory function is adequate as a sole preoperative assessment and (2) evaluation of patients prior to surgery aims to identify patients at increased risk of perioperative morbidity and mortality, allowing resources to be focused to improve their outcome. Respiratory function is assessed in three related areas: respiratory mechanics, gas exchange, and cardiorespiratory interactions. (478)
3. The flow–volume loop for a patient with restrictive or obstructive disease is shown in the figure. Tracing c is from a normal patient, tracing a is from a patient with obstructive disease, and tracing b is from a patient with restrictive lung disease. (478)

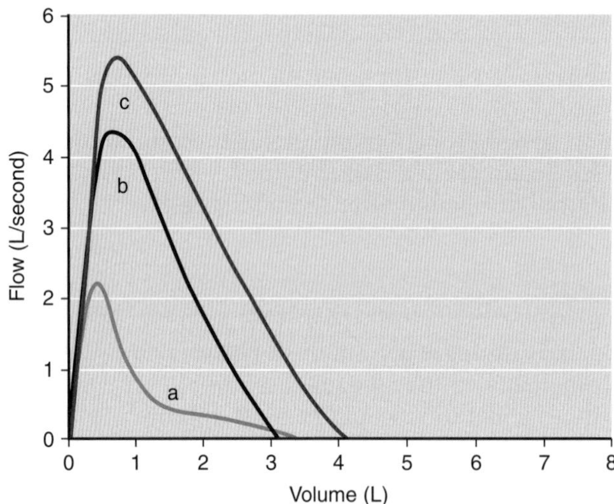

ASTHMA

4. The severity of asthma is defined by the treatment required to control symptoms. The following table represents the stepwise approach for asthma management according to the National Asthma Education and Prevention Program Coordinating Committee. Step 1 is for patients with intermittent asthma only; the remaining steps are for patients with persistent asthma. Alternative management steps and additional treatment recommendations are available. (479)

Step	SABA	ICS	LABA	LAMA	Systemic Corticosteroids
1	PRN				
2	PRN	Daily, low dose			
3		Daily and PRN (combo low-dose ICS-LABA)	Daily and PRN (combo low-dose ICS-LABA)		
4		Daily and PRN (combo medium-dose ICS-LABA)	Daily and PRN (combo medium-dose ICS-LABA)		

Continued

Step	SABA	ICS	LABA	LAMA	Systemic Corticosteroids
5	PRN	Daily medium-high dose ICS-LABA plus long-acting muscarinic antagonist + LAMA	Daily medium-high dose ICS-LABA plus long-acting muscarinic antagonist + LAMA	Daily medium-high dose ICS-LABA plus long-acting muscarinic antagonist + LAMA	
6	PRN	Daily high-dose ICS-LABA plus oral systemic corticosteroids	Daily high-dose ICS-LABA plus oral systemic corticosteroids		Daily high-dose ICS-LABA plus oral systemic corticosteroids

ICS, inhaled corticosteroids; *LABA*, long-acting β_2-agonists (e.g., formoterol); *LAMA*, long-acting muscarinic antagonists (e.g., tiotropium bromide and aclidinium bromide); *SABA*, inhaled short-acting β_2-agonists (e.g., albuterol).

5. Preoperative chest imaging does not need to be ordered for a patient with stable pulmonary disease. It can be considered in patients who may have a recent change in respiratory signs or symptoms, which is not the case for this patient. Inhaled corticosteroids are unlikely to suppress the hypothalamic-pituitary-adrenal axis; perioperative stress-dose steroid supplementation is not necessary for this patient. (479)

CHRONIC OBSTRUCTIVE PULMONARY DISEASE

6. Patients with CO_2 retention cannot be differentiated from patients without CO_2 retention on the basis of history, physical examination, or spirometry. (480)
7. Positive pressure ventilation in a patient with severe COPD can lead to the development of intrinsic positive end-expiratory pressure (auto-PEEP) resulting in dynamic hyperinflation of the lungs, obstruction of venous return and pulmonary blood flow. Patients with severe COPD and associated bullae can also develop a tension pneumothorax with positive-pressure ventilation, particularly with high airway pressures. (480-481)
8. Severe hypercarbia results in central sympathetic stimulation with tachycardia, hypertension, and pulmonary vasoconstriction. (480)

INTERSTITIAL LUNG DISEASE

9. The ventilatory goals in a patient with restrictive lung disease are to optimize oxygenation and ventilation while minimizing the risk of barotrauma and acute lung injury. This includes the use of long inspiratory-to-expiratory ratios (e.g., 1:1), small tidal volumes (e.g., 4–6 mL/kg), and a rapid respiratory rate. PEEP can be safely used in restrictive lung disease. (481)

OBSTRUCTIVE SLEEP APNEA

10. Predisposing clinical characteristics suggestive that a patient has obstructive sleep apnea (OSA) include a BMI ≥35 kg/m², a neck circumference ≥17 inches for men or ≥16 inches for women, craniofacial abnormalities, nasal obstruction, and tonsillar enlargement. History suggestive of OSA includes reported airway obstruction during sleep, e.g., snoring, observed pauses in breathing during sleep, waking from sleep with a choking sensation, or frequent arousals from sleep. Also a history of somnolence is suggestive; for example, fatigue despite adequate sleep or falling asleep easily in a nonstimulating environment despite adequate sleep. (482)
11. Postoperative disposition of a patient with obstructive sleep apnea is influenced by the severity of the OSA, the invasiveness of the surgical procedure and anesthesia, and the predicted postoperative opioid use. (483)

PULMONARY HYPERTENSION

12. Physiologic states that can worsen pulmonary hypertension include hypoxemia, hypercarbia, acidosis, and hypothermia. (484)

13. Hemodynamic goals for a patient with pulmonary hypertension undergoing anesthesia include to avoid or treat the conditions that can worsen pulmonary hypertension, as described in the prior question and answer. Ideally, right ventricular contractility and systemic vascular resistance are maintained while pulmonary vascular resistance is decreased. In addition, conditions that impair right ventricular filling, such as tachycardia and arrhythmias, are not well tolerated in patients with pulmonary hypertension and should be actively managed. (484-485)
14. Vasopressin increases systemic vascular resistance without increasing pulmonary vascular resistance, making it a useful choice for treating systemic hypotension in a patient with pulmonary hypertension. (484)

ANESTHESIA FOR LUNG RESECTION

15. The ppoFEV_1% = preoperative FEV_1% × (100 – % of functional tissue removed)/100. A left upper lobectomy will remove a total of 10 of 42 segments, or 24% of the total lung parenchyma. A patient with a preoperative FEV_1 of 57% undergoing a left upper lobectomy will have a ppoFEV_1% = 57% × ([100 – 24]/100) = 43%. (485)
16. Preoperative respiratory function assessment is via three independent but related areas: respiratory mechanics, cardiopulmonary interaction, and gas exchange. A ppoFEV_1 > 60% would indicate sufficient respiratory mechanics, a VO_2max >20 mL/kg/min, or a stair climb greater than two flights would indicate adequate cardiopulmonary reserve, and a ppoDLCO >60% would indicate sufficient lung parenchymal function to consider a patient low risk for postoperative pulmonary complications after lung resection surgery. (485–486)
17. Atrial fibrillation after thoracic surgery occurs in 12% to 44% of patients, typically on day 2 or 3 postoperatively. Risk factors include male sex, older age, magnitude of lung or esophagus resected, history of congestive cardiac failure, concomitant lung disease, and length of procedure. (486)

OPTIONS FOR LUNG ISOLATION

18. The advantages and disadvantages of using a double-lumen endobronchial tube, a bronchial blocker, an endobronchial tube, and single lumen tube for lung isolation during thoracic surgery are described in the chart below. (487–488)

	Advantages	Disadvantages
Double-lumen tube	• Easy to place • Reposition rarely required • Suction, bronchoscopy, and CPAP to isolated lung • Easy to alternate ventilation between lungs	• Size selection can be challenging • Hard to place in the patient with a difficult airway • Not optimal for postoperative ventilation • Potential for laryngeal and bronchial trauma
Bronchial blocker	• Size selection rarely an issue • Easily added to existing ETT • Easier placement in a patient with a difficult airway • Postoperative TLV easy by removing blocker • Selective lobar isolation possible	• Bronchoscope essential for positioning • More time required for positioning and more likely to require repositioning • Bronchoscopy to isolated lung impossible • Minimal suction to isolated lung
Endobronchial tube	• Easier placement in patients with difficult airways • Short cuff designed for lung isolation	• Does not allow for bronchoscopy, suctioning, or CPAP to isolated lung • Difficult one-lung ventilation to right lung
Endotracheal tube advanced into bronchus	• Easier placement in patients with difficult airways	• Does not allow for bronchoscopy, suctioning, or CPAP to isolated lung • Cuff not designed for lung isolation • Extremely difficult one-lung ventilation to right lung

19. Although there is no consensus as to the optimal method of sizing a DLT, a simplified method based on patient sex and height can be used. Using published guides, a female patient of 165 cm would receive a size 37 Fr DLT, while a male of 168 cm would receive a 39 Fr DLT. It is useful to then check imaging, such as a chest radiograph or CT coronal slice, to exclude aberrant anatomy. For example, an endoluminal obstruction,

significant tracheal deviation, or aberrant right upper lobe takeoff may require an adjustment in the DLT size selected. (488–489)

20. When positioning a left-sided DLT, the endobronchial portion should ideally be positioned in the left main bronchus, with the blue endobronchial cuff approximately 5 to 10 mm below the tracheal carina. Bronchoscopy should also show both the left upper and lower lobes, ensuring the endobronchial portion of the DLT has not advanced into the left lower lobe. (488–489)
21. During one-lung ventilation, perfusion to the nonventilated, nondependent lung decreases due to hypoxic pulmonary vasoconstriction and gravity, thereby favoring perfusion of the ventilated, dependent lung and decreasing shunt. Ventilation of the nondependent lung is stopped by virtue of lung isolation. The application of PEEP to the ventilated lung can compensate for decreased compliance caused by cephalad shift of the diaphragm after induction of anesthesia and muscle relaxation, mediastinal shift after opening of the chest, and surgical pushing and manipulation of the mediastinum. The improved compliance will also improve V/Q matching and oxygenation. (493)
22. A ventilation strategy for a patient undergoing one-lung ventilation is to induce anesthesia and continue with FiO_2 1.0 until lung isolation to speed lung deflation through absorption atelectasis. After the lung is deflated, the FiO_2 can be decreased if tolerated. Ventilate with 6–8 mL/kg of ideal body weight during TLV and 4–6 mL/kg during OLV. A recruitment maneuver before lung isolation decreases hypoxemia during OLV. PEEP 5–10 cm H_2O maintains FRC. A respiratory rate of 12–16 can be used to increase minute ventilation, with permissive hypercapnia to a pH $\geq$7.2. (493)
23. The predictors of hypoxemia during OLV include a higher percentage of ventilation or perfusion to the operative lung on preoperative V/Q scanning, poor PaO_2 during TLV, right-sided surgery, normal or restrictive spirometry, and surgery in the supine position. (493)
24. DLT malposition is the most common cause of desaturation during OLV, with migration inward of the DLT causing obstruction to the left upper lobe in a patient having their left lung ventilated. (493–494)

MEDIASTINOSCOPY

25. Structures that can be compressed or transected during mediastinoscopy include the trachea and bronchi, pleura, great vessels (particularly the innominate artery and vein), lymphatic vessels, phrenic and recurrent laryngeal nerves, and esophagus. (495)
26. Monitoring the pulse of the right hand is useful to detect compression of the innominate artery and therefore hypoperfusion of the right carotid artery and brain. This can be done using an arterial cannula in the right radial artery, a pulse oximeter with plethysmograph, or manual palpation by the anesthesia provider. If there is decreased perfusion of the right arm, a noninvasive blood pressure cuff on the left arm indicating normal blood pressure confirms innominate artery compression. (495)

MEDIASTINAL MASSES

27. The anesthetic management of a patient with a potentially life-threatening lower airway obstruction from a superior mediastinal mass requires careful planning. Maintenance of spontaneous ventilation during the induction of anesthesia avoids a decrease in lung volume associated with anesthesia and maintains a normal transpleural pressure gradient and airway caliber. Fiberoptic intubation allows the tip of a single-lumen endotracheal tube to be placed distal to the obstruction. If this is not possible, the patient can be positioned in an optimal position preinduction based on their symptoms, such as lateral. Rigid bronchoscopy and ventilation distal to the obstruction can be considered as a rescue procedure. (495–496)

Chapter

28 RENAL, LIVER, AND BILIARY TRACT DISEASE

Anup Pamnani

RENAL DISEASE

Physiologic Renal Functions

- Excretion of medications and anesthetics
- Fluid and acid-base balance maintenance
- Regulating hemoglobin levels

- Renal disease is associated with an increased risk of poor postoperative outcomes.
- Multiple preoperative risk factors predict postoperative renal dysfunction.
- Perioperative clinical conditions associated with postoperative renal dysfunction:
  - Major surgery
  - Critical illness
  - Septic shock
  - Exposure to nephrotoxic drugs
  - Radiocontrast

Renal Blood Flow

- Kidneys receive 20% of cardiac output, with about two-thirds of that to the renal cortex.

Autoregulation of Renal Blood Flow

- Renal blood flow (RBF) and the glomerular filtration rate (GFR) are relatively constant at mean renal arterial blood pressures in range of 80 to 180 mmHg.
- Renal afferent arteriolar tone adjusts within this range.
- RBF is pressure dependent outside this range.
- Autoregulation is reset by chronic hypertension and affected by diabetes.
- RBF is influenced by sympathetic nervous system (causes renal vasoconstriction) and renin.

Glomerular Filtration Rate

- The GFR reflects glomerular function.
- Normal GFR is 125 mL/min, which depends on glomerular filtration pressure.
- Glomerular filtration pressure depends on renal artery pressure, afferent and efferent renal arterial tone, and glomerular oncotic pressure.

Humoral Mediators of Renal Function

Renin–Angiotensin–Aldosterone System

- Renin is secreted by kidneys in response to sympathetic nervous system stimulation, decreased renal perfusion pressure, and decreases in sodium delivery to the distal convoluted renal tubules.
- Renin acts on angiotensinogen to form angiotensin I.
- Angiotensin I is converted in the lungs to angiotensin II.
- Angiotensin II, a potent vasoconstrictor, stimulates the release of aldosterone from the adrenal cortex.
- Aldosterone stimulates reabsorption of sodium and water in the distal tubule and collecting ducts.

Prostaglandins

- Released by kidney in response to sympathetic nervous system stimulation, hypotension, and increased angiotensin II levels
- Attenuates the effects on the kidney by arginine vasopressin (AVP), norepinephrine, and the renin–angiotensin system.
- Vasodilates juxtamedullary vessels and maintains cortical blood flow
  - Prostaglandin inhibitors (e.g., aspirin) may inhibit this protective effect.

Arginine Vasopressin

- Secreted from hypothalamus
- Decreases serum osmolality and increases urine osmolality; facilitates water reabsorption

Atrial Natriuretic Peptide

- Secreted when stretch receptors in the atria are stimulated by increased intravascular volume
- Relaxes vascular smooth muscle to cause vasodilation, inhibits the renin–angiotensin system, and stimulates diuresis and natriuresis

- Net effect is a decrease in systemic blood pressure and intravascular volume.

Drug Clearance

- Depends on glomerular filtration, active renal tubule secretion, passive tubule reabsorption.
- Facilitated by alkalinization or acidification of the urine, or drug conjugation

Renal Function Tests

Preoperative Screening Tests of Renal Function

- Renal function tests are not sensitive tests for renal impairment.
- Trends are more useful than a single laboratory measurement.
- >50% decrease in renal function can exist with normal laboratory values.

Serum Creatinine

- Reflects the balance between creatinine production by muscle and its renal excretion
- Is often used as a marker of GFR
- Serum creatinine may falsely reflect normal GFR due to decreased creatinine production, decreased skeletal muscle mass (as in older patients), or nonrenal creatinine excretion.

Blood Urea Nitrogen (BUN)

- Concentrations vary with protein metabolism and changes in GFR.
- The relationship between serum creatinine and BUN levels can help diagnose the cause of renal failure.

Creatinine Clearance

- Measures the ability of the glomeruli to excrete creatinine into the urine
- More accurate measure of GFR but requires a 24-hour urine collection

Proteinuria

- Multiple nonrenal causes including exercise, fever, and congestive heart failure

Urine Indices

- Osmolality, urinary sodium, and the fractional excretion of sodium help differentiate between prerenal and renal tubular causes of azotemia.

Newer Tests of Renal Function

- May provide better markers for GFR and the early detection of kidney injury

Pharmacology of Diuretics

Thiazide Diuretics

- Mobilize edema fluid from renal, hepatic, or cardiac dysfunction
- Inhibit sodium and chloride ion reabsorption from the distal renal tubules
- Hypokalemia is a possible side effect.

Loop Diuretics

- Inhibit sodium and chloride ion reabsorption and augment potassium secretion
- Chronic administration may result in hypochloremic, hypokalemic metabolic alkalosis, and deafness.

Osmotic Diuretics

- Increase osmolarity of the urine
- Redistribute intracellular fluid to extracellular compartments, which decreases intracranial pressure
- May acutely increase intravascular fluid volume prior to diuresis

Aldosterone Antagonists

- Block the renal tubular effects of aldosterone and offset the loss of potassium from administration of thiazide diuretics
- Hyperkalemia is the most serious side effect.

Dopamine and Fenoldopam

- Dilate renal arterioles, increasing renal blood flow and GFR
- May increase urine output at low doses
- A metaanalysis has not demonstrated an impact on postoperative renal replacement therapy or mortality after major surgery.
- Dose-dependent side effects of dopamine include tachydysrhythmias, pulmonary shunting, and tissue ischemia.

Pathophysiology of End-Stage Renal Disease

Cardiovascular Disease

- Cardiovascular disease is the predominant cause of death in patients with end-stage renal disease (ESRD).
- Hypertension can be severe and refractory.
  - Hypervolemia and excess activation of the renin–angiotensin–aldosterone system are the most common causes.
- Uremic toxins and metabolic acids may contribute to poor myocardial performance.

Metabolic Disease

- 30% to 40% of patients with ESRD have diabetes mellitus, and 60% of patients with insulin-dependent diabetes have nephropathy.

Anemia and Abnormal Coagulation

- Normochromic, normocytic anemia due to decreased erythropoiesis and retained toxins
- Platelet function can be affected by uremia in patients with renal failure.

Differential Diagnosis and Management of Perioperative Oliguria

Prerenal Oliguria

- Excretion of concentrated urine that contains minimal amounts of sodium
- Reflects an acute decrease in intravascular fluid volume or decreased cardiac output
- Replacement of intravascular fluid volume should increase urine output.
  - Intrinsic renal disease or renal perfusion causes should be investigated if urine output does not increase in response to intravenous fluids.

Intrinsic Renal Disease

- Causes: acute tubular necrosis, glomerulonephritis, and acute interstitial nephritis
- Urine is poorly concentrated and contains excessive sodium.
- Most severe cause of oliguria and typically difficult to reverse

Postrenal Oliguria

- Usually due to obstruction that is distal to the renal collecting system (e.g., blood clot)
- Frequently reversible once source is identified and removed

Postoperative Acute Kidney Injury

- Clinical syndrome that is usually multifactorial in cause
- Treatment of underlying causes may lead to resolution.

Management of Anesthesia in Patients With ESRD

- Patients with advanced stages of comorbid conditions such as heart failure or symptomatic coronary artery disease may require more extensive monitoring.
- Hemodialysis shunts or fistulas should be periodically monitored to confirm patency.
- Normal saline (NS) administration can cause more acidosis and hyperkalemia than potassium-containing solutions such as lactated Ringer's.
- Patients with uremia or gastroparesis are at increased risk for aspiration of gastric contents.
- Succinylcholine is not contraindicated in patients with ESRD, as the rise in serum potassium is approximately 0.6 mEq/L for patients with renal failure.
- Hypotension may be seen during maintenance of anesthesia, especially if patient was recently hemodialyzed.
- Drugs or their metabolites that depend on renal elimination should be used cautiously or avoided.
  - Morphine has an active metabolite that is renally excreted and can accumulate.
  - Sevoflurane has been safely used in patients with renal failure.

LIVER DISEASE

Physiologic Functions of the Liver
▪ Synthesis of essential plasma proteins
▪ Metabolism and detoxification of drugs
▪ Absorption of clinical nutrients
▪ Carbohydrate, fat, and hormone metabolism
▪ Glucose homeostasis
▪ Bilirubin formation and excretion

Hepatic Blood Flow

- Receives 25% of cardiac output: 70% by the portal vein and 30% by the hepatic artery
- Portal vein flow is not regulated and is susceptible to systemic hypotension and decreases in cardiac output.

Intrinsic Determinants of Hepatic Blood Flow

- Reduction in portal flow (up to a 50% reduction) is compensated for by modulating hepatic artery tone to maintain perfusion to the liver (mediated by adenosine).
- Volatile anesthetics and cirrhosis of the liver attenuate this buffer response and render the liver vulnerable to ischemia.

Extrinsic Determinants of Hepatic Blood Flow

- Splanchnic vascular resistance increases in response to splanchnic nerve stimulation (pain, arterial hypoxemia, surgical stress) and decreases hepatic blood flow.
- Surgical stimulation and the proximity of the operative site to the liver influence the magnitude of the decrease in hepatic blood flow seen during general anesthesia.
- β-Blockers, positive-pressure ventilation, congestive heart failure, and administration of excessive intravascular fluid can cause a reduction of hepatic blood flow.

Glucose Homeostasis

- Hepatocytes store glycogen by extracting glucose via an insulin-mediated mechanism.
- Glucagon-mediated catabolism of glycogen releases glucose back into the systemic circulation to maintain euglycemia, e.g., during times of surgical stress and starvation.

Coagulation

- Hepatocytes synthesize the majority of procoagulant proteins in addition to regulators such as proteins C and S and antithrombin III.
- An important exception is factor VIII, which is partially produced in endothelial cells.
- Most coagulation factors maintain normal function at 20% to 30% of their normal values.

Drug Metabolism

- Hepatic drug metabolism converts lipid-soluble drugs to more water-soluble forms to facilitate renal excretion and transformation to less active substances.
- Three major pathways are used: increasing polarity, conjugation to water-soluble substrates, and elimination by excretion.
- Hepatic enzymes necessary for drug metabolism are affected by many factors.
  - Hepatic enzymes are decreased by cirrhosis or can be inhibited or induced with chronic drug therapy.

Heme Metabolism

- Hepatic hematopoiesis accounts for 20% of adult heme synthesis.
- Heme degrades to form bilirubin, which binds to albumin and is transported to the liver.
- Bilirubin in the liver is mostly conjugated and excreted in bile.
  - A small amount is recirculated to the liver via the enterohepatic circulation.

Cholesterol and Lipid Metabolism

- The liver stores dietary fat as triglycerides, cholesterol, and phospholipids.
  - Free fatty acids are synthesized and released via triglyceride hydrolysis.
- Elimination of cholesterol is achieved by biliary secretion and by excretion of bile acids.

Protein Metabolism

- Numerous biologically active proteins, including albumin, cytokines, hormones, and coagulation factors, are synthesized in the liver.
- Proteins are metabolized and end-products (e.g., ammonia) are converted to urea and excreted by the kidney.

Pathophysiology of End-Stage Liver Disease

Cardiovascular Complications

- Hyperdynamic circulation: normal to low systemic blood pressure, increased cardiac output, and decreased systemic vascular resistance (vasodilation and physiologic shunting)

Portal Hypertension

- High resistance to blood flow through the liver causes blood vessel swelling in vascular beds immediately upstream of the liver, resulting in splenomegaly and esophageal, gastric, and intraabdominal varices.

Pulmonary Complications

- Hepatopulmonary syndrome: caused by intrapulmonary arteriovenous communications, impaired hypoxic pulmonary vasoconstriction, atelectasis, and restrictive pulmonary disease
  - Restrictive pulmonary disease is due to ascites and pleural effusions.
- Portopulmonary hypertension: increased pulmonary arterial pressure in patients with portal hypertension can lead to acute right-sided heart failure.

Hepatic Encephalopathy

- Altered mental state can range from minor changes in brain function to deep coma.
- Mechanism may be multifactorial.
- Treatment: lowering ammonia absorption from intestines (lactulose), antibiotics (neomycin, rifaximin), and other ancillary therapies

Impaired Drug Binding

- Decreased albumin production (usually plasma concentrations <2.5 g/dL) results in increased levels of unbound active fractions of drugs.

Ascites

- End-stage of cirrhosis and associated with significant morbidity
- Ascites can lead to marked abdominal distention, spontaneous bacterial peritonitis, and circulatory instability.
- Contributors: excessive sodium retention, decreased oncotic pressure, and portal hypertension
- Treatments: fluid intake restriction and diuresis, reduced sodium intake, paracentesis, and transjugular intrahepatic portosystemic shunt

Renal Dysfunction and Hepatorenal Syndrome

- Hepatorenal syndrome (HRS) associated with acute kidney injury (AKI) is rapidly progressing

renal failure with poor prognosis in the absence of therapeutic intervention.
  - Characterized by intense renal vasoconstriction
  - Etiologies: decreased intravascular volume (ascites, gastrointestinal hemorrhage), diuretics, nephrotoxic drugs, and sepsis
- Renal dysfunction in patients with end-stage liver disease (ESLD) with a more gradual increase in serum creatinine is considered chronic kidney disease.

Effects of Anesthesia and Surgery on the Liver

Impact of Anesthetics on Hepatic Blood Flow

- Inhaled anesthetics and regional anesthesia decrease hepatic blood flow by 20% to 30% in the absence of surgical stimulation.
- Hepatic autoregulation helps maintain hepatic blood flow under general anesthesia with volatile anesthetics.

Volatile Anesthetic-Induced Hepatic Dysfunction

- Mild: can occur in up to 20% of patients with minimal sequelae
- Life-threatening: occurs rarely, mostly in patients receiving halothane (highly metabolized)
  - Risk factors: prior exposure to halothane, age >40 years, obesity, and female sex
  - Fatality rate is 50% to 70%.

Management of Anesthesia in Patients With End-Stage Liver Disease

Principles of Perioperative Liver Disease Management

- Inhaled anesthetics and regional anesthesia decrease hepatic blood flow 20% to 30%.
- Preoperative Model of End-Stage Liver Disease (MELD) score correlates with postoperative mortality.
- No optimal anesthetic technique has been established for the maintenance of anesthesia.
- Advances in point-of-care coagulation technology allow the clinician to rapidly diagnose and manage coagulopathy.

Preoperative Evaluation of Liver Disease

- Liver function tests: nonspecific, and results can be normal even in a patient with considerable liver damage
- Preoperative MELD score correlates with postoperative mortality.
  - Incorporation of serum sodium into the MELD score (MELD-Na score) improves its accuracy in predicting mortality in liver transplant patients.
- Other risk prediction tools include one from Mayo Clinic that incorporates MELD, age, and American Society of Anesthesiologists (ASA) physical status class.

Intraoperative Management

- Invasive monitoring may be needed for surgeries where significant blood loss is likely.
  - Transesophageal echocardiogram in patients with esophageal varices has an increased risk of bleeding.
  - Correction of coagulopathy should be considered before major surgeries.
  - Blood bank should ensure availability of blood products.
- No optimal anesthetic technique has been established for the maintenance of anesthesia as long as arterial blood pressure, and thus hepatic blood flow, is maintained.

Management of Coagulopathy

- Surgical blood loss due to coagulopathy is managed by administering blood products and factor concentrates as clinically indicated.
- Advances in point-of-care coagulation technology allow the clinician to rapidly diagnose and manage coagulopathy.

Postoperative Jaundice

- Surgical cause is likely if the operation involved the liver or biliary tract.
- Liver function tests can help classify whether the cause of postoperative liver dysfunction is prehepatic, intrahepatic, or posthepatic.

DISEASES OF THE BILIARY TRACT

Bile Metabolism and Secretion

- Bile is an aqueous secretion that originates from hepatocytes.
- Functions to excrete exogenous and endogenous substances, emulsify dietary fats to facilitate intestinal absorption, eliminate cholesterol, assist with immunoprotection, and excrete hormones and pheromones

Pathophysiology of the Biliary Tract

- Gallstones: higher prevalence in women (particularly during pregnancy), patients with obesity, and those >40 years of age
  - Cholangitis and acute cholecystitis are usually associated with fever.

- Gallbladder cancer: linked to chronic infection and environmental, dietary, and genetic factors
  - Typically has delayed presentation of symptoms; difficult to treat
- Gilbert syndrome: benign disorder causing elevation in unconjugated bilirubin
- Dubin-Johnson and Rotor syndromes: congenital disorders leading to elevated conjugated bilirubin levels

Management of Anesthesia for Biliary Tract Surgery

- Anesthetic management should account for the effect of anesthetic drugs on intraluminal pressure in the biliary tract.
  - Opioids can produce spasm of choledochoduodenal sphincter, increasing common bile duct pressure.
    - Can impair passage of contrast medium into the duodenum
    - Can erroneously suggest the presence of common bile duct stones
    - Treatment options include naloxone, glucagon, and nitroglycerin.

Laparoscopic Cholecystectomy

- Anesthetic considerations for laparoscopy apply.
- The anesthetic plan should include monitoring of end-tidal CO_2, avoidance of nitrous oxide, and preparation for the conversion to laparotomy.

QUESTIONS

RENAL DISEASE

1. Name some risk factors for postoperative acute kidney injury.
2. What is the mechanism for renal blood flow autoregulation? What is the range of renal arterial blood pressures through which autoregulation is maintained?
3. Even during normal kidney autoregulatory function, what factor can alter renal blood flow?
4. What are some factors that influence the GFR?
5. Does afferent arteriolar vasoconstriction increase or decrease GFR? What is the mechanism for this effect?
6. For each humoral mediator, name what stimulates its secretion and its effect(s) on renal function.

Humoral Mediator	Secreted in Response to	Renal Effects
Renin		
Angiotensin II		
Aldosterone		
Prostaglandins		
Arginine vasopressin		
Atrial natriuretic peptide		

7. How are drugs excreted into the urine?
8. How sensitive are laboratory tests of renal function?
9. How does the serum creatinine help estimate renal function? What are its limitations?
10. Write the formula to estimate GFR from the serum creatinine.
11. How does the BUN concentration help estimate renal function? What are some causes of increased BUN concentration?
12. How does the serum creatinine help determine the cause of an elevated BUN concentration?
13. Why is the creatinine clearance a more reliable measurement of the GFR than serum creatinine, and what is its disadvantage?
14. How does proteinuria reflect renal function, and what are some nonrenal causes of proteinuria?
15. For a patient with oliguria, what is the use of measuring urine osmolality and urinary sodium and calculating the fractional excretion of sodium?
16. Why might the newly identified markers of renal function (e.g., serum cystatin C, *N*-acetyl-β-D-glucosaminidase, kidney injury molecule-1, and interleukin-18) be beneficial in the perioperative period?
17. What are the differences in site of action of thiazide, spironolactone, loop, and osmotic diuretics?
18. What are the differences in pharmacologic action between dopamine and fenoldopam?
19. Complete the following table by listing the pathophysiologic changes characteristic of chronic renal disease for each organ system.

Organ System	Effects of Chronic Renal Disease
Cardiac	
Vascular	
Metabolic	
Hematologic	

20. Complete the following table comparing prerenal, intrinsic, and postrenal causes of oliguria. For prerenal and intrinsic, indicate whether the laboratory analysis of the urine will result in concentrated or dilute, and minimal or excessive sodium.

Oliguria	Urine	Causes	Management
Prerenal			
Intrinsic			
Postrenal	No clear trends		

21. How is postoperative acute kidney injury defined?
22. What are some anesthetic considerations for the anesthetic management of patients with end-stage renal disease (ESRD)?
23. Should succinylcholine be avoided in patients with ESRD?
24. Is lactated Ringer's solution contraindicated for fluid resuscitation in patients with ESRD?

LIVER DISEASE

25. What is the blood supply to the liver? What percent of the cardiac output goes to the liver?
26. What is the hepatic arterial buffer response, and which anesthetic agent can affect this response?
27. How does sympathetic nervous stimulation affect hepatic blood flow?
28. Name some intraoperative factors that can affect hepatic blood flow.
29. What is the role of the liver in glucose homeostasis?
30. What is the role of the liver in blood coagulation? How is this reflected clinically and in laboratory values for patients with chronic liver disease?
31. What is the role of the liver in drug metabolism, and how is this affected by chronic liver disease?
32. What is the role of the liver in hematopoiesis and heme degradation, and what is the clinical impact for patients with chronic liver disease?
33. What is the role of the liver in cholesterol and lipid metabolism?
34. What is the role of the liver in protein metabolism, and what is the clinical impact for patients with chronic liver disease?
35. Complete the following table by listing the pathophysiologic changes characteristic of end-stage liver disease (ESLD).

Organ System	Effects of End-Stage Liver Disease
Cardiovascular	
Pulmonary	
Neurologic	
Renal	

36. Describe the pathophysiology, symptoms, and potential complications of portal hypertension.
37. Why might a patient with ESLD have arterial hypoxemia? How effective is oxygen supplementation for these patients?
38. What are some causes of, and treatment for, hepatic encephalopathy seen in patients with ESLD?
39. What is the role of the liver in drug binding to serum proteins, and what is the clinical impact for patients with ESLD?
40. Describe the pathophysiology, complications, and treatment for ascites seen in patients with ESLD.
41. Describe the pathophysiology and treatment for hepatorenal syndrome associated with acute kidney injury (HRS-AKI).
42. In the absence of surgical stimulation, how do regional and inhaled anesthetics affect hepatic blood flow?
43. What is halothane hepatitis and its pathophysiology? Which patients are most at risk?

44. What is the use of liver function tests to evaluate liver function in the preoperative period?
45. What is the utility of the preoperative Model of End-Stage Liver Disease (MELD) score?
46. What intraoperative monitoring may be useful for patients with ESLD undergoing surgical procedures?
47. What is the advantage of point of care coagulation testing relative to standard laboratory testing in the perioperative setting for patients with ESLD?
48. What are the most common causes of postoperative jaundice?
49. What laboratory values indicate an intrahepatic cause of liver dysfunction?
50. Complete the table below by listing prehepatic, intrahepatic, and posthepatic causes of postoperative liver dysfunction.

Causes of Postoperative Liver Dysfunction	Prehepatic	Intrahepatic	Posthepatic

DISEASES OF THE BILIARY TRACT

51. How is bile synthesized, and what is its function?
52. What is the role of the gallbladder, and who is at risk for the formation of gallstones?
53. What are the potential etiologies of gallbladder cancer?
54. What is Gilbert syndrome?
55. What is the potential problem with the use of opioids intraoperatively during a cholecystectomy or common bile duct exploration?
56. How can intraoperative spasm of the choledochoduodenal sphincter be treated?
57. What are some anesthetic considerations for patients undergoing laparoscopic cholecystectomy?

ANSWERS

RENAL DISEASE

1. Risk factors for postoperative acute kidney injury are listed in the table below. (498–499)

Risk Factors for Postoperative Acute Kidney Injury	
	GFR <60 mL/min/1.73 m^2
	Diabetes mellitus
	Age >50 years
	Male sex
	Heart failure
	Ascites
	Hypertension
	Emergency surgery
	Intraperitoneal surgery
	Increased number of chronic medications
	Use of ACE inhibitors or ARBs
	High ASA physical status score
	Albuminuria

2. Renal blood flow and the glomerular filtration rate (GFR) remain constant when the mean renal arterial blood pressure is between 80 mmHg and 180 mmHg. This autoregulatory function of the kidneys is accomplished by the afferent arteriolar vascular bed. The afferent arterioles adjust their tone in response to changes in blood pressure, such that during times of higher arterial blood pressure the afferent arterioles vasoconstrict, whereas the opposite occurs during times of lower arterial blood pressure. The ability of the kidneys to maintain constant renal blood flow despite fluctuations in blood pressure ensures continued renal tubular function in the face of changes, especially decreases, in blood pressure. In addition, autoregulatory responses of the afferent arterioles protect the glomerular capillaries from large increases in blood pressure during times of hypertension, as may occur with direct laryngoscopy. When mean arterial blood pressures are <80 mmHg or >180 mmHg, renal blood flow is blood pressure dependent. (498–499)
3. Sympathetic nervous system stimulation can produce renal vasoconstriction and a marked decrease in renal blood flow, even if systemic blood pressure is within the autoregulatory range. (498–499)
4. The glomerular filtration rate (GFR) is dependent on the glomerular filtration pressure (GFP). Factors that influence the GFP (and therefore GFR) include the renal artery pressure, afferent and efferent renal arteriolar tone, and glomerular oncotic pressure. (499)
5. Afferent arteriolar vasoconstriction decreases GFR by decreasing glomerular flow. Conversely, afferent arteriolar dilation and mild efferent vasoconstriction increase GRP and GFR. (499)
6. The precipitating event and renal effects of given humoral mediators are represented in the following table. (499–500)

Humoral Mediator	Secreted in Response to	Renal Effects
Renin	Sympathetic nervous system stimulation Decreased renal perfusion pressure Decreased sodium delivery to the distal renal tubules	Acts on angiotensinogen to form angiotensin I, which then gets converted to angiotensin II Net effect is release of aldosterone from the adrenal cortex
Angiotensin II	Angiotensin I (formed in response to renin) is converted to angiotensin II	Stimulates the release of aldosterone Low levels: increases efferent renal arteriolar tone Higher levels: afferent arteriolar vasoconstriction Inhibits renin (negative feedback loop)
Aldosterone	Angiotensin II (via renin)	Stimulates sodium and water reabsorption in the distal tubule and collecting ducts
Prostaglandins	Sympathetic nervous system stimulation Hypotension Elevated levels of angiotensin II	Attenuates the effects of arginine vasopressin, norepinephrine, and renin-angiotensin system by vasodilating vessels and maintaining cortical blood flow
Arginine vasopressin	Small increases in plasma osmolality Hypotension	Facilitates water reabsorption Decreases serum osmolality Increases urine osmolality
Atrial natriuretic peptide	Increased intravascular volume (stretch receptors in atria)	Inhibits the renin-angiotensin system Stimulates diuresis and natriuresis Decreases systemic blood pressure and intravascular volume

7. The excretion of drugs or their metabolites into the urine depends on three mechanisms: (1) glomerular filtration, (2) active secretion by the renal tubules, and (3) passive reabsorption by the tubules. The liver also plays a role through conjugation of drugs to water-soluble metabolites. (500–501)
8. Most laboratory tests of renal function are not very sensitive; it is estimated that a >50% decrease in renal function may exist before these tests become abnormal. A patient's renal function test result trends may be more useful than an isolated measurement. (501)
9. Serum creatinine reflects the balance of skeletal muscle protein catabolism and renal excretion, serving as a marker for GFR. A limitation of serum creatinine is that patients with low muscle mass, such as elderly patients, may have a normal creatinine level despite a decreased GFR. For this reason, even mild increases in the serum creatinine level of older patients may be an indication of significant renal dysfunction. (501)

10. The GFR can be estimated from serum creatinine using the formula below. (501)

$$\text{GFR} = (140 - \text{age}) \times \text{weight in kg}/(\text{serum creatinine} \times 72)$$

11. The BUN varies with GFR, but other factors unrelated to GFR may also increase the BUN concentration. Factors that may increase the BUN level include increased dietary protein intake, gastrointestinal bleeding, low urinary flow, and increased catabolism as during trauma, sepsis, or febrile illness. During low urinary flow rates, a greater fraction of the urea is reabsorbed by the kidney and the BUN concentration increases. Blood urea nitrogen concentrations >50 mg/dL are almost always a reflection of decreased GFR. (501)
12. The ratio of BUN to creatinine can be helpful to understand the cause of an elevated BUN concentration. During low urinary flow rates, the serum creatinine level remains normal, and the ratio of serum BUN to creatinine is increased. Other causes of a high BUN:creatinine ratio include gastrointestinal bleeding and congestive heart failure. A low BUN:creatinine ratio may reflect low protein intake or advanced liver disease. (501)
13. The creatinine clearance, a measurement of the creatinine excreted into the urine, is a more reliable measurement of GFR than serum creatinine or BUN levels because the clearance does not depend on corrections for age, or the presence of a steady state. A disadvantage of creatinine clearance measurements is the requirement of accurate, timed urine collections. (501–502)
14. The normal kidney filters, then reabsorbs protein. Patients with proteinuria are more likely to have abnormally high filtration rather than impaired renal tubular reabsorption. Healthy individuals may have intermittent proteinuria after standing for long periods of time and after strenuous exercise. Proteinuria may also occur during febrile states and congestive heart failure. (502)
15. Urine osmolality, urinary sodium, and the fractional excretion of sodium help determine if azotemia is due to prerenal or renal tubular causes. (502)
16. The newly identified markers of renal function (e.g., serum cystatin C, *N*-acetyl-β-D-glucosaminidase, kidney injury molecule-1, and interleukin-18) may be beneficial in the perioperative period because they allow earlier detection of kidney injury and are less influenced by variations in muscle mass and nutrition. (502)
17. Thiazide diuretics cause diuresis by inhibition of reabsorption of sodium and chloride ions from the early distal renal tubules. Spironolactone, an aldosterone antagonist, blocks the renal tubular effects of aldosterone. Spironolactone is a potassium-sparing diuretic. Loop diuretics inhibit the reabsorption of sodium and chloride and augment the secretion of potassium primarily in the loop of Henle. Osmotic diuretics, such as mannitol, produce diuresis by being filtered at the glomeruli but not reabsorbed by the renal tubules. The excess osmolarity of the renal tubular fluid leads to excretion of water. (502)
18. Dopamine dilates renal arterioles by its agonist action at the DA-1 receptor and causes adrenergic stimulation leading to an increase in renal blood flow and GFR. Dopamine therapy when used to augment urine output has not been shown to alter the course of renal failure. Dopamine also potentially leads to tachydysrhythmias, pulmonary shunting, and tissue ischemia. Fenoldopam is a dopamine analog that also possesses DA-1 agonist activity but lacks the adrenergic activity of dopamine. (502)
19. Pathophysiologic changes characteristic of chronic renal disease are represented in the following table. (503)

Organ System	Effects of Chronic Renal Disease
Cardiac	Cardiac dysrhythmias Cardiomyopathy Decreased ejection fraction Pericardial effusions
Vascular	Hypertension (can be severe and refractory) Unpredictable intravascular fluid volume Elevated serum triglycerides (progressive atherosclerosis)
Metabolic	Sodium, potassium, calcium, magnesium, and phosphate abnormalities Hyperkalemia is the most life-threatening Metabolic acidosis Diabetes mellitus often accompanies end-stage renal disease
Hematologic	Anemia (normochromic, normocytic from decreased erythropoietin) Decreased platelet adhesiveness (uremia)

20. The following table compares prerenal, intrinsic, and postrenal causes of oliguria. (503, 504)

Oliguria	Urine	Causes	Management
Prerenal	Concentrated Minimal sodium	Decreased intravascular fluid volume Decreased cardiac output Sepsis Liver failure Compression of renal arteries (eg, surgical retraction, clamping)	Fluid volume challenge Drug-related diuresis is controversial (diuretics, dopamine)
Intrinsic	Dilute Excessive sodium	Acute tubular necrosis Glomerulonephritis Interstitial nephritis Renal ischemia Nephrotoxins	Maintain renal perfusion (most difficult to reverse)
Postrenal	**No clear trends**	Obstruction of ureter, bladder, or Foley catheter (eg, blood clots, stones, kinking of catheter)	Removal of the underlying cause (usually reversible)

21. In 2021, a consensus group recommended that postoperative acute kidney injury (AKI) be defined using the criteria established by the Kidney Disease Improving Global Outcomes (KDIGO). Using the KDIGO criteria, the patient is diagnosed with AKI if any of the following are met within 7 days of an operative intervention:
    - Increase in serum creatinine by ≥0.3 mg/dL (≥26.5 μmol/L) within 48 hours
    - Increase in serum creatinine to ≥1.5 times baseline within the prior 7 days
    - Urine volume <0.5 mL/kg/hr for 6 hours
    - (504–505)
22. There are several considerations for the anesthetic management of patients with end-stage renal disease (ESRD). These patients may benefit from extensive monitoring, such as direct arterial blood pressure monitoring and perhaps central venous pressure monitoring depending on the surgical case, comorbidities, and other factors. Hypotension can commonly occur in patients with ESRD, particularly after hemodialysis. Patients with arteriovenous fistulas should have the presence of the thrill monitored during positioning and intraoperatively. Patients with gastroparesis should be considered at increased risk for the aspiration of gastric contents. Electrolytes, especially potassium, may need to be evaluated preoperatively and intraoperatively. Finally, drugs or their metabolites that are renally excreted should be administered judiciously or avoided if possible. (504–505)
23. Succinylcholine is not necessarily contraindicated in patients with ESRD unless the baseline serum potassium level is markedly elevated. The increase in serum potassium after a 1-mg/kg dose of succinylcholine is approximately 0.6 mEq/L for patients both with and without ESRD. This increase can be tolerated without imposing a significant cardiac risk, even in the presence of an initial serum potassium concentration as high as 5 mEq/L. (505)
24. Normal saline (NS) had previously been recommended over lactated Ringer's (LR) solution for fluid resuscitation in patients with ESRD. This was due to the hypothesized risk of hyperkalemia from potassium contained in LR. The concern appears unfounded, however, as prospective randomized clinical trials comparing the two fluid therapies has shown greater hyperkalemia and acidosis with intraoperative therapy using NS. (505)

LIVER DISEASE

25. The liver receives its blood supply via the portal vein (70%) and hepatic artery (30%). Approximately 25% of the cardiac output goes to the liver. While the portal vein supplies 70% of hepatic blood supply, it only contributes 50% of the liver's oxygen supply. The remaining 50% of the liver's oxygen supply comes from the hepatic artery. (505)
26. The hepatic arterial buffer response refers to adjustments in hepatic artery tone to increase hepatic artery blood flow in response to a reduction in portal blood flow. Volatile anesthetics attenuate the response, leaving the liver vulnerable to ischemia. (505)
27. Generalized sympathetic nervous system stimulation, as can occur with arterial hypoxemia or hypercarbia, pain, or surgical stress, results in an increase in the splanchnic vascular resistance. The increase in splanchnic vascular resistance yields a decrease in portal vein blood flow, and therefore hepatic blood flow. (505–506)

28. Multiple intraoperative factors can affect hepatic blood flow. Decreases in arterial blood pressure and surgical retraction can both directly decrease the hepatic blood supply. Positive-pressure ventilation of the lungs, the application of positive end-expiratory pressure, and excessive intravascular volume (e.g., excessive intravenous fluid administration or congestive heart failure) can all increase hepatic venous pressure, decrease the hepatic perfusion pressure, and decrease hepatic blood flow. (506)
29. The liver stores glucose as glycogen in the hepatocytes. Glucose homeostasis is maintained during times of stress (e.g., starvation, surgery) through sympathetic nervous system stimulated breakdown of glycogen stores to glucose for release into the circulation. Prolonged stress that results in the depletion of the glycogen stores requires that the liver convert lactate, glycerol, and amino acids to glucose. This is termed *gluconeogenesis*. Patients with advanced liver disease can have impaired gluconeogenesis and are prone to hypoglycemia in the perioperative period. (506)
30. Hepatocytes synthesize most of the procoagulant proteins, except for factor VIII. Bleeding can be prevented with only 20% to 30% of normal levels of clotting factors, so that abnormal blood coagulation manifests only after significant liver disease. When the patient's prothrombin time, partial thromboplastin time, and fibrinogen levels become impaired it reflects significant hepatic dysfunction. (506)
31. The liver facilitates the renal excretion of lipid soluble drugs by converting the drugs to more water-soluble forms via mechanisms such as conjugation. Chronic liver disease may interfere with the metabolism of drugs because of the decreased number of enzyme-containing hepatocytes or the decreased hepatic blood flow that typically accompanies cirrhosis of the liver. This can be reflected as prolonged elimination half-times for certain drugs, such as morphine or vecuronium. Of note, chronic drug therapy can accelerate some drug metabolism by inducing hepatic enzymes, particularly the cytochrome P isoforms. (507)
32. The liver accounts for 20% of adult heme synthesis. Heme degradation results in bilirubin as an end-product, which is then conjugated in the liver making it water soluble for renal excretion. Chronic liver disease impairs this function of the liver and can lead to increased serum levels of unconjugated bilirubin. (507)
33. The liver regulates both cholesterol and lipids, through a balance of metabolism, uptake, and biliary excretion. (507)
34. Almost all proteins are synthesized in hepatocytes, including albumin, cytokines, hormones, and coagulation factors. The liver also degrades proteins, and via the urea cycle converts the end products of amino acid degradation (e.g., ammonia, nitrogenous waste products), to urea for renal excretion. Severe hepatic dysfunction can lead to the accumulation of serum ammonia, contributing to hepatic encephalopathy. (507–508)
35. Pathophysiologic changes characteristic of end-stage liver disease (ESLD) are represented in the following table. (508–509)

Organ System	Effects of End-Stage Liver Disease
Cardiovascular	Hyperdynamic circulation: low systemic blood pressure, increased cardiac output, and decreased systemic vascular resistance (due to vasodilation and shunting) Portal hypertension: splenomegaly and esophageal, gastric, and intraabdominal varices
Pulmonary	Hepatopulmonary syndrome: intrapulmonary shunting, impairment of hypoxic pulmonary vasoconstriction, atelectasis, and restrictive lung disease due to ascites and pleural effusions Portopulmonary hypertension: increased pulmonary arterial pressure Hepatic hydrothorax (pleural effusion in the absence of cardiopulmonary disease)
Neurologic	Altered mental status (from mild cognitive dysfunction to hepatic encephalopathy)
Renal	Renal dysfunction: chronic intravascular hypovolemia due to diuretics or ascites, nephrotoxic drugs, gastrointestinal hemorrhage Hepatorenal syndrome (HRS) associated with AKI (HRS-AKI) Chronic kidney disease

36. Portal hypertension is caused by the high resistance of blood flow through the liver. This results in an accumulation of blood in the vascular beds that normally drain to the liver, making these vessels dilate and hypertrophy. Vessels draining the esophagus, stomach, spleen, and intestines are affected, resulting in varices. Some of the signs and symptoms of portal hypertension include anorexia, nausea, ascites, esophageal varices, spider nevi, and hepatic encephalopathy. Complications that can occur from portal hypertension include increased susceptibility to infection, renal failure, mental status changes, and massive hemorrhage through the rupture of the engorged dilated submucosal veins. Gastroesophageal varices are at the greatest risk of rupture. (508)

37. Patients with hepatopulmonary syndrome associated with ESLD may have arterial hypoxemia due to intrapulmonary shunting and impaired lung expansion due to ascites and pleural effusions. In the early stages of ESLD supplemental oxygen may improve arterial hypoxemia, but as the disease progresses oxygen therapy may not be effective. (508)
38. The cause of hepatic encephalopathy seen in patients with ESLD is multifactorial. Hepatic encephalopathy is in part due to increased serum concentrations of chemicals normally cleared by the liver, especially ammonia. Other factors include the disruption of the blood–brain barrier, increased central nervous system inhibitory neurotransmission, and altered cerebral energy metabolism. Therapy for hepatic encephalopathy revolves around reducing the production and absorption of ammonia. Neomycin is used to reduce ammonia production by urease-producing bacteria, and lactulose is administered to reduce ammonia absorption. Some symptoms of hepatic encephalopathy are reversible with flumazenil therapy. These therapies are not completely effective because multiple other etiologic factors are associated with hepatic encephalopathy. It is also important to rule out other causes of altered mental status in the patient with ESLD, such as intracranial bleeding, hypoglycemia, or a postictal state. (508)
39. The liver synthesizes albumin, which binds drugs in the plasma to decrease the free, or pharmacologically active, portion of the drug. In patients with ESLD, the synthesis of albumin becomes impaired; with decreased available albumin, there is an increased concentration of free, unbound drug in the plasma. Patients with liver disease may manifest a more pronounced drug effect than patients with normal liver function after an intravenous injection of a specific drug dose. Increased drug effect secondary to a decrease in protein binding is more likely to be seen when the serum albumin concentration is <2.5 g/dL. (508)
40. Ascites affects 50% of patients with ESLD. Ascites is thought to accumulate secondary to a decrease in plasma oncotic pressure, a corresponding increase in the hydrostatic pressure in the hepatic sinusoids, and an increase in sodium retention by the kidneys due to increased circulating levels of antidiuretic hormone. Complications associated with ascites include marked abdominal distention that can lead to atelectasis and restrictive pulmonary disease, spontaneous bacterial peritonitis, and circulatory instability due to compression of the inferior vena cava and right atrium. The treatment for ascites is initially fluid restriction, reduced sodium intake, and diuretic therapy. In severe cases abdominal paracentesis temporarily reduces abdominal distention and restores hemodynamic stability. Patients with refractory ascites may be candidates for a transjugular intrahepatic portosystemic shunt (TIPS) procedure. (508–509)
41. Patients with ESLD tend to have a decrease in arterial blood volume, renal blood flow, and GFR, resulting in chronic, progressive renal disease with gradually rising serum creatinine. In contrast, hepatorenal syndrome associated with acute kidney injury (HRS-AKI) is characterized by intense renal vasoconstriction and presents as rapidly progressing prerenal failure with poor prognosis in the absence of therapeutic intervention. HRS-AKI is amenable to treatment, which includes 20% to 25% albumin administration, withdrawal of diuretics, vasoconstrictors (e.g., terlipressin, norepinephrine, or combined midodrine/octreotide), and reversal of precipitating factors. (509)
42. In the absence of surgical stimulation, regional and inhaled anesthetics decrease hepatic blood flow by 20% to 30%. Changes in hepatic blood flow in response to regional and inhaled anesthetics are believed to result from decreases in cardiac output, mean arterial pressure, or both. Volatile anesthetics may also decrease hepatic blood flow by impairing hepatic autoregulation to varying degrees. (509)
43. There are two different forms of hepatotoxicity that can result from the administration of halothane. Halothane hepatitis typically refers to the extremely rare, but more severe hepatotoxicity that can result in hepatic necrosis and death. Although the exact cause of halothane hepatitis is unclear, it is believed to be due to an immunologic response to a toxic metabolite of halothane. Patients most likely to be affected are middle-aged, obese women who have had repeated administration of halothane anesthesia. (509)
44. Liver function tests may be useful preoperatively in detecting the presence of liver disease. However, liver function tests are nonspecific, and significant liver dysfunction must occur before it is reflected in most tests. Despite this, liver function tests have some utility when incorporated into risk calculators such as the Model of End-Stage Liver Disease (MELD) score. Preoperative measurement of the hematocrit and coagulation status can guide ordering of packed red blood cells, fresh frozen plasma, platelets, or other factors prior to surgery. Preoperative testing may indicate the need for correction of coagulopathy prior to surgery at high-risk for bleeding, or prior to vascular line placement in patients with severe coagulopathy. (509)
45. The preoperative MELD score correlates with postoperative mortality. Incorporation of serum sodium into the MELD score calculation (MELD-Na score) improves its accuracy in predicting mortality in patients listed for liver transplantation. However, the MELD-Na score has not been evaluated as a postoperative surgical risk predictor. (510)
46. Intraoperative monitoring for patients with ESLD should be guided by the surgical procedure. In general, monitoring of the arterial blood pressure with an intraarterial catheter may be useful to ensure arterial blood

pressure, and thus hepatic blood flow, is maintained. This is especially true since patients with cirrhosis are commonly intravascularly depleted and can have low systemic blood pressure during maintenance anesthesia. The intraarterial catheter will allow for closer monitoring and quicker response to fluctuations in arterial blood pressure, as well as monitoring of the arterial blood gases, pH, coagulation status, and glucose. In addition, the urine output should be closely monitored due to the risk of postoperative renal dysfunction that can occur in patients with severe liver disease. Central venous pressure or pulmonary artery catheter monitoring might be useful in the fluid management of patients with cardiomyopathy and congestive heart failure. The intravascular fluid balance of patients with ESLD, especially those with ascites, can be difficult to manage. Finally, the use of an intraoperative transesophageal echocardiogram may be useful to monitor myocardial function and intravascular fluid status, but in patients with esophageal varices there exists a risk of bleeding with its insertion. (510)

47. Recent advances in point of care coagulation technology allow the clinician to rapidly diagnose and manage coagulopathy associated with ESLD in the perioperative setting. Additional information, unavailable through conventional laboratory tests, such as clot strength, platelet function, and hyperfibrinolysis can be assessed rapidly at the bedside with these newer techniques. (511)
48. The most common causes of postoperative jaundice include multiple blood transfusions, drugs, metabolic or infectious causes, and resorption of surgical hematoma. Volatile anesthetics as a cause of postoperative jaundice is much less likely. (511–512)
49. Liver dysfunction may be classified as prehepatic, intrahepatic, or posthepatic through the evaluation of the results of the various liver function tests. Elevated aminotransferase enzymes, decreased albumin, and a prolonged prothrombin time are all indicative of an intrahepatic cause of liver dysfunction. These alterations are reflective of direct hepatocellular damage. (512)
50. This table lists prehepatic, intrahepatic, and posthepatic causes of postoperative liver dysfunction. (512)

Causes of Postoperative Liver Dysfunction	**Prehepatic**	**Intrahepatic**	**Posthepatic**
	Hemolysis Hematoma reabsorption Bilirubin overload from whole blood	Viruses Drugs Sepsis Arterial hypoxemia Congestive heart failure Cirrhosis	Stones Cancer Sepsis

DISEASES OF THE BILIARY TRACT

51. Bile is an aqueous secretion that originates from hepatocytes and is modified distally by absorptive and secretory transport systems in the bile duct epithelium. Bile functions to excrete exogenous and endogenous substances, emulsify dietary fats to facilitate intestinal absorption, eliminate cholesterol, assist with immunoprotection in the intestine, and excrete hormones and pheromones. (512)
52. The gallbladder stores bile, and actively adjusts biliary components during storage. The prevalence of gallstones is between 10% and 15% of the adult population, with a higher prevalence in women (particularly during pregnancy), patients with obesity, and those >40 years of age. (512)
53. Chronic infection, environmental exposure to chemicals, and dietary and genetic factors have all been linked to the development of gallbladder cancer. (512)
54. Gilbert syndrome is a benign disorder causing elevation in unconjugated bilirubin. It is one of the most common causes of jaundice and may occasionally be mistaken for postoperative hepatobiliary dysfunction. (512)
55. Opioids such as morphine, meperidine, and fentanyl may produce spasm in the choledochoduodenal sphincter. This increases the pressure in the common bile duct in a dose-dependent manner and may be painful to an awake patient. The administration of these medications intraoperatively could hinder the passage of contrast medium for exploration of the common bile duct. In clinical practice, however, the administration of opioids to these patients rarely results in difficulty with intraoperative cholangiograms. (512–513)
56. Intraoperative spasm of the choledochoduodenal sphincter can be treated with naloxone, glucagon, or nitroglycerin. (513)
57. Anesthetic considerations for patients undergoing laparoscopic procedures are consistent with other laparoscopic procedures. Included are the insufflation of the abdomen with carbon dioxide and the possible impairment of ventilation of the lungs in the presence of increased ventilatory requirements, the probable placement of the patient in the reverse Trendelenburg position, the risk of puncture of bowel or vessels, and the potential for nitrous oxide to expand bowel gas. (513)

Chapter

29 NUTRITIONAL, GASTROINTESTINAL, AND ENDOCRINE DISEASE

Solmaz Poorsattar Manuel and Sophia Poorsattar

NUTRITIONAL DISORDERS

Obesity

- Characterized by excessive accumulation and storage of adipose tissue
- Measures of obesity
  - Body mass index (BMI) (most commonly used)
  - Abdominal circumference
  - Body fat percentage
  - Waist-to-hip ratio
- Conditions associated with obesity that affect anesthesia care
  - Pulmonary
    - Obstructive sleep apnea
    - Obesity hypoventilation syndrome
    - Restrictive pulmonary physiology (impaired ventilation-perfusion matching)
    - Reduced functional residual capacity (rapid desaturation with apnea)
  - Cardiovascular
    - Hypertension and related structural heart disease
    - Pulmonary hypertension with cor pulmonale
  - Endocrine
    - Insulin resistance and diabetes mellitus

Perioperative Adverse Outcomes Independently Associated With Obesity

- Increased hospital length of stay
- Greater estimated blood loss
- Longer operative times
- Increased surgical site infections
- Increased risk of renal failure
- Prolonged assisted ventilation

- Metabolic syndrome
  - Definition: combination of metabolic risk factors associated with obesity
  - Associated with subsequent development of diabetes mellitus, cardiovascular disease, and surgical morbidity
  - Diagnosed by three of the following five criteria:
    - Abdominal obesity
    - Increased serum triglycerides
    - Decreased high-density lipoproteins
    - Hypertension
    - Increased fasting blood glucose

Perioperative Considerations

- Comorbid conditions must be actively sought and managed perioperatively.
- Use standard preoperative fasting guidelines.
- Sedative premedication
  - May cause increased respiratory depression
  - If used, titrate carefully.
- Anticipate logistical challenges with intravenous access, monitoring, and positioning.
  - May necessitate central venous access
  - Upper arm shape may affect noninvasive blood pressure (NIBP) accuracy.
  - OR table may be narrow relative to patient size.
  - Pressure point padding may be difficult.
- Airway and respiratory concerns
  - Increased risk of difficulty with mask ventilation, tracheal intubation
  - Potential for issues related to respiratory mechanics and gas exchange
  - Remain vigilant for postoperative airway and respiratory issues.

Benefits of Reverse Trendelenburg Positioning for Induction and Intubation in Obese Patients

- Increased functional residual capacity
- Improved ventilation-perfusion matching
- Easier mask ventilation and laryngoscopy

Bariatric Surgery

- Surgically assisted weight loss falls into three categories:
  - Gastric restriction (e.g., gastric banding, sleeve gastrectomy)

- Intestinal malabsorption (e.g., jejunoileal bypass)
- Combination of restriction and malabsorption (e.g., Roux-en-Y gastric bypass)

Malnutrition

- Defined as imbalance between energy expenditure and energy intake
  - Excess intake (e.g., obesity)
  - Deficient intake (e.g., undernutrition)
- Four subforms of undernutrition
  - Wasting (low weight for height)
  - Shunting (low height for age)
  - Underweight (low weight for age)
  - Micronutrient deficient
- Diagnosed by a combination of one phenotype and one etiologic criteria
  - Phenotype criteria: nonvolitional weight loss, low BMI, or reduced muscle mass
  - Etiologic criteria: reduced food intake or absorption, or underlying inflammation
- Organ system effects
  - Central nervous system
    - Cognitive dysfunction, fatigue
  - Cardiovascular
    - Reduced cardiac output, conduction disturbances
  - Respiratory
    - Respiratory muscle weakness, decreased respiratory compliance
  - Gastrointestinal
    - Impaired immune function, delayed gastric emptying
  - Musculoskeletal
    - Myopathy, reduced bone mass
  - Renal
    - Reduced glomerular filtration rate, increased total body water
  - Electrolyte and metabolic
    - Hypokalemia, hypocalcemia, hypoglycemia, metabolic acidosis
- Treatment of malnutrition
  - Aimed at balancing nutritional intake with energy needs
  - Nutritional supplementation may be indicated.
    - Enteral (oral or tube) feeding: preferred because of safety, cost, low complication rate
    - Parenteral (intravenous) feeding: required when gastrointestinal (GI) tract nonfunctional; associated with numerous complications

Perioperative Considerations

- Complications of malnutrition
  - Increased infection rate, poor wound healing, bacterial overgrowth in GI tract
  - Increased intensive care unit (ICU) length of stay and need for mechanical ventilator support
  - Increased hospital length of stay
  - Increased mortality after organ transplant, abdominal, or cardiothoracic surgeries
- Preoperative nutrition assessment
  - Comprehensive history and physical
  - Nutritional risk screening
  - Key laboratory testing
    - Examples: serum albumin, prealbumin, transferrin
- Perioperative optimization and management
  - Parenteral or enteral feedings for 7 to 10 days prior to elective surgery improve outcomes for severely malnourished patients.
  - TPN containing insulin requires regular glucose and electrolyte monitoring.
- Postoperative nutrition assessment
  - Patient's overall clinical course
  - Adequacy of wound healing
  - Trends in lean body mass, calorimetry, laboratory results

Refeeding Syndrome

- Metabolic disturbance that occurs after rapid nutritional repletion in a malnourished patient
- Hallmark: hypophosphatemia
- Potential sequelae
  - Tissue hypoxemia
  - Myocardial dysfunction
  - Respiratory failure
  - Hemolysis
  - Rhabdomyolysis
  - Seizures
- Prevention
  - Titration of nutritional repletion

GASTROINTESTINAL DISORDERS

Inflammatory Bowel Disease

- Inflammatory disorders of the small intestine and colon
  - Two principal types of inflammatory bowel disease (IBD)
    - Ulcerative colitis (mucosal inflammation)
    - Crohn disease (transmural inflammation)
  - Substantial overlap in presentation and characteristics
- Medical therapy aimed at alleviating symptom severity and not curative
- May require surgical intervention in advanced disease

Perioperative Considerations

- Risk for increased morbidity in patients with IBD
  - Patients who are malnourished, aged 60 to 80 years, on long-term immunosuppression, emergent surgery, treated in low-volume centers

- Comorbid conditions and disease complications must be actively sought and managed perioperatively.
  - Nutritional deficiencies
  - Coagulopathy
  - Hypovolemia
  - Electrolyte or acid-base disturbance
- Perioperative medication management
  - Thromboprophylaxis is recommended.
    - Increased risk for venous thromboembolic events in patients with IBD
  - Immunosuppressive medications may need to be held.
  - Glucocorticoids should continue throughout.
    - Supplemental stress dosing before surgery may be necessary.
- Cyclosporine may increase minimum alveolar concentration and enhance the potency of nondepolarizing neuromuscular blocking drugs.

Gastroesophageal Reflux Disease

- Gastroesophageal reflux disease (GERD) symptoms
  - Associated with reflux of gastric contents through lower esophageal sphincter into esophagus
  - Classic symptoms are heartburn and regurgitation
  - Occurs due to an imbalance of symptom-eliciting factors and defensive factors
- Conditions associated with GERD development
  - Hiatal hernia
  - Obesity
  - Pregnancy
  - Obstructive sleep apnea
  - Gastric hypersecretion
  - Gastric outlet obstruction
  - Gastric neuropathy
  - Increased intrabdominal pressure
- Treatment
  - Dietary and lifestyle modification
  - Antacids
  - Mucoprotective drugs
  - Prokinetic agents
  - Histamine$_2$-receptor antagonists
  - Proton pump inhibitors

Perioperative Considerations

- Elevated risk of aspiration at both induction and extubation

Risk Factors for Aspiration Pneumonitis
▪ Gastric fluid pH less than 2.5
▪ Volume of aspirate more than 0.4 mL/kg
▪ Aspirate containing particulate matter
▪ Pregnancy greater than 18 weeks' gestation

- Premedication
  - Consider antacids, histamine$_2$-receptor antagonists, prokinetic agents, proton pump inhibitors.
- Induction of anesthesia
  - Consider rapid-sequence induction and intubation (RSII).
    - If difficult intubation is anticipated, an awake intubation may be indicated.
  - Use of cricoid pressure controversial
- Emergence from anesthesia
  - Consider decompressing stomach with orogastric tube.
  - Elevate head of bed.
  - Ensure intact airway reflexes before extubation.
- Surgical management of GERD
  - For patients unable to tolerate medical therapy or with persistent symptoms requiring long-term therapy
  - Most common procedure is Nissen fundoplication.

ENDOCRINE DISORDERS

Diabetes Mellitus

- Disorder of impaired glucose, fat, and protein metabolism
  - Inadequate supply of insulin
  - Inadequate tissue response to insulin
  - Can be a combination of both
- Hallmark: increased circulating levels of serum glucose
  - Leads to microvascular and macrovascular lesions and end-organ dysfunction
- Four broad categories:
  - Type 1 diabetes mellitus (T1DM)—5%–10% of cases
    - Absent insulin production due to autoimmune destruction of pancreatic beta-cells
  - Type 2 diabetes mellitus (T2DM)—90%–95% of cases
    - Progressive loss of insulin secretion in combination with insulin resistance
    - Substantial overlap in presentation and characteristics of T1DM and T2DM
  - Gestational diabetes mellitus (GDM)
  - Diabetes due to other causes
- Classic symptoms
  - Polyuria
  - Polydipsia
  - Weight loss
  - Blurred vision
- Diagnosis
  - Glycated hemoglobin, or
  - Plasma glucose (fasting, 2-hour, or random)
- Treatment
  - Primary goal is glucose control.
  - Dietary and lifestyle modifications
  - Oral hypoglycemic medications
  - Subcutaneous or intravenous insulin therapy

Perioperative Considerations

- Evaluate for and optimize comorbid conditions prior to elective surgery.
- Perioperative medication management determined on an individual patient basis
- Avoid hypoglycemia and hyperglycemia in the perioperative period.
  - Blood glucose levels should be measured before and after surgery.
  - Intraoperative measurements determined on an individual patient basis
- Prevent ketoacidosis or nonketotic hyperosmolar syndrome.

General Guidelines for Perioperative Diabetic Medication Management
▪ Medication strategies should be determined on a case-by-case basis. ▪ Oral and/or noninsulin injectable hypoglycemic drugs may be held on the morning of surgery. ▪ Insulin dosing the nighttime prior to, or on the day of surgery may be reduced by 20% to 50% to prevent hypoglycemia associated with fasting.

Thyroid Disease

- Thyroid hormones
  - Triiodothyronine (T_3)
  - Thyroxine (T_4)
- Regulation by thyroid-stimulating hormone (TSH)
  - TSH secreted from anterior pituitary gland
- Thyroid disorders
  - Hypothyroidism and hyperthyroidism
  - Thyroid inflammation (thyroiditis)
  - Thyroid enlargement (goiter)

Hypothyroidism

- Deficient secretion of thyroid hormones
- Most common causes
  - Iodine deficiency
  - Autoimmune (Hashimoto thyroiditis)
- Symptoms
  - Unintentional weight gain, fatigue, constipation, heavy menstrual bleeding, hair loss, cold intolerance, bradycardia, and/or depression
  - Severe hypothyroidism manifestations
    - Altered mental status, hypoventilation, hypothermia, hypotension, congestive heart failure, hyponatremia, and/or hypoglycemia
- Laboratory tests
  - Elevated TSH levels and/or
  - Reduced T_4 levels
- Treatment
  - Thyroid hormone replacement
  - Stress dose steroids for severe cases with coexisting adrenal insufficiency

Perioperative Considerations

- Ensure medically euthyroid prior to elective surgeries.
- Continue medical therapy on the day of surgery.
- Screen for coexisting conditions.
  - Adrenal insufficiency, hypoglycemia, anemia, and hyponatremia
- Assess for a goiter.
- Patients with uncontrolled hypothyroidism
  - May be hypersensitive to respiratory depressants
  - May have reduced cardiac output and/or diminished baroreceptor reflexes
  - Anticipate intraoperative issues.
    - Hypothermia
    - Slow drug metabolism
    - Delayed emergence from anesthesia

Preoperative Risk Assessment of Patients With a Goiter
▪ Risks – Difficult intubation – Hemodynamic collapse on induction ▪ Symptoms – Dyspnea – Dysphagia – Hoarseness ▪ Imaging – Tracheal deviation – Tracheomalacia – Compression of great vessels – Retrosternal extension

Hyperthyroidism and Thyroid Storm

- Excess circulating thyroid hormone (T_3 or T_4)
- Most common causes
  - Autoimmune (Graves disease)
  - Toxic multinodular goiter
  - Thyroiditis
- Symptoms
  - Weight loss, muscle weakness, insomnia, heat intolerance, diarrhea, tremor, tachyarrhythmias, and/or anxiety
  - Goiters in severe cases
- Laboratory tests
  - Elevated serum T_4 and T_3
  - Reduced TSH level
- Treatment
  - Rapid management of symptoms with β-blockers
  - Long-term management
    - Thyroid suppression with medications
    - Radioactive iodine destruction
    - Surgical removal (i.e., thyroidectomy)

Perioperative Considerations

- Ensure medically euthyroid prior to elective surgeries.
- Continue medical therapy on the day of surgery.
- Patients with goiters
  - Evaluate for airway compromise or mediastinal extension.
- Patient with uncontrolled hyperthyroidism
  - β-Blockers to control intraoperative adrenergic overactivity
  - Avoidance of sympathomimetic drugs (e.g., ketamine and ephedrine)
  - Treat relative hypovolemia to minimize hemodynamic swings.
  - Look for exophthalmos (associated with increased risk of corneal abrasion).
- Thyroid storm
  - May be precipitated by laryngoscopy or surgical stimulation
  - Symptoms
    - Tachycardia, hemodynamic lability, fever, and/or diaphoresis
    - Lack of rigidity or respiratory acidosis (unlike malignant hyperthermia)
  - Management
    - Supportive care
    - Hydration
    - β-Blockade
    - Antithyroid medication
    - Removal of the precipitating cause

Thyroidectomy Postoperative Complications

- Potential immediate postoperative complications after thyroid surgery
  - Recurrent laryngeal nerve damage
    - Unilateral (hoarseness)
    - Bilateral (stridor)
  - Transient hoarseness
  - Neck hematoma
  - Acute hypocalcemia

Parathyroid Disease

- Major function of parathyroid glands: produce parathyroid hormone (PTH)
  - PTH regulates serum calcium and phosphate levels.
- Parathyroid disorders
  - Hyperparathyroidism
  - Hypoparathyroidism
- Primary hyperparathyroidism
  - Excess levels of PTH and calcium
  - Symptoms
    - Most commonly asymptomatic hypercalcemia
    - Can have bone pain, dehydration, altered mental status
  - Treatment
    - Surgical removal of abnormal parathyroid gland
- Secondary hyperparathyroidism
  - Most commonly from chronic kidney disease or vitamin D deficiency
  - Hospitalized patients
    - PTH-related peptide secretion from malignant tumors is most common cause of hypercalcemia.
- Hypoparathyroidism
  - Most commonly from postsurgical or autoimmune destruction of parathyroid glands
  - Pseudohypoparathyroidism
    - Parathyroid glands produce PTH, but target organs do not respond appropriately.
  - Hypocalcemia is primary manifestation.
    - Symptoms of hypocalcemia: tetany, laryngospasm, stridor, altered mental status, paresthesias, seizures, heart failure
  - Management
    - Calcium supplementation

Perioperative Considerations

- Ensure normalized serum calcium levels prior to elective surgery.
- Rule out concurrent thyroid disease.
- Parathyroidectomy
  - Intraoperative PTH testing to determine when overactive gland removed
- Anticipate postoperative issues
  - Hematoma
  - Vocal cord dysfunction
  - Symptomatic hypocalcemia

Adrenal Cortex Dysfunction

- Adrenal cortex hormones
  - Mineralocorticoids (e.g., aldosterone)
    - Help regulate blood pressure and electrolytes
  - Glucocorticoids (e.g., cortisol)
    - Regulate metabolism and immune function
  - Androgens
- Adrenal medulla produces catecholamines
  - Epinephrine
  - Norepinephrine

Mineralocorticoid Excess

- Primary hyperaldosteronism: causes
  - Hypersecretion of aldosterone by the adrenal cortex (Conn syndrome)
  - Bilateral hyperplasia
  - Adrenal gland carcinoma
- Secondary hyperaldosteronism
  - Occurs with overactivation of the renin-angiotensin-aldosterone system
    - Congestive heart failure

        - Hepatic cirrhosis
        - Nephrotic syndrome
        - Hypertension (certain types)
- Clinical manifestations
    - Result from increased tubular exchange of sodium for potassium and hydrogen ions
        - Hypokalemic alkalosis
        - Hypertension and fluid retention
        - Skeletal muscle weakness
        - Fatigue
- Risks of primary aldosteronism (compared to nonaldosterone hypertension)
    - Higher rates of stroke, myocardial infarction, and atrial fibrillation
    - Patients may require additional workup for cardiovascular disease.
- Perioperative management
    - Monitor intravascular volume and electrolyte status.
    - Treat hypertension and hypokalemia.
        - Aldosterone antagonists
        - Restricting sodium intake
        - Potassium repletion

Glucocorticoid Excess

- Causes
    - Hyperfunction of the adrenal cortex (primary disease)
    - Hypersecretion of ACTH by a pituitary adenoma (Cushing disease)
    - Production of ACTH-like substance by a nonpituitary tumor
    - Exogenous glucocorticoid administration
- Clinical manifestations
    - Hypertension
    - Fluid retention
    - Impaired glucose metabolism
    - Central obesity
    - Hyperlipidemia
    - Hypercoagulability
    - Osteoporosis
    - Altered mental status
    - Muscular weakness
- Perioperative management
    - Assess cardiac risk factors.
    - Control hyperlipidemia and hypertension.
    - Monitor serum glucose.
    - Spironolactone for diuresis and to restore electrolyte balance
    - Careful pressure point padding and positioning due to increased risk of fracture
    - Postoperative glucocorticoid replacement for patients undergoing bilateral adrenal resection

Adrenal Insufficiency

- Causes
    - Primary adrenal insufficiency
        - Inability of adrenal glands to produce adequate hormones
        - May be due to atrophy or destruction of adrenal glands
        - Results in deficiency of both mineralocorticoids and glucocorticoids
    - Secondary adrenal insufficiency
        - Due to low production of ACTH
        - Often due to pituitary dysfunction, traumatic brain injury, or long-term exogenous glucocorticoid use
        - Results in isolated deficiency of glucocorticoids
- Clinical manifestations
    - Depends on the extent of adrenal function loss and physiologic stress
    - May include fatigue, weight loss, abdominal complaints, myalgias, arthralgias, skin hyperpigmentation, salt craving, and/or postural hypotension
- Perioperative management
    - Preoperative electrolyte testing
    - Adrenal crisis (acute adrenal insufficiency)
        - Normal adrenal gland can transiently increase cortisol secretion.
        - Relative lack of cortisol can cause vasodilation, hypotension, shock.
        - Continue maintenance steroid supplementation on day of surgery.
        - Additional "stress dose" steroids for patients with adrenal insufficiency prior to physiologically stressful procedures
        - Treat intraoperative acute adrenal insufficiency with vasopressors, fluid support, and additional rescue steroids.
- Strategies for supplemental steroid dose selection
    - Use rescue dose only if refractory hypotension develops.
    - Additional dose is based on the clinical assessment.
        - Risk of adrenal axis suppression
        - Stress of the surgery

Perioperative Stress Dose Steroid Administration Clinical Examples

High-dose steroid supplementation
- Dose
    - Hydrocortisone 100 mg before incision, then 50 mg every 8 hours for 3 doses
- High risk of adrenal suppression
    - A patient who has been on ≥20 mg/day prednisone for >3 weeks

- High stress of surgery
  - Major surgery, such as cardiac surgery or major trauma

Low-dose steroid supplementation
- Dose
  - No administered dose unless refractory hypotension develops
- Low risk of adrenal suppression
  - A patient who has been on steroids <3 weeks or on <5 mg/day
- Low stress of surgery
  - Minor surgery, such as inguinal hernia repair

Pheochromocytoma and Paraganglioma

- Anatomy
  - Pheochromocytoma
    - Chromaffin cell tumor that occurs inside of the adrenal gland (adrenal medulla)
  - Paraganglioma
    - Chromaffin cell tumor that occurs outside of the adrenal gland
- If hormonally active, can release large amounts of catecholamines and metanephrines
- Clinical manifestations
  - Sympathetic nervous system hyperactivity
    - May be constant or paroxysmal
  - Classic triad: paroxysmal headaches (hypertension), tachycardia, diaphoresis
  - Other symptoms
    - Heat intolerance, weight loss, chest discomfort, nausea, vomiting, orthostatic hypotension, constipation, anxiety, hyperglycemia, and/or hyperresponsiveness to noxious stimuli
- Pheochromocytoma multisystem crisis
  - Rare presentation with hemodynamic instability, hyperthermia (>40°C), neurologic manifestations, and multiorgan failure
  - May not respond to α-antagonism
  - Emergency surgery may be required.
- Diagnosis
  - Gold standard: elevated plasma fractionated metanephrines
  - Anatomic evidence of tumor
- Treatment
  - Surgical resection

Perioperative Considerations

- Primary preoperative goal: minimize catecholamine surges and evaluate for end-organ damage
- Potential end-organ effects
  - Hypovolemia, aortic dissection, myocardial ischemia, toxic myocarditis, catecholamine-induced cardiomyopathy, hypertrophic or dilated cardiomyopathy, congestive heart failure, tachyarrhythmias, and cerebrovascular accidents
- Preoperative testing
  - ECG and echocardiogram
  - Laboratory tests
    - Electrolytes, blood glucose, blood urea nitrogen, creatinine, and complete blood count
- Preoperative management
  - α-Adrenoceptor blockade for 7 to 14 days prior to surgery
  - β_1-Adrenoceptor antagonists to control heart rate after α-blockade has normalized blood pressure
    - β-Blockade with unopposed α-adrenergic stimulation can lead to uncontrolled hypertension.
  - High-sodium diet and adequate fluid intake to prevent hypovolemia prior to surgery
- Intraoperative management
  - Premedicate to minimize anxiety.
  - Ensure adequate depth of anesthesia for intubation, incision.
  - Potential hemodynamic instability
    - First phase: tumor manipulation causes greatest instability
    - Treat hypertension and arrhythmias.
    - After tumor efferent blood supply clamped: hypotension requiring vasopressors is common
    - Need variety of immediate and short-acting pharmacologic agents that target hypertension, hypotension, and tachyarrhythmias
- Perioperative pain management
  - Open procedures: consider epidural analgesia
- Avoid perioperative medications that can trigger catecholamine surges.
  - Sympathomimetic medications
  - Dopamine-blocking medications
  - Arrhythmogenic medications
  - Histamine-stimulating medications
- Postoperative concerns
  - Postresection hypotension due to residual α-adrenoceptor antagonism
  - Postoperative hypertension
  - Blood glucose fluctuations
  - Adrenal insufficiency with bilateral adrenalectomies
  - Acute kidney injury
  - Volume overload
  - Pulmonary complications
  - Thromboembolic events

Pituitary Gland Dysfunction

- Anterior pituitary hormones
  - Human growth hormone, ACTH, TSH, gonadotropic hormones, prolactin

- Posterior pituitary hormones (produced in hypothalamus)
  - Vasopressin, oxytocin

Acromegaly

- Excess growth hormone in adults (after growth plate closure)
  - Most common cause: pituitary adenoma
  - Treatment: transsphenoidal resection
- Clinical manifestations
  - Enlarged hands and feet
  - Enlarged facial features, deepening of the voice, headaches
  - Obstructive sleep apnea
  - Glucose intolerance
  - Hypertension, left ventricular hypertrophy, heart failure, arrhythmias
- Perioperative management
  - Preoperative cardiac evaluation including ECG
  - Blood glucose monitoring
  - Airway management concerns

Airway Management in Patients With Acromegaly

- Upper airway changes associated with acromegaly
  - Macroglossia, enlarged epiglottis, enlarged mandible, subglottic narrowing, and enlarged nasal turbinates
  - Patients are at increased risk for obstructive sleep apnea.
- Advance planning for perioperative airway management
  - Anticipate difficulties with mask ventilation and endotracheal intubation.
  - Noninvasive positive pressure ventilation is relatively contraindicated after transsphenoidal surgery.

Prolactinoma

- Hyperprolactin-secreting tumor of the pituitary gland
  - Most common functional pituitary tumor
  - Size of tumor
    - Microprolactinoma (<10 mm)
    - Macroprolactinoma (>10 mm)
- Clinical manifestations
  - Galactorrhea, amenorrhea, hypogonadism, gynecomastia
  - Tumors with mass effect
    - Headaches, visual field changes, and cranial nerve palsies
- Medical management
  - Dopamine agonists (bromocriptine, cabergoline) to reduce tumor size and normalize prolactin levels
- Surgical management
  - Transsphenoidal resection if medical therapy fails

Hypopituitarism

- Decreased secretion of one or more pituitary hormones
- Check all pituitary hormone levels.
- Replace with endogenous hormone supplements if needed.

Syndrome of Inappropriate Antidiuretic Hormone Secretion

- Characterized by excessive secretion of antidiuretic hormone (ADH)
  - Water retention and volume overload
  - Serum hyponatremia and hypoosmolarity
  - Urine hypernatremia and hyperosmolarity
- Perioperative management
  - Asymptomatic and mild hyponatremia
    - Treat with salt intake and fluid restriction.
  - Symptomatic and moderate hyponatremia
    - Treat with furosemide and normal saline infusion.
  - Severe symptomatic hyponatremia (confusion, seizures, coma)
    - 3% hypertonic saline should be used cautiously.
    - Risk of overrapid correction of serum sodium levels is *osmotic demyelination syndrome*.

Central Diabetes Insipidus

- Decreased ADH production
  - Polyuria, hypernatremia, hypokalemia, and dehydration
- Perioperative management
  - Monitor urine output and serum electrolytes.
  - Preoperative vasopressin analog (desmopressin) or intraoperative vasopressin to prevent significant intraoperative fluid loss

Neuroendocrine Tumors

- Neoplasms that arise from cells of neuroendocrine system
  - Majority are nonfunctional.
  - Functional neuroendocrine tumors
    - Insulinomas, gastrinomas, VIPomas, and carcinoid tumors
- Insulinomas
  - Secrete excess insulin
  - Cause hypoglycemia that can worsen with preoperative fasting
  - Hyperglycemia may occur following insulinoma resection.
  - Perioperative management
    - Close blood glucose monitoring and treatment are required.
- Gastrinomas
  - Secrete excess gastrin causing peptic ulcer disease, diarrhea, and esophageal reflux
  - Perioperative management

        - Treatment with H_2 antagonists and proton pump inhibitors
        - Rapid sequence intubation
        - Rehydration
- VIPomas
    - Secrete excess vasoactive intestinal peptide (VIP) causing watery diarrhea, flushing, hypotension, dehydration, hypokalemia, achlorhydria, and metabolic acidosis
    - Perioperative management
        - Correct preoperative fluid deficits.
        - Start somatostatin analog (octreotide) preoperatively.
- Surgical resection for neuroendocrine tumors
    - Treatment of choice for localized pancreatic neuroendocrine tumors
    - Surgical debulking may be of benefit in metastatic disease.

Carcinoid Tumor

- Carcinoid tumors are neuroendocrine tumors.
    - Secrete excess vasoactive hormones
        - Serotonin, bradykinins, prostaglandins, tachykinins, substance P, and/or histamine
    - Primarily occur in the gastrointestinal tract
        - Most commonly in the midgut (ileum and appendix)
        - Vasoactive substances are metabolized by the liver, preventing significant systemic effects.
    - Metastatic carcinoid tumors
        - Vasoactive substances do not go through hepatic degradation.
        - Symptoms of carcinoid syndrome are seen.
- Clinical manifestations
    - Flushing, tachycardia, hypotension, lacrimation, peripheral edema, abdominal pain, diarrhea, dehydration, electrolyte abnormalities, bronchoconstriction, right-sided valvular heart disease
- Treatment
    - Somatostatin analogs (octreotide) can ameliorate symptoms.
    - Surgical resection is the definitive treatment.
- Perioperative management
    - Cardiac evaluation should include ECG and echocardiogram.
    - Fluid and electrolyte abnormalities should be corrected.
    - Goal is to minimize vasoactive substance release.
        - Octreotide started preoperatively
        - Preoperative benzodiazepines
        - Antihistamines
        - Ondansetron
        - Avoid sympathomimetic agents.
    - Intraoperative hypotension
        - Treat with fluid bolus, octreotide, phenylephrine, and/or vasopressin.
    - Intraoperative hypertension
        - Treat with octreotide or β-adrenergic blockade.

QUESTIONS

NUTRITIONAL DISORDERS

1. What are the potential organ system manifestations of obesity?
2. How is the diagnosis of metabolic syndrome made?
3. What are some anesthetic considerations when caring for an obese patient?
4. What is the definition of malnutrition?
5. Describe the refeeding syndrome. What are the clinical signs of refeeding syndrome?

GASTROINTESTINAL DISORDERS

6. What is the presumed pathogenesis of inflammatory bowel disease (IBD)?
7. What factors increase perioperative morbidity in patients with IBD?
8. How is gastroesophageal reflux disease (GERD) diagnosed? What are the signs and symptoms of GERD?
9. What treatments are used for GERD?
10. What are the perioperative anesthetic goals and management of patients with GERD?

ENDOCRINE DISORDERS

11. How is the diagnosis of diabetes mellitus confirmed?
12. What are the potential end-organ complications of diabetes mellitus?
13. What is the major treatment goal in type 1 diabetes mellitus (T1DM) and type 2 diabetes mellitus (T2DM)?
14. For patients with diabetes mellitus, what blood glucose range should be maintained in the perioperative period?
15. A patient with goiter presents for elective thyroidectomy. What are the implications for preoperative assessment?
16. A patient with thyroid disease requires surgery. What laboratory tests are most useful during preoperative evaluation?
17. After thyroid surgery, what postoperative complications can involve the airway or respiratory system?
18. During total thyroidectomy, a patient has inadvertent surgical resection of all parathyroid glands. What is the most likely presentation and time course of postoperative hypoparathyroidism in this patient?
19. A patient is about to undergo surgery for resection of pheochromocytoma. What measures can be taken to minimize perioperative catecholamine surges?
20. A patient with acromegaly is scheduled for transsphenoidal pituitary adenoma resection. What are the perioperative concerns for this patient and procedure?
21. A patient with carcinoid tumor presents for surgical resection. What are the most common symptoms of carcinoid syndrome?
22. A patient with carcinoid tumor develops a carcinoid crisis during general anesthesia. What is the most appropriate management?

ANSWERS

NUTRITIONAL DISORDERS

1. Obesity is a complex disease with morbidity affecting every organ system, as summarized in the table below. (515–516)

Medical Conditions Associated With Obesity

Organ System	Associated Conditions
Central nervous system	Cognitive decline, dementia Depression
Respiratory system	Obstructive sleep apnea Obesity hypoventilation syndrome Restrictive lung disease
Cardiovascular system	Arrhythmias Systemic hypertension Coronary arterial disease Congestive heart failure Pulmonary hypertension Cor pulmonale Cerebrovascular disease Peripheral vascular disease Venous thromboembolism Hypercholesterolemia Hypertriglyceridemia Sudden cardiac death
Endocrine system	Metabolic syndrome Diabetes mellitus Cushing syndrome Hypothyroidism Infertility
Gastrointestinal system	Hiatal hernia Gastroesophageal reflux disease Nonalcoholic steatohepatitis Fatty infiltration of the liver Cholelithiasis
Musculoskeletal system	Degenerative joint disease Osteoarthritis Joint pain Inguinal hernia
Malignancy	Breast Gastric Pancreatic Liver, gallbladder Kidney Prostate Cervical, uterine, endometrial Colorectal
Other	Kidney failure Hypercoagulable syndromes Shorter life expectancy

2. Metabolic syndrome has six components: abdominal obesity, atherogenic dyslipidemia, hypertension, insulin resistance, proinflammatory state, and prothrombotic state. The diagnosis of metabolic syndrome can be made

with three of the following five criteria: abdominal obesity, increased serum triglycerides, decreased high-density lipoproteins, hypertension, and increased fasting blood glucose levels. (516)

3. There are several anesthetic considerations when caring for obese patients. Preoperatively, attention should be on the evaluation and optimization of any comorbid conditions. Preparation should include standard preoperative fasting guidelines, potential logistical challenges due to body habitus (e.g., monitoring, positioning), and preparation for potential difficulty with airway management (e.g., mask ventilation, endotracheal intubation). The decision on whether to use aspiration prophylaxis techniques should be made on an individual basis. Adequate preoxygenation (in a head-up position, if possible) is important given the risk of rapid desaturation with apnea. Perioperative medications that will minimize the risk of hypoventilation or oversedation are preferred, and the endotracheal tube should be removed only after extubation criteria are met. Postoperatively the patient should be monitored to ensure adequate ventilation. (516–517)
4. Malnourishment refers to an imbalance between energy expenditure and energy intake. Although the term may refer to excessive intake (e.g., individuals with obesity), it more commonly refers to deficient intake, (e.g., individuals with undernutrition). A 2016 global consensus defines malnutrition with a two-step process: (1) one of three phenotypic criteria—nonvolitional weight loss, low BMI or reduced muscle mass; and (2) one of two etiologic criteria—reduced food intake or absorption, or inflammation or disease burden. (518)
5. Refeeding syndrome refers to the metabolic disturbance that occurs following rapid nutritional repletion in a severely malnourished patient. The initial glucose load from feeding can lead to hyperinsulinemia, which promotes movement of extracellular phosphate into the cells. The clinical manifestations are mostly related to hypophosphatemia, which can lead to tissue hypoxia, myocardial dysfunction, respiratory failure, hemolysis, rhabdomyolysis, and seizures. Refeeding syndrome can be avoided by having a cautious approach to nutritional repletion, such as initial under-delivery of calories and careful attention to electrolytes with ongoing refeeding. (519)

GASTROINTESTINAL DISORDERS

6. The pathophysiology of IBD is complex, involving interaction between genetic and environmental factors (e.g., smoking, sedentary lifestyle, sleep deprivation, stress, prior appendectomy, and medications such as antibiotics, oral contraceptives, or nonsteroidal antiinflammatory drugs). Ultimately, these factors trigger an immunologic response resulting in inflammation in the intestine. (519)
7. Increased perioperative morbidity of patients with IBD is more likely in those who are malnourished, aged 60 to 80 years, on long-term immunosuppressive therapy, requiring emergent operation, and treated in low-volume centers. The type of surgical intervention is also related to perioperative morbidity with increased risk in patients undergoing a total proctocolectomy with J pouch compared to ileostomy, a repair for fistulizing disease compared to strictureplasty or stoma revision, and an open compared to a laparoscopic approach. (519)
8. The diagnosis of GERD is based on a combination of symptoms, objective testing (e.g., endoscopy, ambulatory reflux monitoring), and response to empiric antisecretory therapy. The classic symptoms of GERD are heartburn (burning retrosternal sensation) and regurgitation (perception of flow of refluxed gastric contents into the hypopharynx or mouth). Other manifestations of GERD can include dysphagia, globus sensation, chest pain, laryngitis, hoarseness, cough, dental erosions, adult-onset asthma, and aspiration. (520)
9. The initial treatment of GERD typically includes conservative approaches such as lifestyle modification and medication therapy. Lifestyle interventions include weight loss, head-of-bed elevation, smoking cessation, and avoidance of certain eating habits (e.g., late-night meals or foods that can potentially aggravate symptoms). Drug therapies for GERD can be found in the table below. (520–521)

Drug Therapies for GERD

Medication	Mechanism	Comments
Antacids	Neutralize gastric fluid acidity by providing base to react with hydrogen ions	Antacids can be particulate (e.g., TUMS) or nonparticulate (e.g., Bicitra).
Mucoprotective drugs (e.g., sucralfate)	Provide a mucosal barrier from stomach acids	
Prokinetic agents (e.g., metoclopramide)	Promote esophageal and gastric motility through the combined effect of increased muscarinic activity and dopamine and serotonin receptor antagonism	Metoclopramide may cause extrapyramidal side effects, such as tardive dyskinesia.

Medication	Mechanism	Comments
Histamine$_2$-receptor antagonists (e.g., famotidine)	Reduce the secretion of gastric acid	Histamine$_2$-receptor antagonists may cause adverse central nervous system effects, such as confusion, agitation, and psychosis, especially in the elderly.
Proton pump inhibitors (PPIs); e.g., pantoprazole)	Reduce the secretion of gastric acid	PPIs provide faster and more complete symptom relief and wound healing. Certain PPIs have drug–drug interactions, including inhibiting the metabolism and elimination of warfarin, digoxin, phenytoin, and benzodiazepines.

From Katz PO, Gerson LB, Vela MF. Guidelines for the diagnosis and management of gastroesophageal reflux disease. *Am J Gastroenterol.* 2013;108(3):308–329.

10. The perioperative goal for patients with GERD is to reduce the risk of pulmonary aspiration of gastric contents. Proton pump inhibitors should be continued up to the day of surgery. Additional precautions may include premedication with antacids, H_2-receptor antagonists, or prokinetic agents. Rapid sequence induction and intubation will minimize the time of loss of airway reflexes with an unprotected airway. A slight head up position may reduce the risk of passive regurgitation, while cricoid pressure is of questionable value. Finally, airway reflexes should be intact before tracheal extubation. (521)

ENDOCRINE DISORDERS

11. Several different techniques may confirm a diagnosis of diabetes. The diagnostic criteria are outlined in the box below. (522)

Diagnostic Criteria for Diabetes Mellitus

- Glycated hemoglobin (HbA_{1C}) ≥6.5%,
- Fasting plasma glucose ≥126 mg/dL (7.0 mmol/L) after 8 hours of no caloric intake
- Two-hour plasma glucose ≥200 mg/dL (11.1 mmol/L) during an oral glucose tolerance test
- A random plasma glucose ≥200 mg/dL (11.1 mmol/L) in a patient with classic symptoms of hyperglycemia or hyperglycemic crisis

Data from American Diabetes Association. 2. Classification and diagnosis of diabetes: standards of medical care in diabetes—2020. *Diabetes Care.* 2020; 43(Suppl 1):S14–S31.

12. Diabetes mellitus can lead to diffuse microvascular and macrovascular lesions affecting end-organ function, including retinopathy, nephropathy, cardiovascular disease, and cerebrovascular disease. In the US, diabetes mellitus is the seventh leading cause of death. (522)
13. The primary goal of treatment for all forms of diabetes is glucose control, with a reasonable target for HbA_{1C} <7%. While all patients with diabetes receive education regarding lifestyle and dietary interventions, most will require pharmacologic therapy to meet their blood glucose target goals. (522)
14. The general goals of perioperative glucose control include the avoidance of hypoglycemia, the avoidance of hyperglycemia, and the prevention of acute, life-threatening consequences of both extremes, including ketoacidosis or nonketotic hyperosmolar syndrome. There is no consensus on the target glycemic range during intraoperative care. Based mostly on literature from the intensive care setting, most society guidelines suggest maintaining glucose levels between 140 and 180 mg/dL (7.8 to 10 mmol/L) throughout surgery as levels outside this range showed an increase in adverse events, including death. (523–524)
15. Patients with goiters should undergo preoperative evaluation and imaging to assess risk of difficult intubation or hemodynamic collapse on induction. Symptoms of large goiters may include dyspnea, dysphagia, or voice change. Goiters may cause airway or great vessel compression, tracheal deviation, or extend beneath the sternum (which can increase challenges of surgical resection). (524–525)
16. Thyroid function tests should include thyroid-stimulating hormone (TSH), triiodothyronine (T3), and thyroxine (T_4). In uncontrolled hypothyroidism, TSH will be elevated and/or T_4 levels reduced. In uncontrolled hyperthyroidism, TSH will be reduced and T_3/T_4 elevated. Prior to elective surgery, patients should be clinically stable and medically euthyroid. (524–525)

17. There are several immediate postoperative complications after thyroid surgery that involve the airway or respiratory system. Transient hoarseness may develop due to glottic edema. More concerning complications include recurrent laryngeal nerve (RLN) damage, which may present as hoarseness (if unilateral) or as stridor and airway obstruction (if bilateral). Postoperative neck hematoma may also cause airway compromise and require bedside reopening of the surgical incision for hematoma decompression and urgent airway management. Acute hypocalcemia can occur due to unintentional removal of parathyroid glands and present as laryngeal stridor with airway obstruction. (525)
18. Inadvertent surgical removal of the parathyroid glands results in acute hypocalcemia, which most often presents within 12 to 72 hours after surgery. Symptoms of hypocalcemia include tetany (Chvostek sign or Trousseau sign), laryngospasm, stridor, altered mental status, paresthesias, seizures, and congestive heart failure. Hypocalcemia can be confirmed with postoperative serum calcium with or without parathyroid hormone (PTH) levels. (525)
19. Perioperative catecholamine surges may be triggered by a variety of medications, noxious stimuli, or intraoperative tumor manipulation. Preoperative and intraoperative considerations to reduce catecholamine surges and maintain hemodynamic stability are summarized in the box below. (527–528)

Preoperative	Intraoperative
α-Adrenergic blockade: essential	Premedication for anxiety
β-Adrenergic blockade/calcium channel blockade (only after adequate α-blockade)	Open surgery—epidural for analgesia
	Adequate anesthetic depth (especially for intubation, incision)
	Avoid sympathomimetics (e.g., ketamine, ephedrine, meperidine).
	Avoid dopaminergic drugs (e.g., metoclopramide, chlorpromazine, prochlorperazine, droperidol, haloperidol).
	Avoid histamine-stimulating medications (e.g., morphine, atracurium).
	Treat hypertension (e.g., intravenous phentolamine, nitroprusside, nicardipine, clevidipine, labetalol, or esmolol).
	Treat hypotension (e.g., volume resuscitation, phenylephrine, norepinephrine, vasopressin, and/or dopamine).
	Treat tachyarrhythmias (e.g., esmolol, lidocaine, amiodarone).

20. Patients with acromegaly may present with enlarged hands and feet, enlarged facial features, deepening of the voice, headaches, obstructive sleep apnea, hypertension, glucose intolerance, left ventricular hypertrophy, heart failure, and arrhythmias. Preoperative evaluation of patients should include a careful cardiac evaluation. Blood glucose should be monitored and treated perioperatively. An airway management plan should consider the potential for difficult mask ventilation and/or endotracheal intubation due to upper airway changes. For patients with obstructive sleep apnea, postoperative noninvasive positive pressure ventilation is relatively contraindicated after transsphenoidal surgery. (528–529)
21. Carcinoid tumors are neuroendocrine tumors that secrete excess vasoactive hormones. When carcinoid tumors occur in the gastrointestinal tract, released vasoactive substances are largely metabolized by the liver, preventing significant systemic effects. However, when tumors are not located in the gastrointestinal tract (e.g., with metastatic spread), vasoactive substances do not go through hepatic degradation and the symptoms of carcinoid syndrome are seen. Patients with carcinoid syndrome can present with flushing, tachycardia, hypotension, lacrimation, peripheral edema, abdominal pain, diarrhea, dehydration, electrolyte abnormalities, bronchoconstriction, and right-sided valvular heart disease. (529–530)
22. The primary intraoperative goal for patients with carcinoid tumor is to minimize vasoactive substance release, which can occur with anxiety, noxious stimuli, hypercapnia, and hypothermia. Octreotide should be started preoperatively, continued intraoperatively, and only tapered off postoperatively. Other common premedication includes benzodiazepines (anxiolysis), antihistamines, and ondansetron (antiserotonin). Intraoperative hypotension can be treated with a fluid bolus, octreotide, phenylephrine, and/or vasopressin. Sympathomimetic agents (e.g., epinephrine) and histamine-releasing medications should be avoided as they can theoretically stimulate the release of vasoactive substances from the tumor and exacerbate hemodynamic instability. Intraoperative hypertension can be treated with octreotide or β-adrenergic blockade. (529–530)

Chapter

30 CENTRAL NERVOUS SYSTEM DISEASE

Brian P. Lemkuil, Martin Krause, and Piyush Patel

NEUROANATOMY

Supratentorial and Infratentorial Compartments

- Cranial contents are anatomically divided into compartments.
  - Supratentorial
    - Cerebral hemispheres
    - Diencephalon (thalamus and hypothalamus)
  - Infratentorial
    - Cerebellum
    - Brainstem (midbrain, pons, medulla)
- Pathology location has clinical implications.
  - Surgical positioning (supine, prone, lateral, etc.)
  - Anesthetic management (e.g., antiepileptic prophylaxis considered for supratentorial surgery only)
- Intracranial lesions may be classified as
  - Intraaxial
    - Within brain parenchyma
    - Functional preservation (e.g., language, motor, etc.) is a major intraoperative goal.
  - Extraaxial
    - Outside brain parenchyma

Cerebral Vasculature

- Arterial blood supply to the brain
  - Anterior circulation
    - Right and left carotid arteries
  - Posterior circulation
    - Vertebrobasilar system
- Circle of Willis
  - Anastomotic ring between anterior and posterior circulations
  - Provides a collateral network that may limit focal ischemia
  - 50% of individuals may have an incomplete circle of Willis.
    - Collateral cerebral blood flow should not be assumed.
    - The clinical significance of abnormalities should be considered.
    - Preservation of cerebral perfusion pressure (CPP) and avoidance of hypotension are prudent.

Cranial Nerves

- 12 pairs of intracranial nerves (CNs)
  - Each has unique distribution and sensorimotor and autonomic functions.
- Infratentorial surgery can place these nerves at risk.
- CNs can be monitored intraoperatively.
  - Detects reversible injury to potentially prevent permanent deficits
  - Requires close communication and collaboration with neurophysiology team
- Basic anesthetic goals for nerve monitoring
  - Avoid excessive anesthetic depth
  - Maintain normothermia and hemodynamic stability.
- Tailored anesthetic plan to the neurophysiology monitoring modalities
  - Minimal volatile anesthetics during motor and somatosensory evoked potentials (MEP/SSEP)
  - Avoid neuromuscular blocking agents during MEP/electromyography (EMG).
    - Soft bite blocks to protect tongue and soft tissue from induced masseter contraction
  - Monitoring CN IX and XII (glossopharyngeal and hypoglossal nerves)
    - Requires needle electrode placement inside the mouth
    - Caution should be taken at end of surgery until all needles are removed.
  - Monitoring CN X (vagus nerve)
    - Requires a special endotracheal tube (ETT) with electrodes
    - Appropriate ETT placement of the electrodes between the vocal cords
    - Avoid neuromuscular blocking agents.

Blood–Brain Barrier

- The blood–brain barrier (BBB) is capillary endothelial cells that have tight junctions.
  - Prevent the free passage of electrolytes, macromolecules, and proteins
  - Lipid-soluble substances cross easily (e.g., carbon dioxide, anesthetic agents).

- Disruption can be caused by various pathologies.
- Integrity of the BBB is needed to create an osmotic gradient.
  - Efficacy of hyperosmolar therapy (mannitol, hypertonic saline) relies on an intact BBB.

Pathologies That Disrupt the Blood–Brain Barrier
▪ Hypertensive crisis ▪ Trauma ▪ Infection ▪ Tumors ▪ Arterial hypoxemia ▪ Severe hypercapnia ▪ Sustained seizure activity

NEUROPHYSIOLOGY

Regulation of Cerebral Blood Flow

- Normal cerebral blood flow (CBF) is 50 mL/100 g/min.
- The brain has high metabolic demands and limited energy storage capacity.
- Dependence on continuous oxygen delivery necessitates mechanisms to maintain CBF.

Factors That Regulate or Influence Cerebral Blood Flow
▪ Cerebral metabolic rate via neurovascular coupling ▪ Cerebral autoregulation (myogenic regulation) ▪ $PaCO_2$ and PaO_2 ▪ Sympathetic nervous system ▪ Cardiac output ▪ Anesthetic drugs ▪ Vasoactive drugs ▪ Temperature

Cerebral Metabolic Rate and Neurovascular Coupling

- Cerebral metabolic rate of oxygen ($CMRO_2$)
  - Often used as an index of cerebral metabolic activity
  - Changes in $CMRO_2$ result in a proportional change in CBF.
    - Known as *neurovascular coupling*
- Hypothermia and most intravenous anesthetic drugs reduce $CMRO_2$ and CBF.
  - CBF decreases 7% for every 1°C decrease in body temperature below 37°C.
- Seizures increase $CMRO_2$ and CBF substantially.

Cerebral Perfusion Pressure and Cerebral Autoregulation

- Cerebral perfusion pressure
  - Equals mean arterial pressure (MAP) minus intracranial pressure (ICP) or CVP, whichever is greater
  - Can fluctuate with blood pressure changes
- Cerebral autoregulation
  - Changes in vascular resistance to maintain relatively stable CBF during changes in CPP
  - Minutes to take effect
  - Rapid increase (or decrease) in MAP/CPP may be associated with a brief period of cerebral hyperperfusion (or hypoperfusion).
- Cerebral autoregulation curves have three phases (see figure below)
  - Lower limit: vasodilation is maximized, and CBF decreases with decreasing CPP
  - Upper limit: vasoconstriction is maximized, and CBF increases with increasing CPP
  - Plateau: vascular resistance responds to CPP to maintain relatively constant CBF

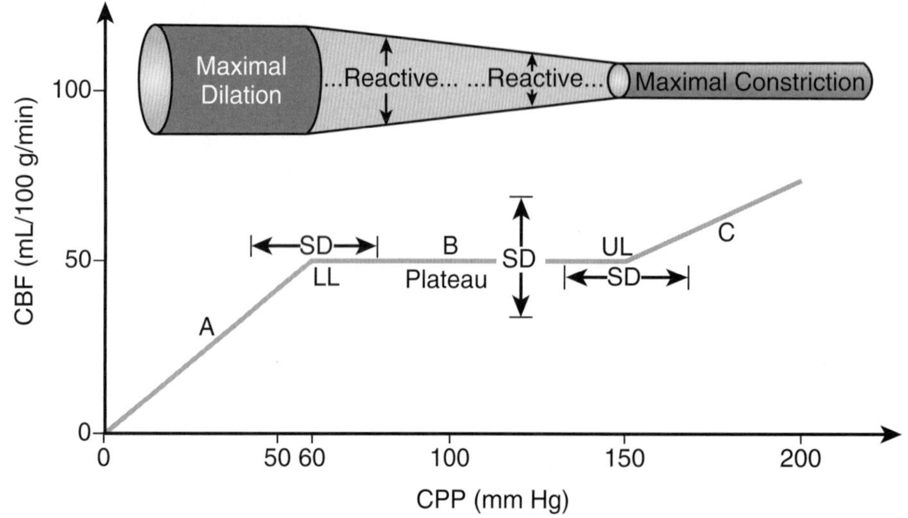

Cerebral autoregulation. CBF, cerebral blood flow; CPP, cerebral perfusion pressure; LL, lower limit of autoregulation; UL, upper limit of autoregulation; SD, standard deviation. (Figure from Meng L, Gelb AW. Regulation of cerebral autoregulation by carbon dioxide. *Anesthesiology.* 2015; 122(1):196-205.)

- The limits of cerebral autoregulation
  - Frequently quoted as CPP between 60 mmHg and 150 mmHg
  - There is great interindividual variation of these limits.
  - Chronic uncontrolled hypertension or sympathetic stimulation is an example.
    - Can shift the autoregulatory curve to the right
    - These patients require a higher CPP to maintain adequate CBF.
- Cerebral autoregulation can be impaired, making control of CPP important.
  - Traumatic brain injury or intracranial surgery
    - Can abolish autoregulation, meaning CBF changes along with CPP
  - Severe hypercapnia (hypoventilation)
  - Inhaled anesthetics
    - Potent vasodilators with dose-dependent effects on autoregulation
- Autoregulatory curves are individualized and dynamic.
- Perioperative blood pressure targets should be individualized to avoid jeopardizing cerebral perfusion.

Cerebrovascular $PaCO_2$ and PaO_2 Reactivity

- $PaCO_2$
  - CBF changes directionally with $PaCO_2$ between 20 mmHg and 80 mmHg.
    - CBF increases when $PaCO_2$ increases above 40 mmHg.
    - CBF decreases when $PaCO_2$ decreases below 40 mmHg.
    - CBF change is by approximately 1 mL/100 g/min or 2% for every 1 mmHg.
  - Mechanism: carbon dioxide–mediated perivascular pH change causes arteriole dilation or constriction
  - $PaCO_2$-related CBF change is sustained for only 6–8 hours.
    - Compensatory change in bicarbonate concentration
  - Extreme hyperventilation and hypoventilation can lead to cerebral hypoperfusion and hyperperfusion, respectively.
  - Prolonged and aggressive hyperventilation after traumatic brain injury (TBI) is associated with worse neurologic outcome.
- PaO_2
  - PaO_2 <50 mmHg increases CBF exponentially.
  - Cerebral oxygen delivery = arterial blood oxygen content (CaO_2) × CBF.
  - If CaO_2 decreases (anemia or desaturation), CBF may increase.

Effects of Anesthetic Agents on CBF

- IV anesthetic agents (e.g., propofol and barbiturates)
  - Simultaneous reduction in $CMRO_2$ and CBF
  - *Neurovascular coupling*: CBF is proportional to $CMRO_2$
- Ketamine
  - Variable effects on $CMRO_2$ and CBF
    - Given alone without control of ventilation: $PaCO_2$, CBF, and ICP all increase
    - Given with other sedative/anesthetic drug AND controlled ventilation: CBF and ICP do NOT increase
    - Ketamine is often avoided in patients with increased ICP.
- Benzodiazepines and opioids
  - Decrease $CMRO_2$ and CBF
    - To a lesser extent than propofol and barbiturates
  - These agents can cause respiratory depression.
    - Ensure $PaCO_2$ is controlled to avoid an increase in CBF and ICP.
- Alpha-2 agonists (e.g., clonidine and dexmedetomidine)
  - Do not cause significant respiratory depression
  - Reduce arterial blood pressure, CPP, and CBF with minimal effects on ICP
  - Intraoperative use
    - Reduce the need for other anesthetics
    - Blunt hemodynamic responses
  - Postoperative use
    - Attenuate postoperative hypertension and tachycardia
- Volatile anesthetic agents
  - Potent cerebral vasodilators
  - Low dose: the reduction of $CMRO_2$ and CBF exceeds direct vasodilation
  - >0.5 MAC: continued dose-dependent vasodilation diminishes the effects of additional $CMRO_2$ suppression
    - Vasodilation may exceed $CMRO_2$ reduction, causing increased ICP
    - Divergent effects on $CMRO_2$ and CBF
- Nitrous oxide
  - Increases CBF and possibly $CMRO_2$ when used in isolation
  - Effects attenuated by coadministration of other anesthetic agents

INTRACRANIAL PRESSURE AND BRAIN RELAXATION

- Intracranial pressure (ICP)
  - Pressure inside of the *closed* cranium
  - When the cranium is open, the ICP equals the atmospheric pressure.

- Brain relaxation
  - Is the volumetric relationship between the brain and intracranial space when the cranium is closed
  - Tactile feeling of the firmness of the brain by the surgeon when the cranium is open
- The ICP can be zero and the brain still not be relaxed.
- Management strategies for ICP and brain relaxation are similar.

Determinants of ICP and the Compensation for an Elevated ICP

- Cranium contains three volumes: brain (cells), CSF, and blood (arterial and venous).
- Increased volume of any component can increase ICP.
- High ICP can decrease CPP and CBF, leading to cerebral ischemia.
- Compensatory mechanisms for elevated ICP
  - Translocation of CSF or venous blood out of cranium
  - Initially can reduce intracranial volume and help minimize ICP elevation
- ICP rises quickly with further intracranial volume increases after compensatory mechanisms are exhausted.
- CBF and cerebral blood volume (CBV) are related but not interchangeable.
  - CBV changes directionally with CBF.
- Elevated ICP is treated by reducing volume of intracranial components.

Effect of Anesthetic Agents on ICP

- Most intravenous agents
  - Reduce $CMRO_2$ and CBF (neurovascular coupling)
  - Decrease CBV
  - Decrease ICP
- For refractory intracranial hypertension, consider deep anesthesia.
  - Propofol-induced burst suppression
  - Barbiturate coma
  - Avoid compromise of cardiac output and cerebral perfusion.
- Etomidate
  - Increased excitatory potentials on EEG compared with thiopental
  - Administer with caution to patients with history of epilepsy.
    - Seizures increase $CMRO_2$, CBF, and ICP
- Opioids and benzodiazepines
  - May reduce ICP (neurovascular coupling)
  - ICP reduction may be offset by respiratory depression/$PaCO_2$ increase.
- Ketamine
  - Often avoided in patients with increased ICP
- Volatile anesthetics
  - Direct cerebral vasodilators causing dose-dependent increase in CBF and ICP
    - Clinical significance of this increase is unclear.
    - Hyperventilation to a $PaCO_2$ <35 mmHg attenuates the increase in ICP.
- No meaningful clinical outcome difference based on anesthesia type
  - Consider intravenous agents if ICP is maximally compensated.
- Neuromuscular blocking drugs
  - No direct effect on ICP
  - Some may induce histamine and cause cerebral vasodilation.
  - Succinylcholine may transiently increase ICP.

NEUROPROTECTION

- Anesthetic agents
  - Potential to reduce $CMRO_2$ and excitotoxicity during ischemia
  - Neuroprotection demonstrated in animal studies
  - Human studies demonstrating efficacy are lacking.
- Hypothermia
  - Animal studies support temperature reduction for ischemic injury.
  - Human studies in aneurysm surgery and TBI failed to show a clinical benefit.
  - More recent studies question benefit of deep hypothermia to 33°C after cardiac arrest.
- Hyperthermia
  - Worsens cerebral ischemia and should be avoided

NEUROPHYSIOLOGIC MONITORING

- Frequently used during neurosurgery
  - Minimal patient risk
  - Potential to reduce the risk of intraoperative neurologic injury
  - Identification of epileptic foci
- Common intraoperative modalities
  - Somatosensory evoked potential (SSEP)
  - Transcranial/transcortical motor evoked potential (MEP)
  - Spontaneous or triggered CN electromyography (EMG)
  - Electroencephalography (EEG) and electrocorticography
- Anesthetic effects on neurophysiologic monitoring
  - Narcotics have minimal impact.
  - Intravenous and volatile anesthetics cause dose-dependent suppression of signals.
    - Volatile anesthetics and nitrous oxide may negatively affect signals more than intravenous anesthetics.

- Avoid major fluctuations of anesthetic level during monitoring.
- Avoid paralysis for EMG or MEP.

ANESTHESIA FOR NEUROSURGERY

Preoperative Assessment

- Clinical evaluation
  - Symptoms of intracranial mass
    - Seizures, altered level of consciousness, headaches, deficits
  - Symptoms of aneurysm or arteriovenous malformation
    - Ruptured: severe "thunderclap" headache
    - Unruptured: focal deficits or visual impairment of optic chiasm compression
  - Signs of increased ICP
    - Positional headache, nausea and vomiting, hypertension and bradycardia, altered patterns of breathing, papilledema
- Imaging studies
  - Midline shift, compressed cerebral ventricles, cerebral edema, hydrocephalus
- Medications
  - CNS medications
    - Antiepileptics (e.g., levetiracetam)
    - Reduce peritumor edema (e.g., dexamethasone)
    - Reduce brain free water (e.g., mannitol, hypertonic saline)
  - Other medications (e.g., anticoagulants, antihypertensives, hypoglycemic)
- Laboratory analysis
  - Coagulation status
  - Electrolytes (e.g., sodium)

Neurologic Exam and Anesthetic Implications

Suspected or Known Increased ICP
- Avoid premedications.
  - Concern for extreme sensitivity
  - May reduce minute ventilation and cause $PaCO_2$/ICP increase
  - May impair airway protection
- May imply difficulty with arousal at the end of the case that may preclude extubation
- May suggest anesthetic sensitivity
  - Reduce anesthetic dose and/or begin emergence early.
- Consider maneuvers to prevent further ICP increase.
  - Head of bed elevated during induction
  - Avoid halogenated anesthetics.
  - Avoid hypercapnia.
- May require aggressive surgical brain relaxation

Motor/Sensory Deficits
- Likely dictates total intravenous anesthetic for neurophysiologic monitoring
- Affects expectations regarding baseline neurophysiologic signals
- Anticipate a more profound deficit postoperatively due to edema/manipulation/residual anesthetics.

Receptive Aphasia
- Affects expectations regarding ability to follow commands prior to extubation

Cranial Nerve Dysfunction
- May dictate which CNs are monitored
- Lower CN involvement at baseline may suggest caution regarding immediate postoperative extubation.

Preoperative Imaging and Anesthetic Implications

Location and Size of Lesion
- Patient positioning
- Dictates need for brain relaxation
- Seizure prophylaxis (if supratentorial)

Proximity to Eloquent Brain Tissue
- Anticipate potential postoperative neurologic deficit
- Unanticipated deficits detected on emergence may require delayed extubation and immediate brain imaging.

Proximity to Vascular Structures
- Anticipate risk of ischemic injury due to vessel injury/vasospasm.
  - Potentially greater need to maintain CPP
- Anticipate neurophysiologic monitoring needs.
- Potential risk of rapid blood loss/intravenous access/blood product availability
- Evaluate risk of venous air embolism.

Superficial vs. Deep Location
- Need for brain retraction
  - Maintain CPP adequate for retractor pressure.
- Brain relaxation required for lesion access/visualization (deep)

Presence of Vasogenic Edema
- Contribution to overall increased parenchymal volume
- Need for brain relaxation to optimize surgical field
- Indication for steroids

Mass Effect (Compressed Ventricle, Midline Shift, Effaced Basal Cisterns)
- Brain relaxation to prevent herniation out of craniotomy site
- Aggressive brain relaxation for patient safety and surgical field optimization
- Potentially greater need to maintain CPP, particularly if neurologic examination at baseline is impaired
- May inform decision on head-of-bed elevation (both during induction and surgery)
- May change induction sequence/premedication use to ensure early control of ventilation to prevent $PaCO_2$ increase

Hydrocephalus
- Brain relaxation until surgeons can place a needle into the ventricle

Monitoring

- Standard monitors
  - Electrocardiogram (ECG)
    - Detection of cardiac dysrhythmias due to surgical manipulation of brainstem, CNs, or dura
  - Capnography
    - Assess and optimize $PaCO_2$ during mechanical ventilation
    - Assess spontaneous breathing in awake or sedated patients.
- Intraarterial catheter
  - Allows for continuous arterial pressure monitoring at level of circle of Willis
  - Intravascular volume assessment by systolic or pulse pressure variation
  - Arterial blood gas sampling for $PaCO_2$ optimization
- Central venous catheter
  - Not routinely used
  - Difficult peripheral venous access
  - Administration of high-dose vasoactive drugs
  - Provides access for high volume resuscitation (e.g., massive transfusion due to an arteriovenous malformation ([AVM]))
- Bladder catheter
  - Long surgery, use of loop or osmotic diuretics
  - Helps guide fluid therapy
- Peripheral nerve stimulator
  - Monitor for neuromuscular blockade
- Continuous ICP monitor
  - Intraventricular and external ventricular device
    - Also allows for drainage of CSF
  - Subarachnoid or subdural bolt
    - Placed via burr hole
    - Can be inserted emergently if necessary

Induction of Anesthesia

- Goals
  - Sufficient anesthesia level to blunt response to laryngoscopy and intubation
    - May require intravenous medications in addition to the induction agent
  - Maintain hemodynamic stability and CPP
- Induction agents
  - Propofol is reliable, prompt, and unlikely to increase ICP.
  - Etomidate is rarely used.
- Hemodynamic support
  - Used when necessary to maintain CPP (e.g., phenylephrine, ephedrine)
- Neuromuscular blockade
  - Prevent coughing during intubation that could cause acute increase in ICP
  - Succinylcholine may transiently increase ICP (likely clinically insignificant).

Positioning

- Limited access to head (table 180 degrees)
  - Ensure ETT is well secured without tension before draping.
  - Cover eyelids with waterproof dressing.
    - Avoids abrasions and chemical injury from prep solutions
  - Soft bite block to prevent tongue injury from MEP monitoring or seizures
- Supratentorial tumors and intracranial vascular lesions
  - Supine, semilateral, or lateral position (axillary roll)
- Posterior fossa/infratentorial tumors
  - Frequently requires prone, sitting, or park bench position
  - Sitting position
    - Facilitates surgical exposure of posterior fossa tumors
    - High risk of venous air embolism (VAE): incidence >25%
    - Risk of upper airway edema: venous obstruction from excessive cervical flexion
    - Risk of quadriplegia: spinal cord compression and ischemia, preexisting cervical stenosis increases risk
  - Park bench position
    - Lateral position rolled slightly forward
    - Head further rotated to "look" at the floor
    - Allows full access to posterior fossa and minimizes risk for VAE
- Avoid extremes in head and neck rotation, flexion, or extension
  - Spinal cord injury risk with cervical spine diseases (e.g., arthritis, stenosis)
  - Can compromise neck vascular structures
    - Impairing cerebral venous drainage can cause poor brain relaxation.
- Secure patients to prevent slipping if operating table is tilted.
- Monitored anesthesia care procedures
  - Surgeries include deep brain stimulator placement and awake craniotomy.
  - Consider patient tolerance and ease of airway instrumentation.
- Head frame using pins
  - Avoid bucking or movement during placement or removal of pins.
  - Propofol or opioids, as well as local anesthesia to pin sites, can be used to blunt hemodynamic response.

Maintenance of Anesthesia

- Provide appropriate levels of hypnosis and analgesia.
  - Propofol and remifentanil infusions are often chosen.
    - Used with/without a low-dose volatile anesthetic.

- Use volatile anesthetic with caution when there are ICP concerns.
- Dexmedetomidine infusions may be added.
  - Excessive depth may impede neurophysiologic monitoring and prolong emergence.
  - Inadequate depth may risk patient movement or coughing.
    - Coughing can cause acute brain swelling and hemorrhage.
    - Neuromuscular blockade avoids movement and coughing, but is not compatible with motor monitoring (EMG, MEP).
- Facilitate brain relaxation and maintain CPP.
  - Direct vasodilators may increase CBF/ICP and are not recommended.
    - Includes hydralazine, nitroglycerin, nitroprusside, and calcium channel blockers
  - Phenylephrine and norepinephrine are commonly used to maintain arterial blood pressure and CPP.
- Facilitate neurophysiologic monitoring (see previous discussion).
- Enable smooth and prompt emergence without coughing, agitation, nausea, or shivering

Anesthetic Goals for Neurosurgery

- Hypnosis and analgesia
- Ensure immobility.
- Maintain CPP.
- Brain relaxation and surgical field optimization
- Prevent coughing and risk of acute brain swelling or hemorrhage.
- Facilitate neurophysiologic monitoring.
- Ensure smooth/prompt emergence without coughing, agitation, and shivering.
- Strict blood pressure control to prevent hemorrhagic complications
- Facilitate an early postoperative neurologic examination.

ICP Reduction and Brain Relaxation

- Osmotic agents (e.g., mannitol, 3% hypertonic saline) reduce cerebral water content.
  - Onset: 5–10 minutes; peak effect: 20–30 minutes; duration: 2–4 hours
  - Mannitol given rapidly can cause short-term peripheral vasodilation and volume expansion.
    - Rapid administration can result in increased ICP and volume overload.
- Furosemide (0.3-0.5 mg/kg IV) is thought to be synergistic with mannitol.
  - May result in profound diuresis
  - Hypovolemia from diuresis may lower cardiac output and tissue perfusion.
  - Fluids should be replaced appropriately.
- Hyperventilation
  - Immediately reduces CBF and ICP, results in brain relaxation
- Intravenous agents
  - May be preferred over volatile agents if reducing cranial volume is critical
  - No clinical outcome data supports one anesthetic technique over another.
- Head-of-bed elevation
  - Increased cerebral venous drainage (avoid constriction around neck)
  - Increased shift in CSF to spinal subarachnoid space

Perioperative Intracranial Volume Management

- Osmotic agents (e.g., mannitol, hypertonic saline) to reduce cerebral water content
- Dexamethasone for vasogenic edema
- Hyperventilation to reduce CBF
- Intravenous GABAergic agents reduce CBF (neurovascular coupling)
- Head-of-bed elevation to augment movement of CSF and venous blood from cranium
- Avoid hyperthermia.

Ventilation Adjustment

- Target $PaCO_2$ 30–35 mmHg after tracheal intubation
  - No evidence for additional benefit below this range
- Minimize high positive end-expiratory pressure (PEEP) or lung recruitment maneuvers
  - May impair cerebral venous drainage
- Raise the head 10–15 cm above level of chest to improve venous drainage.
- Avoid hypoventilation as hypercapnia increases CBF and CBV.
- Current consensus on ventilation
  - Maintain eucapnia during intracranial surgery.
  - Use relative hyperventilation only as temporizing measure.

Fluid Management

- Maintain euvolemia.
- Avoid dextrose solutions.
  - Glucose rapidly distributes throughout the entire body water
  - Reduction of glucose more rapidly in blood than the brain can result in water crossing the BBB and increased brain edema.
  - Hyperglycemia augments ischemic neuronal cell damage.
- Isotonic crystalloid solutions are recommended.
- Colloids are acceptable, no proven outcome benefit compared to crystalloids
  - May be detrimental in patients with TBI

Blood Product Administration and Anticoagulant Management

- Transfusion trigger for red blood cells remains controversial.
- Transfusion threshold should be individualized.
- Coagulopathy and thrombocytopenia should be corrected to avoid risk of intracranial hematoma.
- Anticoagulants and antiplatelets are typically stopped before surgery.

Emergence From Anesthesia and Postoperative Care

- Avoid coughing or straining on the ETT
  - Can increase cerebral venous pressure and cause hemorrhage or edema
- Intravenous lidocaine bolus may help decrease likelihood of coughing during tracheal extubation.
- Early neurologic assessments help identify neurologic injury/complications.
- Delayed return of consciousness or neurologic deterioration should be immediately assessed with imaging.
- Postoperative sympathetic response (hypertension, tachycardia) should be attenuated to avoid risk of intracranial hematoma.
  - Medication options include labetalol, nicardipine, or opioids.
  - Drugs that reduce MAP without cerebral vasodilation are preferred.

Venous Air Embolism

- Neurosurgical procedures are considered high risk for VAE.
  - Head/operative site is often elevated above the heart.
  - Venous structures on cut edge of bone may be "stented" open.
- Mechanism
  - Entrained air acutely increases pulmonary dead space.
  - Air trapping in the right ventricle may cause obstructive heart failure.
  - Microvascular bubbles may cause bronchoconstriction or activate endothelial mediators resulting in pulmonary edema.
  - Death is usually caused by cardiovascular collapse or arterial hypoxemia.
- Paradoxical air embolism
  - Air may reach coronary and cerebral circulation by crossing a patent foramen ovale.
    - Patent foramen ovale is present in 20%–30% of adults.
    - Can result in myocardial infarction or stroke
  - Transpulmonary passage of venous air is an alternative cause.
- Detection
  - Transesophageal echocardiography (most sensitive monitor)
    - Invasive and may be impractical during intracranial surgery
  - Precordial Doppler ultrasound transducer (second most sensitive monitor)
    - Placed over the second or third intercostal space to the right or left of the sternum
    - Practical and noninvasive
  - Carbon dioxide: sudden reduction in end-tidal concentration reflects increased physiologic dead space
  - End-tidal nitrogen concentration increase
    - Rarely monitored
  - Right atrial central venous catheter: aspiration of air is diagnostic and therapeutic
- Signs
  - Early: sudden attempts (gasps) to breathe during controlled ventilation
  - Late: hypotension, tachycardia, cardiac dysrhythmias, hypoxemia, and a "mill wheel" murmur (auscultation or Doppler)
  - Elevated pulmonary artery pressure on pulmonary artery catheter
  - In awake patients: chest pain, coughing, and anxiety
- Management
  - Stop further entrainment and supportive care
  - Notify surgeon immediately.
    - Irrigation of operative site with fluid and application of occlusive material to bone edges (e.g., bone wax)
    - Compression of neck to occlude internal jugular veins
  - Lower the head of the bed
  - 100% inspired oxygen fraction (stop nitrous oxide)
  - Beta-agonist (epinephrine) to support right heart
  - Aspirate from air recovery catheter in the right atrium (if present).
  - Efficacy of PEEP to decrease entrainment of air has not been confirmed.
    - PEEP could reverse the pressure gradient between the left and right atria and predispose to passage of air across a PFO.

COMMON CLINICAL CASES

Intracranial Mass Lesions

- Clinical manifestations may reflect increased ICP.
- Avoid abrupt increases in ICP in patients with large intracranial masses.
- Patient position is determined by mass location and surgical approach.
- Dexamethasone is commonly used to reduce vasogenic edema.
- Intraoperative antiepileptics are typically administered (supratentorial surgery).

- Strategies to improve brain relaxation are frequently required.
- Awake craniotomy considered for lesions near eloquent parenchyma
- Considerations of sitting-position craniotomy for posterior fossa masses (rarely used)
  - Evaluation for PFO (preoperative cardiac echo)
  - Risk of malignant tongue edema due to neck flexion
  - Ensure CPP maintained with arterial line transducer at level of tragus.
  - High risk of VAE: a properly positioned central venous catheter and precordial Doppler are recommended
  - Hydrate adequately to compensate for blood pooling in dependent areas of the body.
  - Stimulation or injury to brainstem respiratory/circulatory centers may cause arrhythmias, hemodynamic instability, and postoperative respiratory failure.
  - CN injury may impair protective airway reflexes.
  - Potential injury to brainstem respiratory center and lower CNs should be considered before extubation.

Sitting Position Craniotomy Considerations

- Preoperative echocardiography to evaluate for PFO
- Limit neck flexion and oral devices (e.g., temperature probes, gastric tubes).
  - Can impair oral venous drainage and contribute to tongue edema
- Transduce arterial line at level of tragus to ensure adequate CPP.
- Consider precordial Doppler and right heart catheter to monitor and treat VAE.
- Hydrate adequately to compensate for blood pooling in lower body.
- Monitor for arrhythmias, hemodynamic instability, and postoperative respiratory insufficiency.
  - Risk increased by manipulation of brainstem respiratory and circulatory centers
- Monitor and evaluate for lower CN injury.
- Decision to extubate based on patient's ability to protect airway and risk of respiratory failure

Intracranial Aneurysms

- Aneurysmal subarachnoid hemorrhage (SAH)
  - Symptoms include sudden-onset severe headache, nausea/vomiting, and neurologic signs.
  - Can result in major complications: rebleeding and death, vasospasm and delayed cerebral ischemia, and hydrocephalus
  - Aneurysmal SAH requires treatment in interventional radiology suites or operating rooms.
    - Unsuitable candidates for endovascular coiling (location/anatomy) require craniotomy for surgical clipping.
  - Early treatment is advocated to reduce rebleeding risk.
    - Surgical clipping after rupture may be associated with technical difficulty due to inflammation and cerebral edema.
- Cerebral vasospasm is a complication.
  - Onset is generally 3–5 days after rupture and is the foremost cause of morbidity and mortality.
  - Transcranial Doppler and cerebral angiography can detect cerebral vasospasm before clinical symptoms.
  - "Triple H" therapy (hypervolemia, hypertension, hemodilution) has fallen out of favor.
    - Induced hypertension is often used to treat *symptomatic* vasospasm if the aneurysm has been secured.
  - Nimodipine decreases morbidity.
  - Other treatment modalities include
    - Selective intraarterial injection of vasodilators
    - Balloon angioplasty of the affected arterial segments
- Other complications of SAH include seizures, hydrocephalus, and intracerebral hematoma.
- Other effects of SAH
  - ECG changes are frequent but rarely clinically significant.
    - Q waves warrant further cardiac workup.
  - Mild elevation of cardiac enzymes is frequent.
    - Does not usually correlate with significant myocardial dysfunction or poor outcome.
  - Hyponatremia is commonly seen after SAH.
    - Correction with sodium supplementation (e.g., 3% hypertonic saline)
- Major anesthetic management goals for intracranial aneurysm clipping
  - Prevent increases in systemic blood pressure and re-rupture
  - Facilitate surgical exposure and access to the aneurysm
- Anesthetic considerations of aneurysm clipping
  - Minimize hypertensive responses to noxious stimulation such as laryngoscopy and head pin placement.
  - Maintain CPP to prevent ischemia during surgical retraction, temporary vessel occlusion, or due to cerebral vasospasm.
  - Hemodynamic control during dissection of the aneurysm to minimize risk of intraoperative rupture
  - Temporary occlusive clips applied to the major feeding artery of the aneurysm can create regional arterial hypotension and cerebral ischemia.
    - Maintain a normal or increased systemic arterial blood pressure to facilitate perfusion through collateral circulations.
    - Achieving burst suppression on EEG monitoring may provide some protection from cerebral ischemia.

- Extubation is the goal in the absence of significant neurologic impairment or major intraoperative complications.
- Postoperative goals
  - Prevention of vasospasm and seizures
  - Maintenance of CPP

Anesthetic Considerations for Aneurysmal Clipping
▪ Prevent sudden increases in arterial blood pressure, which could increase the risk of re-rupture. ▪ Optimize brain relaxation to facilitate surgical exposure to aneurysm. ▪ Maintain CPP to prevent ischemia due to surgical retraction or vasospasm. ▪ During temporary vessel occlusion, maintain a normal or increased blood pressure to facilitate perfusion through collateral circulations.

Arteriovenous Malformations

- Up to 10% of patients diagnosed with an AVM have an associated aneurysm.
- Risk of hemorrhage is related to anatomic features of AVM, including size and characteristics of feeding arteries and draining veins.
- Treatment options:
  - Open resection
  - Endovascular embolization
  - Stereotactic radiosurgery (gamma knife)
- Preoperative embolization is frequently used to reduce blood loss during surgical resection.
- Anesthesia for resection or embolization of AVMs is similar to that of aneurysms with a few distinct considerations:
  - AVMs are unlikely to rupture due to acute arterial hypertension (e.g., during laryngoscopy) due to their flow characteristics (high flow, low resistance).
    - Acute hypertension is still avoided, given the high rate of associated aneurysms.
  - Be prepared for
    - Massive, persistent blood loss
    - Postresection cerebral edema

Carotid Disease

- Stroke is a leading cause of death and disability.
- Carotid atherosclerotic disease is a major cause of stroke.
- Carotid endarterectomy (CEA) remains "gold standard" in treating carotid disease.
  - Perioperative risk of stroke or death is 4%–7%.
- Preoperative assessment includes perioperative risk of cardiac ischemia due to global vascular disease.
- General or regional anesthesia (deep and superficial cervical plexus block) may be used for CEA.
  - No outcome difference has been shown.
- Regional anesthesia
  - Accurate intraoperative assessment of patient's neurologic status
  - Requires a cooperative and motionless patient
- Anesthetic goals
  - Prevent cerebral ischemia by maintaining adequate CPP.
  - Prevent myocardial ischemia by avoiding acute hypertension and tachycardia.
    - Invasive hemodynamic monitoring is indicated.
  - During intraoperative carotid artery clamping, MAP is often maintained above baseline (within 20%) to augment collateral flow.
  - Avoid hypocarbia, given risk of cerebral vasoconstriction and ischemia.
  - Methods to detect intraoperative cerebral ischemia and need for shunting during clamping (none have been shown to definitively improve outcome)
    - EEG
    - Evoked potentials
    - Transcranial Doppler
    - Cerebral oximetry
    - Stump pressure
  - Common postoperative complications
    - Myocardial ischemia
    - Neurologic deficits secondary to intraoperative emboli
  - Postoperative hypertension may lead to complications.
    - Neck hematoma with airway compromise
    - Hyperperfusion syndrome
  - Cerebral hyperperfusion syndrome (rare)
    - Symptoms: severe headache, eye and facial pain, focal neurologic deficits, seizures, and loss of consciousness
    - Mechanism: likely due to impairment of cerebral autoregulation
    - Management: Keep postprocedural blood pressure <140/90 mmHg, or possibly lower based on patient and procedure characteristics.

QUESTIONS

NEUROANATOMY

1. What are the major feeding and distributing vessels for the anterior and posterior cerebral circulations?
2. What is the vascular loop at the base of the brain, and what potential clinical benefit does it provide?

NEUROPHYSIOLOGY

3. Describe cerebral autoregulation.
4. How might you reduce CBF to provide brain relaxation during intracranial surgery?

INTRACRANIAL PRESSURE AND BRAIN RELAXATION

5. If a patient has perioperative ICP elevation or requires additional intraoperative brain relaxation, what are the three volumes contained within the cranium that one must ensure are optimized?

ANESTHESIA FOR NEUROSURGERY

6. What are the principles of perioperative ICP management?

COMMON CLINICAL CASES

7. What are the considerations of a sitting-position craniotomy?
8. What are the considerations for the management of patients undergoing craniotomy for intracranial aneurysm surgery?

ANSWERS

NEUROANATOMY

1. The paired internal carotid arteries and their main distributive vessels (anterior cerebral artery, middle cerebral artery, posterior communicating artery) make up the anterior circulation. The posterior circulation arises from the paired vertebral arteries that join on the anterior surface of the brainstem to form the basilar artery. The basilar artery then gives rise to paired posterior cerebral arteries. (533)
2. The anastomotic vascular loop at the base of the brain is the circle of Willis. It provides potential for collateral blood flow between the left and right vascular territories as well as between anterior and posterior cerebral circulations, which may provide protection during focal ischemia (e.g., carotid clamping during carotid endarterectomy). (533)

NEUROPHYSIOLOGY

3. Cerebral autoregulation describes the vasoconstriction or vasodilation of cerebral blood vessels to maintain a relatively stable cerebral blood flow (CBF) when the cerebral perfusion pressure (CPP) fluctuates. At the lower and upper limits of cerebral perfusion pressure, cerebral autoregulation is not effective, and CBF becomes proportional to CPP. These limits vary among individuals, but generally quoted limits for cerebral autoregulation are CPP 60 mmHg to 150 mmHg. (534)
4. Hyperventilation to moderate hypocapnia ($PaCO_2$ 30–35 mmHg) is a rapid means to reduce ICP or improve intraoperative brain relaxation by reducing CBF. Suppression of the electrophysiologic component of $CMRO_2$ with propofol (GABAergic drugs) causes concomitant CBF reduction via neurovascular coupling. Convert to a total intravenous anesthetic to eliminate the direct cerebral vasodilatory effects of halogenated anesthetics that may be increasing cerebral blood volume. (534–536)

INTRACRANIAL PRESSURE AND BRAIN RELAXATION

5. The three components that make up intracranial volume are brain parenchyma (cells and interstitial fluid), cerebrospinal fluid, and intravascular blood (venous and arterial). (536)

ANESTHESIA FOR NEUROSURGERY

6. Perioperative ICP management includes reducing the volumes of the three intracranial components and avoiding drugs or physiologic changes that may increase volume. Head of bed elevation increases cerebral venous outflow (venous blood) and redistributes CSF from intracranial to spinal subarachnoid space. Hyperosmolar agents (mannitol, hypertonic saline) are used to reduce brain parenchyma volume, and dexamethasone is used to reduce parenchyma volume associated with vasogenic edema. CBF (arterial blood) is reduced as needed with GABAergic drugs (intravenous agents are superior to volatile agents) via neurovascular coupling and moderate hyperventilation ($PaCO_2$ reduction). Avoid poor neck positioning (excessive flexion, rotation, compression) impairing cerebral venous drainage, hyperthermia-induced increases in $CMRO_2$/CBF, vasodilating agents, and hypoxia-induced vasodilation. (540)

COMMON CLINICAL CASES

7. For the patient scheduled for a sitting craniotomy, consider preoperative echocardiography to assess for a PFO that could result in a paradoxical air embolism (ischemic stroke or coronary ischemia). Consider central venous catheter and precordial Doppler due to high risk of venous air embolism. Minimize neck flexion and oropharyngeal devices that may compress the tongue (causing impaired venous drainage or compression ischemia). Intraoperatively, monitor cerebral perfusion accurately by positioning the arterial line transducer at the level of the external auditory meatus. Ensure adequate fluid resuscitation to compensate for venous pooling in the lower body. Monitor for arrhythmias, hemodynamic lability, and potential injury to brainstem and lower

CNs that may impair the respiratory center or the patient's ability to protect their airway postoperatively. Evaluate the safety of extubation in regard to lower CN function, ability of patient to protect their airway, and risk of postoperative respiratory failure. (542)

8. Patients with intracranial aneurysms have several specific considerations for their perioperative management. Preoperatively, assess the patient for neurologic deficits, or evidence of symptomatic vasospasm that can be treated with nimodipine. Changes in the electrocardiogram are frequently present but do not usually correlate with myocardial pathology. The anesthetic plan should be focused on brain relaxation and maintaining cerebral perfusion while avoiding increases in systemic blood pressure that can result in aneurysmal bleeding or rebleeding. During surgical retraction and temporary clipping, normal to increased systemic blood pressure may be necessary, and EEG burst suppression can be considered. Early awakening is usually preferred to evaluate the patient's neurologic status. (543)

Chapter

31 OPHTHALMOLOGY AND OTOLARYNGOLOGY

Steven Gayer and Howard D. Palte

OPHTHALMOLOGY

- Eye surgery among most frequent procedures; majority are cataracts but large variety
  - Typically older or pediatric patients
- Majority are under monitored anesthesia care (MAC) with regional or topical anesthesia

Intraocular Pressure (IOP)

- Intraocular pressure (IOP) range is 10 mmHg to 22 mmHg in normal intact eye
  - Primarily derived from balance between aqueous humor production and drainage
  - Small transient changes occur daily (e.g., eyelid closure, postural changes, mydriasis).

Factors That Influence Intraocular Pressure

- Sustained increased IOP during anesthesia risks acute glaucoma, retinal hemorrhage, retinal ischemia, and permanent visual loss.
- IOP is increased by venous congestion, straining, retching, coughing, and bucking; arterial hypertension has less impact.
  - Bucking during induction of anesthesia can increase IOP by ≥40 mmHg.
- IOP changes significantly more with tracheal intubation than with supraglottic airway.
- IOP increases with hypoxemia and hypoventilation, decreases with hyperventilation and hypothermia

Anesthetic Drugs and Intraocular Pressure

- Most anesthetic agents reduce IOP; succinylcholine produces transient mild increase.
  - Can be mitigated by pretreatment with a nondepolarizing neuromuscular blocking agent (NMBA) or lidocaine

Management of Elevated Intraocular Pressure
▪ Head-up position
▪ Avoid constriction around neck ("tight ties pop eyes")
▪ Consider intravenous mannitol prior to surgery
▪ Consider carbonic anhydrase inhibitor (acetazolamide)
▪ Avoid coughing, retching, straining
▪ Supraglottic airway preferable for GA

Ophthalmic Medications

- Topical ophthalmic agents are readily absorbed systemically via conjunctiva or nasolacrimal duct.
- Phenylephrine drops are associated with significant transient increase in systemic blood pressure (10% >> 2.5%).

Oculocardiac Reflex

- Severe bradycardia or asystole induced by traction of extraocular muscles (strabismus surgery), globe pressure, or during ophthalmic regional anesthetic nerve block
  - May also induce atrioventricular block, ventricular bigeminy, multifocal premature ventricular contractions, or ventricular tachycardia
- Mediated by trigeminal nerve (afferent limb) and vagus nerve (efferent limb)
- Exacerbated by hypoxemia, hypercarbia, acidosis, light anesthesia
- Treatment: prompt removal of instigating stimulus and administration of a parasympatholytic drug if necessary, e.g., atropine or glycopyrrolate
- Avoided with regional eye block, deep anesthesia, or prophylactic anticholinergic (children)

Management of Oculocardiac Reflex
▪ Vigilance – strabismus surgery, pressure on globe
▪ Immediate cessation stimulus ("STOP!")
▪ Assure oxygenation, ventilation, and depth of anesthesia
▪ Consider infiltration of local anesthesia
▪ Recurrences typically attenuated
▪ Consider anticholinergic if symptoms persist

Preoperative Assessment

- Patients at all extremes of age, pediatric syndromes prominent
  - Routine laboratory testing is not indicated.
- Assess risk/benefit of continuing perioperative antithrombotics
- Assessment of the likelihood of intraoperative patient movement is critical.

Anesthetic Options

- General anesthesia, MAC + regional, or topical anesthesia

Needle-Based Ophthalmic Regional Anesthesia

- Regional anesthesia is rarely associated with serious complications, such as convulsions, respiratory arrest, or cardiovascular collapse.

Complications of Regional Anesthesia for Ophthalmic Surgery
▪ Superficial or retrobulbar hemorrhage
▪ Elicitation of oculocardiac reflex
▪ Puncture of the globe
▪ Intraocular injection
▪ Optic nerve trauma
▪ Seizures
▪ Brainstem anesthesia
▪ Central retinal artery occlusion
▪ Blindness

- Intraconal (retrobulbar) block – steeply-angled needle placed within the extraocular muscle cone with tip behind globe
- Extraconal (peribulbar) block – shallow-angle and depth with needle tip outside extraocular muscle cone
  - Safer, but requires larger volumes and more time for diffusion
  - Facial nerve branch innervating orbicularis oculi muscle is also blocked, preventing eyelid squeezing

Cannula-Based Ophthalmic Regional Anesthesia

- Sub-Tenon (episcleral) block – conjunctival dissection with cannula introduced under the capsule of Tenon

Benefits of Ophthalmic Regional Blocks
▪ Analgesia
▪ Akinesia
▪ Suppression of the oculocardiac reflex
▪ Postoperative pain management

Topical Ophthalmic Regional Anesthesia

- Topical – used extensively for cataract surgery; surgeon can supplement with anterior chamber injection of preservative-free local anesthetic

Anesthesia Management of Specific Ophthalmic Procedures

Retina Surgery

- Surgical interventions include scleral buckle, vitrectomy, laser treatment, cryotherapy, and injection of intravitreal gas.
- Diabetic and myopic patients are at higher risk for retina pathology.
- A deep plane anesthesia or dense regional block is required because extensive manipulation of eye risks eliciting the oculocardiac reflex.
- Insoluble intravitreal gas (e.g., sulfur hexafluoride) tamponades retina onto the choroid, slowly resorbed over 10 to 28 days
  - Nitrous oxide can cause permanent loss of vision by diffusing into and expanding the gas bubble.

Glaucoma Surgery

- Sustained increases in IOP affect optic nerve and vision.
- Various forms: acquired vs. congenital, open-angle vs. closed-angle, acute vs. chronic
- Anesthesia management aims to avoid mydriasis and prevent acute increases in IOP.
  - Topical atropine (not intravenous) produces mydriasis and may trigger acute glaucoma crisis.

Strabismus Surgery

- Intraoperative oculocardiac reflex common
- High risk for postoperative nausea and vomiting
- Potential increased risk for malignant hyperthermia and masseter muscle spasm with succinylcholine

Traumatic Eye Injuries

- Avoid increasing IOP such as tight facemask, coughing, Trendelenburg position
- If emergent, patient may be nonfasting and require rapid sequence induction (RSI).
  - Place patient in reverse Trendelenburg position.
  - Consider modified RSI with large dose of NMBA.
  - Succinylcholine may cause transient increase in IOP.

   - Consider pretreatment with a small dose of NMBA or IV lidocaine.
  - Awake endotracheal intubations can greatly increase IOP.
- Regional anesthesia may be an option for select, high-risk patients.

Postoperative Eye Issues

Corneal Abrasion

- Most common cause of postoperative eye pain
- Clinical signs include pain, tearing, foreign body sensation, and photophobia.
- Causes can be general anesthesia–induced loss of blink reflex and diminished tear production, and mechanically by ID tags, anesthesia mask, drapes, or other objects
- Prevention is with eye taping and protective goggles.
  - Ointment can cause postoperative blurring.
- Treated with antibiotic eye ointment and patching for 1 to 2 days

Acute Glaucoma

- Presents as painful, red eye with dilated pupil
- Emergent consult with ophthalmologist is indicated.

Postoperative Visual Loss

- Painless loss of vision following surgery can be ischemic optic neuropathy.
  - Highest-risk surgeries are spine surgery in prone position and cardiac surgery.

OTOLARYNGOLOGY

Issues Related to Otolaryngologic Surgery
▪ Difficult airway ▪ Securing of the endotracheal tube (ETT) ▪ Patient head movement during surgery that can alter ETT placement ▪ ETT occlusion, cuff leaks, disconnections, or dislodgement ▪ Airway compromise by undetected bleeding, edema, or surgical manipulation ▪ Use of posterior pharyngeal packs

Special Considerations for Head and Neck Surgery

The Difficult Airway

- Options to secure the airway include videolaryngoscopy, fiberoptic bronchoscopy, tracheostomy under local anesthesia.
  - Tracheal retention sutures should be placed to recapture airway patency if needed.
- May require postoperative intubation or postoperative nebulized bronchodilators

Laryngospasm

- Mediated by vagal stimulation of superior laryngeal nerve
- Larynx abruptly, completely closes, compromising ventilation.
  - Hypercarbia, hypoxia, and acidosis result in hypertension and tachycardia.
  - Hypoxemia develops rapidly in pediatric patients.
- Causes: instrumentation of the airway, presence of blood or foreign body, inadequate anesthesia
- Treatment: 100% O_2, positive-pressure mask ventilation, oral or nasal airway, deepened anesthesia; consider small-dose succinylcholine
  - Temporal reduction in brainstem firing results in vocal cord relaxation.

Upper Respiratory Infections

- Predisposes children to airway hyperactivity, breath holding, hypoxemia, croup (postextubation airway edema)
- Consider delaying surgery, but may not be needed for uncomplicated URI and brief, non-airway procedure

Epistaxis

- Concealed blood loss due to swallowing; may need rehydration prior to induction of anesthesia
- High risk for aspiration

Obstructive Sleep Apnea

- Symptoms: snoring, sleep disturbance, headache, and daytime somnolence and, in children, behavior and growth disturbances, poor school performance
- Sensitive to hypnotics (sedation) and narcotics (respiratory depression)
- Airway anatomy is often obese with short, thick necks.
- Predictive of difficulty with airway management including mask ventilation, laryngoscopy, and endotracheal intubation

Airway Fires

- Three elements are needed to produce operating room fire.
  - Heat (ignition source) – laser or electrocautery
  - Fuel – paper drapes, endotracheal tube, gauze swabs
  - Oxidizer – oxygen, air, nitrous oxide
- Procedures around head or face during general anesthesia or MAC when electrocautery is used near supplemental oxygen or airway

Anesthesia Management of Specific Otolaryngology Procedures

Ear Surgery

- Nitrous oxide: diffuses into air-filled cavities and increases middle ear pressure

   - Should be avoided or discontinued at least 15 minutes prior to placement of an eardrum graft
- Facial nerve monitoring: when used to avoid surgical injury, NMBAs must be limited to the induction of anesthesia.
- Epinephrine: injections to reduce blood in surgical field may produce dysrhythmias with systemic uptake.
   - Limit concentration of epinephrine to 1:200,000 and consider reverse Trendelenburg position.
- Emergence: movement of head to place bandages can cause ETT movement, airway irritation, coughing, and bucking.
   - Can lead to acute venous bleeding and graft disruption
   - Consider extubation of trachea at a deep plane of anesthesia, if appropriate
- Postoperative nausea and vomiting: common after middle ear surgery
   - Exacerbated by postoperative patient movement and inadequate hydration
   - Apply multimodal antiemetic strategy
- Myringotomy and tube insertion: brief procedure for children, preferably performed with inhalation induction and maintenance with facemask

Tonsillectomy and Adenoidectomy

- Patients frequently have upper airway obstruction, obstructive sleep apnea.
- A cuffed, preformed, curved ETT with air leak at 20 cm H_2O may be used.
- Perioperative issues include airway obstruction, laryngospasm, bleeding, dysrhythmias, croup, and nausea and vomiting.
   - IV dexamethasone may help decrease edema, postoperative pain, and postoperative nausea and vomiting (PONV).
   - In patients <4 years old, postoperative airway obstruction can occur up to 24 hours later.
- Post-tonsillectomy bleeding is associated with occult, swallowed blood loss.
   - Tachycardia, expectoration of red blood, PONV
   - Rehydration and available working suction are critical prior to an RSI.

Epiglottitis

- Cause: most often *Haemophilus influenzae* type B in children 2 to 7 years old with sudden-onset dysphagia and fever
- Clinical signs: agitation, drooling, leaning forward, extended neck, dyspnea
- Management: inhalation induction, spontaneous respiration, availability of an array of anesthesia equipment, and an otolaryngologist prepared for emergent tracheostomy

Foreign Body in Airway

- Mostly occurs in children, requires emergent response
- Clinical signs: dyspnea, dry cough, hoarseness, and wheezing
- Minimize positive-pressure ventilation to avoid distal displacement and complete airway obstruction.
- Surgeon retrieval is via direct laryngoscopy or rigid bronchoscopy while patient is spontaneously breathing.
- For patients <4 years old, airway obstruction can occur up to 24 hours postoperatively.

Nasal and Sinus Surgery

- Functional (endoscopic sinus surgery, polypectomy, septoplasty) or cosmetic (rhinoplasty)
   - Nasal polyps are associated with allergy and reactive airway disease.
   - Significant nasal obstruction may hinder facemask ventilation.
- Topical anesthesia with local anesthetic/vasoconstrictor–soaked pledgets.
   - Cocaine is used less due to cardiovascular and sensorium effects.
- Issues include occult swallowed blood loss into pharynx and stomach, PONV, and dehydration.
   - Extubate trachea after pharyngeal packs removed and airway reflexes return.

Cochlear Implant Surgery

- Majority are done under general anesthesia.

Endoscopic Surgery

- Includes esophagoscopy, bronchoscopy, laryngoscopy, and microlaryngoscopy (with or without laser surgery).
- Possible indications are foreign body, gastroesophageal reflux, papillomatosis, tumors or tracheal stenosis.
- Shared airway with surgeon calls for proactive airway management discussion.
- Techniques may include an anticholinergic agent to decrease secretions, awake fiberoptic endotracheal intubation, and succinylcholine infusion for masseter relaxation.
   - Risk for phase II neuromuscular blockade with succinylcholine infusion
- Consider small-diameter ETT, manual jet ventilator, high-flow nasal O_2.
   - Wall source oxygen supply can result in pneumothorax or pneumomediastinum with manual jet ventilator unless inspiratory pressure is reduced.

Laser Surgery

- Laser energy can cause retinal damage and produce toxic fumes with potential for disease transmission.

- Use a small-diameter ETT to maximize surgical exposure.
- Use smoke evacuator, special masks, protective eyeglasses, and tape patient's eyes.
- Fire hazard precautions must be followed.

Operating Room Precautions for Laser Surgery
Preoperative 1. Avoid accumulation of combustible gases (O_2, N_2O) in surgical drapes. 2. Allow time for flammable skin preparations to dry. 3. Moisten gauze and sponges in vicinity of laser beam.
Intraoperative 1. Alert surgeon and OR personnel about ignition risk. 2. Assign specific roles to each OR member in case of fire. 3. Use appropriate laser-resistant ETT. 4. Reduce inspired O_2 to minimum values. 5. Replace N_2O with air. Wait a few minutes after steps 4 and 5 before activating laser.

Neck Dissection Surgery

- Pulmonary disease is common secondary to smoking history.
  - Consider preoperative pulmonary evaluation, early tracheostomy.
- Challenges can include airway management, radiation changes, intraoperative nerve monitoring, venous air embolism, and carotid sinus traction.
  - Carotid sinus reflex produces prolonged QT interval, bradydysrhythmias, asystole
  - Can be blocked with local anesthetic infiltration
- Postoperative challenges can include unilateral or bilateral vocal cord paralysis (recurrent laryngeal nerve damage), paralysis of ipsilateral diaphragm (phrenic nerve damage), pneumothorax, and bleeding with airway compromise.

Thyroid and Parathyroid Surgery

- Consider armored ETT or a special ETT to facilitate electromyography monitoring of recurrent laryngeal nerve.
- Thyroid storm (massive catecholamine release) can occur with uncontrolled hyperthyroidism.
  - Signs include tachycardia, hypertension, and diaphoresis.
- Postoperative challenges
  - Recurrent laryngeal nerve injury can be unilateral (hoarseness, stridor) or bilateral (airway obstruction).
  - Hypocalcemia – signs include tetany, cardiac dysrhythmias, laryngospasm
  - Bleeding causing airway compression – treat with prompt opening of wound to release accumulated hematoma

Parotid Surgery

- Parotid gland is traversed by facial nerve; monitoring requires avoidance of NMBAs.

Facial Trauma

- Le Fort Classifications I, II, III
- Orotracheal intubation is necessary with possible intranasal injury.

QUESTIONS

1. What are the goals for the anesthesia management of ophthalmic surgery?
2. What are the effects of the various airway management techniques on intraocular pressure?
3. What are the potential systemic side effects of ophthalmic medications?
4. A patient loses consciousness shortly after a retrobulbar block for eye surgery. What is the differential diagnosis and appropriate intervention?
5. A patient who receives sedation for a regional ophthalmic block may develop complications, including oversedation, brainstem anesthesia, or intravascular injection. Complete the following table by indicating whether the listed clinical finding is likely (+), may be present (+/–), or not present (0) with these complications.

Clinical Finding	Oversedation	Brainstem Anesthesia	Intravascular Injection
Loss of consciousness			
Apnea			
Cardiac instability			
Seizure activity			
Contralateral mydriasis			
Contralateral eye block			

6. Your patient in PACU complains of a painful eye. What is the differential diagnosis?
7. What are appropriate precautions for airway laser surgery?
8. What action should you take if your patient has a fire in the airway? Outside the airway?
9. What are potential complications after thyroid surgery?

ANSWERS

1. Goals for the anesthesia management of ophthalmic surgery include safety, analgesia, akinesia, control of intraocular pressure, avoidance of the oculocardiac reflex, awareness and mitigation of possible drug interactions, and awakening without coughing, nausea, or vomiting. (549)
2. Intraocular pressure (IOP) may be exacerbated by difficulty with assisted mask ventilation. Early insertion of an oral or nasal airway may be beneficial. Direct laryngoscopy and endotracheal intubation each increase IOP. Ensure adequate depth of anesthesia and consider intravenous agents such as lidocaine prior to airway manipulation. Similarly, coughing and straining against the endotracheal tube on emergence will provoke acute elevations in IOP. Of note, supraglottic airways are associated with minimal changes in IOP both on insertion and removal. (547)
3. Ophthalmic medications are systemically absorbed through the nasolacrimal duct and nasal mucosa. Phenylephrine drops are commonly used to dilate the pupil to facilitate eye surgery. High concentration (10%) phenylephrine will produce marked and sustained hypertension. Phospholine iodide (echothiopate), a miosis-inducing anticholinesterase, inhibits succinylcholine metabolism and may result in markedly prolonged paralysis. Carbonic anhydrase inhibitors may induce a metabolic acidosis. Intravenous mannitol produces an initial increase in intravascular volume and triggers cardiac decompensation in susceptible individuals. (547)
4. The differential diagnosis for loss of consciousness (LOC) after a retrobulbar block includes oversedation, intravascular injection, and brainstem anesthesia. Excessive sedation may also lead to apnea and cardiac instability. The diagnostic feature of intravascular injection of local anesthesia (LA) is abrupt onset of seizure activity in addition to potential LOC, apnea, or cardiac instability. Brainstem anesthesia results from retrograde spread of LA within the optic nerve dural sheath to the brainstem. In addition to potential LOC, apnea, or cardiac issues, physical signs that may be diagnostic include contralateral mydriasis and ophthalmoplegia. (549)
5. The following table indicates whether the listed clinical finding is likely (+), may be present (+/−), or not present (0) with the corresponding complication. (550)

Clinical Finding	Oversedation	Brainstem Anesthesia	Intravascular Injection
Loss of consciousness	+/–	+	+
Apnea	+/–	+	+/–
Cardiac instability	+/–	+	+/–
Seizure activity	0	0	+
Contralateral mydriasis	0	+/–	0
Contralateral eye block	0	+/–	0

6. The most common reason for a painful eye in the PACU is corneal abrasion. This injury is probably more prevalent than reported and may be caused by a variety of etiologies, such as incomplete eyelid taping, reduced tear production during general anesthesia and direct injury from ID badges. Patients frequently complain of pain, irritation, and photophobia. The application of a drop of ophthalmic local anesthetic will result in immediate relief. The majority of abrasions will heal spontaneously. A more malign cause of unilateral eye pain is acute angle closure glaucoma. The eye is red, and local anesthetic instillation produces no relief. An urgent ophthalmology consult is warranted. (552)
7. Laser surgery around the airway confers potential for severe tissue injury and airway fire. Laser-specific, modified small-diameter endotracheal tubes (ETTs) that carry minimal risk for combustion should be used. Of note, laser beams are injurious to the retina and appropriate eye shielding is needed. Laser treatments are used for a variety of medical conditions such as tumor and viral papillomata. The fumes generated may be toxic and infectious; OR personnel should take suitable precautions. (556)
8. For a fire in the airway or breathing circuit, as fast as possible:
   a. Immediately remove the endotracheal tube.
   b. Stop the flow of all airway gases.
   c. Remove all flammable and burning materials from the airway.
   d. Pour saline or water into the patient's airway.
   e. Reestablish ventilation by mask, avoiding supplemental oxygen if possible.

f. Extinguish and examine the tracheal tube to assess whether fragments were left in the airway. Consider bronchoscopy (preferably rigid) to look for tracheal tube fragments, assess injury, and remove residual debris.
g. Assess the patient's status, and devise a plan for ongoing care.

For a fire elsewhere on or in the patient, as fast as possible:
h. Stop the flow of all airway gases.
i. Remove all drapes, flammable, and burning materials from the patient.
j. Extinguish all burning materials in, on, and around the patient (e.g., with saline, water, or smothering). (556)

9. Thyroid surgery should not be undertaken until medical stabilization of the underlying condition is assured. In the postoperative phase bleeding and tissue edema may directly compromise the airway via external compression. This is a surgical emergency. The parathyroid glands are located in close proximity to the thyroid and may be inadvertently removed at surgery. This may result in an acute hypocalcemic crisis manifest by weakness, tetany, and laryngospasm. Direct injury to the recurrent laryngeal nerve will manifest as hoarseness or stridor. (557)

Chapter

32 ORTHOPEDIC SURGERY

David Furgiuele, Mitchell H. Marshall, and Andrew D. Rosenberg

RHEUMATOLOGIC DISORDERS

Rheumatoid Arthritis

- Chronic inflammatory disease
  - Initially affects joints and adjacent connective tissues
  - Progresses to systemic disease affecting major organ systems
- Causes include genetic, environmental, bacterial, viral, and hormonal factors.
- Systemic manifestation is widespread and can affect every organ system.
  - Pulmonary with interstitial fibrosis and cysts with honeycombing
  - Gastritis and ulcers from aspirin and other analgesics
  - Neuropathy, muscle wasting, vasculitis, and anemia

Airway and Cervical Spine Changes

- The patient's airway should be evaluated for both complexity and risk of endotracheal intubation.
- Mouth opening may be decreased due to temporomandibular arthritis.
- Hypoplastic mandible may fuse early in juvenile rheumatoid arthritis (RA).
  - Can result in noticeable overbite
- Cricoarytenoid arthritis can result in shortness of breath and snoring.
  - May be mistaken for sleep apnea
  - Presents with stridor during inspiration, which may occur after anesthesia
  - Acute subluxation of the cricoarytenoid can be caused by intubation, which does not respond to treatment with racemic epinephrine.
- Cervical spine is abnormal in as many as 80% of patients.
- Sites of potential cervical spine involvement are illustrated in the figure below.

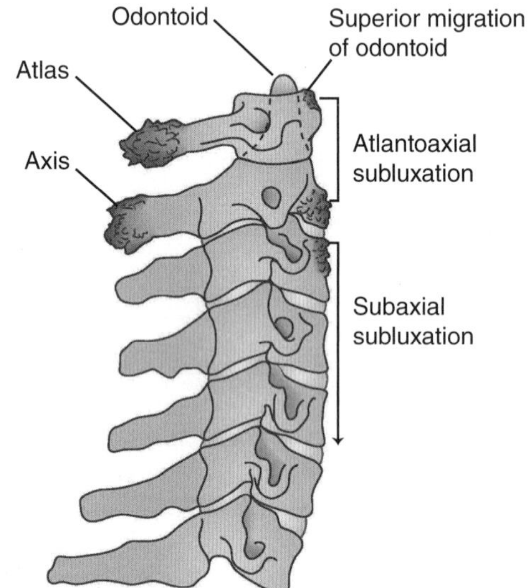

Atlantoaxial Subluxation

- Abnormal movement of C1 vertebra (atlas) on C2 (axis)
  - Result of destruction of the transverse axial ligament (TAL)
  - Movement of the odontoid process (dens) is no longer restricted.
- Dens is the superior projection of C2.
  - C1 vertebra can sublux on the C2 vertebra during flexion and extension
- Can result in impingement of the spinal cord

- The figures below demonstrate normal anatomy (A), and atlantoaxial subluxation (spinal cord impingement) due to destruction of the transverse axial ligament (B).

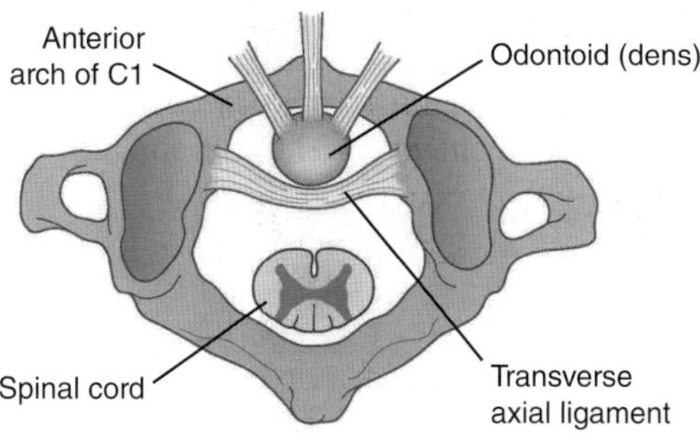

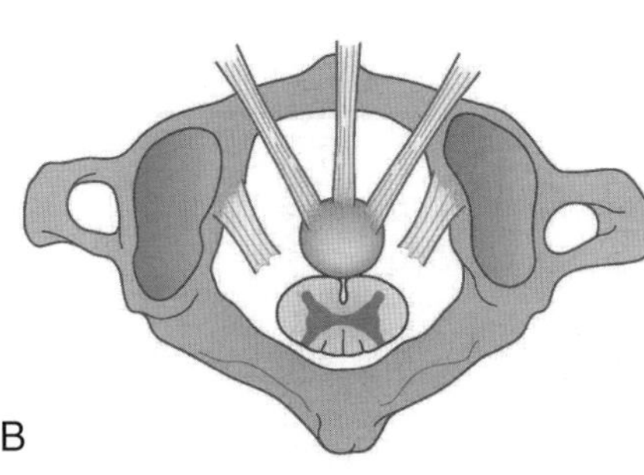

- The degree of subluxation is quantified by the atlas–dens interval (ADI)
  - Flexion and extension radiographs of the cervical spine
  - Determine distance between atlas and dens, and degree of subluxation
- ADI ≥4 mm – instability present, subluxation considered significant, and considered risk for spinal cord injury
- As ADI increases, safe area for the cord (SAC) decreases and higher risk for impingement
- Extension of the head decreases ADI and increases SAC.
- Flexion of the head increases ADI and decreases SAC.

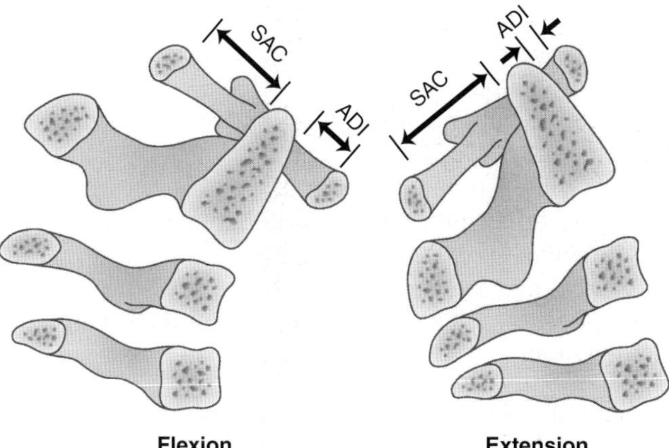

- Asymptomatic patients may have compromised SAC whose instability is compensated by the surrounding musculature while awake.
- Neck motion should be minimized.
- The figures below demonstrate the effects of neck flexion (increased ADI) and extension (decreased ADI) on the safe area for the cord.

Subaxial Subluxation

- Subluxation of ≥15% of cervical vertebra below the level of C2 (axis)
- Can result in significant spinal cord impingement
- C5-C6 level most common
- Neck motion should be minimized.

Superior Migration of the Odontoid

- Inflammation and bone destruction can cause cervical collapse.
- Spared odontoid may project through the foramen magnum into the skull.
  - Can impinge on brainstem resulting in neurologic symptoms, including paralysis or quadriparesis
  - Transoral odontoidectomy decompresses the spinal cord, followed by posterior spinal fusion for stability.
  - This is illustrated in the figure below.

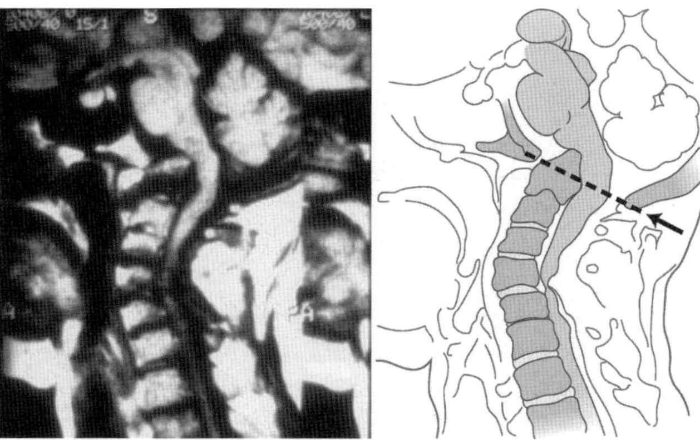

The Trachea in Rheumatoid Arthritis

- The trachea is usually spared in RA.
- Can twist as cervical spine collapses
  - May increase intubation difficulty

Ankylosing Spondylitis

- Inflammatory rheumatologic disorder with repetitive minute fracture and healing
  - Bamboo spine
  - Disease of the sacroiliac joint
  - Fusion of the posterior elements of the spinal column
  - Fixed neck flexion

- Association with *HLA-B27*
- Thoracic and costochondral involvement may cause rapid, shallow breathing.
- Rigid cervical spine may lead to airway management difficulty.
- Cervical spine surgery may return neck to neutral position.
  - Complicated and dangerous procedure
  - Relies on spinal cord monitoring as spine is manipulated

SPINE SURGERY

- Potential for long complex procedures with significant blood loss, fluid shifts, and hemodynamic alterations
- Require in-depth preoperative evaluations to include the assessment for blood products and appropriate monitoring requirements.
- Surgical approach can be posterior or anterior with cervical, thoracic, or abdominal approaches.
- Lung isolation may be necessary for thoracic approach.
  - Double-lumen endotracheal tube (ETT)
    - Exchange with a single-lumen ETT can become difficult due to airway edema.
  - Bronchial blocker
    - Advantageous in that it can be withdrawn when no longer needed
    - Avoids the need to change the ETT from a double to a single lumen
  - CO_2 insufflation can move the lung away from the surgical field.
    - Allows the use of a single-lumen ETT for the entire procedure.

Anesthetic Technique

- Use medications that do not interfere with neurologic monitoring.
- Monitoring of somatosensory evoked potentials (SSEPs)
  - Inhaled anesthetic <50% of 1 MAC
- Transcranial motor evoked potentials (TCMEPs)
  - Volatile anesthetics can interfere with signal acquisition.
    - If used at all, should be discontinued if adequate signals cannot be obtained
  - Paralysis with neuromuscular blockade should not be maintained in continuous TCMEP monitoring.
- Electromyograms (EMGs)
  - Neuromuscular blockade should be discontinued before EMGs performed.

Awareness

- Increased risk due to anesthetic technique that provides for adequate neurophysiologic monitoring
- Brain function monitoring may help avoid awareness, but this has not yet been proved.

Blood Conservation During Spine Surgery

- Predonation, hemodilution, wound infiltration with dilute epinephrine, hypotensive anesthetic techniques, cell salvage, appropriate positioning, and surgical technique are all methods used to mitigate blood loss.
- Antifibrinolytics decrease blood loss.
  - Aprotinin: serine protease inhibitor
    - Withdrawn from market due to negative cardiovascular effects
  - Tranexamic acid and aminocaproic acid: synthetic lysine analogs
    - Tranexamic acid is more effective in decreasing blood loss.

Positioning

- Prone position
  - Neck maintained in neutral position
  - Contact areas padded
  - Face and eyes protected
  - Periodic repositioning may be needed to prevent pressure ulcers.
  - Direct pressure on eyes can result in visual loss.

Intraoperative Spinal Cord Monitoring

- Used to detect and correct adverse effects during the operative period
- Anesthetic technique must be adjusted when certain monitoring techniques are used.

Somatosensory Evoked Potentials

- Signals from cerebral cortex in response to repetitive peripheral nerve stimulation
  - Signals must travel through an intact dorsal column of spinal cord to reach the cerebral cortex.
  - The SSEP waveform is analyzed and monitored for increased latency and decreased amplitude.
- Increased latency >10%, decreased amplitude >60%, or inability to obtain a waveform may indicate spinal cord dysfunction or disruption.
  - Can be from surgical injury, stretching, or blood supply impairment
  - Direct injury is immediate, whereas ischemia can manifest over time.
  - Hypotension, hypothermia, volatile anesthetics, benzodiazepines, hypercarbia, hypocarbia, and anemia can affect SSEPs.
- If a change is noted, arterial blood pressure should be increased while surgical and physiologic causes are sought.

Transcranial Motor Evoked Potentials

- Monitors the ventral column of the spinal cord

- Stimulation over motor cortex generates a waveform down motor pathways and is detected in the arm or leg.
- Loss of wave may indicate neurologic injury.
- Cannot be monitored under neuromuscular blockade
- Stimulation can cause masseter contraction and has resulted in tongue lacerations and ETT damage.
  - A bite block should be placed in the back of the mouth along the teeth line.

Electromyograms

- Electric current can be sent through a pedicle screw to measure EMGs distally.
- Helps determine if screw is too close to a nerve root
- Neuromuscular blockade must be absent for accurate EMGs.

Wake-Up Test

- Traditionally used to assess spinal cord integrity in scoliosis surgery.
- Currently used in cases where monitoring is unobtainable or significant change has been observed
- Wake-up test involves the anesthetic being discontinued, and the patient is asked to move upper extremities (baseline), then lower extremities.
- Risk of self-extubation, increased bleeding, and venous air embolism
- After assessment is completed, medications to rapidly reanesthetize can be given.

Conclusion of the Case

- Patient placed supine
- All lines and tubes secured
- Assess hemodynamic and volume status
- Potential for airway edema; decision on whether to extubate
- Pain management may be complicated.
  - Perioperative multimodal technique should be planned in advance.
  - May include patient-controlled analgesia, ketamine, acetaminophen, gabapentin, and/or other medications
  - Nonsteroidal antiinflammatory agents may interfere with bone formation.

Intraoperative Neurologic Monitoring

- Anesthetic technique should be tailored to surgical case and monitoring being used.
- SSEPs – Avoid volatile anesthetics >0.5 MAC and large doses of benzodiazepines, hypotension, hypothermia, hypocarbia, and hypercarbia.
- TCMEPs – Avoid neuromuscular blockade and volatile anesthetics.
- EMG – Avoid neuromuscular blockade.
- Wake-up test – Discontinue anesthetic to allow for response to commands.

Vision Loss

- Postoperative visual loss (POVL) is rare, but potentially devastating complication after spine surgery
- Risks include long (>6 hours) surgery in the prone position and large (>1 L) amount of blood loss.
  - Multiple additional associated physiologic and patient-related factors
- Ischemic optic neuropathy (ION) is a major cause of POVL.
  - Variations in blood supply to optic nerve
  - Ocular perfusion pressure = mean arterial pressure (MAP) – intraocular pressure (IOP).
  - Venous pressure and edema due to head-down position can contribute.
- Central retinal artery occlusion is second most likely cause.
  - Embolic or from direct pressure on the eye
  - Tends to be unilateral
- Registry created by ASA compared 80 patients with ION to matched controls.
  - Increased incidence seen in males and obese patients who underwent surgery on Wilson frame, with long surgical times and larger blood loss, and who received a small percentage of colloid.

ASA Practice Advisory on POVL

- There is a subset of patients who undergo spine procedures in the prone position and are at increased risk for perioperative visual loss. Patients who may be at increased risk are those having long procedures or substantial blood loss or both.
- Consider informing high-risk patients that there is a small, unpredictable risk of perioperative visual loss.
- The use of deliberate hypotensive techniques during spine surgery is not associated with perioperative visual loss.
- In patients who have substantial blood loss, colloids should be administered in addition to crystalloids to maintain intravascular volume.
- There is no apparent transfusion "trigger" that would eliminate the risk of perioperative visual loss related to anemia.
- When positioning high-risk patients, the head should be level with or higher than the heart when possible. In addition, when possible, the head should be maintained in a neutral forward position (e.g., without significant neck flexion, extension, lateral flexion, or rotation).
- Staged spine procedures should be considered in high-risk patients.

SURGERY IN THE SITTING POSITION

- Sitting, or "beach chair" position, is head of the bed elevated between 30 and 90 degrees.
- Shoulder surgery frequently performed in this position

- Anesthesia is associated with rare complications including stroke and ischemic brain injury.
  - Decreased cerebral perfusion pressure
  - Arterial blood pressure gradient between heart and brain due to positioning
  - Each centimeter of head elevation has a decrease in blood pressure of 0.77 mmHg
- Blood pressure should be recalculated to reflect the blood pressure at the level of the brain.
- Significant hypotension should be avoided.

FRACTURED HIP

- Mortality rates range 14% to 36% in the first year after a fracture.
- The number of preexisting conditions correlates with the risk of death.
- Most common postoperative complications are chest infection and heart failure.
- Medical status should be optimized prior to surgical intervention.
- Operative delay >48 hours is associated with an increased mortality rate.
  - Risk of delay (pneumonia, pulmonary embolism, pain, decubitus ulcers) must be weighed against the risk of proceeding.

Anesthetic Technique

- Choice of general anesthesia vs. spinal anesthesia should be made on a case-by-case basis.
- REGAIN trial showed spinal anesthesia was not superior to general anesthesia with respect to survival and ambulation at 60 days.
- Advantages of regional anesthesia including spinal
  - Avoidance of intubation and airway manipulation
  - Decreases the amount of systemic medications given
  - May play a role in decreasing the risk of thromboembolism
- Spinal anesthetics may result in significant hypotension secondary to hypovolemia and blood loss.
- Peripheral nerve blocks can provide significant analgesia.
  - Lumbar plexus, femoral, and lateral femoral cutaneous nerve blocks
- Intraoperative considerations include patient positioning, blood loss, and maintaining normothermia.
- Postoperatively opioids should be administered judiciously to avoid cumulative effects.

TOTAL JOINT REPLACEMENT

- Hip, knee, and shoulder replacements are frequent in patients with osteoarthritis, rheumatologic disorders, and trauma.
- Concerns include
  - Age and comorbidities
  - Blood loss, proper positioning, and padding
  - Hemodynamic variations and the response to methylmethacrylate cement (MMC)
  - Fat and pulmonary emboli

Tranexamic Acid in Orthopedics

- Antifibrinolytic that prevents clot breakdown, inhibits fibrinolysis
- Shown to be efficacious in decreasing surgical blood loss
- Reviews have shown use does not increase the risk of thromboembolic events.
- Caution must be taken to avoid intrathecal injection.
  - Significant morbidity and mortality
  - Case reports have shown neurologic and cardiac complications.
  - Myoclonic seizures, hypertension, and permanent neurologic injury
  - Delayed supportive treatment can result in death.
- Protocols should be established to prevent avoidable occurrences.

Guideline Recommendations for Tranexamic Acid in Total Hip and Knee Arthroplasty

1. Either IV, topical, or oral administration is effective at reduction of perioperative blood loss.
2. Multiple doses do not have any significant benefit over a single dose in reduction of blood loss and need for transfusion.
3. Administration before incision is more effective than if given after incision.
4. Administration does not increase the risk of venous thromboembolism in patients without a history of venous thromboembolic events.

Total Hip Replacement

- Supine or lateral decubitus position
  - Axillary roll should be used in lateral position to protect the axillary artery and brachial plexus from compression.
  - Lateral positioners can push abdominal contents cephalad and impair respiratory function.
- MMC may be used to secure the implant.
  - Can have cardiopulmonary effects including cardiovascular collapse
    - Hypoxia, bronchoconstriction, hypotension
    - MMC and fat emboli can cross a patent foramen ovale.
    - May be a reaction to the liquid MMC monomer or the result of air, fat, or bone marrow forced into the circulation

- Risk factors include intraoperative hypovolemia or hypotension and significant preexisting cardiac disease.
- Supportive treatment should be started immediately to prevent mortality.
- Multimodal approach should be considered for postoperative pain management.
- Comprehensive protocols exist to optimize management for same-day procedures.

Total Knee Replacement and Tourniquets

- Frequently performed with a tourniquet in place to minimize blood loss.
- Should be inflated 100 mmHg above systolic blood pressure to prevent arterial bleeding
- Tourniquet time should be limited as prolonged ischemia can result in permanent damage.
  - At 2 hours, the tourniquet should be deflated for at least 15 to 20 minutes.
- Recirculation of the ischemic limb can cause a decrease in blood pressure and increase in end-tidal CO_2 as acid metabolites "wash out" and circulate systemically.
- Pain becomes apparent as the tourniquet time increases, reflected as increasing blood pressure and heart rate due to C-fiber firing.
  - Overaggressive treatment can cause hypotension when the tourniquet is released.
- Damage to nerves, vessels, and skin can occur with tourniquets.
- Pulmonary embolism can occur at the time of deflation.
- Observe for hemostasis need after tourniquet deflation is confirmed (i.e., no malfunction).
- Bilateral TKR should be done only after careful patient selection.
- TKR patients have more appreciable pain after surgery compared to THR patients.
  - Multimodal analgesia protocols should be considered.
  - Regional anesthesia may improve pain scores and lead to early ambulation.
    - Adductor canal block potentially spares motor nerves.

Deep Venous Thrombosis and Thromboembolism Prophylaxis

- Use varies by surgeon and institution
- Should be coordinated among providers
- Options include warfarin, low molecular weight heparin, aspirin, and sequential compression boots.
- Medication choice and timing may influence type of anesthetic.
  - Caution needed with DVT prophylaxis and epidural catheters as hematoma can form.
    - Classic signs of epidural hematoma formation are masked by neuraxial anesthesia.
  - Should not perform spinal or epidural anesthetic in a patient who has not discontinued an anticoagulant medication for the appropriate duration.
- Aspirin and NSAIDs do not increase spinal hematoma risk when the patient is receiving a spinal or epidural anesthetic.
- American Society of Regional Anesthesia and Pain Medicine has published guidelines regarding neuraxial procedures and anticoagulant/antiplatelet agents.

QUESTIONS

RHEUMATOLOGIC DISORDERS

1. What are some airway abnormalities that can occur in patients with RA?
2. Can neck movement in patients with RA result in cervical spine injury? What is the clinical implication of this?
3. What are some considerations for the anesthetic management of patients with ankylosing spondylitis?

SPINE SURGERY

4. What are some considerations for the anesthetic management of patients undergoing spine surgery?
5. What are some considerations for patients placed in the prone position?
6. Why are some areas of the spinal cord more prone to ischemia?
7. Complete the following chart describing methods of intraoperative spinal cord monitoring, what portion of the spinal cord is monitored, and the anesthetic implications of each.

Monitor	Area of Spinal Cord Monitored	Anesthetic Implications
Somatosensory evoked potentials		
Transcranial motor evoked potentials		
Electromyogram		
Wake-up test		

8. Which patients are at the greatest risk of postoperative visual loss after spine surgery? What are some other possible factors that contribute to postoperative visual loss?
9. What are the determinants of the ocular perfusion pressure? What is the clinical implication of this?

SURGERY IN THE SITTING POSITION

10. What neurologic postoperative complications have been noted in patients who undergo surgery in the sitting position? How can this risk be mitigated?

FRACTURED HIP

11. Describe the risks and benefits of proceeding with surgery in the patient with acute hip fracture and recent myocardial infarction.
12. Does choice of anesthetic technique—regional or general anesthesia—play a role in the outcome of patients who have fractured a hip?
13. What are some advantages of regional anesthesia for patients undergoing repair of a hip fracture?

TOTAL JOINT REPLACEMENT

14. What are some anesthetic considerations for patients undergoing total joint replacement?
15. What are the potential effects of inadvertent intrathecal injection of TXA?
16. What are risk-reduction strategies to prevent the injection of TXA into the spinal space?
17. What are some potential effects of the use of methylmethacrylate cement?
18. Describe the physiologic changes and risks associated with tourniquet use during total knee replacement.
19. What are some approaches to postoperative pain management in the patient undergoing total knee replacement?
20. What is the concern with the administration of thromboembolism prophylaxis in patients undergoing neuraxial anesthesia for total knee replacement?

ANSWERS

RHEUMATOLOGIC DISORDERS

1. Some airway abnormalities that can occur in patients with RA include decreased mouth opening, a hypoplastic mandible, cricoarytenoid arthritis, and cervical spine abnormalities. (559)
2. Yes, movement of the neck in patients with RA can result in cervical spine injury. The patient with RA must be carefully evaluated for both the complexity and the risk of endotracheal intubation. Many cervical spine abnormalities may occur in patients with RA, making visualization of the airway difficult and placing the cervical spinal cord at risk. Normal endotracheal intubation maneuvers with neck movement may result in an increased risk of cervical spine injury because of destruction of the bones and ligaments of the cervical spine. (560)
3. Patients with ankylosing spondylitis typically have a rigid cervical spine and neck fused in flexion, which makes endotracheal intubation difficult. Airway manipulation should be performed only after careful assessment, and an intubation assist device can help secure the airway. Some patients with ankylosing spondylitis also develop thoracic and costochondral involvement, which may result in a rapid shallow breathing pattern. (563)

SPINE SURGERY

4. There are several considerations for the anesthetic management of patients undergoing spine surgery, and much depends on the level of the spine in which the surgery will take place, as well as the surgical approach. Preoperative assessment of the patient for underlying neurologic deficits and chronic pain issues is important. For patients in whom the approach may be thoracic, pulmonary function tests may be indicated. In general, spine surgery can be long and complex, with significant blood loss and hemodynamic alterations. Intravascular access and intraoperative monitoring should be adjusted accordingly, and blood products may need to be ordered. If there will be intraoperative monitoring of the spinal cord with evoked potentials, the anesthesia administered for the surgery may need to be modified so as not to interfere with the acquisition of waveforms. (563)
5. Spine surgery is often performed with the patient in the prone position, and careful positioning avoids injury. Movement to the prone position should be performed in a carefully coordinated manner with the surgical team. The neck should not be hyperextended or hyperflexed but placed in the neutral position. The endotracheal tube is positioned so it is not kinked, contact areas are padded, and the face and eyes are protected. Pressure and stretch on nerves are avoided by proper padding and preventing any extension over 90 degrees. The abdomen needs to be hanging free to avoid increased venous pressure and thereby increased venous bleeding. The prone position alters pulmonary dynamics, so pulmonary function must be reassessed in this position. (565)
6. Some areas of the spinal cord are more vulnerable and therefore more prone to ischemia because their blood supply is dependent on watershed blood flow. (565)
7. The following chart describes methods of intraoperative spinal cord monitoring, what portion of the spinal cord is monitored, and the anesthetic implications of each. (565–567)

Monitor	Area of Spinal Cord Monitored	Anesthetic Implications
Somatosensory evoked potentials	Dorsal column	Volatile anesthetics >0.5 MAC and benzodiazepines avoided or used minimally
Transcranial motor evoked potentials	Ventral column	No neuromuscular blockade or volatile anesthetics
Electromyogram	Nerve root	No neuromuscular blockade
Wake-up test	Spinal cord – mostly motor but can be sensory	All inhaled anesthetics and intravenous infusions must be terminated Care to avoid excessive head movement causing extubation

8. Although the cause is unclear, patients undergoing prolonged spine surgery (>6 hours) in the prone position who have large blood loss (>1 L) are particularly at risk for postoperative visual loss. In fact, in the ASA visual loss registry blood loss of >1 L and procedures of ≥6 hours were present in 96% of cases. Yet patients with small blood loss and short procedures also have had visual loss. Other possible etiologic perioperative factors include anemia, hypotension, and prone positioning, as well as systemic diseases such as diabetes, hypertension, and vascular disease. (568)

9. The ocular perfusion pressure (OPP), or the blood pressure supplying blood flow to the optic nerve, is a function of the mean arterial pressure (MAP) and intraocular pressure (IOP) such that OPP = MAP − IOP. Increases in IOP or decreases in MAP can have a negative impact on the ocular perfusion pressure. (568)

SURGERY IN THE SITTING POSITION

10. Postoperative complications that have been noted in the patient undergoing surgery in the sitting position are rare but significant and devastating. These neurologic complications include stroke, ischemic brain injury, and vegetative states. A contributing factor is the decrease in cerebral perfusion pressure causing insufficient blood supply to the brain. One way to mitigate this risk is to recalculate target blood pressures accounting for the height differential between the blood pressures at the heart and the brain. For example, a 20-cm height differential calculates to an approximate 15 to 16 mmHg gradient. (569)

FRACTURED HIP

11. The mortality rate after hip surgery ranges from 14% to 36% in the first year after fracture. Several studies have been conducted regarding risks of hip fracture repair, particularly in older patients with comorbid conditions. Patients who are admitted to the hospital immediately after fracture and who have surgery within 48 hours tend to have a better outcome. An especially difficult decision is when to proceed with repair of acute hip fracture in the patient who has had a recent myocardial infarction, weighing the risks of delaying the procedure (pneumonia, pulmonary embolism, pain, loss of ability to walk, decubitus ulcers) with the cardiac risk of proceeding (extension of infarcted myocardium). Factors to be considered include the extent of the myocardium affected and at risk, the presence of ongoing angina, and the presence of congestive heart failure. A pharmacologic stress test may be necessary to facilitate the decision of whether to proceed. For example, if the patient had a small subendocardial myocardial infarction with minimal increase in cardiac enzymes, normal echocardiogram, and cardiac stress test, they may be able to proceed safely with the fractured hip repair. (569)
12. A long-standing issue has been whether one anesthetic technique, regional or general, is associated with better outcomes in patients undergoing hip fracture repair. In general, the data accumulated over many years and many different studies have not documented a clear advantage of one technique over another. Choice of anesthesia technique should be made on a case-by-case basis. (569)
13. Advantages of regional anesthesia for patients undergoing repair of a hip fracture are that 1) it avoids endotracheal intubation and airway manipulation and the medications that need to be administered to accomplish this, 2) it decreases the total amount of systemic medication the patient receives throughout the procedure, and 3) it may play a role in decreasing the risk of thromboembolism. The vasodilatory effect of the spinal anesthetic may help the patient with congestive heart failure (CHF). However, intravascular fluid still should be given cautiously because CHF may worsen as the intravascular vasodilatory effect of the spinal anesthesia recedes. (570)

TOTAL JOINT REPLACEMENT

14. Anesthetic considerations for patients undergoing total joint replacement include the patient's age, concurrent medical conditions, blood loss, proper positioning and padding, hemodynamic variations during the procedure, the use of methylmethacrylate cement, and the risk of fat and pulmonary emboli. (570)
15. Intrathecal injection of TXA could cause disastrous effects, including seizures, arrhythmias, permanent neurological injury, and death. (571)
16. Risk-reduction measures to reduce the risk of accidental intrathecal injection of TXA include having the pharmacy provide non-vial preparations of TXA, two-person verification of medications to be injected into the intrathecal space, and having TXA made available for intravenous injection only after spinal anesthesia has been performed. (571)
17. Methylmethacrylate cement use can cause systemic reactions including hypoxia, bronchoconstriction, hypotension, cardiovascular collapse, and even death. The mechanism for these effects can be due to the monomer itself or as a result of air, fat, or bone marrow elements being forced into the circulation. (572)
18. A tourniquet is often used on the upper thigh, inflated to approximately 100 mmHg above systolic blood pressure, during total knee replacement. Physiologic changes associated with tourniquet use include limb ischemia, pain, and cardiovascular changes. The tourniquet has a limit of 2 hours to prevent ischemia causing

permanent leg damage. At the 2-hour mark, the tourniquet needs to be deflated for a minimum of 15–20 minutes before reinflation (if reinflation is necessary). Pain associated with the tourniquet manifests as an increase in heart rate and blood pressure. When the tourniquet is deflated, "wash-out" and systemic circulation of the acidic metabolites in the ischemic limb can cause hypotension and an increase in end-tidal CO_2. Complications from tourniquet use include pulmonary embolism, and nerve, vessel, and skin damage. (572–573)

19. Patients undergoing total knee replacement experience more postoperative pain than patients undergoing a total hip replacement. A postoperative pain management plan may include oral and intravenous pain medications, as well as nerve blocks. Preoperative oral pain medications such as acetaminophen, gabapentin, or NSAIDs (with cardiovascular risk considered) are employed by some as part of a total knee pain pathway. With postoperative ambulation as early as the postanesthesia care unit becoming popular, there is a need to provide adequate pain relief for mobilization. Peripheral nerve blocks such as a femoral or an adductor canal block can supply such pain relief. The adductor canal block potentially spares motor components of the femoral nerve, preserving motor strength in the femoral nerve distribution; it is not clear that use of femoral or adductor canal blocks results in a higher incidence of falls. Postoperative pain relief may also include patient-controlled analgesia, continuous infusions through catheters, individual nerve blocks of the lower extremities, and intravenous or oral medications. (573)
20. Thromboembolism prophylaxis is often administered to patients undergoing total knee replacement, although the medication type, dose, and timing vary by surgeon and institution. The anesthesia provider should understand the thromboembolism prophylaxis plan, as this will influence anesthesia technique. The concern is particularly for epidural anesthesia and the risk of developing an epidural hematoma with the manipulation of an epidural catheter while a patient is anticoagulated. Additionally, the classic findings of an epidural hematoma (severe pain and onset of numbness and weakness) may be masked by epidural analgesia, delaying diagnosis and treatment. (573)

Chapter

33 OBSTETRICS

Christine Warrick and Mark D. Rollins

PHYSIOLOGIC CHANGES IN PREGNANT WOMEN

Causes of Physiologic Changes in the Pregnant Patient
▪ Altered hormonal activity ▪ Biochemical changes associated with increasing metabolic demands of a growing fetus, placenta, and uterus ▪ Mechanical displacement by an enlarging uterus

Cardiovascular System Changes

Intravascular Fluid and Hematology

- Plasma volume increases by 50%, and erythrocyte volume increases by 25% at birth.
  - Accounts for the relative anemia of pregnancy
  - Offsets blood loss during delivery
    - Blood loss is 300–500 mL for vaginal delivery, and 800–1000 mL for cesarean section.
    - Uterus contracts and autotransfuses about 500 mL of blood after delivery.
- Decreased plasma protein concentration decreases osmotic pressure from 27 to 22 mmHg.
- Increases in coagulation factors make pregnancy a hypercoagulable state.

Cardiac Output

- Increases by 40% to 50% at third trimester, by an additional 25% to 40% in labor, and by 80% after delivery
  - Cardiac output increase is secondary to increases in both stroke volume (mostly) and heart rate.
  - Cardiac output changes with pregnancy, labor, and delivery can put patients with coexisting cardiac disease at unique risk.
- Cardiac output reaches prelabor values 48 hours postpartum and prepregnant values after 2 weeks.

Systemic Vascular Resistance

- Decreases by about 20% during pregnancy
  - Systemic, mean, and diastolic blood pressures also decrease during pregnancy.

Aortocaval Compression

- Vena cava compression in supine position decreases preload and cardiac output.
  - Blood returns through epidural, azygos, and vertebral veins.
  - Can contribute to lower extremity edema, varices, and increased risk of venous thrombosis
- Supine hypotension syndrome occurs in supine position in about 15% of pregnant patients at term.
  - Hypotension, with diaphoresis, nausea, vomiting, and changes in cerebration

Echocardiography Changes

- Heart is displaced anteriorly and leftward.
- Heart chamber volume on both the right and left increase, with associated left ventricular hypertrophy.
- One in four pregnant patients have mitral regurgitation.

Compensatory Responses and Anesthetic Implications

- Systemic vascular resistance increases to compensate for decrease in preload when supine.
  - Regional anesthesia impairs this compensation.
  - Left lateral tilt (30 degrees) displaces the gravid uterus off the vena cava.
- Abdominal aorta compression by gravid uterus for >15 minutes can decrease uterine blood flow (UBF) and cause fetal acidosis.
- Increased venous pressure diverts blood flow via the paravertebral veins to the azygos veins.
  - Epidural veins can become dilated, increasing the risk of intravascular epidural catheter placement.

Pulmonary System Changes

Upper Airway

- Increased capillary engorgement, tissue edema, and friability
  - Vocal cords and arytenoids are affected.
  - Exacerbated by preeclampsia and active pushing during labor
- Mask ventilation and intubation may be more problematic.

Minute Ventilation and Oxygenation

- Minute ventilation increases about 50% above prepregnancy levels during first trimester.
  - Primarily by increased tidal volume, with a small increase in respiratory rate
  - Stimulus is elevated CO_2 levels caused by elevated progesterone levels.
  - Resting maternal $PaCO_2$ decreases from 40 mmHg to 30 mmHg.
  - Resting maternal pH is only mildly alkalotic (renal compensation).
- Maternal hemoglobin is right-shifted (P_{50} increases).
  - Fetal hemoglobin is left-shifted, facilitating oxygen delivery across the placenta.
- Maternal oxygen consumption increases by 20% at term, and up to an additional 75% during labor.

Lung Volumes

- Functional residual capacity (FRC) decreases by 20%, leading to atelectasis.

Anesthetic Implications

- During induction of anesthesia, PaO_2 decreases rapidly due to decreased FRC and increased metabolic rate.

Gastrointestinal Changes

- Beyond 20 weeks' gestation, risk of aspiration of gastric contents increases.
  - Stomach and pylorus are displaced cephalad.
  - Lower esophageal sphincter becomes incompetent due to positioning.
  - Progesterone levels reduce esophageal sphincter tone.
- During vaginal delivery, gravid uterus and lithotomy position increase gastric pressure.
- Gastrin, secreted by the placenta, lowers gastric pH.

Anesthetic Implications

- Pregnant patients should be considered as having a full stomach with increased aspiration risk regardless of the interval of time that has passed since last oral intake.
  - Timely administration of nonparticulate antacids, intravenous (IV) H_2-recepter antagonists, and/or metoclopramide is recommended prior to induction.

Nervous System Changes

- Pregnant patients may have reduced volatile anesthetic requirements and more sensitivity to local anesthetics.
  - Decreased local anesthetic doses are needed for epidural or spinal anesthesia.

Renal Changes

- At term, renal blood flow and glomerular filtration are increased by about 50%.
- Serum creatinine and blood urea nitrogen levels are decreased, and urinary excretion of protein and glucose are increased.

Hepatic Changes

- Both plasma protein and plasma cholinesterase activity are decreased.

PHYSIOLOGY OF THE UTEROPLACENTAL CIRCULATION

Uteroplacental Circulation

- Maternal (two) uterine arteries: deliver blood to the uterus and placenta
- Fetal (one) umbilical vein: nutrient-rich, waste-free blood from the placenta to the fetus
- Fetal (two) umbilical arteries: fetal blood returns to the placenta

Uterine Blood Flow

- At term is 700 mL/min, about 10% of cardiac output
  - 80% supplies the placenta, 20% supplies the myometrium.
- Uterine blood flow (UBF) is dependent on uterine perfusion pressure.
  - Decreases due to hypotension, hypovolemia, aortocaval compression, and Valsalva maneuver
- Uterine blood flow is not directly affected by spinal or epidural anesthesia.
- Norepinephrine, phenylephrine, or ephedrine do not increase uterine vascular resistance at standard clinical doses.

Placental Exchange

Factors Affecting Maternal–Fetus Oxygen Transfer

- Ratio of maternal UBF to fetal umbilical blood flow
- Oxygen partial pressure gradient
- Respective hemoglobin concentration gradients and affinities
- Placental diffusing capacity
- Acid-base status of the fetal and maternal blood (Bohr effect)

- Oxygen: fetal hemoglobin has greater affinity than maternal hemoglobin
  - Facilitates oxygen transfer
  - Fetal PaO_2 is normally 20 to 40 mmHg, but can reach up to 60 mmHg.
- Carbon dioxide: readily crosses the placenta, limited only by blood flow
- Drugs: substances <1000 Daltons diffuse across the placenta
  - Factors that affect diffusion of substances across the placenta
    - Maternal–fetal concentration gradient
    - Maternal protein binding
    - Molecular weight
    - Lipid solubility
    - Degree of ionization

Fetal Uptake

- Fetal blood has lower pH than maternal blood.
  - Slightly basic drugs that cross the placenta in nonionized form can become ionized after crossing to fetal circulation.
  - Once ionized, they become "trapped."
  - This effect is more pronounced when fetus is acidotic, as in times of fetal distress.
  - Accidental maternal intravascular local anesthetic injection can lead to local anesthetic "ion trapping" in the fetus, with fetal bradycardia, ventricular arrhythmia, acidosis, and severe cardiac depression.

Characteristics of the Fetal Circulation

- About 75% of fetal umbilical venous blood passes through the liver before reaching fetal circulation.
  - Most drugs are metabolized before they reach the fetal heart and brain.

STAGES OF LABOR

- Progression of labor is reliably unpredictable.
- There are three stages of labor.
  - First stage starts with onset of uterine contractions to full cervical dilation.
    - Latent phase is onset of maternal contractions to slow cervical dilation and can last for hours to days.
    - Active phase is during significant acceleration of cervical dilation, usually after 5-cm dilation.
  - Second stage is from full cervical dilation to birth.
  - Third stage is from birth to delivery of the placenta.
- Active-phase arrest: if cervical dilation slows or stops in the active phase of labor
- Arrest of descent: neonate cannot be born vaginally during the second stage of labor
  - May require operative vaginal delivery if neonate is sufficiently low in pelvis

ANATOMY OF LABOR PAIN

- First stage of labor: nerve fibers from the uterus and cervix send pain signals to the dorsal root ganglia of levels T10–L1.
- Second stage of labor: in addition to pain perception at T10–L1, nerve fibers from the vagina and perineum now send pain signals to the dorsal root ganglia of levels S2–S4.
- Maternal sympathetic nervous system response to pain causes maternal tachycardia and hypertension and can decrease UBF.
- Neuraxial anesthesia onset can decrease maternal epinephrine levels, affecting the uterus.
  - Uterine effects include uterine hyperstimulation (tachysystole), a period of uterine quiescence, or conversion from dysfunctional to a more regular pattern of contractions.

METHODS OF LABOR ANALGESIA

Nonpharmacologic Techniques

- Based on three theoretical models that act on endogenous pain pathways
  - Gate control provides tactile stimulation to an area of pain.
  - Diffuse noxious inhibitory control works by causing pain at sites remote from labor pain.
  - CNS control model diverts attention away from labor pain.
- Hydrotherapy, massage, position changes, transcutaneous electrical nerve stimulation (TENS), acupuncture/acupressure, sterile water injections, Lamaze, meditation, hypnosis, relaxation, expectation management, and music are all nonpharmacologic techniques.
- Perceived patient autonomy and control contribute to a patient's satisfaction.
- A support individual (e.g., family member, doula) is associated with fewer analgesics, decreased length of labor, higher likelihood of vaginal delivery, and less likelihood of feeling negatively about childbirth.

Systemic Medications

- Systemic analgesics are limited by both dose and timing due to concerns about maternal and neonatal effects.

Opioids

- Cross placenta; can cause decreased fetal heart rate variability and neonatal respiratory depression
- Maternal side effects include nausea, vomiting, pruritus, and delayed gastric emptying.
- Fentanyl is preferred because it lacks active metabolites and has a short duration of action.
  - With small maternal IV doses, neonates have unchanged Apgar scores or respiratory effort.
- Meperidine is long-acting, has active metabolites, and has a prolonged neonatal half-life.
  - Associated with decreased Apgar scores, respiratory effort, and oxygen saturation in neonates
- Morphine is long-acting, has active metabolites, and causes profound maternal sedation.
  - No longer commonly used
  - Occasionally administered intramuscularly (IM) with promethazine to provide 2.5 to 6 hours of labor analgesia, termed *morphine sleep.*
- Remifentanil: rapid onset and fast elimination by plasma and tissue esterases
  - Has minimal neonatal side effects
  - Typically used for patients with contraindications to neuraxial techniques, but the patient must be closely monitored (e.g., continuous pulse oximetry, 1:1 nursing)

Nitrous Oxide

- Typically administered in fixed mixture of 50% with oxygen, at all stages of labor
- Rapid onset, rapid elimination, and no effect on uterine contractility
- Maternal side effects include nausea, dysphoria, and dizziness.
- Coadministration of opioids is not recommended.

Neuraxial (Regional) Analgesia

- Administration of local anesthetics in combination with opioid analgesics into the epidural and/or intrathecal space

Local Anesthetics

- Bupivacaine and ropivacaine are most common and safe when appropriately dosed.

Neuraxial Opioids

- Fentanyl and sufentanil are most used.
- Improve quality of labor analgesia and allow a reduction in local anesthetic concentration
- Intrathecal opioids may cause fetal bradycardia.

NEURAXIAL TECHNIQUES

- Provide effective labor analgesia, without sedation, and the patient can actively participate during labor
- Negative experience can occur: if poor communication, or if pain relief is delayed or inadequate

Preoperative Assessment

- Assess the patient's history and physical examination; discuss risks, benefits, and alternatives; and obtain consent before initiation of any neuraxial blockade.
- Healthy laboring patients may have modest amounts of clear liquids.
  - Anesthesia provider may consider restricting oral intake in a patient with complicated labor.

Timing and Placement of Epidural

- A laboring patient's request for pain relief is sufficient justification for epidural placement regardless of cervical dilation.
- Studies have shown no difference in the progression of labor between neuraxial labor analgesia and those receiving only opioids.

Epidural Technique

- Labor pain relief via a catheter-based technique
- Aseptic technique with typical placement at L3-L4
- The epidural space is found using a tactile technique called *loss of resistance.*
- Local anesthetics and opioids are administered via the epidural catheter.

Combined Spinal Epidural and Dural Puncture Epidural Techniques

- Technique: after accessing epidural space, a spinal needle is inserted into the epidural needle, using a needle-through-needle technique
  - *Dural puncture epidural (DPE)*: once cerebrospinal fluid (CSF) is visualized in the spinal needle hub, the spinal needle is removed, and the epidural catheter is placed
    - Benefits: fewer one-sided blocks, less sacral sparing, slightly faster onset
  - *Combined spinal epidural (CSE)*: intrathecal dose of local anesthetic and/or opioid is administered through the spinal needle before removal
    - Benefits: quick onset, fewer one-sided blocks, less sacral sparing, and fewer catheter failures
    - Drawbacks: increased risks of opioid-based pruritus, uterine tachysystole, and fetal bradycardia

Neuraxial Dosing and Delivery Techniques

- Epidural catheters allow infusion or bolus administration of local anesthetic with or without opioid drugs

- Programmable infusion pumps allow two methods of epidural medication delivery:
  - *Patient-controlled epidural analgesia* (PCEA) allows patient-controlled epidural boluses with or without a continuous background infusion.
  - *Programmed intermittent epidural bolus* (PIEB) administers automated fixed epidural boluses at scheduled intervals.
- Opioids (e.g., fentanyl or sufentanil) are added to augment analgesia and decrease local anesthetic requirements.
  - Dose-dependent side effects include pruritus, nausea, and sedation.
- Dilute concentrations of epinephrine can be added to augment analgesia.
- For CSEs, initial intrathecal dose includes a local anesthetic and/or opioid.
- Epidural test dose: commonly lidocaine and epinephrine are administered to evaluate catheter placement
  - If intravascular: increased heart rate and blood pressure >20% above baseline
  - If intrathecal: rapid analgesia and lower extremity block
- To dose catheter, aspirate then inject incremental boluses, followed by direct observation and monitoring of the patient for at least 20 minutes.

Spinal Labor Analgesia

- Intrathecal medications provide rapid analgesia.
- Useful for instrumented (forceps/vacuum) delivery, management of retained placenta, or repair of high-degree perineal lacerations in patients without an epidural catheter

CONTRAINDICATIONS OF NEURAXIAL ANESTHESIA

- Include patient refusal, infection at needle insertion site, coagulopathy, hypovolemic shock, increased intracranial pressure, and inadequate provider expertise

COMPLICATIONS OF NEURAXIAL ANESTHESIA

- Inadequate labor analgesia occurs in 7–12% of epidurals.
- Unintended dural puncture occurs in 1–2% of epidural placements; about half of these will result in severe headache.
- Side effects include pruritus, nausea, shivering, urinary retention, motor weakness, low back soreness, and prolonged block.
- Serious complications of epidural abscess, meningitis, epidural hematoma, and neurologic injury from placement are exceedingly rare.

Systemic Toxicity and Excessive Blockade

- Unintended IV administration has dose-dependent side effects.
  - Minor: tinnitus, perioral tingling, mild blood pressure and heart rate changes
  - Major: seizures, loss of consciousness, severe arrhythmias, cardiovascular collapse
  - Bupivacaine has higher affinity for sodium channels than lidocaine and has high protein affinity.
    - Toxicity characterized by more difficult and prolonged cardiac resuscitation
  - Minimize risk by test dosing, aspiration before injection, and incremental dosing.
  - Allow enough time for excretion of local anesthetic from fetus if possible.
    - Neonate has limited ability to metabolize local anesthetics.
- High or total spinal
  - Unrecognized subdural epidural catheter placement, migration of catheter during use, or an overdose of local anesthetic in the epidural space
  - Severe maternal hypotension, bradycardia, loss of consciousness, and blockade of respiratory muscles

Treatment

- Goal: to restore maternal and fetal oxygenation, ventilation, and circulation
- Maternal uterine displacement, intravenous fluids, vasopressors, intubation, lipid emulsions, and ACLS may be required.
  - For ACLS: remove fetal and uterine monitors before defibrillation
  - For fetus ≥20 weeks' gestational age, emergent delivery if patient is not resuscitated before 5 minutes

Hypotension

- Hypotension due to decreased systemic vascular resistance is the common complication after neuraxial analgesia.
- Left uterine displacement and prehydration can help prevent it, and treatment may require vasopressor administration.

Increased Core Temperature

- Fever develops in a subset of patients receiving epidural labor analgesia and is not associated with an infectious process.

ANESTHESIA FOR CESAREAN DELIVERY

- Neuraxial anesthesia has advantages over general anesthesia.
  - Avoids the risks of maternal aspiration and difficult airway
  - Less anesthetic exposure to neonate
  - Patient is awake.
  - Neuraxial opioids can be given for postoperative pain.
- General anesthesia may be necessary.
  - Need for rapid and reliable anesthesia, e.g., conditions of fetal bradycardia or uterine rupture
  - Secure airway, controlled ventilation, and potentially less hemodynamic instability (no neuraxial block-related sympathectomy)

Spinal Anesthesia

- Rapid and reliable without systemic toxicity risk
- Low rate of postdural puncture headache (PDPH) with smaller-diameter, noncutting spinal needles
- Higher rate of hypotension
  - Prophylactic infusion of phenylephrine, crystalloid infusion, and left uterine displacement
  - Maintain maternal blood pressure within 80% of baseline
  - Ephedrine or glycopyrrolate for low maternal heart rate maintains cardiac output.
- Typically, a hyperbaric solution is used to facilitate control of block distribution, combined with opioids for postoperative pain.
- Continuous spinal anesthesia with an intrathecal catheter is reliable and titratable.
  - Can be used after accidental dural puncture
  - Increased risks of high spinal, and possibly meningitis and neurologic impairment

Epidural Anesthesia

- Used if the patient has an indwelling catheter and/or cannot tolerate sudden onset of sympathectomy (e.g., cardiac disease)
- Compared to spinal anesthesia: less reliable block, slower onset, and greater risk of maternal systemic toxicity
- Sensory level to T4 is needed for cesarean section.
- Failure to convert from a labor analgesia block to surgical epidural block can range from 2% to 20%.
  - Risks include placement by a nonspecialist, an increased number of manual doses for labor analgesia, and the urgency of the cesarean delivery.
  - May require conversion to general endotracheal anesthesia

Combined Spinal Epidural Anesthesia

- Rapid, reliable dense block with the ability to extend block level or duration if needed

General Anesthesia

- Used for emergencies or if neuraxial anesthesia is contraindicated
- Risk of mortality is 1.7 times that of neuraxial anesthesia.
  - Induction/intubation failure and postoperative airway obstruction and/or hypoventilation are all causes.
- Nonparticulate antacid administration and confirmation of surgical readiness should precede a rapid sequence induction.
- Typically, benzodiazepines and opioids are administered after neonate delivery.
- Time to incision and delivery is usually prior to a sufficient depth of anesthesia from halogenated agents, making the induction agent the primary anesthetic.
  - If intubation fails, successful mask ventilation may be sufficient until neonate delivery.
- Total intravenous anesthesia after delivery reduces the risk of uterine atony caused by halogenated agents.

Induction Drugs

- Propofol is frequently used for induction and has no significant effect on neonatal behavior at standard doses.
  - Can cause maternal hypotension
- Etomidate has minimal effects on cardiovascular system.
  - Painful on injection
  - Can increase the risk of seizures and nausea and vomiting
  - Decreases neonatal cortisol production usually <6 hours, with unknown significance
- Ketamine is useful in patients with hemodynamic compromise due to its sympathomimetic effects.
  - High doses can lower seizure threshold and increase uterine tone, risking uterine hypoperfusion.
  - Associated undesirable psychomimetic side effects can be lessened by coadministration of benzodiazepines.

Neuromuscular Blocking Drugs and Reversal Agents

- Succinylcholine is the neuromuscular blocking drug of choice because of its rapid onset and short duration of action.
  - Highly ionized and poorly lipid soluble so only small amounts cross the placenta
  - Requires extremely high doses to cause neonatal neuromuscular blockade

- Maternal decreases in pseudocholinesterase associated with pregnancy have minimal clinical effect.
- Rocuronium is an acceptable alternative with longer duration of action.
  - Sugammadex provides rapid reversal if provider cannot intubate or ventilate the patient.
  - Neuromuscular blocking drugs do not affect uterine smooth muscle.
  - Nondepolarizing drugs in large doses over long periods can cause neonatal neuromuscular blockade, for which treatment is respiratory support for up to 48 hours.
- Sugammadex is not recommended in pregnant patients undergoing nonobstetric surgery.
  - Reduces unbound progesterone and theoretically can affect the length of pregnancy
- Neostigmine more readily crosses the placenta than glycopyrrolate.
  - Reports of profound fetal bradycardia in pregnant patients undergoing nonobstetric surgery
  - Atropine (crosses the placenta) is recommended for coadministration with neostigmine in these patients.

Maintenance of Anesthesia

- Volatile anesthetics rapidly cross the placenta but do not appear to have long-term effects on neonatal outcome.
- Time from uterine incision to delivery is an important variable for neonatal outcome.
  - Fetal asphyxia can result from compromised UBF.
  - The neonate may be lightly anesthetized resulting in flaccidity and respiratory depression, which should rapidly improve with assisted ventilation.

ABNORMAL PRESENTATIONS AND MULTIPLE BIRTHS

Multiple Gestations

- Comprise about 3% of live births in the US
- Risks include preterm labor, hypertensive disorders, gestational diabetes, hyperemesis gravidarum, anemia, premature rupture of membranes, intrauterine growth restriction, and fetal demise.
- Twin pregnancies have a threefold increase of perinatal mortality over singleton pregnancies; planned cesarean does not decrease the risk.
  - Epidural placement is advised for vaginal delivery.
  - Second twin may be in breech position or have bradycardia and require emergent cesarean delivery or perineal relaxation for extraction.
  - Rapid uterine relaxation (e.g., IV nitroglycerin) may be required to improve vaginal delivery conditions and reduce the risk of head entrapment for the second twin.

Abnormal Presentations

Breech Presentation

- Most parturients with breech presentation have a planned cesarean delivery.
  - If attempting vaginal delivery, epidural catheter placement is encouraged.
- *External cephalic version* (ECV): rotating the fetus into a cephalic position through external palpation and pressure, while continuously monitoring the fetus
  - ECV under neuraxial anesthesia increases the success rate for ECV.
  - Terbutaline relaxes the uterus and increases likelihood for success.
- Risks of ECV include placental abruption, fetal bradycardia, and rupture of membranes.

Shoulder Dystocia

- When expulsion of the infant after delivery of the fetal head is obstructed by the fetal shoulders within the maternal pelvis
- Risk factors: macrosomia, maternal diabetes, history of dystocia, and instrumented delivery
- Risks: postpartum hemorrhage, fourth-degree laceration, neonatal injuries/mortality
- Treatment: obstetric maneuvers to deliver the infant with the final maneuver of pushing the fetal head back into the pelvis and proceeding with emergent cesarean delivery
- Fetal injuries: brachial plexus injury, asphyxia, fractured clavicle or humerus

HYPERTENSIVE DISORDERS OF PREGNANCY

Types of Hypertensive Disorders of Pregnancy

- *Preeclampsia-eclampsia*
- *Chronic hypertension*: elevated blood pressure predating pregnancy or occurring before 20 weeks' gestation (higher risk for superimposed preeclampsia)
- *Chronic hypertension with superimposed preeclampsia*
- *Gestational hypertension*: new-onset elevated blood pressure occurring after 20 weeks' gestation

- Hypertensive disorders of pregnancy are associated with increased future risk of cardiovascular disease, including stroke and hypertension.

Preeclampsia

- Preeclampsia is a pregnancy-specific, progressive disease with multiorgan system involvement.
- Highest risk factors: chronic hypertension and previous eclampsia
- Diagnosis: systolic blood pressures ≥140 mmHg or diastolic ≥90 mmHg on two separate occasions at

least 4 hours apart after 20 weeks of gestation AND new onset of any of the following:
  - Proteinuria (≥300 mg in 24 hours OR protein/creatinine ratio ≥0.3)
  - Thrombocytopenia (platelets <100,000/μL)
  - Renal insufficiency (creatinine ≥1.1 mg/dL or doubling)
  - Impaired liver function (liver transaminases twice normal)
  - Pulmonary edema
  - Headache (unresponsive to medication) or visual disturbances
- May progress to eclamptic seizures that can occur before, during, or after labor and delivery
  - Many parturients do not display signs of preeclampsia prior to seizure onset.
- HELLP syndrome: hemolysis, elevated liver enzymes, and low platelet count
- Treatment: definitive treatment of preeclampsia is with delivery
  - Timing of delivery depends on severity of symptoms and gestational age.

Intrapartum Management

- Use of invasive monitoring is guided by the severity and treatment of preeclamptic symptoms.
- Magnesium
  - Decreases eclampsia rates and reduces placental abruption risk
  - Increases efficacy and duration of depolarizing and nondepolarizing muscle relaxants
  - Increases uterine and smooth muscle relaxation
  - Should be started prior to vaginal delivery or cesarean section through 24 hours after delivery
  - Therapeutic range: 6 to 8 mg/dL for seizure prophylaxis
  - Monitor for magnesium toxicity by deep tendon reflexes, respiratory and neurologic status, and electrocardiogram findings.
    - Can lead to respiratory arrest and asystole
    - Treat with IV calcium and IV furosemide.
    - Dose should be adjusted in patients with renal dysfunction.
- Antihypertensives
  - For acute severe hypertension (systolic blood pressure ≥160 mmHg or diastolic blood pressure ≥110 mmHg)
  - Should be started expeditiously to prevent sequelae while monitoring fetus
  - First-line agents: IV labetalol or hydralazine, and oral nifedipine
  - Second-line agents: IV continuous infusions (e.g., nicardipine)
  - Goal blood pressure: 10% to 20% below the severe thresholds (e.g., 130/85)
- Neuraxial analgesia considerations
  - Neuraxial analgesia is the preferred analgesic method for labor or cesarean delivery.
  - Advantage of possibly avoiding general anesthesia for urgent or emergent cesarean delivery
  - Platelet levels should be assessed before placement of neuraxial block.
    - Risk of epidural hematoma is considered low for platelets ≥70 × 10^9/L.
    - Recommendation is to evaluate coagulation status for platelets <100 × 10^9/L in the setting of preeclampsia.
    - Platelet levels can continue to decrease after delivery and should be checked before removal of catheter.
- General anesthesia may be necessary under urgent conditions.
  - Airway edema may be exaggerated in patients with preeclampsia.
  - Sympathetic response to direct laryngoscopy can increase risk of stroke.
    - Sympathetic response can be attenuated with IV nitroglycerin or esmolol.
  - Postpartum uterine atony is common with magnesium sulfate infusion.
    - Oxytocin and prostaglandins may be used to treat uterine atony.
    - Methylergonovine is contraindicated due to risk of hypertensive crisis.

HEMORRHAGE IN PREGNANT WOMEN

Morbidity and Mortality in Obstetric Hemorrhages
▪ Poor quantification of blood loss ▪ Unrecognized associated risk factors for hemorrhage ▪ Delayed initiation of treatment ▪ Inadequate readiness and resources including insufficient transfusion of appropriate blood products in a massive hemorrhage situation

Placenta Previa

- Uterine implantation of the placenta in front of the presenting fetus
- Risk factors: advanced age, multiparity, assisted reproductive techniques, prior hysterotomy, and prior placenta previa
- A trial of labor is acceptable with placental edge >2 cm from cervical os.

Massive Hemorrhage

- Hemorrhage requires large bore access, massive transfusion protocol, need for transfusion based on point-of-care testing or clinical judgment.

- Ketamine can be used for induction.
- Tranexamic acid can reduce risk of mortality if administered within 3 hours of delivery.
- Uncontrolled hemorrhage may require obstetric interventions such as uterine artery ligation, embolization, or hysterectomy.
- Neonate is likely to be acidotic and hypovolemic, requiring resuscitation.

Abruptio Placentae

- Separation of the placenta after 20 weeks' gestation but before delivery
- Risk factors: advanced age, hypertension, trauma, smoking, cocaine use, chorioamnionitis, premature rupture of membranes, previa, and history of prior abruption
- Increased risk of perinatal and maternal mortality
- Maternal risks: hemorrhage, coagulopathy, thromboembolism, and acute kidney injury
- Large volumes (>2 L) of blood can be concealed within the uterus.
  - Chronic abruption with clotting can lead to disseminated intravascular coagulation.
- Epidural analgesia can be used for labor and vaginal delivery if no signs of maternal hypovolemia, active bleeding, clotting abnormalities, or fetal distress

Uterine Rupture

- Ranges from scar dehiscence to catastrophic uterine wall rupture
- Risk factors: presence of a prior uterine scar, rapid delivery, trauma, excessive oxytocin stimulation, and a large or malpositioned fetus
- Signs and symptoms may include fetal bradycardia, persistent abdominal pain, vaginal bleeding, cessation of contractions, loss of station, maternal hypotension, and breakthrough pain with epidural analgesia
  - Abnormal fetal heart rate (FHR) pattern is often the first sign of uterine rupture.
- A trial of labor after previous low transverse uterine incision for cesarean delivery often includes neuraxial analgesia, which should not mask the signs of uterine rupture

Retained Placenta

- Retained placenta has significant risk of hemorrhage and need for transfusion.
- Manual removal of placenta may be necessary.
- Analgesia may be provided by intravenous opioids and uterine relaxants, neuraxial analgesia with an indwelling or newly placed epidural catheter, or general anesthesia (rarely).

Uterine Atony

- Common cause of postpartum hemorrhage; can be immediate or delayed by several hours
- Risk factors: retained products, long labor, high parity, macrosomia, polyhydramnios, excessive oxytocin augmentation, and chorioamnionitis
- Management: oxytocin, uterine massage, umbilical cord traction
- Additional uterotonics: methylergonovine, prostaglandin $F_{2\alpha}$, and prostaglandin E_1

Placenta Accreta Spectrum

- Range of pathologic placental growth and adherence to the uterus
  - *Placenta accreta vera*: abnormal implantation and adherence to the myometrium
  - *Placenta increta*: implantation into the myometrium
  - *Placenta percreta*: placental growth through the myometrium, can adhere to pelvic organs (e.g., bowel, bladder, ovaries)
- Most common cause of peripartum hysterectomy in the United States
- Risk factor: previous uterine incisions
- Massive, rapid intraoperative blood loss (2000–5000 mL, and more) with coagulopathies in about 20% of patients
- Choice of anesthetic technique considers multiple factors.
- Preparation for massive hemorrhage, including intraoperative cell salvage and tranexamic acid

AMNIOTIC FLUID EMBOLISM

- Incidence is 1 to 6 cases per 100,000 deliveries
- Clinical presentation: sudden hypotension, respiratory distress, altered mental status, coagulopathy (DIC), cardiopulmonary arrest, absence of fever
- Typically occurs during labor or within 30 minutes of delivery of the placenta
- Differential diagnosis: venous air embolism, pulmonary thromboembolism, hemorrhage, peripartum cardiomyopathy, sepsis, anaphylaxis, local anesthetic toxicity, high spinal, and aspiration of gastric contents
- Echocardiography findings include right ventricular systolic dysfunction, D-shaped septum, and acute pulmonary hypertension.
- Treatment: supportive, usually requiring tracheal intubation and hemodynamic support

ANESTHESIA FOR NONOBSTETRIC SURGERY DURING PREGNANCY

- Most frequent indications: trauma, appendicitis, cholecystitis, and malignancy

Timing of Nonobstetric Surgery During Pregnancy

- Elective procedures should always be delayed until after pregnancy.
- Early in pregnancy risk of spontaneous abortion is a concern.
- Later in pregnancy, premature labor is a concern.
- If surgery is required, the second trimester is often preferred.
- Indicated surgery should never be denied or delayed.

- Anesthetic considerations are physiologic changes associated with pregnancy and the prevention of intrauterine fetal hypoxia and acidosis.
  - Anesthetic plan should optimize the maternal and fetal condition.
- There is no difference in outcomes between open and laparoscopic procedures.
  - For laparoscopic procedures, low pneumoperitoneum pressures should be used if possible.
- The decision of regional or general anesthesia technique should be made independent of the patient's pregnancy.
- Surgery should be done at an institution with obstetric and neonatal care readily available.

Avoidance of Teratogenic Drugs

- Critical period of organogenesis is between 15 and 56 days of gestation.
- Pregnancy testing may be offered to female patients of childbearing age and for whom the result would alter the patient's management.
  - Routine pregnancy testing before elective surgery remains controversial.
- No currently used anesthetic drugs have known teratogenic effects in humans at standard dosing, except cocaine.

Avoidance of Intrauterine Fetal Hypoxia and Acidosis

- Maintain UBF with left uterine displacement and prevent maternal hypotension
- Prevent arterial hypoxemia and excessive changes in $PaCO_2$ (which affects UBF)
  - The PaO_2 of the fetus doesn't exceed 60 mmHg even if maternal PaO_2 exceeds 500 mmHg.
- FHR monitoring decision should be based on gestational age, type of surgery, and facilities available.
  - Interpretation can be difficult since most anesthetics reduce variability, and signal acquisition and interpretation can be challenging.
- At 25 to 27 weeks of gestation, FHR variability can be reliably used as a marker of well-being.
  - Continuous FHR monitoring allows for optimization of the fetal condition if fetal compromise is detected.
- At 16 to 18 weeks' gestational age, FHR monitoring via Doppler is possible.
  - Preprocedure and postprocedure FHR assessment is generally considered sufficient when the fetus is considered previable.

Prevention of Preterm Labor

- The need for surgery increases the risk of preterm labor, independent of the anesthetic.
  - Risk is increased with intraabdominal procedures.
- FHR and uterine activity should continue to be monitored postoperatively.
  - Postoperative analgesia can alter the perception of contractions.
- If uterine activity is noted, tocolytics (e.g., nifedipine, indomethacin) can be used.
- Magnesium sulfate can be administered to reduce the risk of cerebral palsy.
- For severely preterm delivery, corticosteroid administration is recommended to decrease neonatal respiratory morbidity.

Management of Anesthesia

- Preoperative discussion with the surgeon, obstetrician, and perinatologist regarding fetal monitoring, potential maternal arrest, and possible emergent cesarean delivery
- Postoperative issues include deep venous thrombosis prophylaxis, FHR and uterine activity monitoring for at least 24 hours, and postoperative analgesia plan.

DIAGNOSIS AND MANAGEMENT OF FETAL DISTRESS

Overview

- FHR monitoring was developed as a basic, nonspecific method of tracking fetal oxygenation and distress.
- Monitors can be external; internal fetal scalp electrode provides more accurate continuous monitoring.

Key Evaluation Components

Uterine Contractions

- External monitors: contraction frequency
- Internal monitors: contraction frequency and intra uterine pressure
  - Uterine contractions can decrease UBF and oxygen delivery by constricting the spiral arteries.

  - A tonic contraction or period of tachysystole can be treated with subcutaneous terbutaline or IV nitroglycerin to briefly relax the uterus and restore fetal perfusion.

Baseline FHR

- Reflects the mean FHR rounded to increments of 5 beats per minute (bpm) during a 10-minute window
- Normal FHR ranges from 110 to 160 beats per minute (bpm).
  - Fetal bradycardia is <110 bpm.
  - Fetal tachycardia is >160 bpm.

Variability

- Examination of irregular fluctuations in amplitude and frequency during a 10-minute window
- Variability of amplitude range can be *absent*, *minimal* (≤5 bpm), *moderate* (6 to 25 bpm), or *marked* (>25 bpm).

Accelerations

- An increase from onset to peak in >30 seconds; peak must be ≥15 bpm and last ≥15 seconds from onset to return
  - Before 32 weeks' gestation, peak must be ≥10 bpm and last ≥10 seconds.

Decelerations

- Prolonged deceleration is decreased in FHR from baseline ≥15 bpm, lasting ≥2 minutes.
- *Late decelerations* result from uterine contractions causing uteroplacental insufficiency and fetal brain hypoxia.
  - Bradycardia is a reflex to sympathetic-mediated increased fetal blood pressure.
  - More severe drop in FHR can indicate myocardial depression due to worsening hypoxia.
- *Variable decelerations* indicate umbilical cord compression.
- *Sinusoidal FHR* is an ominous sine wave pattern cycling 3 to 5/min for ≥20 minutes.
  - Can be associated with placental abruption
- Severe decelerations (<70 bpm for >60 seconds) indicate fetal acidemia; extremely ominous when there is also absence of variability

FHR Categories

- FHR tracing is a nonspecific assessment of fetal acidosis and should be interpreted over time in relation to the clinical context and fetal and maternal factors.

Fetal Heart Rate Categories

Category I FHR tracing: predicts a normal fetal acid-base state
- Baseline FHR of 110 to 160 bpm
- Moderate baseline FHR variability
- No late or variable decelerations
- Early decelerations may be present or absent.
- Accelerations may be present or absent.

Category II FHR tracing: indeterminate
- Includes all FHR tracings not in categories I or III
- Fetal tachycardia
- Prolonged decelerations between 2 and 10 minutes
- Recurrent late decelerations with moderate baseline variability

Category III FHR tracing: abnormal fetal acid-base status
- A sinusoidal FHR pattern
- Absent FHR variability with recurrent late decelerations, recurrent variable decelerations, or bradycardia

EVALUATION OF THE NEONATE AND NEONATAL RESUSCITATION

- Umbilical cord gases measured at delivery provide fetal assessment.
  - Umbilical artery values reflect fetal well-being.
  - Umbilical vein values are a reflection of maternal status and uteroplacental perfusion.
- Apgar scoring system provides a simplified method for rapid neonatal assessment
  - Identifies neonates who need resuscitation
  - Assessed at 1, 5, and 10 minutes after delivery
  - Assesses five parameters: heart rate, breathing, reflex/irritability, muscle tone, color
- Most newborns only need suctioning of nose and mouth, tactile stimulation to promote breathing, and to be wiped dry, wrapped in blankets, and kept warm.

Cardiopulmonary Resuscitation

- Management of neonates in the delivery room falls into 30-second evaluations and interventions.
- Evaluation of tone, breathing, and crying occur in the first 30-second evaluation.
- Evaluation for apnea/breathing and heart rate occur at 1-minute Apgar score.
  - Possible interventions include positive pressure ventilation (PPV), placement of pulse oximetry, and ECG monitoring.
- For heart rate <100, evaluate PPV efficacy by checking for chest movement, optimize PPV delivery, and consider the need for intubation or supraglottic airway placement.
- If the heart rate drops below 60, then chest compressions, intubation, and ventilation with 100% oxygen should commence with ECG monitoring and preparation for umbilical vein cannulation.
- If meconium is present, emphasis is on ventilation by clearing the airway and use of PPV if necessary.
  - Routine intubation for tracheal suction in this setting is no longer suggested.

Epinephrine

- Indicated if heart rate remains <60 despite PPV

Hypovolemia

- Volume expansion may be indicated in situations of placental abruption, placenta previa, or vasa previa.
- If neonate has not responded to other resuscitative measures, blood or isotonic saline may be administered in 10-mL/kg aliquots.

Glucose

- Hypoglycemic risk factors: severe asphyxia, intrauterine growth restriction, or maternal diabetes
- Heelstick can determine blood glucose level.

QUESTIONS

PHYSIOLOGIC CHANGES IN PREGNANT WOMEN

1. Describe the expected changes in the cardiovascular system of the pregnant patient in an uncomplicated pregnancy at term, compared to nonpregnant values, by completing the following table.

Cardiovascular Parameter	Expected Change at Term
Intravascular fluid volume	
Plasma volume	
Erythrocyte volume	
Coagulation status	
Blood pressure	
Systemic vascular resistance	
Central venous pressure	
Cardiac output	
Stroke volume	
Heart rate	

2. How does maternal cardiac output change during labor, delivery, and postpartum?
3. Describe factors pertaining to supine hypotension syndrome by completing the following table.

Cause	
Symptoms	
Clinical implications	
Compensatory mechanisms	
Significance in anesthesia practice	
Anesthetic management	

4. What are some echocardiographic changes during pregnancy?
5. Describe the expected changes in the pulmonary system of the pregnant patient in an uncomplicated pregnancy at term, compared to nonpregnant values, by completing the following table.

Pulmonary Parameter	Expected Change at Term
Minute ventilation	
Tidal volume	
Respiratory rate	
Expiratory reserve volume	
Residual volume	
Functional residual capacity	
Vital capacity	
Total lung capacity	
Maternal $PaCO_2$	
Oxygen consumption	

6. How does oxygen consumption change during labor?
7. What are some physiologic changes of the upper airway that occur in pregnancy, and their associated clinical implications?
8. Why does the pregnant patient desaturate rapidly with apnea?
9. What are the gastrointestinal changes in pregnancy that render the patient vulnerable to gastric reflux?
10. Describe the clinical management of the pregnant patient with regard to the risk of gastric reflux.
11. Does the minimum alveolar concentration of anesthesia with volatile anesthetics change in pregnancy?
12. How do renal blood flow, glomerular filtration rate, and the normal upper limits of serum creatinine and blood urea nitrogen change in pregnancy?
13. How do hepatic blood flow, plasma protein concentrations, and plasma cholinesterase activity change during pregnancy?

PHYSIOLOGY OF THE UTEROPLACENTAL CIRCULATION

14. What is the uterine blood flow rate at term?
15. What are the determinants of uterine blood flow?
16. What factors affect the transfer of oxygen between the patient and fetus?
17. How are the fetal and maternal hemoglobin dissociation curves shifted? What is the effect of this?
18. What is normal fetal $Pa{O_2}$?
19. What factors affect placental exchange of drugs and other substances? What is the most reliable way to minimize fetal transfer of a drug?
20. Which drugs commonly used in anesthesia have limited ability to cross the placenta?
21. How does the pH of fetal blood affect the transfer of drugs? What is ion trapping?
22. What characteristics of the fetal circulation are protective against the distribution of large doses of drugs to vital organs?

STAGES OF LABOR

23. Name the stages of labor and the events that define each stage.
24. What is an “active-phase arrest”? What is an “arrest of descent”?

ANATOMY OF LABOR PAIN

25. In the first stage of labor, from which organs do afferent nerve impulses originate, and what are the associated sensory levels?
26. In the second stage of labor, from which organs do afferent nerve impulses originate, and what are the associated sensory levels?

METHODS OF LABOR ANALGESIA

27. Describe the various nonpharmacologic techniques used for labor analgesia.
28. What are some limitations of systemic medications for labor pain?
29. List the different opioid medications used for labor analgesia, their active metabolites, and what limits their utility. Which opioid is used most frequently?
30. What is *morphine sleep*?
31. Can inhaled nitrous oxide be administered safely for labor and delivery analgesia?

NEURAXIAL TECHNIQUES

32. What are some local anesthetics used for neuraxial labor analgesia and their potential complications?
33. What are some advantages and disadvantages of the coadministration of an opioid for neuraxial labor analgesia?
34. What are some advantages and disadvantages of the coadministration of clonidine and epinephrine for neuraxial labor analgesia?

35. What are the benefits of neuraxial techniques for labor analgesia?
36. During what stage of labor should neuraxial labor analgesia be administered?
37. Does neuraxial analgesia affect the progress of labor or the rate of cesarean delivery?
38. What preparations should be made prior to the administration of neuraxial labor analgesia?
39. Should laboring patients remain NPO ("nothing by mouth") after placement of an epidural or combined spinal-epidural?
40. What is the combined spinal epidural (CSE) technique, and what are some benefits of this technique?
41. Can a "test dose" be used with a CSE?
42. What is programmed intermittent epidural boluses (PIEB) and some advantages of its use?
43. What is a "saddle block," and when is it utilized during labor and delivery?

CONTRAINDICATIONS OF NEURAXIAL ANESTHESIA

44. What are the contraindications to neuraxial procedures?

COMPLICATIONS OF NEURAXIAL ANESTHESIA

45. List the possible complications of a neuraxial block.
46. What are some effects of an unintended intravascular injection of local anesthetic?
47. What is the treatment for systemic bupivacaine toxicity?
48. What physiologic effects do you expect to see with a high spinal or high epidural?
49. What are the important differences in performing ACLS (advanced cardiac life support) for the pregnant patient compared to a nonpregnant patient?
50. What is the rate of hypotension after neuraxial blockade for labor analgesia?
51. How does labor epidural analgesia affect maternal body temperature?

ANESTHESIA FOR CESAREAN DELIVERY

52. For cesarean delivery, compare and contrast the advantages of epidural versus spinal anesthesia and regional versus general anesthesia by completing the following tables.

Epidural Anesthesia	Spinal Anesthesia

Regional Anesthesia	General Anesthesia

53. What dermatomal level for spinal and epidural anesthesia is needed for cesarean delivery?
54. Which local anesthetics and dose are typically administered to achieve an adequate density and dermatomal level of spinal and epidural anesthesia for cesarean delivery?
55. What is the advantage and some potential negative effects of the administration of preservative-free morphine into the epidural space for cesarean delivery?
56. What are some indications for general anesthesia for cesarean delivery?
57. What is the approach to general anesthesia for cesarean delivery with respect to preparation, induction, maintenance, and emergence?
58. What is the level of exposure of the fetus to propofol after the administration of induction doses for general anesthesia?
59. What are some of the advantages and disadvantages of etomidate for the induction of general anesthesia for cesarean delivery?
60. What are some of the advantages and disadvantages of ketamine for the induction of general anesthesia for cesarean delivery?
61. Which neuromuscular blocking drugs are typically used for cesarean delivery under general anesthesia, and what are the effects on uterine muscle tone and the fetus?

ABNORMAL PRESENTATIONS AND MULTIPLE BIRTHS

62. What are some complications that can develop with multiple gestations?
63. What are the modes of delivery for twin pregnancies? What anesthetic techniques can be used to optimize delivery?
64. What is external cephalic version, and what are the associated risks?
65. What is a shoulder dystocia, risk factors associated with its development, and risks to the fetus?

HYPERTENSIVE DISORDERS OF PREGNANCY

66. What are the four classifications of hypertensive disorders in pregnancy? What distinguishes gestational hypertension from chronic hypertension?
67. What are the risk factors associated with developing preeclampsia?
68. What are the criteria for the diagnosis of preeclampsia?
69. What is preeclampsia with severe features?
70. What is HELLP syndrome?
71. Does a preeclampsia diagnosis always require immediate delivery?
72. What is the clinical use of magnesium sulfate in the treatment of preeclampsia? What are some considerations when using this treatment?
73. What are the clinical signs of magnesium sulfate toxicity? What is the treatment?
74. Which antihypertensive drugs are commonly used in preeclampsia?
75. What are some anesthetic considerations in the urgent or emergent delivery in patients with preeclampsia?

HEMORRHAGE IN PREGNANT WOMEN

76. What are some causes of hemorrhage in the pregnant patient? When do these typically manifest?
77. What is placenta previa? What are the associated risk factors?
78. What is abruptio placentae? What are some risk factors for abruptio placentae?
79. What are the clinical presentation and anesthetic considerations for the management of abruptio placentae?
80. What are some risk factors for uterine rupture? What is the incidence of uterine rupture associated with vaginal birth after a previous cesarean delivery?
81. What approximate percent of vaginal deliveries are associated with some amount of retained placenta, and what are the anesthetic management options?
82. What are some risk factors for postpartum uterine atony?
83. Which medications are used to manage uterine atony? What are their side effects?
84. Define placenta accreta, increta, and percreta.
85. In a patient with known placenta previa, how does the risk of placenta accreta spectrum change with the number of prior cesarean deliveries?

AMNIOTIC FLUID EMBOLISM

86. What is the clinical presentation of an amniotic fluid embolism? What are some conditions that may mimic amniotic fluid embolism?
87. How is the definitive diagnosis of an amniotic fluid embolism made?

ANESTHESIA FOR NONOBSTETRIC SURGERY DURING PREGNANCY

88. What are common nonobstetric surgeries that occur during pregnancy?
89. When should nonobstetric surgeries be performed during pregnancy?
90. What are some considerations for the anesthetic management of pregnant patients undergoing nonobstetric surgery?
91. Which anesthetics are teratogenic?
92. How can intrauterine fetal hypoxia and acidosis be prevented during nonobstetric surgery?
93. When should fetal heart rate monitoring be done during nonobstetric surgery?

DIAGNOSIS AND MANAGEMENT OF FETAL DISTRESS

94. Describe the frequency of normal uterine contractions and tachysystole. What is the treatment for tachysystole?
95. What is the normal baseline fetal heart rate (FHR)?
96. Define FHR variability in terms of absent, minimal, moderate, and marked.
97. What is the definition of a FHR acceleration?
98. What is a late deceleration indicative of in the fetus?
99. What is a variable deceleration indicative of in the fetus?
100. Complete the table below detailing the categories in the three-tier FHR classification system for general fetal assessment.

Fetal Heart Rate Classification System			
Category	**Interpretation**	**Criteria**	**Fetal Status**
I			
II			
III			

101. How should category III FHR tracings be managed?

EVALUATION OF THE NEONATE AND NEONATAL RESUSCITATION

102. Define the neonate characteristics evaluated by the Apgar score, and how the score values are assigned.
103. What are normal blood gas values for the umbilical artery and vein?
104. When is it appropriate to give positive-pressure ventilation and chest compressions during neonatal evaluation and resuscitation?
105. What is the dose of epinephrine given for neonatal resuscitation?
106. In neonates delivered with meconium-stained amniotic fluid, when should suctioning below the cords be instituted?

ANSWERS*

PHYSIOLOGIC CHANGES IN PREGNANT WOMEN

1. The table describes the expected changes in the cardiovascular system of pregnancy in an uncomplicated pregnancy at term, compared to nonpregnant values. The relative *physiologic anemia of pregnancy* is explained by changes described in the table. (578–579)

Cardiovascular Parameter	Expected Change at Term
Intravascular fluid volume	Increases by 35 to 45% (about 1000 mL to 1500 mL above the nonpregnant state)
Plasma volume	Increases by approximately 50%
Erythrocyte volume	Increases by approximately 25%
Coagulation status	Hypercoagulable: increases in factors I, VII, VIII, IX, X, and XII and von Willebrand factor and decreases in factors XI and XIII and antithrombin III. Prothrombin time (PT) and partial thromboplastin time (PTT) decrease about 20%. Platelets may remain normal or decrease 10%.
Blood pressure	Systolic, mean, and diastolic blood pressures may all decrease 5% to 15% by 20 weeks of gestational age and gradually increase toward prepregnant values at term.
Systemic vascular resistance	20% reduction
Central venous pressure	No change, despite the increased plasma volume because venous capacitance increases
Cardiac output	Increases by 45%
Stroke volume	Increases 25% to 30%
Heart rate	Increases 15% to 25%

2. Labor further increases maternal cardiac output by 10% to 25% during the first stage and 40% in the second stage. The largest increase in cardiac output occurs just after delivery, when it increases as much as 80% above prelabor values. This is the maximal change in cardiac output in the parturient. Cardiac output decreases to prelabor values about 48 hours after delivery and has substantial further decreases toward prepregnant values by 2 weeks postpartum. (578–579)
3. Factors pertaining to supine hypotension syndrome are described in the following table. (579)

Cause	Supine hypotension syndrome is the decrease in blood pressure seen when a pregnant patient lies supine Gravid uterus compresses the inferior vena cava, decreasing venous return, cardiac preload, and cardiac output by approximately 10% to 20% Gravid uterus also compresses the lower abdominal aorta leading to lower extremity arterial hypotension and a decrease in uterine blood flow
Symptoms	Diaphoresis, nausea, vomiting, and possible changes in cerebration
Clinical implications	Decrease in uterine blood flow can lead to fetal compromise Compression of the vena cava may contribute to venous stasis and increased risk of venous thrombosis
Compensatory mechanisms	Diversion of blood flow from the inferior vena cava to the paravertebral venous plexus, then to the azygos vein, to return to the heart via the superior vena cava Increase in peripheral sympathetic nervous system activity and peripheral vascular tone
Significance in anesthesia practice	Regional anesthesia can interfere with these compensatory mechanisms by causing sympathetic nervous system blockade, making the pregnant patient at term more susceptible to decreases in blood pressure Dilation of the epidural veins may make unintentional intravascular placement of an epidural catheter more likely
Anesthetic management	Uterine displacement, typically with displacement being to the left (accomplished by table tilt (30°) or the placement of a wedge or folded blanket under the right hip, elevating the hip by 10 to 15 cm) Have the patient lie in the lateral position

4. Echocardiographic changes during pregnancy include anterior and leftward displacement of the heart, increases in right (20%) and left (10%) heart chamber sizes, and associated left ventricular hypertrophy and increase in ejection fraction. About 1 in 4 pregnant patients have mitral regurgitation. In addition, small pericardial effusions may be present. (579)
5. The table below describes the expected changes in the pulmonary system in an uncomplicated pregnancy at term, compared to nonpregnant values. (580–581)

Pulmonary Parameter	Expected Change at Term
Minute ventilation	Increased 45–50%
Tidal volume	Increased 40–45%
Respiratory rate	Increased 0–15%
Expiratory reserve volume	Decreased 20–25%
Residual volume	Decreased 15–20%
Functional residual capacity	Decreased 20%
Vital capacity	No change
Total lung capacity	Decreased 0–5%
Maternal $PaCO_2$	Decreases from 40 mmHg to 30 mmHg
Oxygen consumption	Increases by 20%

6. During labor, oxygen consumption increases by 40% above prelabor rates during the first stage and by 75% during the second stage. (580)
7. There is significant capillary engorgement of the mucosal layer of the upper airway and increased tissue friability during pregnancy. This results in an increased risk of obstruction from tissue edema and bleeding with instrumentation of the upper airway. Additional care is needed during suctioning, placement of airways (avoid nasal instrumentation if possible), direct laryngoscopy, and intubation. In addition, because the vocal cords and arytenoids are often edematous, smaller cuffed endotracheal tubes (6.0- to 6.5-mm internal diameter) may be a better selection for intubation of the trachea for pregnant patients. The presence of preeclampsia, upper respiratory tract infections, and active pushing with associated increased venous pressure further exacerbate airway tissue edema, making both intubation and ventilation more challenging. (580)
8. There are at least three physiologic contributions for more rapid desaturation observed during pregnancy. First, a decreased FRC leads to subsequent decreased oxygen reserve. Second, maternal oxygen consumption is increased by 20% at term, with further increases noted during labor. Third, aortocaval compression (and decreased venous return) leads to decreases in cardiac output in the supine intubating position. This decrease in cardiac output would lead to an increase in overall oxygen extraction and therefore decrease the level of oxygenation of blood returning to the heart. (580–581)
9. Multiple gastrointestinal changes render the pregnant patient significantly vulnerable to the regurgitation of gastric contents beyond 20 weeks of gestation. The enlarged uterus acts to displace the stomach and pylorus cephalad from its usual position. This repositions the intra-abdominal portion of the esophagus into the thorax and leads to relative incompetence of the physiologic gastroesophageal sphincter. The tone of the gastroesophageal sphincter is further reduced by the higher progesterone and estrogen levels of pregnancy. Gastric pressure is increased by the gravid uterus. Gastrin secreted by the placenta stimulates gastric hydrogen ion secretion, decreasing the pH of the gastric fluid. During labor, gastric emptying is delayed, and intragastric fluid volume tends to be increased as a result. The administration of opioids can further decrease gastric emptying. (581)
10. Regardless of what amount of time has elapsed since the last ingestion of solids, the pregnant patient is at increased risk of regurgitation and aspiration of gastric contents. Clinical management includes the routine use of nonparticulate antacids, rapid-sequence induction, cricoid pressure, and cuffed intubation as part of general anesthesia induction sequence in a pregnant patient after approximately 20 weeks of gestational age. American Society of Anesthesiologists (ASA) guidelines recommend the "timely administration of oral nonparticulate antacids, intravenous (IV) H_2-receptor antagonists, and/or metoclopramide for aspiration

prophylaxis" prior to the induction of anesthesia in pregnant patients, and this is common practice. Nonparticulate antacids such as 30 mL sodium citrate work rapidly, metoclopramide can significantly decrease gastric volume in as little as 15 minutes in the absence of prior opioid administration, and H_2-receptor antagonists can increase gastric fluid pH in approximately 1 hour. (581)

11. The minimum alveolar concentration of anesthesia with volatile anesthetics is decreased within the first trimester of pregnancy by up to 40% in animal studies and 28% in human studies. However, electroencephalographic monitoring studies did not reflect these results, but rather showed the effects of sevoflurane on the brain are similar in pregnant and nonpregnant patients. (581)
12. Renal blood flow and glomerular filtration rate both increase by about 50% to 60% before the third month of pregnancy. This results in a decrease in what is considered the normal upper limit of both the blood urea nitrogen and serum creatinine concentrations during pregnancy to about 50% of what it was in the prepregnancy state. Renal blood flow and glomerular filtration rate return to prepregnancy values around 3 months postpartum. (582)
13. Hepatic blood flow does not change significantly with pregnancy. Plasma protein concentrations are reduced in pregnancy, which can create increased blood levels of highly protein-bound drugs. Plasma cholinesterase, or pseudocholinesterase, decreases in activity by about 25% to 30% by about the 10th week of pregnancy, and persists for as long as 6 weeks postpartum. The clinical manifestation from this change in plasma cholinesterase activity is minimal but return of muscle strength should always be verified. (582)

PHYSIOLOGY OF THE UTEROPLACENTAL CIRCULATION

14. Uterine blood flow increases during gestation from approximately 100 mL/min before pregnancy to 700 mL/min at term. About 80% of the uterine blood flow perfuses the placenta, and 20% supports the myometrium. (582)
15. During pregnancy uterine blood flow has limited autoregulation, and the uterine vasculature is essentially maximally dilated under normal pregnancy conditions. Uterine blood flow is proportional to the mean blood perfusion pressure to the uterus and inversely proportional to the resistance of the uterine vasculature. Decreased perfusion pressure can result from systemic hypotension secondary to hypovolemia, aortocaval compression, or decreased systemic resistance from either general or neuraxial anesthesia. Uterine blood flow also decreases with increased uterine venous pressure. This can result from vena caval compression (supine position), uterine contractions (particularly uterine tachysystole as may occur with oxytocin administration), or significant abdominal musculature contraction (Valsalva maneuver during pushing). Additionally, extreme hypocapnia ($Paco_2$ <20 mmHg) associated with hyperventilation can reduce uterine blood flow to the point of fetal hypoxemia and acidosis. Epidural or spinal anesthesia does not alter uterine blood flow as long as maternal hypotension is avoided. Although high doses of exogenous vasopressors have the capability of increasing uterine arterial resistance and decreasing uterine blood flow, use of phenylephrine, ephedrine, and norepinephrine in standard clinical doses to correct maternal hypotension does not adversely affect fetal well-being. (582)
16. Factors affecting the transfer of oxygen between the patient and the fetus include the ratio of maternal to fetal umbilical blood flow, the oxygen partial pressure gradient, the respective hemoglobin concentrations and affinities, the placental diffusing capacity, and the acid-base status of the fetal and maternal blood (Bohr effect). (582)
17. The fetal oxyhemoglobin dissociation curve is left-shifted (greater oxygen affinity), whereas the maternal hemoglobin dissociation curve is right-shifted (decreased oxygen affinity), resulting in facilitated oxygen transfer to the fetus. The maternal hemoglobin P_{50} increases from 27 to approximately 30 mmHg. (580, 582)
18. The fetal Pao_2 is normally 20 to 40 mmHg and not more than 60 mmHg, even if the pregnant patient is breathing 100% oxygen. Placental exchange from the pregnant patient to the fetus represents exchange from more of a maternal venous rather than arterial blood. (582)
19. The relative transfer of drugs and other substances <1000 Da from the maternal circulation to the fetal circulation and vice versa is determined primarily by diffusion. Factors that affect the exchange of substances from the maternal circulation to the fetus include the concentration gradient of the substance across the placenta, maternal protein binding, molecular weight, lipid solubility, and degree of ionization of the substance. The most reliable way to minimize the amount of drug that reaches the fetus is by minimizing the concentration of the drug in the maternal blood. (582)
20. Nondepolarizing neuromuscular blocking drugs have a high molecular weight and low lipid solubility. These two characteristics together limit the ability of nondepolarizing neuromuscular blocking drugs to cross the

placenta. Succinylcholine is highly ionized, preventing it from diffusing across the placenta despite its low molecular weight. Additionally, heparin, insulin, and glycopyrrolate have significantly limited placental transfer. Conversely, placental transfer of local anesthetics, benzodiazepines, and opioids is facilitated by the relatively low molecular weights of these substances. (582–583)

21. Fetal blood is slightly more acidic than maternal blood, with a pH about 0.1 unit less than maternal blood pH. The lower pH of fetal blood facilitates the fetal uptake of drugs that are basic. Weakly basic drugs, such as local anesthetics and opioids that cross the placenta in the nonionized state become ionized in the fetal circulation. This results in an accumulated concentration of drug in the fetus for two reasons. First, once the drug becomes ionized it cannot readily diffuse back across the placenta. This is known as *ion trapping.* Second, a concentration gradient of nonionized drug is maintained between the patient and the fetus. For example, if the fetus was distressed and acidotic, and lidocaine was maternally administered in sufficient doses, lidocaine may accumulate in the fetus. This can be particularly harmful to the fetus if direct maternal intravascular local anesthetic injection occurs. Decreased neonatal tone and potential bradycardia can result from significant fetal local anesthetic toxicity. (583)
22. The fetal circulation protects against the distribution of large doses of drugs to vital organs in two ways. First, about 75% of the blood that is coming to the fetus via the umbilical vein first passes through the fetal liver. Despite decreased liver enzyme activity in comparison to adults, fetal/neonatal enzyme systems are adequately developed to metabolize most drugs. This allows for a significant amount of drug metabolism to take place before entering the fetal arterial circulation and delivery to the heart and brain. Second, drug within umbilical vein blood enters the inferior vena cava via the ductus venosus. This blood is diluted by drug-free blood returning from the lower extremities and pelvic viscera of the fetus, resulting in a decrease in the concentration of drug in the inferior vena cava. (583)

STAGES OF LABOR

23. Labor is a continuous process divided into three stages. The first stage is the onset of labor until the cervix is fully dilated. This first stage is further divided into latent and active phases. The latent phase can persist for many hours. The active phase begins at the point when the rate of cervical dilation increases (often between 5- and 6-cm dilation). The second stage of labor begins when the cervix is fully dilated and ends when the neonate is born. This stage is referred to as the "pushing and expulsion" stage. The third and final stage begins with birth of the neonate and is completed when the placenta is delivered. (583)
24. If dilation slows or stops in the active phase of labor despite pharmacologic interventions, this is considered active-phase arrest and cesarean delivery will likely be considered by the obstetrician. Arrest of descent occurs during the second stage of labor, when the neonate cannot be born vaginally. If the neonate is low enough in the pelvis, the obstetrician can perform an instrumented vaginal delivery (also known as an operative vaginal delivery) via vacuum or forceps. If the neonate remains too high in the pelvis, then the patient will likely need a cesarean delivery. (583)

ANATOMY OF LABOR PAIN

25. During the first stage of labor (cervical dilation) the majority of painful stimuli results from afferent nerve impulses from the lower uterine segment and cervix. This pain is typically visceral in nature (dull, aching, poorly localized). The nerve cell bodies are located at the dorsal root ganglia of the T10–L1 levels. (583)
26. In the second stage of labor, pain additionally originates from afferents of the vagina, perineum, and pelvic floor that travel primarily via the pudendal nerve to the dorsal root ganglia of the S2–S4 levels. This pain is typically somatic in nature (sharp and well localized). (584)

METHODS OF LABOR ANALGESIA

27. There are many nonpharmacologic techniques for labor analgesia including hydrotherapy, massage, position changes, transcutaneous electrical nerve stimulation (TENS), acupuncture/acupressure, sterile water injections, Lamaze breathing techniques, meditation, hypnosis, relaxation, expectation management, music therapies, and many others. A meta-analysis noted that parturients with a support individual used fewer pharmacologic analgesia methods, had decreased length of labor, were more likely to have a vaginal birth, and were less likely to have negative feelings about childbirth. (584)

28. Systemic medications for labor pain are dose-limited secondary to their potential effects of maternal sedation, respiratory compromise, loss of airway protection, and effects on the neonate. Sedatives, anxiolytics, and dissociative drugs are rarely used for labor pain. Systemic opioid use is common, particularly in the early stages of labor, but must be administered judiciously. All opioids readily cross the placental barrier and can cause decreased fetal heart rate (FHR) variability and dose-related neonatal respiratory depression. (584)
29. Fentanyl, commonly used for labor analgesia, has a short duration with no active metabolites. When administered in small IV doses of 50 to 100 μg per hour, there are no clinically significant differences in neonatal Apgar scores and respiratory effort compared to patients who have not received fentanyl. Morphine, which currently is rarely used, has an active metabolite with a prolonged duration of analgesia. The half-life of morphine is longer in neonates compared to adults, and it produces significant maternal sedation. Meperidine is still one of the most frequently used opioids worldwide. The maternal half-life of meperidine is 2 to 3 hours, with half-life in the fetus and newborn significantly greater (13–23 hours) and more variable. In addition, meperidine is metabolized to an active metabolite (normeperidine) that can significantly accumulate after repeated doses. With increased dosing and shortened time between doses there are increased neonatal risks of decreased Apgar scores, lowered oxygen saturation, and prolonged time to sustained respiration. Remifentanil causes minimal neonatal side effects due to its rapid onset and fast elimination by plasma and tissue esterases. Although remifentanil patient-controlled analgesia (PCA) does not provide superior pain relief compared with epidural labor analgesia, remifentanil provides better pain relief with improved patient satisfaction compared with other opioids and does not appear to adversely affect neonatal outcomes. Because of maternal safety concerns (specifically related to respiratory effects), remifentanil use in labor is typically reserved for patients with contraindications to neuraxial techniques. When remifentanil is used for labor analgesia, continuous pulse oximetry, end-tidal CO_2 monitoring, oxygen supplementation, and 1:1 nursing are recommended. (585)
30. In latent labor, obstetric providers may administer intramuscular (IM) morphine combined with promethazine for analgesia, sedation, and rest termed *morphine sleep.* This produces analgesia for approximately 2.5 to 6 hours with an onset of 10 to 20 minutes. (585)
31. An inhaled mixture of 50% nitrous oxide blended with 50% oxygen may be used for labor analgesia but should be self-administered after appropriate patient instruction. Side effects are mild, with nausea, dizziness, and drowsiness most common. Maternal cardiovascular and respiratory depression is minimal, uterine contractility is not affected, and neonatal depression does not occur regardless of the duration of nitrous oxide administration. Out of concern for maternal respiratory depression and loss of airway reflexes with deeper levels of sedation, coadministration of systemic opioids or other sedating medications is not recommended. (585)

NEURAXIAL TECHNIQUES

32. The local anesthetics most used for neuraxial labor analgesia are bupivacaine and ropivacaine. These are both amide-linked and are degraded by the P450 enzymes in the liver. When administered appropriately they are safe, but an accidental intravascular injection can result in significant maternal morbidity (seizures, loss of consciousness, severe arrhythmias, and cardiovascular collapse), maternal fatality, and the potential for fetal accumulation (ion trapping). (586)
33. The coadministration of an opioid augments the neuraxial labor analgesia provided by local anesthetics by improving the quality and allowing local anesthetic–sparing effects. Neuraxial opioids alone can be administered but are not as effective. Disadvantages of neuraxial opioids include dose-dependent maternal side effects of pruritus, sedation, and nausea. In addition, administration of intrathecal opioids can result in fetal bradycardia independent of hypotension. (586)
34. Clonidine inhibits the release of substance P in the dorsal horn and increases the level of acetylcholine in the cerebral spinal fluid. Neuraxial clonidine can augment analgesia, but sedation and hypotension are associated with its use. The Food and Drug Administration (FDA) has issued a "black box" warning regarding the possibility of significant hypotension with neuraxial clonidine in obstetrics, and caution should be used. Epidural epinephrine has been shown to decrease the dose of local anesthetic required for labor analgesia. (585–586)
35. Benefits of neuraxial techniques for labor analgesia include the most effective labor analgesia, the highest rates of maternal satisfaction, minimal sedative side effects, reduced maternal catecholamine concentrations, the facilitation of maternal active participation during labor, and the avoidance of hyperventilation. (586)
36. Maternal request for relief of labor pain is sufficient justification for epidural placement for labor analgesia according to current ASA and American College of Obstetricians and Gynecologists (ACOG) guidelines, regardless of cervical dilation. A single-shot spinal analgesic has a finite analgesic time depending on the local anesthetic and should be considered when utilizing this technique (e.g., it is ideal if the obstetrician is

performing an instrumented vaginal delivery in a patient without previous neuraxial block). Epidural catheter delivery techniques can be extended throughout the length of the labor. (586)

37. A Cochrane review of studies up to 2017 comparing use of labor epidural with either no epidural or systemic opioid labor analgesia found no difference in rates of cesarean delivery, but a modest increase in the length of the second stage (about 15 minutes) and an increased rate of instrumented vaginal delivery in patients using neuraxial analgesia for labor. However, a secondary analysis of only trials conducted after 2005 found there was no longer an association between use of labor epidural and need for instrumented vaginal delivery. This increase in the second stage duration is not harmful to the infant or patient, provided the fetal status remains reassuring and there is ongoing progress towards delivery. (586)
38. Prior to the administration of neuraxial labor analgesia the patient's history and physical examination should be performed, the airway assessed, informed consent obtained, and the confirmation of the availability of resuscitative equipment should be established. Patient and fetus should be closely monitored with maternal vital signs and FHR during the initiation of neuraxial blockade. The ASA recommendations regarding aseptic technique during neuraxial procedures should be followed. (586–587)
39. Otherwise healthy laboring patients may have modest amounts of clear liquids throughout labor. However, in complicated labors (e.g., by morbid obesity, difficult airway, concerning fetal status), the decision to restrict oral intake should be individualized. (586)
40. In the CSE technique a spinal needle is placed through the epidural needle, and an intrathecal dose of local anesthetic and/or opioid is administered prior to placing the epidural catheter. A 24- to 27-gauge pencil-point spinal needle is commonly selected to reduce the risk of postdural puncture headache (PDPH). Benefits of this technique are its quicker onset of analgesia and no motor blockade if opioids (e.g., 15 μg fentanyl) are used alone in the intrathecal space. (587)
41. A test dose can be and should be utilized with the CSE technique. The test will confirm whether the catheter is intravascular (an intravascular invection will increase heart rate and blood pressure in response to 3 mL of 1:200,000 epinephrine), and unintended intrathecal catheter placement can still be assessed as the patient should still be able to move their lower extremities after typical analgesic spinal doses of local anesthetic (e.g., 2.5 mg bupivacaine). For example, use of 3 mL of 1.5% lidocaine administered through an intrathecal catheter will result in lower extremity motor blockade. (587)
42. The programmed intermittent epidural boluses (PIEB) technique administers fixed epidural boluses at scheduled intervals. This technique can be used alone or with a patient-controlled epidural analgesia (PCEA) technique. The PIEB technique may slightly reduce local anesthetic usage, improve maternal satisfaction, and decrease the need for rescue boluses. (589)
43. If primarily perineal anesthesia is needed (i.e., forceps delivery, perineal laceration repair), the patient may be left in the sitting position for approximately 3 minutes after the administration of hyperbaric local anesthetic to concentrate the sensory block toward the sacral fibers ("saddle block"). A true saddle block anesthetic (requiring more time in the sitting position) does not produce complete uterine pain relief because the afferent fibers (extending to T10) from the uterus are not blocked. (590)

CONTRAINDICATIONS OF NEURAXIAL ANESTHESIA

44. Certain conditions contraindicate neuraxial procedures, including (1) patient refusal, (2) infection at the needle insertion site, (3) significant coagulopathy, (4) hypovolemic shock, (5) increased intracranial pressure from mass lesion, and (6) inadequate provider expertise. Other conditions such as systemic infection, neurologic disease, and mild coagulopathies are relative contraindications and should be evaluated on a case-by-case basis. (590)

COMPLICATIONS OF NEURAXIAL ANESTHESIA

45. Possible complications of neuraxial analgesia include inadequate block, hypotension, intravascular catheter placement, systemic toxicity of local anesthetic, unintentional intrathecal catheter placement, excessive blockade, PDPH, epidural hematoma, epidural abscesses, meningitis, and nerve or spinal cord injury. Other side effects include pruritus, nausea, shivering, urinary retention, motor weakness, low back soreness, and a prolonged block. (590)
46. If accidental intravascular injection of local anesthetic occurs, dose-dependent effects can be mild (tinnitus, perioral tingling, mild arterial blood pressure and heart rate changes) or major (seizures, loss of consciousness, severe arrhythmias, cardiovascular collapse). (590)
47. If systemic bupivacaine local anesthetic overdose occurs, in addition to following standard ACLS algorithms for pregnancy, consider use of a 20% IV lipid emulsion to bind the drug and decrease toxicity. (590)

48. A high spinal (total spinal) can result from an unrecognized epidural catheter placed subdural, migration of the catheter during its use, or an overdose of local anesthetic in the epidural space (i.e., high epidural). Both high spinals and high epidurals can result in severe maternal hypotension, bradycardia, loss of consciousness, and blockade of the motor nerves to the respiratory muscles. (590)
49. ACLS guidelines for pregnancy include use of left uterine displacement, avoidance of lower extremity vessels for drug delivery, chest compressions positioned slightly higher on the sternum, and no modifications to the defibrillation protocol except removal of fetal and uterine monitors prior to shock, unless it would result in a significant delay. In any situation of maternal cardiac arrest with unsuccessful resuscitation, the fetus should be emergently delivered if the patient does not have return of spontaneous circulation (ROSC) within 5 minutes of the arrest. This guideline for emergent cesarean delivery increases the chances of survival for both the patient and neonate. The use of checklists and prior simulation can improve health care provider performance in these rare but critical events. (590–591)
50. Hypotension (decrease in systolic blood pressure >20%) secondary to sympathetic blockade is the most common complication of neuraxial blockade for labor analgesia, with rates of approximately 14%. Treatment of hypotension includes additional left uterine displacement, and the administration of intravenous fluids and vasopressors. (591)
51. Labor epidural anesthesia can be associated with a rise in maternal body temperature. Interestingly, only about 20% of parturients with labor epidurals develop a fever, and the remaining 80% have no body temperature increase. The cause of the temperature increase remains uncertain but appears associated with noninfectious proinflammatory cytokines. The temperature rise is not associated with an increase in maternal white blood cell count or the incidence of neonatal sepsis. (591)

ANESTHESIA FOR CESAREAN DELIVERY

52. For cesarean delivery, the advantages of epidural versus spinal anesthesia and regional versus general anesthesia are compared in the following tables. (591–592)

Epidural Anesthesia	Spinal Anesthesia
Ability to extend duration and control block height Can slowly titrate dose to control maternal hemodynamics	Technical ease of administration Rapid onset and more reliable Low levels of systemic medication (less systemic toxicity and fetal effects) Low failure rate

Regional Anesthesia	General Anesthesia
Avoid risks of general anesthesia Decreased neonatal depression due to anesthetic exposure Placement of neuraxial opioids for postoperative pain Maintenance of maternal awareness	Rapid and dependable onset Secure airway and controlled ventilation Potential for less hemodynamic instability

53. Anesthesia with a sensory level of T4 is usually sufficient for patient comfort during cesarean delivery. (592)
54. For spinal anesthesia, a T4 sensory level can be achieved with the administration of hyperbaric bupivacaine 10 to 15 mg. For epidural anesthesia, an approximate volume of 15 to 20 mL of 2% lidocaine or 3% 2-chloroprocaine is administered in the epidural space to achieve the T4 level of anesthesia. These should be administered in increments to minimize the risk of accidental IV administration of toxic levels of local anesthetic. The addition of epinephrine (1:200,000) and fentanyl (50–100 μg) can enhance the intensity and duration of the block. Exteriorization of the uterus or traction of the abdominal viscera may still lead to discomfort in the patient. (592)
55. The epidural administration of preservative-free morphine (e.g., 2 mg) during cesarean delivery decreases postoperative pain requirements up to 24 hours after the operation. Side effects of epidural morphine include pruritus, nausea and vomiting, and, on rare occasions, delayed respiratory depression. (592)
56. Indications for general anesthesia for cesarean delivery include fetal distress and required emergent delivery to prevent poor fetal outcome, maternal hemorrhage, and contraindications to regional anesthesia such as maternal coagulopathy or maternal refusal. (592)

57. Prior to the induction of general anesthesia for cesarean delivery a nonparticulate antacid should be administered, standard monitors placed, uterine displacement maintained, adequate preoxygenation performed, and surgical readiness confirmed. A rapid-sequence induction is typically performed. Maintenance of anesthesia is achieved with a combination of a volatile anesthetic, propofol, and nitrous oxide. Opioid and benzodiazepine administration is usually delayed until after delivery of the baby to avoid placental transfer of these drugs. Following delivery, halogenated anesthetics should be partially or completely replaced with other anesthetics to decrease uterine atony. Extubation of the trachea is done once the patient is awake and airway reflexes have returned. (592–593)
58. The level of exposure of the fetus to propofol after its administration to the pregnant patient for the induction of general anesthesia is generally low. No significant effects on newborn behavior scores and markers of well-being are noted with typical induction doses of 2.5 mg/kg, but large doses of 9 mg/kg are associated with neonatal depression. (593–594)
59. Like propofol, etomidate has a quick onset because of its high lipid solubility. The rapid redistribution results in a relatively short duration of action. At typical induction doses (0.3 mg/kg), unlike propofol, etomidate has minimal cardiovascular effects, making it a suitable choice for the induction of anesthesia in the pregnant patient who is hemorrhaging, has uncertain intravascular fluid volume status, and is at risk for hypotension. Etomidate is painful on injection, can cause muscle tremors, has higher rates of nausea and vomiting, has increased risk of seizures in patients with decreased thresholds, and decreases neonatal cortisol production. (594)
60. Ketamine induction (1–1.5 mg/kg) produces a rapid onset of anesthesia, but unlike propofol, ketamine typically maintains arterial pressures, heart rate, and cardiac output through central stimulation of the sympathetic nervous system. This makes it advantageous in patients with hemodynamic compromise, such as the pregnant patient who is actively hemorrhaging. If administered in an amount greater than a typical induction dose, ketamine can increase uterine tone, reduce uterine arterial perfusion, and lower seizure threshold. (594)
61. Succinylcholine (1–1.5 mg/kg IV) remains the neuromuscular blocking drug of choice for obstetric anesthesia because of its rapid onset and short duration of action. Because it is highly ionized and poorly lipid-soluble, only small amounts cross the placenta. It is normally hydrolyzed in maternal blood by the enzyme pseudocholinesterase and does not generally interfere with fetal neuromuscular activity. If large doses are administered (2–3 mg/kg) it results in detectable levels in umbilical cord blood, and extreme doses (10 mg/kg) are needed for the transfer to result in neonatal neuromuscular blockade. Rocuronium is an acceptable alternative. It provides adequate intubating conditions in approximately 60 seconds at doses of 1.2 mg/kg. Unlike succinylcholine, rocuronium has a much longer duration of action, potentially decreasing maternal safety in the event the anesthesia provider is unable to intubate or ventilate the patient. However, a large intravenous dose of sugammadex (16 mg/kg) can rapidly reverse the neuromuscular block. Under normal circumstances, the poorly lipid-soluble, highly ionized, nondepolarizing neuromuscular blockers do not cross the placenta in amounts significant enough to cause neonatal muscle weakness. This placental impermeability is only relative, and when large doses are administered over long periods, neonatal neuromuscular blockade can occur. Uterine smooth muscle is not affected by neuromuscular blockade. (594–595)

ABNORMAL PRESENTATIONS AND MULTIPLE BIRTHS

62. Around 3% of live births in the United States are from multiple gestation pregnancy, with 97% of these being twins. Multiple gestation pregnancies carry increased risks of preterm labor, hypertensive disorders of pregnancy, gestational diabetes, hyperemesis gravidarum, anemia, preterm premature rupture of membranes, intrauterine growth restriction, and intrauterine fetal demise. (595–596)
63. The majority of twin pregnancies are vertex-vertex positioning of the fetuses and can be delivered vaginally. If the second twin is breech, it is important to discuss the mode of delivery with the obstetricians and perinatologists. If a vaginal delivery is attempted, an emergent cesarean delivery might be required if the second twin changes position after delivery of the first or develops fetal bradycardia. Placement of an epidural can facilitate delivery and extraction of the second twin if it becomes necessary for the obstetrician to perform an instrumented delivery. At the late second stage of delivery a more concentrated local anesthetic will optimize the perineal anesthesia. Drugs that provide quick uterine relaxation (e.g., IV nitroglycerin) also improve delivery conditions. At this time, the potential for head entrapment or fetal bradycardia is highest, and a denser block allows for possible transition to urgent cesarean delivery. (595–596)
64. Singleton breech presentation is uncommon (3–4% of all pregnancies). External cephalic version (ECV) is a procedure that involves rotating the fetus into a cephalic position via external palpation and pressure of the fetal parts. Ultrasound and fetal heart rate monitoring can help assess for fetal distress during ECV. ECV has

been shown to decrease the cesarean delivery rate. Terbutaline is a tocolytic that facilitates uterine relaxation and nearly doubles success rates for ECV. In a meta-analysis, ECV under neuraxial anesthesia had significantly higher odds of decreased pain, improved satisfaction, and successful fetal version compared with control. Risks of ECV include placental abruption, fetal bradycardia, and rupture of membranes. Although these risks are low, ECV should be performed in a facility where cesarean delivery can occur and an anesthesia provider is immediately available in case an urgent or emergent cesarean delivery is needed. (596)

65. A shoulder dystocia occurs when, after delivery of the fetal head, further expulsion of the infant is prevented by obstruction of the fetal shoulders within the maternal pelvis. Shoulder dystocia occurs in up to 3% of vaginal deliveries and is an obstetric surgical emergency. Risk factors include macrosomia, maternal diabetes, history of dystocia, and instrumented delivery. Once shoulder dystocia is diagnosed, a set of maneuvers is performed to deliver the infant; if delivery is unsuccessful then the final maneuver (Zavanelli maneuver) requires pushing the fetus back into the pelvis and proceeding to emergent cesarean delivery. Cases of shoulder dystocia 7 minutes or longer have a significant increase in risk of neonatal brain injury. Among the fetal injuries and sequelae of shoulder dystocia are brachial plexus injury, neurologic injury from asphyxia, and fractured clavicle or humerus. Often these neurologic injuries improve over time with roughly <10% having permanent Erb palsy. (596)

HYPERTENSIVE DISORDERS OF PREGNANCY

66. The four classifications of hypertensive disorders in pregnancy are preeclampsia-eclampsia, chronic hypertension, chronic hypertension with superimposed preeclampsia, and gestational hypertension. Gestational hypertension is diagnosed in previously normotensive patients who develop elevated blood pressure (SBP >140 mmHg or DBP >90 mmHg) after 20 weeks of gestational age. Chronic hypertension is elevated blood pressures predating pregnancy, occurring prior to 20 weeks of gestation, or persisting for more than 12 weeks postpartum. (596)
67. Preeclampsia affects 3–5% of all pregnancies. The greatest risk factors for developing preeclampsia include a history of preeclampsia and chronic hypertension. Other risk factors include nulliparity, multigestation pregnancy, pregestational diabetes, systemic lupus erythematosus or antiphospholipid antibody syndrome, renal disease, body mass index >30 kg/m^2, maternal age <17 or >35 years, and use of assisted reproductive technologies. (596)
68. The criteria for the diagnosis of preeclampsia are SBP >140 mmHg or DBP >90 mmHg (on two separate occasions at least 4 hours apart) that occurs after 20 weeks of gestation or during the postpartum period in a previously normotensive parturient. This increase in blood pressure is either associated with excess protein in the urine or the new development of thrombocytopenia (platelets <100,000 /μL), renal insufficiency, impaired liver function, cerebral or visual disturbances, or pulmonary edema. Proteinuria is defined as urinary excretion of 300 mg protein or higher in a 24-hour urine specimen. (597)
69. Preeclampsia with severe features is diagnosed if one or more of the following criteria are present in addition to preeclampsia:
    - SBP >160 mmHg or DBP >110 mmHg on two occasions at least 4 hours apart
    - Thrombocytopenia (platelet count <100,000/μL)
    - Impaired liver function as indicated by abnormally elevated blood concentrations of liver enzymes (to twice normal concentration), severe persistent right upper quadrant or epigastric pain unresponsive to medication
    - Renal insufficiency (serum creatinine concentration >1.1 mg/dL or a doubling of the serum creatinine concentration in the absence of other renal disease)
    - Pulmonary edema
    - New-onset headache (unresponsive to medications) or visual disturbances (597)
70. A subcategory of severe preeclampsia is HELLP syndrome, which is a constellation of **H**emolysis, **E**levated **L**iver enzymes, and **L**ow **P**latelet count. (597)
71. The definitive treatment of preeclampsia is delivery. If the pregnancy is remote from term in the presence of severe preeclampsia, a determination must be made whether to deliver or expectantly manage. This requires repeated evaluation of the patient and fetus. It is critical for the anesthesia provider on labor and delivery to be aware of these patients and their clinical course, as they can rapidly deteriorate and require urgent or emergent delivery. (597)
72. Magnesium sulfate is used for seizure prophylaxis in preeclamptic patients with severe features. The infusion is usually performed by loading 4 to 6 g over 20 to 30 minutes, then a continued magnesium sulfate infusion

of 1 to 2 g/h until 24 hours after delivery. Considerations of the use of magnesium sulfate infusions in this patient population include its potentiation of neuromuscular blockade of both depolarizing and nondepolarizing muscle relaxants, its effect on uterine and smooth muscle relaxation, and that magnesium sulfate is excreted renally and may have prolonged effects in patients with decreased renal function. (597–598)

73. Magnesium sulfate toxicity can be seen clinically as loss of deep tendon reflexes, respiratory depression, and neurologic compromise. The therapeutic blood level range for seizure prophylaxis is between 6 and 8 mg/dL. Loss of deep tendon reflexes occurs at 10 mg/dL with prolonged PQ intervals and widening QRS complex on the electrocardiogram. Respiratory arrest occurs at 15 to 20 mg/dL, and asystole occurs when the level exceeds 20 to 25 mg/dL. If toxicity occurs, IV calcium chloride (500 mg) or calcium gluconate (1 g) should be administered. (598)
74. Current guidelines recommend treating pregnant patients with an SBP >160 mmHg to prevent intracerebral hemorrhage. Initial therapeutic agents normally include IV labetalol, IV hydralazine, and oral nifedipine. (598)
75. Anesthetic considerations in the urgent or emergent delivery in patients with preeclampsia include their increased risk for upper airway edema and difficult intubation, the potential for exaggerated hypertension associated with laryngoscopy, possible uterine atony secondary to magnesium sulfate, and the relative contraindication of methylergonovine for the treatment of uterine atony as its administration can precipitate a hypertensive crisis in this patient population. (598)

HEMORRHAGE IN PREGNANT WOMEN

76. Placenta previa, abruptio placentae, and uterine rupture are major causes of bleeding in the third trimester and during labor. Postpartum hemorrhage occurs in 3% to 5% of all vaginal deliveries and is typically due to uterine atony. Morbidity can be reduced through recognition of the risk of hemorrhage, quantification of blood loss, preparation, and prompt treatment. (598–599)
77. Placenta previa is an abnormal uterine implantation of the placenta in front of the presenting fetus. The incidence is approximately 1 in 200 pregnancies. Risk factors include advanced age, multiparity, assisted reproductive techniques, prior hysterotomy, and prior placenta previa. Placenta previa classically presents as painless vaginal bleeding that usually occurs preterm in the third trimester, although most previas are now diagnosed antenatally by ultrasonography with delivery by scheduled cesarean. (599)
78. Abruptio placentae is separation of the placenta after 20 weeks of gestation but before delivery. The incidence is approximately 1 in 100 pregnancies. Risk factors include advanced age, hypertension, trauma, smoking, cocaine use, chorioamnionitis, premature rupture of membranes, and history of prior abruption. (599)
79. The patient with abruptio placentae often has painful, frequent uterine contractions. When the separation involves the placental margin, it can present as vaginal bleeding with associated uterine tenderness. Abruptio placentae can also occur without vaginal bleeding in which blood can accumulate in large volumes (>2 L) and be entirely concealed within the uterus. Therefore the degree of vaginal bleeding may not reflect the total amount of blood loss from the placenta. Chronic bleeding and clotting between the uterus and placenta can cause maternal disseminated intravascular coagulopathy (DIC). Severe hemorrhage and fetal distress frequently necessitate emergent cesarean delivery and use of general anesthesia. (599)
80. Risk factors for uterine rupture include prior uterine scar, rapid spontaneous delivery, motor vehicle trauma, trauma from instrumented vaginal delivery, large or malpositioned fetus, and excessive oxytocin stimulation. After previous cesarean delivery, vaginal birth is associated with a ≤1% incidence of uterine rupture. The presentation of uterine rupture is variable but may include vaginal bleeding, cessation of contractions, fetal bradycardia, loss of station, and persistent abdominal pain normally not masked by neuraxial analgesia. Unfortunately, none of these findings is 100% sensitive. An abnormal FHR pattern represents the most common associated sign of uterine rupture. Although persistent abdominal pain between contractions is highly correlated with uterine rupture, it is not always present. (599–600)
81. Approximately 2% to 3% of all vaginal deliveries are associated with some retained placenta. The treatment involves manual exploration of the uterus for the removal of retained placental parts. The anesthetic goals of patients with retained placenta involves uterine relaxation as well as decreasing the pain and anxiety of the patient. Anesthetic methods that may be used to initially accomplish this typically include IV sedation (keeping airway reflexes intact) or dosing of a preexisting epidural catheter. If uterine relaxation is necessary for assisted placental removal, nitroglycerin (administered in 200-μg IV boluses) is normally effective. Additionally, relocation to the operating room and placement of neuraxial analgesia may be beneficial for thorough evaluation. Rarely, induction of general anesthesia with tracheal intubation and administration of a volatile anesthetic to provide uterine relaxation will be necessary. (600)

82. Risk factors for postpartum uterine atony include retained products, long labor, high parity, macrosomia, polyhydramnios, excessive oxytocin augmentation, and chorioamnionitis. Uterine atony can occur immediately after delivery or several hours later. (600)
83. The treatment of uterine atony involves the administration of agents that increase uterine tone. Oxytocin (20–40 IU/L as an IV infusion or with algorithms that bolus 3 IU at a time) is normally the initial treatment. This dilute solution of oxytocin exerts minimal cardiovascular effects, but rapid IV injection is associated with tachycardia, vasodilation, and hypotension. Methylergonovine (0.2 mg IM) is an ergot derivative. Because it produces significant vasoconstriction, it is relatively contraindicated in patients with cardiac disease or preeclampsia. The prostaglandin $F_{2}\alpha$ (0.25 mg IM) is associated with nausea, tachycardia, pulmonary hypertension, desaturation, and bronchospasm. It should be avoided in patients with asthma. Prostaglandin E_1 (600 μg oral/sublingual/rectal) has no significant cardiac effects but may cause hyperthermia. (600)
84. Placental accreta spectrum refers to a range of pathologic placental growth and adherence. Placental implantation beyond the endometrium gives rise to (1) placenta accreta vera, which is implantation and adherence onto the myometrium; (2) placenta increta, which is implantation into the myometrium; and (3) placenta percreta, which is penetration through the full thickness of the myometrium. With placenta percreta, implantations may occur onto bowel, bladder, ovaries, or other pelvic organs and vessels. (600)
85. In patients with placenta previa and no previous cesarean delivery, the incidence of placenta accreta spectrum (PAS) is approximately 3%. However, the risk of PAS associated with placenta previa increases with the number of previous cesarean deliveries. With one previous uterine incision, the incidence of placenta accreta has been reported to be 11%, with two previous uterine incisions the rate is 40%, and with three or more prior uterine incisions the incidence rises to above 60%. Patients with both placenta previa and PAS can have rapid and massive intraoperative blood loss, with a reported median blood loss ranging from 2000 mL to 5000 mL. (601)

AMNIOTIC FLUID EMBOLISM

86. The incidence of amniotic fluid embolism (AFE) is estimated between 1 and 6 cases per 100,000 deliveries. Clinical features of AFE include the sudden onset of hypotension, respiratory distress, hypoxia, disseminated intravascular coagulopathy, altered mental status, and eventual maternal collapse. These signs must be differentiated from other more common morbidities of pregnancy and delivery, such as acute hemorrhage, inhalation of gastric contents, air embolism, pulmonary thromboembolism, high spinal, anaphylaxis, peripartum cardiomyopathy, and local anesthetic toxicity. (601)
87. The diagnosis of AFE is a clinical diagnosis of exclusion because no diagnostic laboratory test for AFE currently exists. Although in the past it had been believed that aspirating amniotic fluid debris such as fetal squamous cells from the maternal pulmonary circulation was diagnostic, the presence of fetal squames has been demonstrated in asymptomatic pregnant patients. Point-of-care echocardiography is a valuable aid in the diagnosis and management of AFE. Echocardiography findings include right ventricular systolic dysfunction, D-shaped septum, and acute pulmonary hypertension. (576)

ANESTHESIA FOR NONOBSTETRIC SURGERY DURING PREGNANCY

88. The most common nonobstetric surgeries that occur during pregnancy are trauma, appendicitis, cholecystitis, and malignancy. The incidence is as high as 1% to 2% of pregnancies. (602)
89. Elective procedures for the pregnant patient should be delayed until at least 6 weeks postpartum. The second trimester is considered the optimal time for surgical intervention during pregnancy. Regardless of trimester, a pregnant patient should never be denied a surgical procedure. In the case of acutely urgent surgical procedures, their timing should mimic that of nonpregnant patients. (602)
90. Considerations for the anesthetic management of pregnant patients undergoing nonobstetric surgery include maternal awareness, hemodynamics, respiration, deep venous thrombus prophylaxis, postoperative analgesia, the prevention of intrauterine fetal hypoxia and acidosis, the concern for spontaneous abortion or preterm labor, and monitoring of FHR and uterine activity. For these reasons the anesthesia provider should consult with an obstetrician and perinatologist to determine a plan for unexpected events, determine if FHR monitoring is appropriate, and discuss a plan for cesarean delivery should it become necessary for a maternal or fetal indication. There is no evidence that regional techniques provide better outcomes to either parturient or fetus compared to general anesthesia for these patients. (602)

91. Because the critical gestational period for organogenesis occurs between 15 and 56 days of gestation, teratogenic drugs administered during this time will exert their most disastrous effects. In animal studies most drugs, including anesthetics, have been demonstrated to be teratogenic in at least one animal species. Most data regarding the administration of anesthetics to pregnant patients in the first trimester are retrospective. There is no evidence that any of the currently used local or systemic anesthetics are teratogenic (with the exception of cocaine) when administered during pregnancy. Neurodegeneration and widespread apoptosis following exposure to anesthetics has been clearly established in developing animals, and a few studies demonstrate cognitive impairment in adult animals after neonatal anesthetic exposure. No specific anesthetic agent is known to be safer than another. There is no evidence that in utero human exposure to anesthetic drugs has an effect on the developing fetal brain. (602)
92. Intrauterine fetal hypoxia and acidosis has been associated with maternal hypotension, arterial hypoxemia, and excessive changes in the $PaCO_2$. During surgery, the goals are maintenance of normocarbia and adequate uterine perfusion pressure using fluids, vasopressors, and uterine displacement if after 20 weeks of gestational age. High oxygen consumption of the placenta, uneven distribution of maternal and fetal blood flow in the placenta, and specific hemoglobin binding characteristics prevent fetal PaO_2 from exceeding about 60 mmHg even with high maternal arterial oxygen levels. (602)
93. FHR monitoring via Doppler is possible at 16 to 18 weeks of gestational age, but variability as a marker of fetal well-being is not established until 25 to 27 weeks. Fetal monitoring can display fetal compromise and allows further optimization of the maternal and fetal condition with in utero resuscitation maneuvers. Currently there is no evidence for the efficacy of FHR monitoring. In addition, interpretation is difficult as most anesthetics reduce FHR variability, placement and signal acquisition may be challenging, and a trained person is needed for interpretation. The decision of whether to monitor the FHR during nonobstetric surgery should be individualized case by case in discussion with an obstetrician and other perioperative team members. (602–603)

DIAGNOSIS AND MANAGEMENT OF FETAL DISTRESS

94. Uterine activity is defined in the table below. If a tonic contraction or period of tachysystole occurs during labor, treatment with IV nitroglycerin or subcutaneous terbutaline can briefly relax the uterus and assist in restoring fetal perfusion. (603–604)

Uterine Activity Terminology	
Normal	≤5 contractions in 10 minutes averaged over a 30-minute window
Tachysystole	>5 contractions in 10 minutes averaged over a 30-minute window

95. The normal baseline FHR is between 110 and 160 beats per minute. (604)
96. Baseline variability is determined by examining fluctuations that are irregular in amplitude and frequency during a 10-minute window excluding accelerations and decelerations. Variability is classified as follows:
   a. Absent FHR variability: amplitude range undetectable
   b. Minimal FHR variability: amplitude range detectable, and ≤5 beats/min
   c. Moderate FHR variability: amplitude range 6 to 25 beats/min
   d. Marked FHR variability: amplitude range >25 beats/min (604)
97. A FHR acceleration is an abrupt increase in FHR defined as an increase from the acceleration onset to the peak in <30 seconds. In addition, the peak must be ≥15 beats/min and last ≥15 seconds from the onset to return. Before 32 weeks of gestation, accelerations are defined as having a peak >10 beats/min and duration of ≥10 seconds. (604)
98. Late decelerations are a result of uteroplacental insufficiency causing relative fetal brain hypoxia during a contraction. The change results in sympathetic response and increased peripheral vascular resistance in the fetus, elevating the fetal blood pressure, which is detected by the fetal baroreceptors and results in a slowing in the FHR. In addition, the relative hyperemia causes a chemoreceptor-mediated stimulation of the vagus nerve and decrease in FHR. Another type of late deceleration is decompensation of the myocardial circulation and fetal myocardial failure in the presence of worsening hypoxia. (604)
99. Variable decelerations are generally synonymous with umbilical cord compression. (579)
100. A three-tiered FHR classification system is used for a more general fetal assessment and is shown in the table below. (604–606)

Fetal Heart Rate Tracing Criteria for Fetal Status			
Category	**Interpretation**	**Criteria**	**Fetal Status**
I	Normal	Baseline FHR between 110 and 160 beats/min Moderate baseline FHR variability No late or variable decelerations Early decelerations may be present or absent Accelerations may be present or absent	No acidemia
II	Indeterminate	All tracings not categorized as I or III FHR >160 beats/min FHR <110 without absent variability FHR 110–160 with: • Minimal or marked variability • Absent variability without recurrent decelerations • No accelerations • Periodic decelerations • Recurrent variable decelerations with minimal/moderate variability • Prolonged decelerations more than 2 minutes but <10 minutes • Recurrent late decelerations with moderate variability	Not predictive of fetal acid–base status
III	Abnormal	Sinusoidal FHR pattern Absent FHR variability with • Recurrent late decelerations • Recurrent variable decelerations • Bradycardia	Evidence of actual or impending damaging fetal asphyxia

101. Category III FHR tracings require prompt patient evaluation and efforts to improve the fetal condition. Interventions may include intrauterine resuscitation, which involves changing maternal position, treatment of hypotension, use of supplemental oxygen, and treatment of tachysystole if present. If the FHR tracing doesn't improve despite these interventions, expeditious delivery of the fetus should proceed. (604)

EVALUATION OF THE NEONATE AND NEONATAL RESUSCITATION

102. Below is a table describing the characteristics and values assigned when evaluating a neonate using the Apgar scoring system. (606)

Characteristic	Score = 0	Score = 1	Score = 2
Heart rate (bpm)	Absent	<100	>100
Breathing	Absent	Slow	Irregular, crying
Reflex irritability	No response	Grimace	Cry
Muscle tone	Limp	Flexion of the extremities	Active
Color	Cyanotic	Body pink, extremities cyanotic	Pink

103. The table below describes normal umbilical cord blood gas values (606)

Parameter	Mean Artery	Mean Vein
pH	7.27	7.34
PCO_2 (mmHg)	50	40
PO_2 (mmHg)	20	30
Bicarbonate (mEq/L)	23	21
Base excess (mEq/L)	−3.6	−2.6

104. During neonatal evaluation, American Heart Association guidelines are followed to determine neonatal status and need for resuscitation, as highlighted in the figure below. In the event of apnea or heart rate <100 beats/min, positive-pressure hand ventilation should be provided with 21% oxygen or up to 100% oxygen using a properly fitted face mask (avoiding excessive inspiratory pressure >30 cm H_2O). Chest compressions, intubation, and positive-pressure ventilation with 100% oxygen become indicated in the event the heart rate drops to <60 beats/min. (606–607)

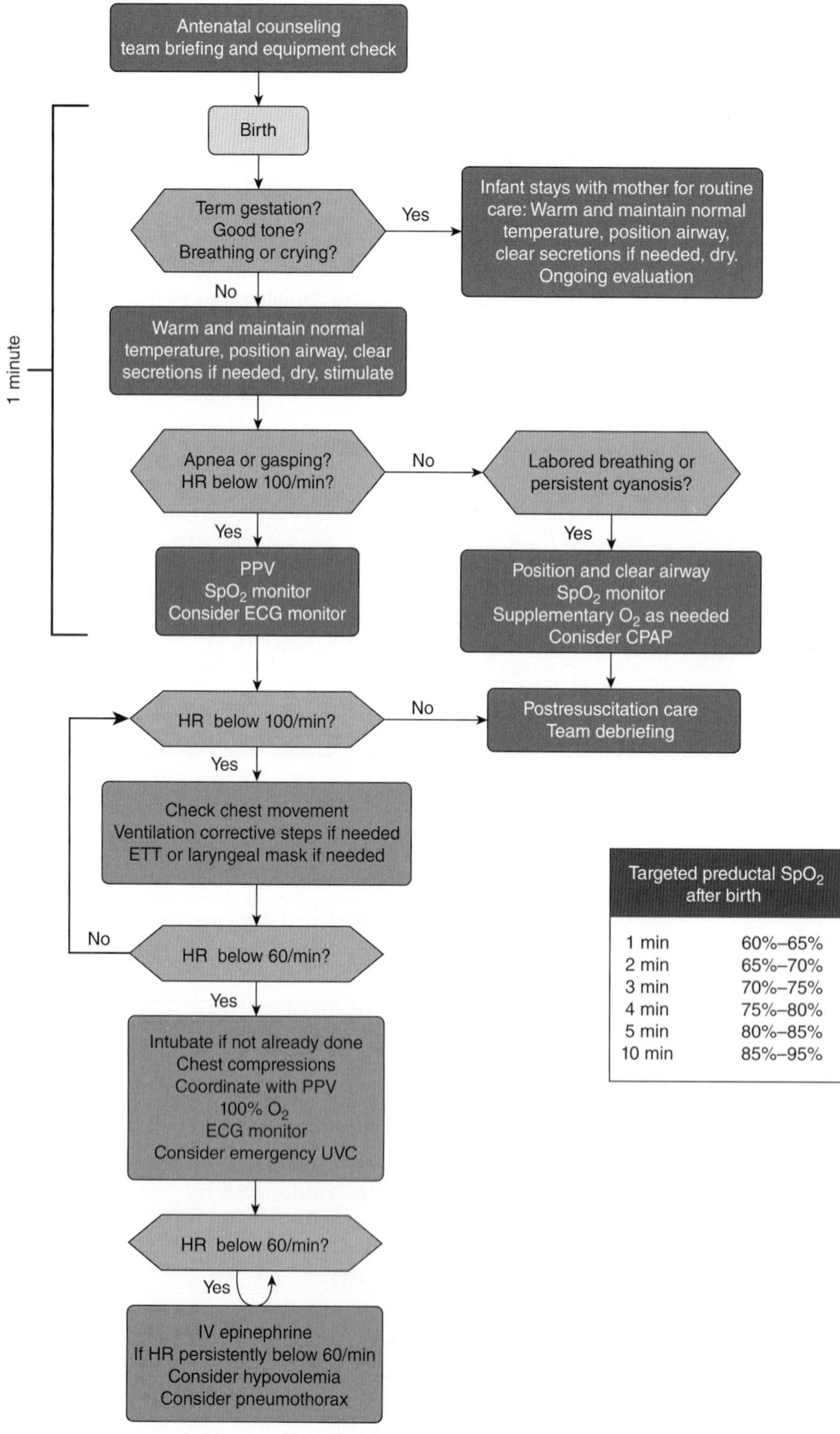

Targeted preductal SpO_2 after birth	
1 min	60%–65%
2 min	65%–70%
3 min	70%–75%
4 min	75%–80%
5 min	80%–85%
10 min	85%–95%

Based on a figure from Neonatal resuscitation: 2020 American Heart Association Guidelines update for cardiopulmonary resuscitation and emergency cardiovascular care. Circulation. 2020;142:S524–S550.

105. The dose of epinephrine for neonatal resuscitation is 0.01–0.03 mg/kg administered intravenously through an umbilical artery catheter inserted just below the abdominal skin (preferred) or other IV access point. The dose may be repeated every 3 to 5 minutes, if necessary. (606)
106. If meconium is present, an individual skilled in tracheal intubation should be present at the time of birth. No significant interventions are needed if the infant is vigorous with good respiratory effort and muscle tone after delivery. However, if poor muscle tone and inadequate breathing efforts are present, resuscitation should commence with positive-pressure ventilation (PPV) if the infant is not breathing and the heart rate is <100 beats/min. Routine intubation for tracheal suction in this setting is no longer suggested. Instead, emphasis is made on initiating ventilation within the first minute of life in a nonbreathing or ineffectively breathing infant by clearing the airway and use of PPV. (608)

Chapter

34 PEDIATRICS

Erin A. Gottlieb

INTRODUCTION

- Age-related differences in physiology, pharmacokinetics and pharmacodynamics, and types of procedures create challenges in caring for pediatric patients.
- Special considerations
  - Neonates: fetal circulation, neonatal procedures, and emergencies
  - Congenital heart disease (CHD): recognition of high-risk lesions, understanding diagnoses and management

DEVELOPMENTAL PHYSIOLOGY

Respiratory System

Lung Development

- 24 weeks of gestation: type II pneumocytes produce surfactant
- 26 weeks of gestation: extrauterine survival becomes possible
- 36 weeks of gestation: alveoli start to form

Chest Wall and Respiratory Muscles

- In infants, ineffective accessory muscles and cartilaginous ribs commonly result in paradoxical chest movement during spontaneous ventilation.
- Low percentage of type I muscle fibers in the diaphragm results in earlier respiratory failure in neonates.
  - The term infant diaphragm muscle has 25% type I fibers compared to 50% in adult diaphragm

Respiratory Variables

- Total lung capacity (TLC): much smaller per kilogram in neonates because adults have stronger, more efficient muscles
- Functional residual capacity (FRC): is similar across ages on a per-kilogram basis
  - Expiratory time is prolonged in infants through *laryngeal braking* (reduced expiratory flow from laryngeal activity).
- Lung volumes: in infants, apneic lung volume is lower than FRC causing more rapid desaturation with apnea
- Closing capacity (lung volume at which small airway closure begins): larger than FRC in infants, causing airways to collapse and trap air on exhalation

Factors Affecting Respiration

- PaO_2, $PaCO_2$, and pH control respiration (similar to adults).
- High FiO_2 depresses respiratory drive in neonates; low FiO_2 stimulates it.
- Hypoglycemia, anemia, and hypothermia depress respiratory drive.
- Metabolic demand increases minute ventilation by increasing the respiratory rate.

Respiratory Demand Is Higher in Neonates than in Adults

- The total oxygen consumption of the neonate is 6 to 8 mL/kg vs. 3 to 4 mL/kg for adults.
- This increased metabolic rate is associated with increased CO_2 production.
- Respiratory airway resistance is higher in neonates.
- Lung compliance is lower, and chest wall is floppy.
- Accessory muscles are ineffective in neonates due to the horizontal angle of the ribs.
- Work of breathing is increased in neonates.
- Increasing respiratory rate is primary method of increasing minute ventilation.
- The diaphragm is more susceptible to fatigue due to fewer type I muscle fibers.

Breathing Patterns

- Newborns exhibit periodic breathing characterized by pauses of <10 seconds.
- Apnea is defined as ventilatory pauses associated with desaturation and bradycardia.
- Postanesthetic apnea in former preterm infants is a potential risk that must be considered in surgical planning.

Cardiovascular System

Fetal Circulation

- High pulmonary vascular resistance (PVR) due to unventilated lungs
- Low systemic vascular resistance (SVR) due to the placental unit
- Right-to-left blood flow through the foramen ovale and ductus arteriosus

Changes in the Circulatory System at Birth

- PVR decreases due to breathing (expansion of lungs and increased oxygen partial pressure).
- SVR increases due to removal of the placenta (a low-resistance unit).
- Closure of the foramen ovale, ductus arteriosus, and ductus venosus
  - Foramen ovale closes in response to increased left atrial pressures and is probe patent in 30% of adults.
  - Ductus arteriosus constricts in response to increased oxygenation and decreased prostaglandins.
  - Ductus venosus closes with umbilical vein clamping or can become access pathway for umbilical venous catheter placement in inferior vena cava.
- Closure of these structures leads to the separation of the pulmonary and systemic circulations.

- Persistent fetal circulation (right-to-left shunt) can occur secondary to hypoxemia, acidosis, or pulmonary hypertension in the first few days of life.
  - Treatment: decrease PVR

Neonatal Myocardium

- Immature myocytes are dependent on ionized calcium concentration.
- Cardiac output increases predominately due to increases in heart rate; stroke volume is relatively fixed.

Autonomic Innervation of the Heart

- Parasympathetic nervous system predominates early in life.
- Bradycardia or asystole can occur with laryngoscopy, tracheal suctioning, or orogastric tube placement.
- Pretreatment with an anticholinergic medication can attenuate the bradycardic response to these procedures.

Newborn Cardiovascular Assessment

- Similar to adults including checking blood pressure (in all extremities) and auscultation for presence of murmurs

Renal System

- Glomerular filtration rate (GFR) is 15% to 30% of adult values at birth.
- GFR reaches adult values at 1 year.
- Creatinine level at birth reflects maternal level.

Hematologic System

- Blood volume is 82 to 93 mL/kg in the term neonate and 90 to 105 mL/kg in the preterm neonate.
- Hemoglobin F (HgF) makes up 70% to 80% of hemoglobin at birth.
- HgF has a higher affinity for oxygen than adult hemoglobin.
- Physiologic nadir in hemoglobin occurs at 9 to 12 weeks of life (10–11 g/dL).
- Vitamin K–dependent factors are 20% to 60% of adult levels.
  - All newborns receive vitamin K at birth.

PHARMACOLOGIC DIFFERENCES

Pharmacokinetics

- Decreased protein binding in neonates compared with adults results in a higher concentration of free drug and an increase in drug effect.
- Increased total body water in preterm/term neonates results in a larger volume of distribution.
  - Larger initial dose required to reach therapeutic drug levels
- Decreased percentage of fat and muscle in small infants leads to prolonged effect of drugs that rely on redistribution to fat and muscle for termination of effect.

Hepatic Metabolism

- Neonatal hepatic metabolism is approximately 50% of adult levels.
- Hepatic metabolism is fully mature at 1 to 2 years of age.
- Reduced activity of hepatic enzymes and reduced hepatic blood flow in the neonate result in a longer duration of action of drugs that rely on hepatic metabolism.

Renal Excretion

- Renal function is nearly mature at 20 weeks of life and is fully mature at 2 years.
- Immature renal function results in prolonged elimination half-times.

Pharmacology of Inhaled Agents

- F_A/F_i increases more rapidly in neonates than in adults, resulting in faster inhaled induction.

- Increased cardiac output in neonates and small children slows the rate of an inhaled anesthetic induction.

Effect of Shunt on Inhaled Induction of Anesthesia

- Right-to-left shunts slow inhaled induction.
  - Blood bypasses the lungs, where inhaled anesthetic uptake occurs.
- Left-to-right shunts have no real effect on the rate of induction.

Minimum Alveolar Concentration

- The minimum alveolar concentration (MAC) of inhaled anesthesia is highest at 1 to 6 months of age.
- MAC is reduced by prematurity, cerebral palsy, and development delay.

FLUID AND ELECTROLYTES

Intraoperative Fluid Administration

- Non–glucose-containing isotonic solutions (Plasmalyte-A, lactated Ringer's) are generally used in the operating room.
- Most commonly used colloid is 5% albumin.

Replacement of Preoperative Fluid Deficits

- Calculated by hourly maintenance fluid requirement multiplied by the number of hours of nil per os (NPO)
- Deficit may be higher for patients with vomiting, bleeding, and third-space losses.
- Deficit replacement is generally 50% in the first hour of anesthesia, with the remaining 50% replaced in the following 2 hours.
- Use warmed fluids to avoid hypothermia.

Maintenance Fluids

- Maintenance fluids administered using the 4-2-1 rule, usually isotonic fluids

The 4-2-1 Rule for Calculating Maintenance Fluids

Hourly fluid requirements are estimated to be the sum of
- 4 mL/kg for children up to 10 kg
- 2 mL/kg for each kilogram from 11 kg to 20 kg
- 1 mL/kg for each kilogram above 20 kg

For example, a child weighing 24 kg would require 40 mL + 20 mL + 4 mL = 64 mL per hour maintenance fluids as a baseline.

Ongoing Fluid Losses

- Blood loss replaced 3:1 with crystalloid or 1:1 with blood or colloid
- Third-space or evaporative losses vary widely with type of procedure.

Calculating Replacement of Ongoing Losses

How invasive is the surgery?

Noninvasive (e.g., inguinal hernia repair):	0–2 mL/kg/hr
Mildly invasive (e.g., ureteral reimplantation):	2–4 mL/kg/hr
Moderately invasive (e.g., elective bowel reanastomosis):	2–8 mL/kg/hr
Significantly invasive (e.g., bowel resection for necrosis):	>10 mL/kg/hr

Treatment of Hypovolemia

- 10 to 20 mL/kg bolus of fluid can be given if hemodynamic variables suggest hypovolemia.

Glucose Administration

- Usually not required in patients >1 year of age or >10 kg
- Neonates are at risk for hypoglycemia.
- Neonates and patients on total parenteral nutrition or continuous tube feeds should be monitored closely for hypoglycemia.

TRANSFUSION THERAPY

Maximum Allowable Blood Loss

- The maximum allowable blood loss (MABL) should be calculated preoperatively to plan for intraoperative transfusion.
- Blood loss should be replaced with crystalloid or colloid until MABL is reached; after this, red blood cells should be used.
- Transfusion triggers should be determined based on patient comorbidities.

Transfusion of Blood Products

Packed Red Blood Cells

- Irradiation of blood products is indicated in young infants and patients with immunosuppression, transplant or potential transplant recipients, components from blood relatives, and all designated donors.

Leukocyte Reduction and Irradiation of Blood Products

- Leukocytes can cause febrile, nonhemolytic transfusion reactions, human leukocyte antigen (HLA sensitization), and transmission of cytomegalovirus.
- Irradiation reduces the risk of graft versus host disease; irradiated directed-donor blood from family members should be given to children who share an HLA haplotype, including children with normal immunity.

Platelets

- Indications for platelet transfusion include platelet number, platelet function, and presence of bleeding.
- May require irradiation per same criteria as packed red cells

Fresh Frozen Plasma

- Prothrombin concentrates contain vitamin K–dependent factors; can be used for emergent reversal of anticoagulation or coagulopathy after cardiopulmonary bypass surgery

Cryoprecipitate and Fibrinogen Concentrate

- Cryoprecipitate: contains concentrated fibrinogen and factors VIII, XIII, and von Willebrand factor
- Fibrinogen concentrate: used for fibrinogen replacement in complex surgeries such as cardiac surgery, cranial remodeling, and scoliosis repair

Pediatric Transfusion Dosing Guidelines

Packed Red Blood Cells
- 10 to 15 mL/kg increases the hemoglobin by 2 to 3 g/dL.

Platelets
- 5 to 10 mL/kg increases the platelet count by 50,000 to 100,000.

Fresh Frozen Plasma
- 10 to 15 mL/kg increases coagulation factors by 15% to 20%.

Cryoprecipitate
- 1 unit/5 kg to a maximum of 4 units usually corrects coagulopathy.

Antifibrinolytics

- Used in cases associated with large blood losses or severe coagulopathy

Recombinant Factor VIIa

- Indicated for factor VII deficiency and for certain hemophilias; off-label use for trauma and postcardiopulmonary bypass bleeding have been reported
- Thromboembolic complications are a concern.

PEDIATRIC AIRWAY

Airway Assessment

- Examine for micrognathia, midface abnormalities, small oral aperture, limited cervical spine mobility
- Question about loose teeth or orthodontic appliances

Airway Management Techniques

- Important airway differences in infants and neonates include larger occiput, large tongue, and soft, omega-shaped epiglottis.
- Anesthesia via face mask is commonly used for short procedures such as myringotomy tube placement.
- Supraglottic airways are also commonly used and have been reported to be associated with fewer respiratory complications than tracheal intubation.
- Endotracheal intubation is common; considerations include the use of uncuffed, cuffed, or Microcuff tubes.

Difficult Pediatric Airway

- Difficult laryngoscopy is associated with craniofacial syndromes (e.g., Pierre-Robin, Klippel-Feil, Goldenhar).
- Management techniques include the use of a videolaryngoscope, optical stylet, fiberoptic bronchoscope, supraglottic airway, or as an *ex utero* intrapartum therapy (EXIT) procedure (using the placenta as a source of oxygenation).

ANESTHETIC CONSIDERATIONS

Preoperative Evaluation and Preparation

- Age and weight are critically important as equipment and dosing are dependent on the size of the patient.
- Past medical history: prematurity, the presence of a genetic or dysmorphic syndrome, and signs and symptoms of obstructive sleep apnea
- Family history: malignant hyperthermia, muscular dystrophies, or a family history of problems related to anesthesia

Preoperative Laboratory Testing

- Routine testing is usually not warranted in healthy patients.
- Urine pregnancy testing protocols for children and adolescents exist but remain controversial.

Recent Upper Respiratory Tract Infection

- Increased risk of airway hyperreactivity with recent or current upper respiratory tract infection (URI)
  - Laryngospasm, bronchospasm, and postoperative arterial desaturation
- Exclude a lower respiratory infection through signs, symptoms, and exam
- Perioperative decision making remains controversial for patients with URI.

- Elective major surgery should be postponed 2 to 6 weeks if possible.
- For minor surgery, risks associated with anesthetizing a patient with URI are usually manageable.

Preoperative Fasting Guidelines

- NPO guideline adherence minimizes the risk of the aspiration of gastric contents.

Pediatric NPO Guidelines

- Minimizing the fasting period improves patient and family satisfaction and lowers the likelihood of hypovolemia during the induction of anesthesia.
- Fasting prior to the induction of anesthesia:
  - Solids: 6 to 8 hours
  - Formula: 6 hours
  - Breast milk: 4 hours
  - Clear fluids: 2 hours
- These times may be modified in patients with gastroesophageal reflux, gastrointestinal obstruction, and conditions associated with delayed gastric emptying.

- A 1-hour fasting period for clear fluids has been adopted by multiple global pediatric anesthesia societies.
- Hypovolemia leads to perioperative hemodynamic instability in patients with high-risk congenital heart lesions (e.g., left ventricular outflow tract obstruction, systemic-to-pulmonary artery shunt).
- Fasting can lead to hypoglycemia in patients receiving continuous tube feeds.

Premedication

- Midazolam is most commonly used.
  - Administration can be oral, intranasal, rectal, or intramuscular (IM).
  - Oral (0.5–0.75 mg/kg, max 20 mg) or intranasal (0.2–0.3 mg/kg, max 10 mg) administration will have effect in about 20 minutes.
- Ketamine can be a useful adjunct.
  - Delivered orally (often in combination with midazolam) or IM
  - IM ketamine is especially useful for agitated or uncooperative patients.
  - Associated with excessive salivation, nystagmus, and nausea and vomiting, but airway tone and spontaneous respiration are maintained.
- α_2-Agonists can be used for premedication, with effects comparable to midazolam.
  - Clonidine, given orally, reduces requirements for anesthesia and postoperative pain medications, but has an onset time of about 1 hour.
  - Dexmedetomidine, given intranasally, has an onset of action that is slightly longer than midazolam and reduces postoperative agitation, delirium, shivering, and pain medication requirements.
- Parental presence at induction can be comforting for the patient, but parental anxiety and physiologic response (e.g., syncope) can be problematic.

Perioperative Considerations

Thermoregulation and Heat Loss

- Hypothermia is a concern in small infants as they have a larger surface area–to-weight ratio; they lose heat rapidly by both radiation and convection.
- Small infants use nonshivering thermogenesis and metabolize brown fat to produce heat.
- Creating a warm environment, warmed fluids, forced air warming, radiant warmers, and airway humidification are all helpful for maintaining temperature.

Monitoring

- Standard American Society of Anesthesiologists monitors are used in children, including temperature.
- Invasive arterial and central venous pressure monitoring are used in complex, invasive surgeries, and in patients with significant comorbidities.
- Cerebral oxygenation monitoring can be used in cardiac surgery.

Routes of Induction of Anesthesia

- Inhalation induction is usually carried out with sevoflurane in oxygen with or without nitrous oxide.
  - After the patient has passed through stage 2 (excitement phase), intravenous (IV) access is established in most cases.
    - Involuntary movement, coughing, vomiting, and laryngospasm are all possible during the excitement phase.
    - Laryngospasm that occurs before IV access can be treated with continuous positive airway pressure or IM succinylcholine.
- IV induction (usually propofol) is used in patients with an IV line, who desire IV induction, who are at risk for aspiration, or who are at cardiopulmonary risk.
- IM induction is commonly used in uncooperative children who will not accept a face mask and in children with severe burns, poor veins, and/or a difficult airway.
  - IM ketamine induction with an antisialogogue helps to maintain airway tone and spontaneous respiration while IV access is established.

Maintenance of Anesthesia

- Inhaled anesthetics and/or IV drugs
- Neuromuscular blockade to facilitate operative exposure is used less frequently in children compared with adults.

Emergence

- Deep extubation is performed while the patient is deeply anesthetized before regaining airway reflexes, often with less coughing and bucking.
  - The patient passes through stage 2 without an airway in place, risking laryngospasm or potential aspiration in the operating room, in the hallway, or in the postanesthesia recovery unit.
- Awake extubation decreases the risk of laryngospasm or aspiration but can be associated with coughing or bucking.

Pain Management

- Opioids
  - Fentanyl and morphine are the most commonly used opioids in pediatric patients.
  - Side effects include itching, nausea, and respiratory depression.
- Acetaminophen
  - Can be given orally, rectally, or intravenously
  - Communication is important to avoid accidental duplicate dosing and hepatotoxicity.
- Nonsteroidal antiinflammatory drugs (NSAIDs) and ketorolac
  - Used for pain control without excessive sedation or respiratory depression
  - Concerns about postoperative bleeding due to platelet dysfunction and renal impairment can limit their use.

Regional Anesthesia

- Caudal analgesia can be administered as a single-shot or as an infusion via a catheter.
  - Most commonly used for surgery below the umbilicus
- Lumbar or thoracic epidural catheter placement is also possible.
- Other regional and field blocks are regularly performed.
- Spinal anesthetics can be used as the sole anesthetic or in combination with sedation or a general anesthetic.
  - Useful as sole anesthetic to avoid postoperative apnea in former preterm infants undergoing inguinal hernia repair

The Postanesthesia Care Unit

Airway Monitoring

- Emergence after deep extubation without an endotracheal tube in place has risks.
- Laryngospasm and airway obstruction must be quickly identified and treated.
  - Laryngospasm management
    - Jackson-Rees bag and mask, oxygen source for CPAP and positive pressure ventilation
    - Succinylcholine should be readily available.
  - Postintubation croup or stridor can occur from airway swelling.
    - Management includes humidified oxygen, dexamethasone, or nebulized racemic epinephrine.
- Hypoventilation or apnea may also require support.

Postoperative Nausea and Vomiting

- Risk factors: age $\geq$3 years, strabismus surgery, longer duration of surgery, and previous history of postoperative nausea and vomiting (PONV) in a parent or sibling
- Risk reduction: liberal fluid administration, total IV anesthesia, opioid-sparing regional anesthesia, use of IV acetaminophen or α_2-agonist.
  - Prophylaxis with ondansetron and dexamethasone has a relative risk reduction of 80%.
  - Aprepitant may be substituted if there is a contraindication to ondansetron or dexamethasone.

Emergence Agitation and Delirium

- Can be disturbing to families, PACU caregivers, and anesthesia providers
- The Pediatric Anesthesia Emergence Delirium Scale (PAED) can help to differentiate emergence agitation (EA) and emergence delirium (ED) from pain.
- Decreased incidence with propofol, fentanyl, clonidine, and dexmedetomidine, but they may prolong emergence
  - Ketamine and nalbuphine decrease the incidence without prolonging emergence.

Pediatric Anesthesia Emergence Delirium Scale

Behavior	None	Some	Modest	Much	Extreme
Makes eye contact with caregiver	4	3	2	1	0
Actions are purposeful	4	3	2	1	0
Aware of surroundings	4	3	2	1	0
Restless	0	1	2	3	4
Inconsolable	0	1	2	3	4

A PAED score of $\geq$10 is the minimum score that is required to diagnose ED; a score $<$10 rules out a diagnosis of ED.

Pain Control

- Difficult to assess due to the age, developmental stage of the patient, and the ability to communicate
- Use vital signs and scales for pain assessment in children, which include the FLACC (face, legs, anxiety, cry, and consolability) and Wong-Baker Faces Pain Scales.
- Pain can be difficult to differentiate from EA/ED, anxiety, and anger in pediatric patients.

Discharge Criteria

- Phase I recovery: after transfer from operating room where vital signs and airway are carefully monitored
  - Patients are treated for pain and PONV.
- Phase II recovery: after patients are awake, comfortable, and stable from an airway standpoint until discharge
- The modified Aldrete Score is commonly used to determine discharge readiness.

Behavioral Recovery

- Negative behavioral changes can occur after surgery, including sleep and feeding disturbance, separation anxiety, new-onset enuresis, and others.
- Influenced by parental anxiety, presence at induction or in PACU, and premedication
- Behaviors seldom last beyond 3 days; however, avoidance of these behaviors is associated with a better perioperative experience and higher patient/family satisfaction.

MEDICAL AND SURGICAL DISEASES AFFECTING THE NEONATE

Necrotizing Enterocolitis

- The most common neonatal surgical emergency, usually seen in premature infants
- Pathophysiology involves intestinal mucosal ischemia, infection, and inflammation from reduced perfusion.

Clinical Manifestations

- Comorbidities associated with prematurity including respiratory distress syndrome, patent ductus arteriosus (PDA), and cardiorespiratory instability.
- Clinical signs: abdominal distention and bloody stools, temperature instability, sepsis with dilated loops of bowel, pneumatosis intestinalis, and possible perforation on radiograph
- Intestinal perforation is a surgical emergency, and the patient may have sepsis with hypotension, thrombocytopenia, and disseminated intravascular coagulation.

Medical and Surgical Treatment

- Medical treatment without perforation includes antibiotics, gastric decompression, serial abdominal and radiographic examinations, and careful monitoring for cardiorespiratory instability.
- Surgery may involve less invasive peritoneal drainage or more extensive open laparotomy with resection of the perforated segment of bowel and the creation of ostomies; reconstructive surgery may be required later.

Management of Anesthesia

- Surgery for necrotizing enterocolitis (NEC) is often emergent.
- Preoperative assessment should focus on hemodynamic instability, fluid and electrolyte abnormalities, coagulation derangements, and antibiotic requirements.
- Surgery is in the operating room or at the bedside in the NICU.
- Invasive arterial blood pressure monitoring and central venous access are helpful.
- Anesthesia maintenance with fentanyl in divided doses with muscle relaxant
  - Vasodilatory properties of volatile anesthetics are often not tolerated.
- Volume loss and resuscitation are often very large.
  - Volume replacement with 5% albumin, packed red blood cells, fresh frozen plasma, and platelets
  - Vasoactive support with dopamine, epinephrine, calcium chloride, and vasopressin may be required.
- Temperature monitoring and management is critical; these small neonates have significant exposure and temperature loss through the exposed bowel.
  - Warmed environment, forced air warming, and administration of warmed fluids and blood products to maintain core temperature

Abdominal Wall Defects: Gastroschisis and Omphalocele

- Gastroschisis is an abdominal wall defect where the intestines are exposed usually to the right of the umbilical cord without a sac or umbilicus involvement.
  - Usually not associated with other congenital defects or chromosomal abnormalities
- Omphalocele is a midline defect with the intestines covered by a peritoneal sac and the umbilicus incorporated into the defect.
  - Commonly associated with other congenital defects including congenital heart disease

Medical and Surgical Treatment

- Prenatal diagnosis is common; after birth, the defect is temporarily covered with plastic, intravascular volume is monitored carefully, and the bowel is assessed for ischemia and volvulus.

- Abdominal closure is achieved through a staged approach to gradually reduce the defect; surgical closures of the peritoneum and skin take place at the end.
  - Immediate surgical correction can lead to a sudden increase in intraabdominal pressure, difficulty ventilating, and abdominal compartment syndrome, leading to gut ischemia and renal compromise.

Management of Anesthesia

- For one-stage reduction and closure, it may be difficult to ventilate, and abdominal compartment syndrome may result.
  - Muscle relaxant is required, invasive arterial and central venous pressure monitoring are suggested, ventilator parameters should be monitored closely, and vasoactive infusions should be available.
- In a staged approach, the initial surgical procedure is to suture the Silastic silo and partially reduce the viscera.
  - Subsequent reductions can be done at bedside under sedation.
- Volume replacement and temperature management are critical with the viscera exposed.

Tracheoesophageal Fistula

- Classified into five anatomic types, with the most common (type C) having esophageal atresia and a distal tracheoesophageal fistula (TEF)), as illustrated in the figures below.

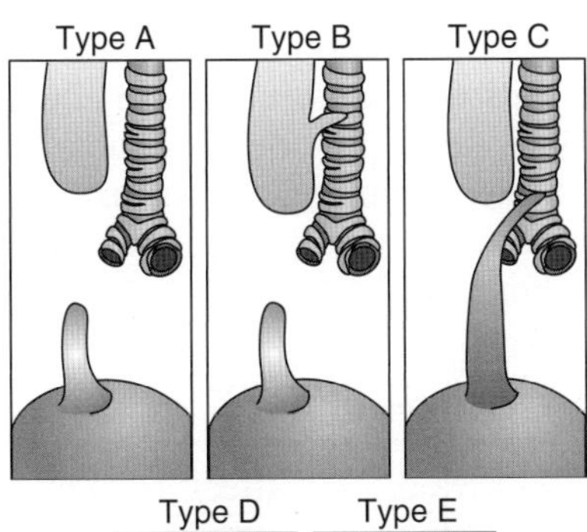

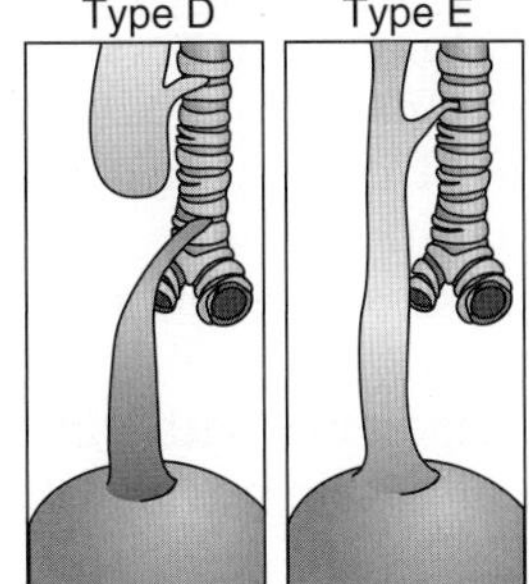

Figure from Gross RE: Atresia of the esophagus. In The Surgery of Infancy and Childhood. Philadelphia: Saunders, 1953, pp. 75–102.

- Diagnosis: neonate has choking and cyanosis when attempting oral feeds
  - Radiographs reveal an inability to pass an orogastric tube (curls in the blind esophageal pouch) and gas-filled intestines from the distal TEF.
- Associated with VACTERL: Vertebral defects, imperforate Anus, Cardiac defects, TracheoEsophageal fistula, Renal and Limb anomalies
- Patients may be very ill due to continued aspiration of gastric contents through the fistula and abdominal distention from gas filling the stomach and intestines.
- Perioperative morbidity and mortality risk factors include complex congenital heart disease, weight <2 kg, poor pulmonary compliance, large pericarinal fistulas, and those scheduled for thoracoscopic repair.

Surgical Approaches

- A one-stage approach with ligation of the fistula and primary surgical repair of the esophagus is done in 80% to 90% of patients.
- Staged approach for critically ill patients
  - Gastrostomy placed under local anesthesia for pulmonary function improvement
  - Right thoracotomy with ligation of the fistula and possible repair of the esophageal atresia done later
- Another approach includes a cervical esophagostomy to drain the upper esophageal pouch and prevent aspiration.
- Outcomes vary; the full-term neonate without other problems has an operative survival rate approaching 100%.

Anesthetic Management

- Emergent TEF repair can be required for the sick neonate with high ventilatory pressures and gastric distention.
  - Tidal volume can be mostly lost through the fistula.
  - Manual ventilation, vasoactive support, and boluses of emergency drugs may be needed until the fistula is ligated and the stomach is decompressed.
  - Intraarterial blood pressure monitoring is essential.
- Vigilance is critical to ensure the endotracheal tube does not migrate into the TEF.
  - A large TEF located near the carina can predict difficulties with ventilation.
- These patients are rarely extubated at the end of the procedure.

Congenital Diaphragmatic Hernia

- Herniation of the intestines, and sometimes stomach, liver, or spleen into the thorax through the diaphragmatic defect, and resulting pulmonary hypoplasia
  - Defect is most commonly on the left through the foramen of Bochdalek and is often evident early in gestation.
- Patient presents after birth with a scaphoid abdomen, bowel sounds in the chest, respiratory distress, and cyanosis.
- Pulmonary hypertension from lung hypoplasia and the postnatal elevation in PVR
  - Right-to-left shunting through the patent foramen ovale and ductus arteriosus
  - Can cause profound cyanosis and hemodynamic instability from persistent fetal circulation
    - High-frequency oscillatory ventilation (HFOV), inhaled nitric oxide, or ECMO may be necessary to stabilize the patient prior to repair.
- Repair of the diaphragmatic defect removes the viscera from the thorax but does not fix the pulmonary hypoplasia or pulmonary hypertension, which may be chronic problems.

Management of Anesthesia

- These patients may be critically ill; transport may be difficult, and the patient may need to be transitioned from HFOV to conventional ventilation.
  - Inhaled nitric oxide should be continued to reduce pulmonary artery pressures.
- High-dose opioids, benzodiazepines, and ketamine are best tolerated anesthetics.
- Invasive arterial and central venous pressure monitors are essential.
  - Inotropes and vasopressors should be available.
  - Frequent arterial blood gas analysis to optimize oxygenation, ventilation, and pulmonary artery pressures.
- Repair while on ECMO has the benefits of cardiorespiratory support.
  - Significant blood loss due to anticoagulation is possible.
  - Blood products should be readily available.

Patent Ductus Arteriosus

- Causes pulmonary overcirculation through a left-to-right shunt
  - Pulmonary edema, respiratory distress, and ventilator dependence can occur.
  - Can cause difficulty weaning from ventilator, congestive heart failure, and NEC
- Bounding pulses and widened pulse pressures caused by the low diastolic pressure
  - There is diastolic runoff from the aorta to the pulmonary artery through the PDA.
- PDA is most common in premature infants with diagnosis by echocardiography.
- Medical closure attempted using indomethacin, ibuprofen, or acetaminophen
  - May affect renal and platelet function
  - This effect should be considered in surgical patients after failed medical treatment

Management of Anesthesia

- Neonates are often premature, weighing 500 to 1000 g, hemodynamically unstable, and ventilator dependent.
- Ductal ligation via left thoracotomy is often performed in the NICU.
- Arterial blood pressure monitoring is useful, and lower extremity pulse oximetry and noninvasive blood pressures
- Anesthesia is typically opioid, muscle relaxants, and avoidance of high Fio_2 to prevent worsening of retinopathy of prematurity (ROP).
  - Small doses of ketamine and benzodiazepines can also be used.
  - Volatile anesthetics are generally not well tolerated.
- Duct ligation results in an increase in blood pressure, especially diastolic blood pressure.
  - Loss of lower extremity blood pressure or pulse oximeter reading may suggest that the surgeon has ligated the descending aorta instead of the PDA.
- Transcatheter closure of the PDA in the cardiac catheterization laboratory has become a useful approach with few complications.
- Some patients with congenital heart disease depend on a PDA to either provide systemic or pulmonary blood flow (depending on the lesion).
  - In these cases, ductal patency is maintained with prostaglandin E_1.

Retinopathy of Prematurity

- Vasoproliferative disease affecting premature or low-birth-weight infants, especially those ventilated with cardiopulmonary instability
- One cause of ROP is high oxygen tension in the vessels of the retina.
  - The Spo_2 in premature infants is targeted from 88% to 93%.
- ROP has five stages; in stages 4 and 5, retinal detachment occurs with possible permanent blindness.
- Premature infants are examined for ROP, and if high-risk ROP is diagnosed, urgent surgical therapy is undertaken to maximize visual outcomes.

- The treatment of choice is retinal ablative therapy with indirect laser photocoagulation of the proliferating vessels.

Management of Anesthesia

- Patients for urgent ROP surgery may not be NPO.
- These cases may be of long duration.
  - Maintenance of the patient's temperature and blood glucose during surgery
  - Patients are usually ventilated postoperatively due to the need for narcotic pain control and the risk for postoperative apnea.

Myelomeningocele

- Defect of the neural tube resulting in an open neural placode covered by a thin membrane and cerebrospinal fluid
- Myelomeningocele (MMC), often diagnosed prenatally, varies in size and location.
  - Most common presentation is a full-term neonate with a lumbosacral MMC.
- It is critical to avoid sac rupture.
  - Infants are nursed prone with moist gauze covering the defect.
- Surgery is emergent and consists of dissection of nerve roots and coverage of the defect with fascia and skin.
- Over 75% of these infants have hydrocephalus, and many have Arnold-Chiari malformation.
  - These patients will require a ventriculoperitoneal shunt after recovery from the MMC repair.

Management of Anesthesia

- Extreme care to protect the sac from rupturing during transport and positioning
  - Anesthetic induction and intubation are performed with the patient in the left lateral decubitus position or supine.
  - Defect on a doughnut that prevents the sac from resting on the operating room bed.
- Muscle relaxant is generally avoided so that motor function can be assessed.
- Latex-free environment as patients are at high risk for developing latex allergy.
- Extubation in the same positioning as intubation to avoid pressure on the defect
- MMC can now be repaired during fetal life.

Pyloric Stenosis

- Pyloric muscle hypertrophy resulting in gastric outlet obstruction
- The typical presentation occurs 2 to 8 weeks of age with persistent projectile vomiting.
  - 5:1 male predominance
  - Hypochloremic, hypokalemic metabolic alkalosis, weight loss, and hypovolemia
  - Patients may develop severe dehydration, lethargy, skin turgor, sunken eyes and fontanel, and poor urine output.
  - An olive-shaped mass is palpable in the epigastrum, and the definitive diagnosis is made by ultrasound.
- Repair is not a surgical emergency.
  - Preoperative rehydration and electrolyte corrections can take 12 to 72 hours.

Management of Anesthesia

- In the operating room, the stomach is evacuated with a large-bore orogastric tube before inducing anesthesia.
- Anesthesia induction can be with propofol, cricoid pressure, and a nondepolarizing muscle relaxant (preferred) or succinylcholine.
  - Awake tracheal intubation, favored in the past, has largely been abandoned.
  - Modified rapid sequence technique with gentle mask ventilation to prevent hypoxemia or an inhalation induction
- After intubation, anesthesia is usually maintained with volatile anesthetic.
  - Opioids are largely avoided because of the risk of postoperative apnea.
- Surgery is performed through either an epigastric incision or laparoscopically.
- A nasogastric tube is often left in place, and the patient is extubated awake.
- Resumption of spontaneous ventilation can be difficult.
  - CSF pH changes from the metabolic alkalosis and subsequent reduced ventilatory drive
  - Patients are at risk for postoperative apnea and should be monitored for 12 to 24 hours after surgery.

CONGENITAL HEART DISEASE

- Present in 1 in 100 live births
  - In the first year of life, CHD is the most common indication for surgery or invasive catheter treatment.
- Preoperative planning may include an echocardiogram, CT, MRI, and cardiac catheterization.
- Knowledge of the lesion, previous repair or palliation, and presence of residual defects is important prior to anesthetic care.

Left-to-Right Shunts

- Left-to-right shunts arise from communications between the atria, the ventricles, or the great arteries.

- Atrial septal defects, ventricular septal defects (VSDs), and PDA are the most common CHD lesions.
- Severity of disease is related to the degree of left-to-right shunting.
  - The size and position of the defect
  - The pressure gradient between chambers
  - The relative pulmonary and systemic vascular resistances
- Large shunts lead to pulmonary overcirculation and a heart that is volume loaded.
  - Patients develop pulmonary edema, tachypnea, poor feeding, and intercostal retractions.
- Longstanding pulmonary overcirculation leads to changes in the pulmonary vasculature.
  - Pulmonary hypertension and reversal of the shunt (Eisenmenger syndrome) can result.
  - Early repair of the left-to-right shunt lesion has largely eliminated Eisenmenger syndrome in developed countries.

Right-to-Left Shunts

- Right-to-left shunt lesions result from right ventricular outflow tract obstruction and shunting across a VSD from the right to the left ventricle, leading to arterial desaturation.
  - The degree of cyanosis is related to the degree of right ventricular outflow tract obstruction, the size of the VSD, and the SVR.
- Tetralogy of Fallot (TOF) is the most common right-to-left shunt lesion, making up 6% of CHD patients.
  - TOF: RV outflow tract obstruction, RV hypertrophy, a large VSD, and an overriding aorta

Obstructive Lesions

- Obstructive lesions can be seen at multiple locations in the heart and great vessels.
  - Most common are pulmonary stenosis (13% of CHD), coarctation of the aorta (7% of CHD), and valvar aortic stenosis (5% of CHD).
- Left-sided obstruction is less well tolerated than right-sided obstruction.
  - Left ventricular hypertrophy, ischemia, ventricular arrhythmias, and death can result.
  - All adverse sequelae may be exacerbated by anesthetic care.

Transposition of the Great Arteries

- Dextro-transposition of the great arteries (d-TGA) occurs when the aorta arises from the right ventricle and the pulmonary artery arises from the left ventricle.
- d-TGA is about 4% of CHD lesions and, without mixing, results in profound cyanosis.
  - Survival depends on mixing after birth at the ventricular, atrial, or PDA levels.
- Patients with d-TGA who have a VSD (15%–20%) have less cyanosis.
  - Patients without a VSD are started on prostaglandin E_1 to maintain ductal patency.
  - Many patients undergo a balloon atrial septostomy to allow mixing at the atrial level prior to surgery.
- The arterial switch operation is usually performed in the first few weeks of life and accounts for about 10% of all neonatal cardiac surgeries.

Single-Ventricle Lesions

- Single-ventricle lesions result from severe obstruction or atresia of structures on the left or right side of the heart.
  - These lesions make up about 4% of CHD.
- Prostaglandin E_1 is needed to maintain ductal patency.
  - Provides pulmonary blood flow in cases of right-sided lesions like pulmonary atresia or tricuspid atresia
  - Provides systemic blood flow in left-sided lesions like hypoplastic left heart syndrome
- Hypoplastic right heart lesions are often better tolerated than hypoplastic left heart due to the presence of a left ventricle as the systemic ventricle.
- Stage I palliation for hypoplastic left heart syndrome is also a common neonatal heart surgery, making up about 10% of neonatal cardiac operations.

Conclusion

- The anesthesia provider is increasingly likely to encounter patients with CHD during everyday practice due to improvements in survival.

SPECIAL ANESTHETIC CONSIDERATIONS

Anesthesia for the Former Premature Infant

- Often need anesthetic care for procedures including inguinal herniorrhaphy, circumcision, eye examination, and strabismus surgery
- Sequelae of prematurity may persist, including bronchopulmonary dysplasia, apnea and bradycardia, anemia, hydrocephalus, developmental delay, and visual impairment.
- The postconceptual age of the patient (the gestational age of the patient added to the age of the patient) affects the risk of the anesthetic, need for postoperative monitoring, and hospital admission.
  - Postanesthetic apnea is a major risk factor and can be fatal.
  - Infants <50 weeks postconceptual age who are anesthetized are admitted for apnea monitoring for 24 hours after the procedure.

Anesthesia for Remote Locations

- Anesthesia and sedation cases in nonoperating room locations are increasing.
- Locations include MRI and CT scanners, interventional radiology, cardiac catheterization laboratories, and endoscopy suites.
- Standards for preoperative evaluation, monitoring, and postprocedural recovery must be maintained to ensure safety.

Ex Utero Intrapartum Therapy Procedure and Fetal Surgery

- The EXIT procedure allows the airway of the neonate to be secured by laryngoscopy, rigid bronchoscopy, or tracheostomy while the placental unit is still oxygenating the baby.
  - The EXIT procedure can be used for patients with neck masses and airway obstruction.
  - For other patients with thoracic or cardiac diagnoses, placental bypass can be used while the patient is cannulated for ECMO.
- Open fetal surgery has been used to address myelomeningocele, congenital cystic adenomatoid malformation, and sacrococcygeal teratoma.
  - Usually performed under maternal general anesthesia with volatile anesthetic, anesthetizing both the mother and the fetus while also relaxing the uterus
- Minimally invasive fetal surgery has been used to address congenital diaphragmatic hernia, bladder outlet obstruction, hypoplastic left heart syndrome, and twin-twin transfusion syndrome.
  - Performed under general, regional, sedation, and local anesthesia
- Anesthetic medications, muscle relaxants, and resuscitative drugs can be delivered directly to the fetus.
  - Anesthetic requirements for the procedure should be discussed with proceduralists preoperatively.
- Obstetric principles to resuscitate the fetus should be considered and used.
  - These include left lateral uterine displacement, oxygen delivery, and the treatment of maternal hypotension with volume and vasopressors.

Anesthetic Neurotoxicity and Neuroprotection in the Developing Brain

- Neonatal rat studies using prolonged anesthesia with GABA agonists (e.g., isoflurane, midazolam, propofol) and NMDA antagonists produce apoptosis in the developing brain
  - Concerns exist about whether this occurs in human neonates and infants.
- Human studies include the GAS study, the PANDA study, and the MASK study, which have reported no effect on cognitive neurodevelopmental testing.
- Currently, there is insufficient evidence to change the approach to anesthesia in the infant.

QUESTIONS

DEVELOPMENTAL PHYSIOLOGY

1. What are some of the physiologic variables that account for respiration being less efficient in infants than adults?
2. What is the difference between periodic breathing and apnea in newborns?
3. Describe the changes in circulatory physiology that occur at birth. What are some causes of persistent fetal circulation?
4. Explain why atropine may be used for premedication on induction in neonates.

PHARMACOLOGIC DIFFERENCES

5. Complete the following table by indicating whether the pharmacokinetic property is increased or decreased in infants compared with adults.

Pharmacokinetic Property	Infants Compared With Adults
Plasma protein concentration	
Total body water percent	
Percent fat and muscle	
Hepatic metabolism	
Renal excretion	

6. How are the uptake and distribution of inhaled anesthetics different in neonates and infants compared with adults?

FLUIDS AND ELECTROLYTES

7. You are scheduled to anesthetize an otherwise healthy ex-premature infant for a colostomy takedown. The infant weighs 8.5 kg, has a hematocrit (Hct) of 35, and has been NPO for 3 hours. Describe the following: fluid deficit replacement volume, type, and timing; maintenance fluid type and rate.

TRANSFUSION THERAPY

8. You are scheduled to anesthetize an otherwise healthy ex-premature infant for a colostomy takedown. The infant weighs 8.5 kg, has an Hct of 35, and has been NPO for 3 hours. The parent has donated blood for the procedure. Calculate the maximum allowable blood loss. Does the blood need to be irradiated?

PEDIATRIC AIRWAY

9. What are some of the characteristics of the pediatric airway that differ from the adult airway?
10. What has the classic teaching been to use uncuffed tubes in children under the age of 8 years and why has this changed?
11. What are some of the indications for cuffed endotracheal tubes in infants and small children?
12. What is the general approach to the difficult pediatric airway, and how does it differ from the adult difficult airway?

ANESTHETIC CONSIDERATIONS

13. How does an existing or recent upper respiratory infection affect anesthetic care?
14. What are some pharmacologic and nonpharmacologic methods of reducing preoperative anxiety in the pediatric patient?
15. Why are infants at an increased risk for perioperative hypothermia, and how can this risk be mitigated?
16. What is deep extubation? Describe some advantages and disadvantages.
17. What are some important aspects of pediatric care in the postanesthesia care unit (PACU)?

MEDICAL AND SURGICAL DISEASES AFFECTING THE NEONATE

18. Match the disease on the left with the letter of the appropriate description on the right.

Disease	Letter	Description
Necrotizing enterocolitis		a. Associated with VACTERL; patients may have abdominal distension and aspiration of gastric contents
Gastroschisis and omphalocele		b. Often in ventilator-dependent premature infants; treatment may be urgent and surgery prolonged
Tracheoesophageal fistula		c. Lower extremity blood pressure and/or pulse oximetry monitoring is indicated during surgical repair
Congenital diaphragmatic hernia		d. Most common neonatal surgical emergency; patients may have sepsis, bloody stools, and coagulopathy
Patent ductus arteriosus		e. Endotracheal intubation may need to be in lateral position in a latex-free environment
Retinopathy of prematurity		f. Repair may be staged; single surgery repair can lead to abdominal compartment syndrome and renal compromise
Myelomeningocele		g. Surgery should be delayed for hydration and correction of electrolytes
Pyloric stenosis		h. Scaphoid abdomen, bowel sounds in chest, respiratory distress, cyanosis

CONGENITAL HEART DISEASE

19. What are the three basic locations of left-to-right shunt lesions, and what is a determinant of the severity of disease in left-to-right shunt lesions?
20. What are right-to-left shunt lesions, and how do they lead to cyanosis?
21. What are obstructive lesions, and how are they tolerated?

SPECIAL ANESTHETIC CONSIDERATIONS

22. An infant who was born premature undergoes a minor surgical procedure. Can this patient be discharged home on the day of surgery?
23. What is the *ex utero* intrapartum therapy (EXIT) procedure?

ANSWERS

DEVELOPMENTAL PHYSIOLOGY

1. Respiration is less efficient in infants than adults for multiple reasons. The infant's chest wall is more compliant and cannot effectively maintain negative intrathoracic pressure. The airways are narrow, small, and collapsible. Finally, the infant's diaphragm has fewer type I muscle fibers and therefore tire more easily. Neonates and infants develop respiratory failure earlier than older patients. (613)
2. Periodic breathing is normal in newborns and is characterized by pauses in respiration of less than 10 seconds and periods of increased respiratory activity. Apnea is a ventilatory pause associated with desaturation and bradycardia. When a neonate or infant is apneic, the lung volume is smaller than the FRC, so an apneic infant has a disproportionally smaller store of intrapulmonary oxygen than an adult. Hypoxemia quickly ensues if the airway is inadequately maintained. (613)
3. Fetal circulation is characterized by high PVR and very little pulmonary blood flow and low SVR with the placenta as the major low resistance vascular bed. There is right-to-left blood flow through the foramen ovale and the ductus arteriosus. At birth, the baby takes a breath, expands the lungs, and increases the PaO_2 which decreases PVR. The placenta is removed from the circulation which increases the SVR. The ductus arteriosus is functionally closed in 98% of neonates at 4 days of life. The ductus venosus closes with the clamping of the umbilical vein. The increase in left atrial pressure from the blood returning from the lungs functionally closes the foramen ovale between 3 and 12 months of age. About 30% of adults have a probe-patent foramen ovale. Persistent fetal circulation occurs when the PVR fails to drop after birth due to hypoxemia, acidosis, and/or pulmonary hypertension. Blood continues to shunt right to left at the foramen ovale and the ductus arteriosus, creating a cycle of hypoxemia, cyanosis, and pulmonary hypertension. (613-614)
4. The parasympathetic nervous system predominates early in life while the sympathetic nervous system is still developing. This can manifest as bradycardia during maneuvers that are associated with vagal stimulation such as laryngoscopy or the placement of a nasogastric tube, nasal temperature probe, or transesophageal echocardiography probe. Bradycardia can result in a marked fall in cardiac output. Some anesthesia providers pretreat with atropine or glycopyrrolate before laryngoscopy. (615)

PHARMACOLOGIC DIFFERENCES

5. The following table indicates whether the given pharmacokinetic property is increased or decreased in infants compared to adults. (616-617)

Pharmacokinetic Property	Infants Compared to Adults
Plasma protein concentration	Decreased
Total body water percent	Increased
Percent fat and muscle	Decreased
Hepatic metabolism	Decreased
Renal excretion	Decreased

6. The uptake and distribution of inhaled anesthetics are more rapid in neonates than in adults. This is most likely due to the smaller functional residual capacity per body weight in neonates, as well as to greater tissue blood flow to the vessel-rich group. The higher blood flow to the vessel-rich group increases the partial pressure of agent in the blood and speeds the increase in FA/FI. The vessel-rich group of tissues includes the brain, heart, kidneys, and liver and comprises 22% of the total body volume in neonates, compared with the 10% of total body volume in adults. (617)

FLUIDS AND ELECTROLYTES

7. The preferred crystalloid solution for replacing a preexisting deficit and ongoing losses is non-glucose-containing isotonic solutions such as lactated Ringer solution or Plasma-Lyte A. Using the 4-2-1 rule, the fluid deficit is calculated to be 34 mL x 3 hours, or 102 mL. Fifty percent, 51 mL, is replaced in the first hour of anesthesia, and the remaining 50% is replaced in the subsequent 2 hours. For fluid maintenance the intravenous rate would be 34 mL/hour, plus an additional 34 to 68 mL/ hour (4-8 mL/kg/hr) for ongoing losses. (617-618)

TRANSFUSION THERAPY

8. The formula for maximum allowable blood loss (MABL) may be used by the anesthesia provider to help guide blood loss replacement. This formula should be applied to the pediatric patient prior to surgery so that when the threshold is reached, it is immediately recognized, and the transfusion is initiated.

   MABL (mL) = EBV (mL) × (patient Hct – minimum acceptable Hct)/patient Hct

   EBV is the estimated blood volume, which is between 100 mL/kg in the premature newborn and 70 mL/kg at about 5 years of age. The transfusion trigger varies greatly according to the patient's underlying physiology, age, nature of surgery, and anticipated ongoing blood loss. For patients with cyanotic heart disease, a hemoglobin threshold of 12-13 g/dL is often used. For healthy, acyanotic patients, a lower threshold of 7-8 g/dL is often used. Transfusion of 10-15 mL/kg of packed red blood cells should increase the hemoglobin concentration by 2-3 g/dL. In this case, the MABL can be calculated using EBV= 75 mL/kg, and minimum acceptable Hct = 22%. This gives us an MABL of 237 mL. Yes, the blood needs to be irradiated since it is a designated donation from blood relatives. (618-619)

PEDIATRIC AIRWAY

9. There are multiple differences between the pediatric and adult airway. Pediatric patients tend to have a larger tongue relative to the size of their mouths. Particularly true in neonates is that the occiput is larger, so that placing the head in a neutral position naturally places the head in a position favorable for direct laryngoscopy. Extending the head can make direct laryngoscopy difficult. The larynx is more cephalad in pediatric patients, with the cricoid cartilage opposing the C4 vertebra rather than the C6 vertebra in adults. The larynx is also more anterior. The epiglottis is longer, floppier, more omega-shaped, and has more of a horizontal lie in the infant. The narrowest part of the airway is at the level of the cricoid cartilage in the presence of neuromuscular blockade. MRI studies, however, suggest that the narrowest part in infants might be at the glottis, which is also the narrowest part in adults. The difference between the pediatric and adult airway are present until about age 8 years, after which the difference between the pediatric and adult airway is mainly just a difference in size. (620)
10. Because the narrowest point of the pediatric airway is at the level of the cricoid cartilage, it was believed that an endotracheal tube that passes easily through the larynx may cause ischemia or damage to the trachea distally. However, recent imaging studies challenge this notion, and the difference in diameter between the larynx and subglottis in younger children is minimal. Historically, uncuffed tubes were the standard of care in children younger than 8 years of age owing to concerns about subglottic stenosis and postextubation stridor. However, with the introduction of high-volume/low-pressure cuffs, recent studies suggest that there is no increased risk of airway edema with cuffed endotracheal tubes and that the use of cuffed endotracheal tubes may decrease the number of laryngoscopies and intubations due to inappropriate tube size. The risk of postintubation tracheal edema is greatest in children between 1 and 4 years of age, whether a cuffed or uncuffed tube is used. Postintubation croup can be treated with humidified gases, aerosolized racemic epinephrine, and intravenous dexamethasone. (620)
11. Cuffed endotracheal tubes are especially useful when poor ventilatory compliance exists or when a change in ventilatory compliance is anticipated. In patients with chronic lung disease, a cuffed endotracheal tube may be the most efficient way to deliver breaths requiring high pressures on the ventilator. If an uncuffed tube is used, the leak may be excessive. Cuffed tubes may also be indicated in cases in which compliance may change, such as the complete reduction of gastroschisis or an omphalocele. With the increase in intraabdominal pressure, higher pressures may be needed to ventilate, and a large leak can develop. If a cuffed tube is used, the cuff can be inflated until the leak disappears. Cuffed tubes are also useful when transesophageal echocardiography is planned, as compliance often changes with probe placement. Cuffed tubes are often advised when

reliable oxygenation and ventilation are critical, as when caring for a patient with severe pulmonary hypertension or when separating from cardiopulmonary bypass with high pulmonary artery pressures; trying to manage a leak in this situation can negatively impact hemodynamic status. (620)

12. The approach to the difficult pediatric and adult difficult airway is generally similar: maintain spontaneous respiration; use adjuncts such as a supraglottic airway, videolaryngoscope, or fiberoptic bronchoscope to secure the airway; awaken the patient if the airway cannot be secured; avoid neuromuscular blockade until the airway is secured; and have surgical backup for emergency tracheostomy for particularly difficult cases. The major difference between managing the pediatric versus adult airway is that young pediatric patients will not tolerate an "awake" intubation with topical anesthesia of the airway; they must have some level of moderate to deep sedation or general anesthesia. Also, cricothyrotomy is technically difficult in small patients, and ventilation via this method is ineffective. (621)

ANESTHETIC CONSIDERATIONS

13. An ongoing or recent URI may complicate anesthetic care. It predisposes the patient to airway hyperreactivity that can be manifest as laryngospasm or bronchospasm. Patients may have excess secretions and have an oxygen requirement or require hospital admission postoperatively. If the procedure is elective, it should be postponed 2-6 weeks to decrease the risk of airway-related complications. If a procedure is urgent, airway issues should be anticipated, and the patient should be cared for in such a way that airway hyperreactivity is minimized and that they are closely monitored for compromise. (622)
14. Midazolam is the most used premedication in children. It is usually given by mouth (0.5-0.75 mg/kg, max 20 mg) or intranasally (0.2-0.3 mg/kg, max 10 mg). Ketamine can be a useful adjunct and can be delivered orally, usually in conjunction with midazolam, or intramuscularly. Intramuscular ketamine is useful for uncooperative or agitated patients. Unfortunately, it is associated with excessive salivation, nystagmus, and nausea/vomiting; however, airway tone and spontaneous respiration are usually maintained. Alpha-2 agonists clonidine and dexmedetomidine can be used for premedication with effects comparable to midazolam. Clonidine is given orally and has an onset of action of about an hour. Dexmedetomidine can be given intranasally and has an onset of action of about 20-30 minutes. Nonpharmacologic techniques for allaying anxiety include parental presence at induction in well-selected cases, the use of a tablet or phone, preparation and facilitation by a child life specialist, and video games. (622-623)
15. Hypothermia is a concern in small infants as they have a larger surface area to weight ratio. They lose heat to the environment through radiation and convection. Small infants use nonshivering thermogenesis and metabolize brown fat to produce heat. Strategies for maintaining normothermia in infants include maintaining a warm room, using warmed IV fluids or blood, forced air warming, "French fry" lights, and airway humidification. (623)
16. It is common practice in pediatric anesthesia to extubate the trachea during deep anesthesia. The advantage of a deep extubation is that emergence occurs without an endotracheal tube in place, avoiding coughing, bucking, and straining on surgical suture lines. Potential risks of deep extubation are those associated with emergence with an unprotected, anesthetized airway. The patient may aspirate blood or secretions, vomit, have laryngospasm, hypoventilate, or experience airway obstruction. The patient who has undergone deep extubation should be monitored closely. A face mask and a device for delivering positive pressure should be readily available, and anesthesia providers and recovery room personnel should be ready to intervene. (623-624)
17. Airway monitoring is an important aspect of PACU care of the pediatric patient. As patients who experienced a deep extubation emerge, they may obstruct, hypoventilate, vomit, aspirate, or have laryngospasm. Other patients may need monitoring for postextubation stridor or croup. PACU care also involves the treatment of postoperative nausea and vomiting and the assessment and treatment of postoperative pain. In addition, PACU care involves the assessment and treatment of emergence delirium. (624-625)

MEDICAL AND SURGICAL DISEASES AFFECTING THE NEONATE

18. The table below matches the disease to the appropriate corresponding description. (625-632)

Disease	Letter	Description
Necrotizing enterocolitis	d	Most common neonatal surgical emergency; patients may have sepsis, bloody stools, and coagulopathy
Gastroschisis and omphalocele	f	Repair may be staged; single surgery repair can lead to abdominal compartment syndrome and renal compromise
Tracheoesophageal fistula	a	Associated with VACTERL; patients may have abdominal distension and aspiration of gastric contents
Congenital diaphragmatic hernia	h	Scaphoid abdomen, bowel sounds in chest, respiratory distress, cyanosis
Patent ductus arteriosus	c	Lower extremity blood pressure and/or pulse oximetry monitoring is indicated during surgical repair
Retinopathy of prematurity	b	Often in ventilator-dependent premature infants; treatment may be urgent and surgery prolonged
Myelomeningocele	e	Endotracheal intubation may need to be in lateral position in a latex-free environment
Pyloric stenosis	g	Surgery should be delayed for hydration and correction of electrolytes

CONGENITAL HEART DISEASE

19. Left-to-right shunt lesions arise from communications between the atria (atrial septal defect), ventricles (ventricular septal defect), or the great arteries (patent duct arteriosus, aortopulmonary window). The severity of disease is related to the degree of left-to-right shunt which depends on several factors including the size of the defect, the pressure gradient between chambers, and the relative pulmonary and systemic vascular resistances. Large shunts lead to pulmonary overcirculation and a heart that is volume-loaded. The patient can develop signs of heart failure including tachypnea, pulmonary edema, poor feeding, intercostal retractions, and failure to thrive. Longstanding pulmonary overcirculation leads to changes in the pulmonary vasculature and can result in pulmonary hypertension. If the shunt goes untreated, this can lead to reversal of the shunt and cyanosis. This is known as Eisenmenger syndrome. Fortunately, early repair of left-to-right shunt lesions has largely eliminated Eisenmenger syndrome in developed countries. It is still seen where there is uncertain access to care. (632)
20. Right-to-left shunt lesions result from obstruction to the right ventricular outflow tract and shunting across a ventricuar septal defect (VSD) from the right to the left ventricle. This results in arterial desaturation. The degree of cyanosis is related to the degree of right ventricular outflow tract obstruction and the size of the VSD. The most common right-to-left shunt lesion is tetralogy of Fallot, making up 6% of CHD patients. Other examples include transposition of the great arteries, truncus arteriosus, and tricuspid atresia. (633).
21. Obstructive lesions can be seen at multiple locations in the heart and great vessels. The most common obstructive lesion is pulmonary stenosis, accounting for 13% of CHD. Coarctation of the aorta makes up 7% of CHD. Valvar aortic stenosis makes up 5% of CHD. Left-sided obstruction is less well-tolerated than right-sided obstruction. Lesions like subaortic stenosis, aortic stenosis, and supravalvar stenosis can lead to ischemia, ventricular arrhythmias, and death, all of which may be exacerbated by anesthetic care. (633)

SPECIAL ANESTHETIC CONSIDERATIONS

22. Former premature infants who present for surgery are at an increased risk for postanesthetic apnea. This risk increases with increased prematurity at birth and younger age at the time of the anesthetic. Apnea spells that result in the cessation of breathing for 20 seconds or longer can lead to cyanosis and bradycardia. Especially at risk are preterm infants younger than 50 weeks' postconceptual age. Is estimated that 20% to 30% of

preterm infants have apnea spells during their first month of life. Apnea spells may be increased in the postoperative period secondary to the residual effects of inhaled and injected anesthetics that affect the control of breathing. The recommendation for these patients is that apnea and bradycardia monitors be used after surgery. These patients are not candidates for outpatient surgery because of the risk of apnea occurring at home where health care workers are not available to respond. Treating anemia and administering a single dose of intravenous caffeine citrate will reduce the incidence and severity of postanesthetic apnea in this population. The current recommendation is that former premature infants should have their surgery delayed until after 50 weeks postconceptual age or greater to minimize the risk. Prior to this, and on a case-by-case basis, infants may need to be admitted postoperatively for 24 hours of apnea monitoring. (637)

23. The *ex utero* intrapartum therapy (EXIT) procedure involves partial delivery of the head, chest, and arms of the fetus to manage a severe airway or pulmonary anomaly. The fetus remains connected to the placental circulation to provide oxygenation and carbon dioxide removal during the procedure to secure the airway or manage the airway or lung mass. Indications include large airway, neck, or chest masses such as cystic hygroma, teratoma, and congenital adenomatoid malformation. Two anesthesia providers are required, one for the mother and one for the fetus. The mother requires deep inhalational general anesthesia to reduce uterine tone during the fetal procedure to prevent placental separation. The fetus receives intravenous or intramuscular fentanyl or morphine for analgesia. Resection of the mass or securing the airway by rigid bronchoscopy or tracheostomy is the primary goal. Then the fetus is delivered. (639)

Chapter

35 GERIATRICS

Tyler Seth Chernin

INTRODUCTION

- Critical perioperative considerations often relevant in the elderly patient
  - Frailty
  - Cognitive function
  - Nutritional status
  - Functional independence
- Physiologic changes of aging
  - Affects most organ systems
  - Affects pharmacokinetics and pharmacodynamics of most anesthetic agents

THE PHYSIOLOGIC CHANGES OF AGING

- Homeostenosis
  - The ability to respond to physiologic stressors and return to a state of homeostasis diminishes with age
- Frailty
  - A predisposition to disease states with decreasing physiologic reserve
  - Commonly accompanies the aging process
- Aging versus disease
  - Must distinguish normal physiologic aging from disease states common in the elderly
  - Disease is *not* a normal part of aging

Cardiovascular System

- Reduced compliance in venous and arterial system
  - Due to decrease in elastin production
  - Diminished ability to adequately respond to drops in preload
    - Decreased compliance of venous capacitance vessels
- Reduced endothelial nitric oxide (NO production) leads to:
  - Vasoconstriction
  - Platelet aggregation
  - Endothelial dysfunction
- Blood pressure and SVR changes
  - *Increase* in systolic blood pressure (SBP), systemic vascular resistance (SVR), and pulse pressure (PP)
  - *Decrease* in diastolic blood pressure (DBP)

Induction of Anesthesia in Geriatric Patients

- Geriatric patients often have labile BP
  - Partly because of decreased compliance in both venous and arterial vessels
  - Especially during induction
- To avoid hypotension on induction
  - Reduce the dosages of most anesthesia induction agents.
  - Consider administering slowly in divided doses.
- Preemptive, low-dose vasopressor infusions (phenylephrine, norepinephrine)
  - Can be helpful to offset the vasodilatory effects of anesthetic drugs
- Short-acting β-blockers (esmolol)
  - Helpful to mitigate exaggerated hemodynamic responses to laryngoscopy

- Increased risk of dysrhythmias
  - Progressive calcific deposits within valvular structures
  - Fibrosis within the cardiac conduction system
- Left ventricular hypertrophy (LVH) increases with aging
  - Caused by progressive increases in afterload
  - Leads to reduced LV compliance, impaired early ventricular filling, and higher filling pressures
  - Predisposition to diastolic dysfunction
  - LVH predisposes to myocardial ischemia in the setting of hypotension, especially in the subendocardial layer
- Resting ejection fraction (EF) and cardiac output (CO) remain stable.
  - Reduced ability to *augment* EF and CO during physiologic stress
- Resting heart rate (HR) and maximum HR steadily decline.
  - Loss of pacemaker cells
  - Fibrosis within sinoatrial (SA) node
- Sympathetic nervous system (SNS) response is reduced.
  - β-Receptor downregulation and reduced receptor responsiveness
  - Diminished HR component of baroreceptor reflex
  - Even with higher levels of circulating norepinephrine and epinephrine

- Parasympathetic nervous system (PNS) regulation decreases
  - Blunting of resting HR variability
  - Less robust HR increase with anticholinergic medications

Pulmonary System

- Lung function starts to decline by the third decade of life.
  - Loss of elastin in lung parenchyma
  - Progressive anatomic changes
- Changes in lung volume and mechanics
  - Closing capacity (CC) = residual volume (RV) + closing volume (CV)
    - CC increases with age so smaller airways more prone to collapse at steadily higher lung volumes
    - Age 45: CC exceeds supine functional residual capacity (FRC)
    - Age 65: CC exceeds sitting FRC
    - Leads to increased shunting and lower resting arterial partial pressure of oxygen (PaO_2)
  - Lung compliance increases and air trapping occurs (functional emphysema).
- Progressive changes to chest wall, respiratory muscles, and airway
  - Stiffening of thoracic muscles and joints
  - Diaphragm flattens and becomes less efficient
  - Fewer type 2 fast-twitch fibers (more muscle fatigue)
- Loss of alveolar and pulmonary capillary surface area
  - Worsening V/Q mismatch
  - Increased anatomic dead space
  - Resting PaO_2 declines, A-a gradient widens.
- Blunting of compensatory responses to hypoxemia and hypercarbia
- Effects on pulmonary function tests
  - Total lung capacity (TLC): relatively unchanged, balanced by chest wall (reduced compliance) and lung parenchyma (increased compliance)
  - RV: increases 5% to 10% per decade
  - FRC: increases 1% to 3% per decade
  - Vital capacity (VC): decreases 40% between ages of 20 and 70
  - Forced VC (FVC) and forced expiratory volume in 1 second (FEV_1): decreases
  - Oxygen diffusing capacity (DL_{CO}): decreases 5% per decade
- Blunting of pharyngeal reflexes and muscle tone
  - Predisposition toward pulmonary aspiration

Renal System

- Renal function progressively declines with aging
  - Renal blood flow (RBF) decreases 10% per decade over age of 40
  - Glomerular filtration rate (GFR) decreases 1 mL/year over age 50
  - Renal cortical atrophy, fewer functioning nephrons, more renal cysts/tumors
  - Decreased activity of renin-angiotensin-aldosterone systems (RAAS)
  - Prone to renal ischemia and subsequent renal failure
- Prone to electrolyte disturbances (hypo- and hypernatremia, hyperkalemia)
  - Decreased ability to reabsorb and excrete sodium and free water
  - Decreased GFR and RAAS activity predispose to hyperkalemia
- Changes in ability to excrete and reabsorb many common medications

Nervous System

- Progressive loss of brain mass and neuronal function
  - Most pronounced in prefrontal cortex and medial temporal lobes
    - Volume loss of 5% per decade over age 40
    - Impairments in attention, executive function, and short-term memory
  - Increased cerebrospinal fluid (CSF) volume
  - Decreased cerebral blood flow (CBF)
  - Fewer neurons and lower neurotransmitter levels (dopamine, serotonin, acetylcholine, glutamate, brain neurotrophic factor)
- Blood brain barrier (BBB) becomes more permeable
- Arteriosclerosis of intracerebral vessels
- Impairment in processing sensory inputs
  - Increased risk of falls, postoperative delirium, cognitive impairment

Gastrointestinal System

- Prone to pulmonary aspiration
  - Reduced esophageal muscle compliance and lower esophageal sphincter tone
  - Prolonged gastric emptying
- Reduction in gastric prostaglandin and bicarbonate synthesis
  - Higher risk of gastritis and irritation from nonsteroidal antiinflammatory drugs (NSAIDs)
- Liver atrophy—20% to 40% reduction of mass by age 80
  - Hepatic blood flow (HBF) – 50% decrease between ages of 30 and 100
  - Prone to hepatic ischemia
  - Liver function also declines
    - Decreased serum albumin
    - Cytochrome P450 metabolism less effective
    - Increased plasma levels of some acidic drugs

Hematologic System

- Bone marrow mass decreases
  - Leads to decline in hematopoietic reserves
- Tendency toward prothrombotic state
  - Higher rates of deep venous thrombosis (DVT)
- Immunosenescence
  - Immune system becomes less effective at mounting robust responses to novel foreign antigens.

PHARMACOLOGIC CONSIDERATIONS

- In general, geriatric patients are more sensitive to most anesthetic agents.
  - Due to both pharmacodynamic (PD) and pharmacokinetic (PK) changes
- Pharmacokinetic changes
  - Decrease in total body water (TBW) by 10% to 15%
  - Decreased muscle mass
  - Increase in fat mass (20% to 40%)
  - Volume of distribution (Vd)
    - Increases for lipophilic agents
    - Decreases for hydrophilic agents
- Plasma protein changes
  - Serum albumin decreases (binds acidic drugs)
  - α_1-Acid glycoprotein increases (binds basic drugs)
- Reductions in RBF, HBF, and hepatic metabolism
  - Can prolong action of drugs that depend on renal or hepatic clearance
- Anesthetic drug doses
  - Nearly all drug doses should be initially reduced.
  - Potentially use longer time between repeat doses.
  - Titrate to clinical effect.

Pharmacokinetic Properties Affected by Aging

- Absorption
- Volume of distribution
- Metabolism
- Clearance

Pharmacology of Specific Anesthetic Medications in the Elderly

- Volatile anesthetics
  - Minimum alveolar concentration (MAC) decreases 6% per decade over age 40
  - For nitrous oxide, decrease is 8% per decade over age 40
- Propofol
  - Reduce induction dose by at least 20%.
  - Reduce maintenance infusions by 30% to 50% (while always titrating to clinical effect).
    - Reduced clearance due to reduction in hepatic metabolism
- Etomidate
  - Reduce induction dose (by up to 50% to 66% in patients over age 80).
    - Reduced drug clearance and Vd
- Ketamine
  - Reduce induction and maintenance dosing (exact guidelines lacking).
  - Mixed data supporting a pro-delirium effect in elderly
  - Produces less hypotension on induction
  - Increased SNS output can be problematic in patients with coronary artery disease (CAD) or significant stenotic valvular lesions.
- Benzodiazepines
  - Reduce doses.
    - PD-related changes increase sensitivity.
    - PK-related changes prolong their effect.
  - Concerns for causing/worsening delirium
  - Synergistic effect on respiratory depression when used with opioids
- Opioids
  - Generally, reduce doses by 50%.
    - Increased sensitivity to analgesic and respiratory effects
    - Changes related to PD and PK
  - Avoid morphine and meperidine
    - Active metabolites that are renally cleared and may accumulate
    - Meperidine has central anticholinergic effects
- Dexmedetomidine
  - Reduce dose (33% reduction by some sources).
    - Lower albumin levels may increase amount of free drug in plasma.
- Acetaminophen
  - No specific adjustments necessary in geriatric population
- Nonsteroidal antiinflammatory drugs (NSAIDs)
  - Reduce doses by 25–50%.
  - Avoid in patients with GFR < 60 ml/min
  - Potential for increasing cardiac risk, acute renal failure, and gastrointestinal bleeding
- Local anesthetics (LAs)
  - Reduce dose of amide LAs due to hepatic metabolism.
  - Reduced vascularity of neuraxial space may help to limit systemic absorption.
  - Elderly are at greater risk for local anesthetic systemic toxicity (LAST).
- Neuromuscular blocking agents
  - Potential for prolonged effects
    - Due to reductions in renal and hepatic metabolism

- No specific PD-related changes
- Sugammadex may have slower onset of action

PREOPERATIVE ASSESSMENT AND RISK MANAGEMENT

- Several issues arise more frequently in this population
  - Consider their impact on the anesthesia plan
- Cognitive function
  - Multiple validated assessment tools
    - E.g., Mini Mental State Examination, Mini-Cog
  - Establish a preprocedural baseline
    - Cognitive deficits correlate with postoperative delirium and even mortality
  - Assess medical decision-making capacity
  - Screen for mood disorders and substance use disorder

Assessing Medical Decision-Making Capacity

The patient must demonstrate proficiency in four major areas:

1. *Understanding* the various treatment options
2. *Appreciating* the disease type, severity, and consequences
3. The ability to *reason* between the various treatment options offered
4. The ability to make an *informed choice*

- Functional capacity
  - Evaluate ability to carry out activities of daily living (ADLs) and instrumental activities of daily living (IADLs)
  - Preoperative deficits correlate with perioperative morbidity.
  - Assess deficits in hearing, vision, swallowing as well as fall risk
    - Design recovery plan specific to these needs.
    - E.g., nutritional support, physical therapy and rehabilitation, fall prevention
- Nutritional status
  - Risk factors
    - Albumin <3 g/dL
    - Body mass index <18.5 kg/m^2
    - Unexplained 10% to 15% weight loss within 6 months
  - Patients with poor nutritional status
    - Increased risk of surgical site infections, pneumonia, and urinary tract infection
- Frailty
  - Defined by global reduction in physiologic reserve
    - Limits ability to respond to physiologic stressors
    - Reduced ability to return to state of homeostasis
  - Multiple validated assessment tools
    - E.g., Fried Index, Modified Frailty Index, Edmonton Frail Scale
  - Associated with higher periprocedural morbidity and mortality
- Polypharmacy
  - Very common issue in the elderly
    - E.g., 40% of patients over 65 years old use five or more medications
  - Risks of polypharmacy
    - Falls, adverse drug reactions, increased hospital length of stay, and increased mortality
  - Consider compliance with, and appropriateness of, all prescribed and over-the-counter medications.
  - Provide clear and simple instructions whether certain medications should be held or discontinued before procedure
- Preoperative optimization can be challenging
  - Many, sometimes competing, factors in the geriatric patient
    - E.g., complex medical comorbidities vs. urgency of a procedure
- Preoperative testing requirements
  - No specific laboratory or diagnostic studies are indicated solely on basis of age
- Consider obtaining a Comprehensive Geriatric Assessment (CGA).
  - Formalized, global assessment by a geriatrician
  - Can offer pre-, intra-, and postsurgical recommendations for optimization
  - E.g., by using targeted interventions specific to the geriatric patient

INTRAOPERATIVE CONSIDERATIONS

- Anesthetic plan should involve special considerations to avoid delirium and cardiopulmonary complications
- Choice between regional anesthesia (RA) and general anesthesia (GA)
  - No conclusive evidence of superiority of GA vs. RA
  - RA potential advantages
    - Can be opioid-sparing and help avoid polypharmacy
    - Potential for improved hemodynamic stability, though neuraxial procedures can be associated with significant hypotension
- Neuraxial and/or peripheral nerve blocks
  - Can be more challenging due to anatomic changes
  - Elderly are more sensitive to effects of LAs with a higher risk of LAST
  - Concurrent use of anticoagulant/antiplatelet medications often contraindicates neuraxial techniques

- Airway techniques
  - Can be complicated by anatomic changes
    - Reduced neck range of motion
    - Edentulous patients can be difficult to ventilate
  - Exaggerated hemodynamic responses to laryngoscopy
    - Can be attenuated with short-acting β-blockers

POSTOPERATIVE MANAGEMENT

Acute Pain

- Pain is often underreported and undertreated in the elderly
- Can be challenging to assess in patients with cognitive impairment
  - Information from family or caregivers often valuable
  - Critical Care Pain Observation Tool (CPOT) and Faces Pain Scale designed for patients with cognitive impairment
- Implications of PK- and PD-related changes of aging
  - Geriatric patients more susceptible to adverse effects from many common analgesic medications (e.g., respiratory depression, falls)
- Uncontrolled pain
  - Can lead to delirium, chronic pain syndromes, or adverse cardiovascular events
- Use multidisciplinary approach.
  - Involve geriatric expertise
  - Use multimodal regimens that include regional anesthesia

Hypoxemia

- Hypoxemia is common postoperatively
  - V/Q mismatch and shunting more common in the aging pulmonary system
- Diminished hypoxic ventilatory drive and higher risk of aspiration
- Maintain vigilance
  - Judicious pulse oximetry use and supplemental oxygen
  - Encourage incentive spirometry

Fluid Management

- Renal system
  - Decreased ability to compensate for conditions of hyper- and hypovolemia, as well as alterations in serum sodium levels
- Monitor fluid status carefully
  - Clinical
    - E.g., mucous membranes, orthostatic blood pressure
  - Laboratory
    - E.g., lactate, electrolytes
  - Imaging
    - E.g., bedside transthoracic echocardiography

CHRONIC PAIN IN THE ELDERLY

- Chronic pain is common in the elderly
  - Often due to degenerative processes, cancer, and neuropathy
  - But is *not* a normal part of aging process
- Challenge of assessing chronic pain patients with cognitive impairment
  - Consider coexisting mood disorders as contributors to pain syndromes.
- Multimodal approach to treatment
  - Pharmacotherapy
    - Make sure chronic medications (including antidepressants) are maintained throughout the perioperative period
    - Gabapentinoids should be titrated slowly, can cause respiratory depression, and contribute to fall risk
  - Physical therapy and rehabilitation programs
    - Consider benefits to functional status as well as improving pain scores
  - Interventional pain procedures
    - E.g., epidural steroid, facet joint, and sacroiliac joint injections

PERIOPERATIVE NEUROCOGNITIVE DISORDERS

- Nomenclature revised in 2018 to better align terminology among various disciplines (psychiatry, neurology, geriatrics, surgery, and anesthesiology)
  - The older term *postoperative cognitive dysfunction (POCD)* has been replaced
- *Preoperative neurocognitive disorder* (NCD)
  - Present before surgery, defined as mild and major
    - Mild: 1 to 2 standard deviations from normal with intact ADLs
    - Major: > 2 standard deviations plus objective impairment in ADLs
  - "Cognitive concern" must be present in both cases
    - Subjective cognitive dysfunction raised by patient, caregiver, or provider
- *Delayed neurocognitive recovery* (dNCR)
  - New impairment that resolves by postoperative day 30
- *Postoperative neurocognitive disorder* (referred to here as pNCD)
  - New impairment that persists beyond postoperative day 30 but resolving by 12 months
  - Defined as mild or major, as above

- *Neurocognitive disorder*
  - Defined as deficits beyond 12 months, similar to preoperative time period
  - Defined as mild or major, as above
- *Postoperative delirium*
  - Distinct clinical entity
  - Categorized as *emergence* or *postoperative* based on timing

Postoperative Delirium

- Definition of postoperative delirium (POD)
  - Acute, fluctuating disturbance in consciousness
    - Characterized by alterations in awareness, attention, cognition
    - Develops over a short period of time
    - Not from a previous cognitive disorder
  - Very common in elderly (26% to 35%)
- Emergence vs. postoperative delirium
  - Distinction based on timing
  - Emergence delirium: very early onset before or at arrival in PACU
- Several assessment tools available
  - E.g., Confusion Assessment Method (CAM) or Riker Sedation Agitation Scale
- Types of delirium
  - Hyperactive, hypoactive, or mixed
    - Based on perceived level of agitation
    - Hypoactive delirium associated with worst prognosis
- Predictors of POD
  - Preexisting cognitive impairment one of the strongest risk factors
  - Other risk factors
    - Advanced age, number of comorbidities, frailty, higher ASA score, prolonged mechanical ventilation, uncontrolled pain
  - Exacerbating factors
    - Certain medications (i.e., benzodiazepines, anticholinergics, steroids)
    - Deeper planes of general anesthesia
- Biologic basis for delirium
  - Exact cause unknown
  - Neuroinflammatory state with permeable blood-brain barrier caused by surgical stress
- Adverse outcomes in patients with POD
  - Associated with increased morbidity and mortality
  - Predictor of future, permanent cognitive dysfunction/dementia
- Prevention strategies
  - Frequent reorientation, timely provision of visual/hearing aids, maintain sleep/wake cycles
  - Avoid deep planes of anesthesia
  - Avoid urinary catheters and restraints
  - Proactive geriatric consultation
- Treatment strategies
  - Address underlying causes
    - Pain, physiologic derangements, polypharmacy, withdrawal
  - Pharmacologic medications when risk of harm to self or others

Postoperative Neurocognitive Disorders

- Postoperative neurocognitive disorders – dNCR and pNCD
- Characterized by deficits in memory, language, motor, and executive functions
  - Requires dedicated, sophisticated neuropsychiatric testing for diagnosis
  - Historically, diagnosis has been challenging.
    - Lack of consistency in diagnostic criteria
    - Lack of baseline preoperative measurements
    - Confounded by inherent risk of developing dementia in any elderly patient
  - Incidence described between 16% to 60% postoperatively
- Risk factors
  - Similar to those described for POD, including POD itself
  - Cerebrovascular disease, lower educational level
- pNCDs associated with higher rates of morbidity and mortality
  - Does not seem to be associated with any particular intraoperative insults (e.g., hypotension, hypoxemia) or type of anesthesia
- Pathophysiology
  - Similar to POD, likely caused by a neuroinflammatory state triggered by surgical stress
  - Compounded by patient-specific risk factors
- Prevention strategies
  - Prehabilitation programs for high-risk patients
  - Educational programs for patients and caregivers
  - Avoid POD and its triggers

SUMMARY

- Elderly patients are increasingly presenting for surgery across all settings
- Anesthesia providers must understand normal physiology of aging as well as common comorbidities often seen in the elderly
- Future research is needed to elucidate causes of, and best practices to avoid, perioperative neurocognitive disorders.

QUESTIONS

THE PHYSIOLOGIC CHANGES OF AGING

1. Explain the term *frailty* and why it is relevant to the aging patient.
2. What are the main changes to the aging cardiovascular system? In the table below, describe the impact of aging on the listed cardiovascular parameters. Why are these changes relevant during anesthesia care?

Parameter	Change With Aging
Left ventricular (LV) compliance	
LV afterload	
Ejection fraction (EF) and cardiac output (CO)	
Heart rate (HR)	
Blood pressure	

3. What are the main changes to the aging pulmonary system? Why is the geriatric patient more prone to hypoxemia?

PHARMACOLOGIC CONSIDERATIONS

4. In general, what are the main physiologic changes of aging that affect the pharmacokinetic (PK) and pharmacodynamic (PD) profiles of many drugs and anesthetics?

PREOPERATIVE ASSESSMENT AND RISK MANAGEMENT

5. During preoperative evaluation, how can functional capacity be assessed in an elderly patient? What are ADLs and IADLs?
6. How can frailty be measured during preoperative evaluation before a major surgery?

INTRAOPERATIVE CONSIDERATIONS

7. In the categories listed in the table below, describe some of the main pros and cons of general anesthesia (GA) versus regional anesthesia (RA, including neuraxial) in the geriatric patient.

	General Anesthesia	Regional Anesthesia
Technical considerations		
Risk of deep venous thrombosis		
Polypharmacy		
Risk of perioperative neurocognitive disorders		
Hemodynamic stability		
Perioperative use of anticoagulant/antiplatelet medications		
Pain control		

POSTOPERATIVE MANAGEMENT

8. What are some of the challenges in assessing acute and chronic pain in the geriatric population? How do treatment approaches differ from younger patients?

PERIOPERATIVE NEUROCOGNITIVE DISORDERS

9. What are some risk factors for, and clinical implications of, postoperative delirium (POD) in the geriatric patient? How can POD best be avoided?

ANSWERS

THE PHYSIOLOGIC CHANGES OF AGING

1. Frailty is a state characterized by diminished physiologic reserve, which leads to a predisposition to disease states. It is not exclusive to the elderly population, but is more common as one ages since organ systems become less adaptable to physiologic stressors. Apart from aging, other factors that contribute to the frail state include genetics, environment, nutritional status, physical inactivity, mood, and social support structures. Once an elderly person enters a frail state, they are at risk of a number of negative outcomes, including falls, cognitive decline, and increasing healthcare needs. The figure below provides a framework for considering the relationship between physiologic reserve, functional capacity, and frailty. (643–644)

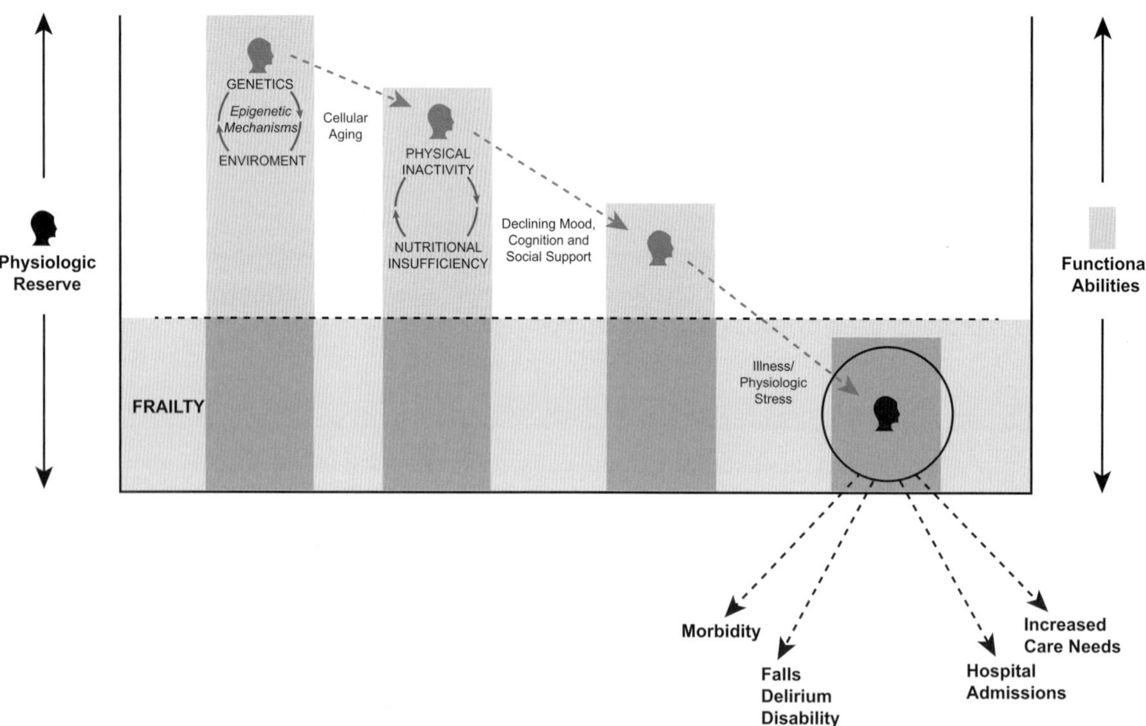

Physiology of Aging. Figure depicts a conceptual model of physiologic reserve, functional ability, and frailty. As the aging process occurs (*dashed, arrowed line*), physiologic reserves and functional abilities normally decline. A multitude of other factors and processes (genetics, environment, cellular aging, nutritional status, physical inactivity, mood and social support) may hasten or slow down this process. At a certain point, the aging process or an acute physiologic stressor causes the individual to enter into a state of frailty (*dashed, horizontal line*), at which point they are at risk of poor outcomes, such as morbidity, falls, cognitive decline, and increased health care needs. These outcomes may further worsen the conditions of frailty. (Reproduced with permission from Khan KT, Hemati K, Donovan AL. Geriatric physiology and the frailty syndrome. *Anesthesiol Clin.* 2019;37[3]:453–474.)

2. Beginning around the fourth decade of life, elastin production begins to decrease; this leads to fibrosis within the media of the aorta and other large muscular arteries and veins. The table below highlights some of the implications of these changes.

Parameter	Change With Aging
Left ventricular (LV) compliance	Reduced (predisposing to diastolic dysfunction)
LV afterload	Increased (leading to LV hypertrophy)
Resting ejection fraction (EF) and cardiac output (CO)	Unchanged (though reduced ability to augment with stress)

Parameter	Change With Aging
Heart rate (HR)	Decreased heart rate variability at rest Decreased maximum heart rate achievable Decreased effectiveness of HR response to the baroreceptor reflex
Blood pressure	Increased systolic blood pressure Decreased diastolic blood pressure Widened pulse pressure

During anesthesia care, elderly patients are more prone to hypotension since the reduced compliance of the venous capacitance vessels makes them unable to effectively respond to conditions of reduced preload. Also, the baroreceptor reflex is less effective because the HR response is often blunted in the setting of hypotension. (643–646)

3. Lung function begins to decline around the third decade of life, partly caused by a reduction in elastin fibers within the lung parenchyma as well as loss of alveolar and capillary surface area. This leads to a progressive increase in closing capacity (CC), which is the lung volume at which small airways begin to close due to a loss of elastic recoil. CC tends to exceed supine functional residual capacity (FRC) by age 45 and sitting FRC by age 65. When this occurs, shunt fraction increases and hypoxemia worsens. As such, resting PaO_2 declines with age accompanied by a widened A-a gradient. The loss of elasticity also leads to air trapping and a state of functional emphysema. Compensatory responses to hypoxemia and hypercarbia are also blunted in the elderly. Geriatric patients are thus very prone to hypoxemia during the perioperative period. They are more sensitive to the respiratory depressant effects of many common anesthetics. In addition, shunting and V/Q mismatch are especially common during controlled mechanical ventilation regardless of age, which only further predisposes them to hypoxemia given the effects of aging mentioned above. (646–647)

PHARMACOLOGIC CONSIDERATIONS

4. During the aging process, total body water (TBW) decreases by 10% to 15%, muscle mass decreases, and fat content increases by 20% to 40%. This increases the volume of distribution (Vd) for lipophilic agents and decreases Vd for hydrophilic agents. Serum albumin decreases, which increases the unbound fraction of acidic drugs. α_1-Acid glycoprotein increases, which decreases the unbound fraction of basic drugs. The absorption and systemic effects of oral drugs are affected by changes in gastric pH and gastric emptying as well as reductions in hepatic blood flow (HBF). Due to reduced HBF and hepatic enzymatic activity, certain drugs may reach higher plasma concentrations and display prolonged effects. The same phenomenon occurs for drugs that depend on renal clearance due to a normal decline in renal function and GFR with aging. From a pharmacodynamic standpoint, many anesthetics have higher potency due to changes at the receptor level. (648–649)

PREOPERATIVE ASSESSMENT AND RISK MANAGEMENT

5. A broad assessment of functional capacity can begin with evaluation of a patient's ability to carry out activities of daily living (ADLs) and instrumental ADLs, as noted in the box below.
The presence of poor preoperative functional capacity correlates with development of postoperative complications. (652)

Activities of Daily Living and Instrumental Activities of Daily Living

Activities of Daily Living
- Bathing
- Dressing
- Toileting
- Transferring
- Eating

Instrumental Activities of Daily Living
- Use of telephone
- Use of public transportation
- Shopping
- Preparation of meals
- Housekeeping
- Taking medications properly
- Managing personal finances

From Barnett SR. Elderly patients. In Pardo MC, Miller RD, eds. *Basics of Anesthesia*. 7th ed. Philadelphia: Elsevier; 2018:610.

6. While there is no universally accepted tool for defining frailty, multiple scoring systems exist, such as the Modified Frailty Index and the Edmonton Frail Scale. The table below describes several approaches to assessing frailty in the perioperative setting. (652–653)

Selected Frailty Assessment Methods in the Perioperative Setting

Name	Description	
Modified Frailty Index (mFI)[a]	Compilation of deficits/impairments into an index based on symptoms, signs, laboratory values, disease states, and disabilities based on NSQIP database	mFI-11—11 factors used mFI-5—5 factors used
Hopkins Frailty Score[b]	Five domains: weight loss, grip strength/weakness, exhaustion, low physical activity, slowed walking speed	Score: 0, nonfrail; 1–2, prefrail; 3–5, frail
Edmonton Frail Scale[c]	Standardized assessment of cognition, general health, functional independence and performance, social support, medication usage, nutritional status, mood, continence	Scored out of 17, higher scores associated with increasing frailty
FRAIL Scale[d]	Five domains: fatigue, resistance, ambulation, illnesses, weight loss	Score: 0, nonfrail; 1–2, prefrail; 3-5, frail
Groningen Frailty Indicator[e]	15-item questionnaire, 8 indicators: mobility, physical fitness, vision, hearing, nutrition, morbidity, cognition, psychosocial	Score out of 15, 4 or greater indicative of frailty

NSQIP, National Surgical Quality Improvement Program.
Reproduced with permission from Khan KT, Hemati K, Donovan AL. Geriatric physiology and the frailty syndrome. *Anesthesiol Clin.* 2019;37(3):453–474.
[a]Farhat JS, Velanovich V, Falvo AJ, et al. Are the frail destined to fail? Frailty index as predictor of surgical morbidity and mortality in the elderly. *J Trauma Acute Care Surg* . 2012;72(6):1526–1530 and Subramaniam S, Aalberg JJ, Soriano RP, et al. New 5-Factor Modified Frailty Index using American College of Surgeons NSQIP data. *J Am Coll Surg.* 2018;226(2):173–181.e8.
[b]Fried LP, Tangen CM, Walston J, et al. Cardiovascular Health Study Collaborative Research Group. Frailty in older adults: Evidence for a phenotype. *J Gerontol A Biol Sci Med Sci.* 2001;56(3):M146–M156.
[c]Rolfson DB, Majumdar SR, Tsuyuki RT, et al. Validity and reliability of the Edmonton Frail Scale. *Age Ageing.* 2006;35(5):526–529.
[d]Morley JE, Malmstrom TK, Miller DK. A simple frailty questionnaire (FRAIL) predicts outcomes in middle aged African Americans. *J Nutr Health Aging.* 2012;16(7):601–608.
[e]Steverink N, Slaets JPJ, Schuurmans H, et al. Measuring frailty: Development and testing of the Groningen Frailty Indicator (GFI). *Gerontologist.* 2001;41(special issue 1):236–237.

INTRAOPERATIVE CONSIDERATIONS

7. There is no conclusive evidence of the superiority of one anesthesia approach in the elderly patient. The table below highlights considerations regarding anesthesia choice for the elderly patient. Ultimately, the decision should be guided by a detailed risk/benefit assessment of both approaches in the context of surgical requirements and patient preferences. (654–655)

Considerations Regarding Regional Versus General Anesthesia in the Elderly

	General Anesthesia	Regional Anesthesia
Technical considerations	Difficult mask ventilation in edentulous patients Neck stiffness reducing ROM Exaggerated hemodynamic response to laryngoscopy	Neuraxial techniques may be challenging; ligament ossification, positioning Greater LA spread in neuraxial space
Risk of deep venous thrombosis (DVT)	Variable	May be reduced with neuraxial techniques
Polypharmacy	May contribute to drug–drug interactions perioperatively	Regional techniques are often opioid-sparing Fewer systemic medications needed Elderly patients at higher risk of LAST
Risk of perioperative neurocognitive disorders	No conclusive evidence of one technique being superior. May be confounded by depth of sedation used during regional anesthetics.	

	General Anesthesia	Regional Anesthesia
Hemodynamic (HD) stability	Variable	Hypotension common with neuraxial techniques PNBs under sedation may provide superior HD stability
Perioperative use of anticoagulant/ antiplatelet medications	May present surgery-specific contraindications	Frequently contraindicates neuraxial and certain PNB procedures Epidural catheters may complicate postoperative DVT prophylaxis/anticoagulation
Pain control	Variable	Often superior

LA, Local anesthetic; *LAST,* local anesthetic systemic toxicity; *PNB,* peripheral nerve block; *ROM,* range of motion.

POSTOPERATIVE MANAGEMENT

8. Acute and chronic pain are both underreported and undertreated in the elderly. This is partly explained by the erroneously held belief that pain is a normal part of the aging process. In addition, assessing pain in patients with cognitive dysfunction can be more challenging. In such situations, it is helpful to engage closely with family and other caregivers who can offer more insight into a patient's subjective pain experience. This may manifest in the form of behavioral changes that are more likely to be underappreciated by a provider in a clinical setting. There are also a number of pain scoring systems designed to be used in patients with cognitive impairment, as noted in the table below.

Common Pain Scoring Tools

Tool	Assessment	Ideal Population
Visual Analog Scale	Patient places mark on graded line representing pain scale	Cognitively intact patients with difficulty speaking
Numeric Rating Scale	Pain score of 0–10	Cognitively intact, but validated in mild to moderate cognitively impaired patients
Verbal Descriptor Scale	Patient describes pain as "mild, moderate or severe"	Cognitively intact, but validated in mild to moderate cognitively impaired patients
Faces Scale	Patient chooses face that describes level of pain (frowning to smiling)	Validated in mild to moderate cognitively impaired patients
Pain Assessment Checklist for Seniors With Limited Ability to Communicate (PACSLAC)[a]	Observer scored assessment on a wide variety of scales of behavior, movement, facial expression	Validated in severe cognitively impaired patients
Pain Assessment in Advanced Dementia (PAINAD)[b]		
Doloplus-2[c]	Observer-scored assessment of somatic, psychomotor, and psychosocial parameters	

Data from Falzone E, Hoffmann C, Keita H. Postoperative analgesia in elderly patients. *Drugs Aging*. 2013;30(2):81–90; and Gagliese L, Katz J. Age differences in postoperative pain are scale dependent: A comparison of measures of pain intensity and quality in younger and older surgical patients. *Pain*. 2003;103(1–2):11–20. Modified from McKeown JL. Pain management issues for the geriatric surgical patient. *Anesthesiol Clin*. 2015;33(3):563–576.

[a]Fuchs-Lacelle S, Hadjistavropoulos T. Development and preliminary validation of the pain assessment checklist for seniors with limited ability to communicate (PACSLAC). *Pain Manag Nurs*. 2004;5(1):37–49.

[b]Warden V, Hurley AC, Volicer L. Development and psychometric evaluation of the Pain Assessment in Advanced Dementia (PAINAD) scale. *J Am Med Dir Assoc*. 2003;4(1):9–15.

[c]Lefebvre-Chapiro S. The DOLOPLUS 2 scale—Evaluating pain in the elderly. *Eur J Palliat Care*. 2001;8:191–194.

Treatment plans should focus both on reducing pain and improving functional capacity. Unlike their younger counterparts, elderly patients with dementia will be unlikely to benefit from patient-controlled analgesia (PCA) in the acute care setting. In addition, elderly patients are more sensitive to most of the analgesic effects of common pain medications, as well as their side effects, which can lead to life-threatening complications (e.g., respiratory arrest, falls). The best approach is often a multidisciplinary, multimodal approach (emphasizing nonopioid analgesics whenever possible) along with the use of regional techniques and interventional pain procedures that both treat pain and enhance functional capacity and quality of life. (655–657)

PERIOPERATIVE NEUROCOGNITIVE DISORDERS

9. Risk factors for the development of POD include preexisting cognitive impairment, advanced age, extent of comorbidities, higher ASA score, prolonged mechanical ventilation, uncontrolled pain, and medication effects. Benzodiazepines, drugs with central anticholinergic effects, and steroids are some of the more commonly implicated agents. Additionally, deeper planes of anesthesia also appear to contribute to POD. While POD is common (estimates ranging from 26% to 35%), it carries an increased risk of morbidity and mortality and is a strong predictor of developing dementia. Providers should use a multidisciplinary approach to preventing and treating POD, including frequent reorientation, maintenance of healthy sleep-wake cycles, provision of adequate visual and hearing aids as well as avoidance of urinary catheters and restraints whenever possible. Pharmacologic treatment should be reserved for severe cases when a patient is at risk of harm and typically include antipsychotic medications (e.g., haloperidol). At all times, providers should start by addressing any potentially serious underlying causes, such as hypoxemia, hypercarbia, electrolyte imbalances, or acute cerebral processes. (657–658)

Chapter

36 ORGAN TRANSPLANTATION

Randolph H. Steadman and Victor W. Xia

INTRODUCTION

- Donor death must be declared before organ procurement.
  - Donation after brain death is the most common.
  - Donation after cardiac death (DCD) is increasing due to organ shortages.
    - There are some ethical considerations with DCD, including respecting the end-of-life wishes of a potential donor and avoiding the potential for conflicts of interest.

CONSIDERATIONS FOR ORGAN TRANSPLANTATION

- Organ shortages have led to prolonged waits, typically 1 year or longer.
  - Some transplant candidates may not survive to organ transplantation.
  - Prelisting assessments may need to be updated and/or supplemented.

Contraindications for Organ Transplantation

- Systemic infection
- Incurable malignancy
- Untreated substance use disorder
- Insufficient social support to comply with posttransplant care

- Donor and recipient procedures must be coordinated, often at different hospitals.
  - Recipient operation should not begin until organ suitability is confirmed.
  - Recipient may need preoperative optimization, e.g., dialysis, laboratory values.

KIDNEY TRANSPLANTATION

- The kidney is the most frequently transplanted solid organ.
  - Improved quality-of-life benefit
  - Cost savings over dialysis for the management of renal failure
- Five-year posttransplant survival rates are 92% for live donor graft recipients and 83% for deceased donor recipients.
- The Kidney Donor Risk Index (KDRI), calculated from several donor characteristics, is used to assess the quality of a graft.

Preoperative Assessment

- Prolonged wait times make it challenging to maintain up-to-date preoperative assessments.
  - Over half of deceased donor kidney transplant candidates wait >5 years for an organ.
  - Living donor kidney transplants account for one-third of organ transplants and have shorter recipient waiting times.
- Diabetes, hypertension, and glomerulonephritis are the causes of renal failure in two-thirds of patients.

Key Points in Kidney Transplant Preoperative Assessment

Dialysis
- Review dialysis route and frequency.

Diabetes
- Most common cause of renal failure
- Medically manage to treatment goals.

Cardiovascular Disease
- Leading cause of death in dialysis patients and often undertreated
- Manage hypertension and hyperlipidemia to treatment goals.
- Assess for ischemic heart disease.
- Consider coronary angiography and intervention for significant lesions/risk.
- Cardiovascular risk decreases from 10 to 2 times normal after transplantation.

Congestive Heart Failure
- Medical management of intravascular fluids
- Ejection fraction typically improves after transplantation.

Key Points in Kidney Transplant Preoperative Assessment—Continued
Anemia ▪ Erythropoietin treatment to hemoglobin goal 12 g/dL decreases the risk of blood transfusion. **Hyperkalemia** ▪ Mild increases may reflect normal hemostasis. ▪ Potassium levels of 5.0 to 5.5 mEq/L are acceptable. ▪ Dialysis immediately before transplant corrects hyperkalemia but also reduces intravascular central volume.

Intraoperative Management

- Donor kidneys are usually implanted in the iliac fossa with vascular anastomoses to the iliac artery and veins, and the ureter directly to the bladder.
- Decreased protein binding increases the free fraction of protein-bound drugs, which increases the volume of distribution and clearance.
- Neuromuscular blocking drugs (NMBs), even those hepatically metabolized, may have prolonged durations of action in patients with renal failure.
  - Cisatracurium has a more predictable duration of action because of its spontaneous breakdown.
- Sugammadex–NMB complexes are renally excreted, leading to concerns of recurring paralysis if the complex dissociates.
  - Sugammadex has been safely administered to patients with end-stage renal disease (ESRD).
- Volatile anesthetics can be used in patients with renal failure, but produce dose-dependent decreases in renal blood flow.
- Balanced salt solutions are preferred for volume expansion.
  - Examples include lactated Ringer's solution and Plasma-Lyte.
  - Balanced solutions are associated with a reduced requirement for renal replacement in critically ill patients, compared with high-chloride solutions such as 0.9% saline.
  - Paradoxically, potassium-containing balanced salt solutions do not increase serum potassium as much as potassium-free hyperchloremic solutions (e.g., normal saline), which generate a hyperchloremic acidosis.
- Invasive arterial blood pressure monitoring is used sparingly to preserve arterial access for dialysis in some centers.
- Central venous catheters (CVCs) should be reserved for immunosuppression induction drugs or other drugs that need to be administered in a large-flow vein.
- Delayed graft function and acute tubular necrosis can lead to the need for posttransplant renal replacement therapy.
  - Outcomes are influenced by donor and recipient hemodynamics, adequate hydration, and graft warm ischemia time.
  - Osmotic diuretics, such as mannitol, may also be helpful.
    - Other diuretics are also variably administered.

Postoperative Management

- Maintaining renal perfusion is important and best accomplished by maintaining adequate intravascular volume.
  - Dopamine and diuretics postoperatively are of no proven benefit.
- Avoid nonsteroidal antiinflammatory drugs.
- Enhanced recovery after surgery (ERAS) pathways may help decrease length of stay.

LIVER TRANSPLANTATION

- The liver is the second most frequently transplanted solid organ.
- The median time to transplant for wait-listed candidates is 11 months.
  - Wait-listed patients: 25% are >65 years old, and >25% are hospitalized with comorbid conditions
- There is an ongoing shortage of organs.
  - Marginally viable grafts may be accepted, which include donors with advanced age, obesity, steatotic livers, malignancy, bacterial infections, DCD, prolonged ICU stays, on multiple vasopressors, or who had suffered cardiac arrest.

MELD Scores and Liver Transplantation
Factors for Calculation ▪ Dialysis (in the last week) ▪ Creatinine ▪ Bilirubin ▪ International normalized ratio (INR) ▪ Sodium **Scores of ≥35** ▪ One-fifth of transplant patients ▪ Median wait time to transplant is 7 days

Preoperative Assessment

- End-stage liver disease affects nearly every organ system.
- The most common indications for liver transplantation are nonalcoholic steatohepatitis (NASH, associated with metabolic syndrome) and alcohol-associated liver disease, followed by malignancy, cholestatic disease, hepatitis C, and acute liver failure.
- Patients have varying symptoms.

Key Points in Liver Transplant Preoperative Assessment

Encephalopathy
- Sensitivity to sedatives and analgesics
- Increased risk of aspiration of gastric contents, need for endotracheal intubation

Cardiovascular Disease
- Assess for ischemic heart disease through testing or cardiac catheterization.
- Commonly have hyperdynamic circulation
  - High cardiac output and low systemic vascular resistance (SVR)
  - Likely due to circulating vasoactive substances

Portopulmonary Hypertension (PPHTN) Screening
- Echocardiography, then right-sided heart catheterization if indicated
- Moderate PPHTN is associated with increased perioperative mortality and warrants consideration of pretransplant treatment.
- Severe PPHTN is a contraindication to transplant in some centers.

Hepatopulmonary Syndrome
- Pao_2 <70 mmHg on room air with intrapulmonary shunt on bubble echocardiography; typically resolves posttransplant
- Pao_2 <50 mm Hg is associated with longer hospital stays and higher mortality.

Hepatorenal Syndrome
- Renal disease is common due to excessive volume, acidosis, and/or hyperkalemia.
- May resolve after transplantation depending on chronicity

Coagulopathy
- Multifactorial; may not need correction unless there is active bleeding
- Endogenous anticoagulants may also be reduced, leading to thrombosis risk.

Acute Liver Failure
- Less than 5% of liver transplant patients
- Potential for cerebral edema and death

Gastrointestinal
- Variceal bleeding history
- Ascites

Intraoperative Management

- Considerations for drug and anesthetic choices include how liver failure may affect their metabolism, effects in encephalopathic patients, and their effect on SVR.
- Intraoperative monitoring varies by center.
  - An arterial line and large-bore central venous access are typically placed.
  - Pulmonary artery catheter (PAC) may be placed.
  - Transesophageal echocardiography (TEE) is gold standard for cardiac preload monitoring but can only be used intraoperatively and is operator dependent.
- Venovenous bypass is used in some cases to reroute blood from the inferior vena cava and portal venous systems to the upper body.
- The operative course is divided into preanhepatic, anhepatic, and neohepatic phases.

Operative Phases of Liver Transplantation

Preanhepatic
- Prepares for native hepatectomy
- Associated with blood loss, especially with varices or previous surgery

Anhepatic
- Clamping of the inferior vena cava (IVC), portal vein, and hepatic artery (vascular isolation)
- Excision of the native liver
- Implantation of the donor graft (two approaches)
  - Anastomosis of suprahepatic IVC, infrahepatic IVC, and the portal vein ("full caval clamp")
  - Anastomosis of donor hepatic veins to recipient vena cava, then portal anastomosis ("piggyback" technique); typically, venous return is better preserved with piggyback technique compared to full caval clamp

Neohepatic
- Reperfusion: release of cold acidotic effluent from the graft and lower extremities
- Associated with reperfusion syndrome, fibrinolysis
- Most precarious phase, which can be life-threatening
- Signs of liver function include improvement of acidosis, increased core temperature, decreasing calcium requirement, and increased urine output in previously oliguric patients.

Postoperative Management

- Posttransplant survival rates are 89% at 1 year and 77% at 5 years.
- Thrombosis of the hepatic artery usually necessitates retransplantation.
- Infection is a major threat to survival in the initial months after transplant.

HEART TRANSPLANTATION

- Indication for 90% of transplants is ischemic and idiopathic dilated cardiomyopathy.
- 1-year survival is about 90%.

Preoperative Evaluation

- Detailed preanesthetic evaluation is challenging owing to the urgent nature of the surgery, the complex clinical presentation, and multiple comorbid conditions.

Key Points in Heart Transplant Preoperative Assessment

The review should include
- Medications, especially inotropes and anticoagulants
- Cardiac status, including pacemakers, defibrillators, and mechanical devices
- Function of other organs
  - Pulmonary hypertension should be excluded.
  - Multiple organ failure may result in combined transplant (e.g., liver, kidney, or lung).
- Active infection should be excluded.

Intraoperative Management

- An arterial line, CVC, and PAC are routinely used.
  - PAC is withdrawn to the jugular vein before the native heart is excised.
- TEE is used for assessment of intravascular volume status, contractility, valvular function, and potential thromboembolism.
- Maintenance of anesthesia is often by a combination of a volatile anesthetic and an opioid.
- Anesthetic technique is selected to minimize hemodynamic changes.
  - Maintain systemic blood pressure and coronary filling
  - Optimize preload and reduce afterload to improve ejection fraction
  - Avoid pulmonary vasoconstriction
  - Support contractility
- Weaning from cardiopulmonary bypass includes rewarming, electrolyte and acid-base correction, ensuring cardiac chambers are free of air, and ventilating with 100% oxygen.

Intraoperative Issues Unique to Cardiac Transplant

The transplanted heart is denervated.
- Heart rate does not respond to hemodynamic changes or indirect-acting drugs.
- Bradycardia after reperfusion must be treated by pacing or chronotropic drugs.

Failure to wean from cardiopulmonary bypass is often caused by right-sided heart failure.
- Preexisting pulmonary hypertension can worsen during reperfusion, and the right ventricle is prone to ischemia/reperfusion injury.
- Causes: increases in cardiac output, pulmonary vessel spasm, and blood or air embolism are all possible
- Treatment goals are to decrease pulmonary artery (PA) resistance with selective vasodilators and increase right ventricular contractility.
  - Medical management can include inhaled nitric oxide, aerosolized iloprost, and inhaled or infused sildenafil.
  - Mechanical right ventricular support may be necessary.

Postoperative Management

- Postoperative management targets adequate oxygenation, ventilation, intravascular volume, pulmonary and systemic pressures, coagulation, and body temperature.
- Inotropic and chronotropic support are commonly needed postoperatively for a few days.
- Some patients require permanent pacemaker implantation for sinus node function loss.
- Nonfunctional graft and posttransplant bleeding can be life-threatening emergencies.
- Graft vasculopathy and immunosuppression-related side effects affect long-term survival.

LUNG TRANSPLANTATION

- Chronic obstructive lung disease, bronchiectasis, and interstitial lung disease are common indications for lung transplantation in adults.
- Cystic fibrosis is the most common indication in children.
- Bilateral lung transplant constitutes 75% of lung transplants.
  - Use of two sequential single lung transplants during the same surgery avoids cardiopulmonary bypass.

Preoperative Evaluation

- The focus is on the lung disease severity, baseline function of other vital organs, the airway, and any interval changes since the last examination.

Key Points in Lung Transplant Preoperative Assessment

- Avoid sedatives or uncontrolled anxiety that can worsen pulmonary hypertension.
- Supplemental oxygen should be administered cautiously; most lung transplant patients depend on their hypoxic drive.
- Consider epidural analgesia for postoperative pain control.

Intraoperative Management

- Monitoring includes arterial catheter, CVC, and PAC (often with mixed venous O_2 sampling and cardiac output monitoring), and TEE.
- Induction of anesthesia balances the risk of aspiration of gastric contents with hypoxia and hemodynamic instability.
- Positive-pressure ventilation can cause decreased venous blood return (even cardiac arrest), further damage to diseased lungs, and worse hypoxia and hypercarbia.

Intraoperative Issues Unique to Lung Transplant
Endobronchoscopy is a necessary monitor used to ▪ Assess the position of the double-lumen endotracheal tube ▪ Examine the airway anastomoses ▪ Examine for bleeding and obstruction secondary to blood or sputum **Protective ventilation strategies should be used.** ▪ Small tidal volumes, avoidance of air trapping and barotrauma **Ventilation-reperfusion mismatch** ▪ Hypoxia is a challenging issue and managed similarly to thoracic surgery. **Pulmonary artery (PA) hypertension** ▪ PA hypertension is challenging, and PA pressure increases further with PA clamping. ▪ PA pressure can be decreased by intravascular fluid restriction and administration of selective and nonselective pulmonary vasodilators (inhaled and intravascular). **Noncardiogenic pulmonary edema** ▪ Develops frequently in lung transplant patients ▪ Excessive intravascular fluid administration should be avoided.

Postoperative Management

- Denervation of the transplanted lungs leads to a loss of normal cough reflexes, predisposing to infection.
- Special care in the postoperative period is provided to avoid barotrauma, volutrauma, and anastomotic dehiscence during positive-pressure mechanical ventilation.
- Post-lung transplantation mortality is primarily due to anastomotic dehiscence and respiratory failure caused by sepsis or rejection.

PANCREAS TRANSPLANTATION

- The most common indication for pancreas transplantation is type 1 diabetes.
- Endogenous insulin, normoglycemia, and the glucagon response are restored.
- Most pancreas transplants are performed simultaneously with kidney transplants.

Key Points in Pancreas Transplant Preoperative Assessment
▪ Diabetes mellitus affects cardiovascular, autonomic, nervous, renal, gastrointestinal, and metabolic systems. ▪ Neuropathy and silent ischemia make coronary artery disease difficult to diagnose. ▪ Evaluation may need to include a preoperative stress test or coronary angiogram. ▪ Renal function, acid-base status, electrolytes, and hemoglobin should be checked.

- Pancreas transplantation can be performed under general or regional anesthesia.

Intraoperative Issues Unique to Pancreas Transplant
▪ Diabetic autonomic nervous system dysfunction risks should be considered. ▪ Glucose levels should be closely monitored intraoperatively and postoperatively. – Severe intraoperative hyperglycemia may adversely affect islet function and promote posttransplant infection. – Graft function after reperfusion can lead to hypoglycemia.

CONCLUSION

- Patients presenting for organ transplantation have end-stage disease of one or more organs, and many are critically ill.
- Anesthetic management tailored to the patient's comorbid conditions is vital for successful transplant.

QUESTIONS

CONSIDERATIONS FOR ORGAN TRANSPLANTATION

1. What defines donation after brain death (DBD) and donation after cardiac death (DCD)?

KIDNEY TRANSPLANTATION

2. What is the kidney donor risk index?
3. You are doing a preoperative evaluation for a patient who is scheduled to undergo a deceased donor renal transplant. The patient has end-stage renal disease (ESRD) secondary to diabetes mellitus, is dialysis-dependent, and has a hemoglobin of 9.8 and a potassium of 5.4. What are some preoperative considerations?
4. What are some intraoperative considerations for the anesthetic management of patients undergoing renal transplantation?
5. For each drug listed below, describe the considerations specific for patients undergoing renal transplantation.

Drug	Consideration for Patients With Renal Failure
Pancuronium	
Vecuronium Rocuronium	
Cisatracurium	
Atracurium	
Succinylcholine	
Sugammadex	
Morphine	
Meperidine	
Sevoflurane	
Desflurane	

6. Why should intravascular fluid balance be maintained in patients undergoing renal transplantation? Which crystalloid and colloid are preferred?
7. Which diuretics are commonly used during renal transplantation?
8. How is maintenance of renal perfusion best accomplished postoperatively?

LIVER TRANSPLANTATION

9. What are common indications for liver transplantation in the United States?
10. What is the clinical application of the MELD (Model for End-Stage Liver Disease) score?
11. What are some preoperative considerations for patients undergoing liver transplantation?
12. Describe the characteristic hemodynamic pattern commonly seen in patients with end-stage liver disease.
13. What is the best screening test for portopulmonary hypertension? What is its clinical significance?
14. What is hepatopulmonary syndrome? What is its clinical significance?
15. What is the most common cause of death in acute liver failure?
16. What are the goals of the anesthetic plan for liver transplantation?
17. For each drug listed below, describe the considerations specific for patients undergoing liver transplantation.

Drug	Consideration for Patients With Liver Failure
Anxiolytics	
Vecuronium and Rocuronium	
Cisatracurium	

Drug	Consideration for Patients With Liver Failure
Meperidine	
Morphine	
Fentanyl	
Volatile anesthetics	

18. What is the rationale for venovenous bypass use in liver transplantation?
19. Complete the following chart defining the three operative phases of liver transplant and the operative portion of liver transplant that defines each stage.

Phase of Liver Transplant	Operative Portion of the Liver Transplant
Preanhepatic	
Anhepatic	
Neohepatic	

20. What are the characteristic physiologic derangements of the preanhepatic stage of liver transplantation?
21. What are the characteristic physiologic derangements of the anhepatic stage of liver transplantation?
22. What are the classic and "piggy-back" techniques in liver transplantation?
23. What are the characteristic physiologic derangements that occur with reperfusion of the donor graft during the neohepatic phase of liver transplantation? How can it be managed?
24. What signs of liver function can be assessed intraoperatively after graft reperfusion?

HEART TRANSPLANTATION

25. What are some preoperative considerations when assessing the patient undergoing heart transplantation?
26. What are some perioperative goals for the anesthetic management of heart transplant patients?
27. Which vessels are transected and anastomosed during heart transplant surgery? What does this mean with regard to a central venous or pulmonary artery catheter?
28. A patient has become bradycardic during reperfusion during heart transplantation. What effect would you expect from the administration of atropine? What are some other treatment options?
29. A patient who is undergoing heart transplantation develops right-sided heart failure during reperfusion. What are some possible causes and treatment options?
30. What are some possible causes of pulmonary hypertension during heart transplantation, and how can it be treated?
31. Name the physiologic conditions that should be optimized prior to weaning from cardiopulmonary bypass.
32. What are some postoperative considerations in the management of heart transplant patients?

LUNG TRANSPLANTATION

33. What are some preoperative considerations for the patient undergoing lung transplantation?
34. Why are double-lumen endotracheal tubes used for intubation of the trachea during lung transplantation?
35. In addition to standard monitors and transesophageal echocardiography (TEE), why is endobronchoscopy necessary during lung transplantation?
36. What are some challenges and strategies in the anesthetic management of patients undergoing a lung transplantation?
37. What are some postoperative management considerations in the lung transplant patient?

PANCREAS TRANSPLANTATION

38. What are some preoperative considerations in patients undergoing pancreas transplantation?
39. Why should intraoperative hyperglycemia be avoided in patients undergoing pancreas transplantation?
40. What other organ is often transplanted simultaneously along with the pancreas?

ANSWERS

CONSIDERATIONS FOR ORGAN TRANSPLANTATION

1. Organ procurement occurs most frequently in the setting of donation after brain death (DBD). Brain death is the irreversible loss of clinical function of the brain, including the brain stem. Because of organ shortages, the number of grafts from donation after cardiac death (DCD) is increasing, although it remains a minority of donors. Candidates for DCD are patients who have irreversible brain injury but do not meet brain death criteria and who are not expected to survive once life-preserving measures such as mechanical ventilation are withdrawn. In DCD, life support is withdrawn, cardiac death is confirmed, and then the organs are procured. For DCD, there is a period of warm ischemia that does not occur in DBD. (661)

KIDNEY TRANSPLANTATION

2. The kidney donor risk index (KDRI) provides an assessment of risk associated with donor kidneys using several donor characteristics. The following donor characteristics are used to calculate the kidney donor profile index. (662)
   - Age
   - Height
   - Weight
   - Ethnicity
   - History of hypertension
   - History of diabetes
   - Cause of death
   - Serum creatinine
   - Hepatitis C virus status
   - Donation after circulatory death status
3. Preoperative considerations for the patient scheduled to undergo a renal transplant procedure are similar to those for any other surgical procedure in which the patient has chronic renal failure. This includes scheduling of hemodialysis prior to surgery to optimize the patient's volume status, electrolytes, and acid-base balance. Patients who are potential renal transplant recipients should have a preoperative assessment for ischemic heart disease since the cardiovascular risk in patients requiring dialysis is increased tenfold compared to that of normal patients. In addition, ischemic heart disease may be silent, particularly in patients with diabetes. As a result of preexisting vasodilation, stress echocardiography is probably better than thallium imaging in predicting postoperative cardiac events. Coronary angiography should be considered in high-risk patients. The preoperative serum glucose levels of the patient with diabetes mellitus should also be evaluated and treated if necessary. Potassium levels of 5.0 to 5.5 mEq/L are acceptable in patients scheduled to undergo renal transplantation; mild increases in potassium may reflect normal homeostasis for patients with renal failure. Anemia is common in patients with renal failure but may increase cardiovascular risk in patients who also have ischemic heart disease. Erythropoietin treatment (if time allows) or blood transfusion may be considered after assessing the severity of anemia, hemodynamics, and other patient comorbidities. (662)
4. Some intraoperative considerations for the anesthetic management of patients undergoing renal transplantation include drug excretion, management of intravascular volume and adequate hemodynamics, appropriate monitoring, and minimizing the risk of renal dysfunction in the transplanted kidney. (663)
5. Choice of drugs during anesthesia for renal transplantation should consider drug metabolism and duration of action, and the potential for the buildup of toxic metabolites. (663)

Drug	Consideration for Patients With Renal Failure
Pancuronium	Prolonged duration of action
Vecuronium	Prolonged duration of action
Rocuronium	Prolonged duration of action
Cisatracurium	Metabolism is independent of both the kidney and liver and an attractive choice for these patients.
Atracurium	Metabolite laudanosine is renally excreted and has seizure-inducing potential in high concentrations. At clinical doses, laudanosine concentrations are unlikely to cause seizures.

Drug	Consideration for Patients With Renal Failure
Succinylcholine	Can be used provided that the serum potassium is not acutely elevated Renal failure is not a contraindication.
Sugammadex	Sugammadex–neuromuscular blocker complex is renally excreted. Concern for recurring paralysis if the complex dissociates Has been safely administered to patients with renal failure
Morphine	Metabolite (morphine-6-glucoronide) is renally cleared and active, resulting in a prolonged clinical effect.
Meperidine	Metabolite (normeperidine) is renally cleared and has seizure-inducing potential.
Sevoflurane	Produces a nephrotoxic metabolite (compound A) in rat models Fluoride levels produced through metabolism are negligible. Causes dose-dependent decrease in renal blood flow and glomerular filtration rate Is clinically safe to use in patients with renal failure
Desflurane	Dose-dependent decrease in renal blood flow and glomerular filtration rate Is clinically safe to use in patients with renal failure

6. Intravascular fluid balance should be maintained during renal transplantation to improve renal perfusion; adequate intravascular fluid balance has been shown to reduce the incidence of acute tubular necrosis in the transplanted kidney. In an intensive care unit (ICU) population, balanced salt solutions (e.g., lactated Ringer's, Plasma-Lyte) are preferred over hyperchloremic crystalloid such as normal saline because they are associated with a lower incidence of acute kidney injury. Paradoxically, balanced salt solutions (which contain potassium) elevate serum potassium levels less than potassium-free crystalloids because the potassium-free crystalloids (e.g., 0.9% saline) elevate potassium levels by generating a hyperchloremic acidotic state. Albumin is the colloid of choice in these patients. (663)
7. The diuretics mannitol and furosemide are often administered intraoperatively during renal transplant procedures to facilitate diuresis and decrease the risk of delayed graft function and acute tubular necrosis. Controlled studies supporting an improved outcome in graft function are lacking, although the administration of osmotic diuretics, such as mannitol, may be helpful. (663–664)
8. Maintaining renal perfusion in the postoperative period is best accomplished by maintaining intravascular volume status. Dopamine, large-dose diuretics, and osmotic diuretics provide no proven benefit. (664)

LIVER TRANSPLANTATION

9. Currently the most common indications for liver transplantation in the United States are nonalcoholic steatohepatitis (NASH) and alcohol-associated liver disease, followed by malignancy, cholestatic disease, hepatitis C, and acute liver failure. NASH, a diagnosis associated with metabolic syndrome and obesity, is an increasingly prevalent indication for liver transplantation. Hepatitis C, the most common indication for transplantation over the previous decade, has decreased significantly due to antiviral agents. (664)
10. The MELD score, derived from calculation of three laboratory values (the international normalized prothrombin time, creatinine, and bilirubin), is an index of severity of liver disease. Recently, sodium was added into the calculation to create the MELD-Na score. The MELD, or MELD-Na score, predicts 90-day mortality risk in the absence of liver transplantation and thus is used to allocate organs for liver transplantation. (664)
11. Preoperative considerations for the patient undergoing liver transplantation include screening for ischemic heart disease, portopulmonary hypertension, hepatopulmonary syndrome, variceal bleeding, ascites, renal disease, acid-base abnormalities, coagulopathy, anemia, and encephalopathy. Encephalopathy, even if not clinically overt, can lead to sensitivity to sedative and analgesic medications. (664–665)
12. The hyperdynamic circulation commonly seen in liver transplant recipients is characterized by a high cardiac output and low systemic vascular resistance. The decreased afterload contributes to the elevated cardiac output. This hyperdynamic state can be confused with sepsis. (664–665)
13. Resting echocardiography is a highly sensitive screening test for portopulmonary hypertension; however, it is not specific. Therefore patients with an elevated estimated right ventricular systolic pressure should undergo right-sided heart catheterization to confirm or rule out the diagnosis. Mean pulmonary artery pressures higher than 35 mm Hg are associated with increased perioperative complications, and treatment prior to transplantation should be considered. (665)
14. Hepatopulmonary syndrome (HPS) consists of arterial hypoxemia (Pa_{O_2} <70 mmHg on room air) in the presence of an intrapulmonary shunt. Liver transplantation cures HPS, albeit over a variable time course.

A preoperative Pa_{O_2} <50 mmHg is associated with greater postoperative morbidity and, in some studies, postoperative fatality. (629)

15. Cerebral edema is the most common cause of death in acute liver failure. Acute liver failure accounts for approximately 5% of liver transplantations. (665)
16. The goals of the anesthetic plan for liver transplantation are to maintain systemic vascular resistance and to avoid intravenous agents that undergo extensive hepatic metabolism. In addition, rapid transfusion of fluids and products should be possible. There should be availability of vasopressors, laboratory analysis, and intraoperative monitoring with arterial and central venous catheters, and possibly transesophageal echocardiography (TEE). (665)
17. Choice of drugs during anesthesia for liver transplantation should consider drug metabolism and duration of action, and the potential for the buildup of toxic metabolites, as highlighted in the table below. (665)

Drug	Consideration for Patients With Liver Failure
Anxiolytics	Use sparingly in patients with a history of encephalopathy.
Vecuronium and Rocuronium	May have prolonged duration of action After reperfusion, metabolism may improve once the newly implanted liver functions.
Cisatracurium	Metabolism is independent of the liver.
Meperidine	Hepatically metabolized, can have a prolonged effect The metabolite, normeperidine, has seizure-inducing potential and can accumulate if patients have renal insufficiency.
Morphine	Hepatically metabolized, can have a prolonged effect The metabolite, morphine-6-glucoronide, is active and can have prolonged effect in patients with renal insufficiency.
Volatile anesthetics	Mild decreases in hepatic blood flow but is frequently used clinically

18. When the vena cava is fully clamped (classic caval interruption), venous return decreases markedly and can cause hemodynamic instability. Some centers use extracorporeal venovenous bypass, in which blood is rerouted from the inferior vena cava to the superior vena cava in order to augment venous return. (665–666)
19. (666)

Phase of Liver Transplant	Operative Portion of the Liver Transplantation
Preanhepatic	Dissection of the portal venous structures and mobilization of the native liver for resection
Anhepatic	Vascular isolation of the native liver by cross-clamping of the inferior vena cava, portal vein, and hepatic artery Excision of the native liver Implantation of the donor graft and vascular anastomoses
Neohepatic	Reperfusion, usually via the vena cava and portal vein

20. The preanhepatic stage of liver transplantation is characterized by cardiovascular instability because of sudden decreases in the intraabdominal pressure and the exacerbation of chronic hypovolemia due to loss of ascites and hemorrhage. Metabolic and electrolyte abnormalities can occur during this stage, including metabolic acidosis, and hypocalcemia resulting from citrate toxicity. Hemorrhage, often requiring the rapid infusion of fluids and blood products, is related to the degree of portal hypertension and adhesions from prior abdominal surgery. (666)
21. The anhepatic stage of liver transplantation is characterized by decreases in venous return and cardiac output. For this reason, sympathomimetic drugs are often administered during this portion of the procedure to maintain cardiac output. Hypocalcemia and metabolic acidosis commonly occur during this stage as a result of citrate toxicity and decreased renal perfusion pressure, respectively. The anhepatic stage is the most hemodynamically quiescent stage of liver transplantation. (666)
22. The classic surgical technique involves dissection and anastomoses of the suprahepatic IVC, the infrahepatic IVC, and the portal vein. The "piggy-back" technique, an alternative to the classic caval-interruption technique, involves the anastomosis of the donor hepatic veins to the recipient vena cava. In general, venous return is better preserved during the anhepatic phase with the piggyback technique unless venovenous bypass is used. (666)

23. The neohepatic stage of liver transplant procedures is characterized by the potential for precipitous hyperkalemia, acidosis, and hypothermia due to the cold, acidotic effluent from the graft and lower extremities entering the central circulation. The systemic vascular resistance drops, and emboli of blood or air can occur. Hyperkalemia is exacerbated by the washout of the potassium-containing solution used to preserve the liver, in addition to unclamping of the inferior vena cava and portal vein. Fibrinolysis can also occur, leading to ongoing oozing due to microvascular bleeding. Antifibrinolytic drugs may need to be administered if the fibrinolysis is not self-limited. Hypotension, arrhythmias, and cardiac arrest may potentially occur during this time. *Reperfusion syndrome* is a term used to describe these physiologic changes. Insulin (effective if given in advance), calcium, adrenergic agonists, and alkalizing agents are often administered to treat hyperkalemia and maintain systemic vascular resistance and pH during this period. Warm saline with peritoneal lavage can help rewarm the patient. (666, Box 36.5)
24. Signs of liver function after graft reperfusion include improvement in metabolic acidosis (due to metabolism of citrate to bicarbonate), a reduced calcium requirement (due to the metabolism of citrate), and a rising body temperature (due to exothermic reactions in the liver). In some cases, an increase in urine output may reflect the resolution of hepatorenal syndrome. (666)

HEART TRANSPLANTATION

25. Preoperative considerations when assessing the patient undergoing heart transplantation include current cardiac status, inotropic and anticoagulant drugs, and mechanical support required, such as an intraaortic balloon pump or ventricular assist device. Patients should not have severe, irreversible pulmonary hypertension or active infection. Finally, because of the urgency of the procedure, heart transplant patients often have a full stomach. (666–667)
26. Perioperative goals for the anesthetic management of heart transplant patients include maintaining systemic blood pressure and coronary filling, optimizing preload, reducing afterload to improve ejection fraction, supporting contractility, correcting acid-base abnormalities, and avoiding pulmonary vasoconstriction, hypercapnia, and high tidal volumes. The induction and maintenance of anesthesia should provide favorable endotracheal intubating conditions while preserving cardiac function. Selection of drugs is dictated by underlying heart condition and assessment of benefits and risks of each drug. (667)
27. Vessels and structures that are transected and anastomosed during heart transplant procedures include the aorta, pulmonary artery, and left and right atria. These steps are done during cardiopulmonary bypass. A central venous or pulmonary artery catheter that is in place at the onset of surgery must be pulled back into the internal jugular vein when the patient's heart is excised. (667)
28. Bradycardia may be seen after reperfusion in the donor heart because it is denervated and not responsive to hemodynamic changes. Atropine and other indirect-acting drugs that work via the autonomic nervous system are ineffective because of denervation of the graft. The transplanted heart reacts better to direct-acting catecholamines. Bradycardia can be treated by pacing (usually 90–110 beats/min) or chronotropic drugs such as isoproterenol. Isoproterenol maintains myocardial contractility and heart rate in the denervated donor heart and decreases pulmonary vasculature resistance. (667)
29. While undergoing heart transplantation, right-sided heart failure may be seen during reperfusion because of pulmonary hypertension or ischemia of the right ventricle. The primary treatment goals of right-sided heart failure during heart transplantation are to increase contractility of the right ventricle and decrease pulmonary vascular resistance. Failure to respond to treatment may necessitate mechanical right ventricular support. (667)
30. Pulmonary hypertension during heart transplantation can be due to an increase in cardiac output, pulmonary vessel spasm, and emboli. It is exacerbated by hypoxemia and hypercarbia. Treatment of pulmonary hypertension can be with nonselective vasodilators, such as nitroglycerin and sodium nitroprusside, but these drugs can also decrease systemic vascular resistance and result in systemic hypotension. Selective pulmonary vasodilators, such as inhaled nitric oxide, aerosolized iloprost, and sildenafil, may be helpful. (667)
31. Prior to weaning from cardiopulmonary bypass, patients should be normothermic and free from acid-base and electrolyte disturbances. The lungs should be ventilated, and the cardiac chambers should be free from air. (667)
32. Postoperative considerations in heart transplant patients include management of oxygenation, ventilation, intravascular volume, pulmonary and systemic pressures, coagulation, and body temperature. Inotropic and chronotropic support is often required in the few days following heart transplant. Permanent pacemaker implantation may be necessary because of the loss of sinus node function. Patients should be monitored for postoperative bleeding and graft function, which can require emergent intervention. (667-668)

LUNG TRANSPLANTATION

33. Preoperative considerations for the patient undergoing lung transplantation include the severity of the pulmonary disease, controlling anxiety without oversedation, cautious use of supplemental oxygen so as not to abolish the hypoxic drive, and possible epidural placement for postoperative pain management. (668)
34. Double-lumen endotracheal tubes are used for intubation of the trachea for lung transplantation to allow for isolated ventilation of either the left or right lung. One lung may be ventilated while the other is being transplanted. (668)
35. Endobronchoscopy is necessary during lung transplantation not only to assess the position of the double-lumen endotracheal tube, but also to examine airway anastomoses for stenosis, bleeding, or obstruction secondary to blood or sputum. (668)
36. Challenges in the anesthetic management of patients undergoing lung transplantation are multiple. The onset of positive-pressure ventilation can cause a precipitous decrease in venous return and potential cardiac arrest in patients with severe pulmonary hypertension. Positive-pressure ventilation further damages diseased lungs and worsens hypoxemia and hypercarbia, air trapping, barotrauma, and ventilation-perfusion mismatch during one-lung ventilation. It also contributes to pulmonary hypertension during pulmonary artery clamping, particularly in patients with preexisting elevation of pulmonary artery pressure. Strategies for the management of patients undergoing lung transplant include preparation for emergent cardiopulmonary bypass during the induction of anesthesia, ventilation with low tidal volumes, intravascular fluid volume restriction, and the use of nonselective and selective pulmonary vasodilators. (668)
37. Some postoperative management considerations in the lung transplant patient include the avoidance of barotrauma, volutrauma, and anastomotic dehiscence during positive-pressure ventilation. Lung transplant patients are also predisposed to pneumonia in the transplanted lung due to disruption of lymphatic drainage, poor mucociliary function, obstruction of bronchi from clots in the bronchial suture lines, and loss of the cough reflex. Immunosuppression exacerbates the risk of infection. (668)

PANCREAS TRANSPLANTATION

38. Preoperative considerations in patients undergoing pancreas transplantation are similar to those undergoing kidney transplant for end-stage renal disease secondary to diabetes. They include assessment of the effects of diabetes on cardiovascular, autonomic, nervous, renal, gastrointestinal, and metabolic systems. (668)
39. Intraoperative hyperglycemia should be avoided in patients undergoing pancreas transplantation because it may adversely affect islet function and promote posttransplant infection. (669)
40. Pancreas transplant procedures are often performed simultaneously with kidney transplantation because of the advanced nature of the diabetes, which is associated with renal failure. Simultaneous pancreas-kidney transplant recipients experience the best graft survival rates. The success of a pancreas transplant is measured by monitoring blood glucose levels after surgery; blood glucose concentrations may return to normal within hours. (669)

Chapter

37 OUTPATIENT ANESTHESIA

Jeremy Juang

INTRODUCTION

- Ambulatory anesthesia involves three distinct areas.
  - Outpatient anesthesia
  - Office-based anesthesia (OBA)
  - Nonoperating room anesthesia (NORA)
- History
  - Over 100 years ago, the first ambulatory surgical center (ASC) opened in Iowa.
  - In 1970 the first modern ASC opened in Phoenix, Arizona.
  - In 2014 more than half of hospital visits that included surgeries were performed in ambulatory settings.
- Society for Ambulatory Anesthesia (SAMBA)
  - Founded in 1985 as a resource for providers working in ambulatory settings
  - Issues statements and an evidence-based guide for ASCs
- The American Society of Anesthesiologists (ASA) issued guidelines for ambulatory anesthesia and surgery in 2003, reaffirmed in 2018.

Ambulatory Anesthesia Settings

- Patient flow for ambulatory surgery includes the following steps:
  - Arrive at the facility
  - Undergo the surgery or invasive procedure
  - Discharge home on the same day (or within 23 hours)
- Ambulatory surgery can be performed in a variety of facilities.
  - Outpatient office
  - Freestanding ASC
  - ASC with extended stay (<23 hours)
  - ASC within a hospital
  - Hospital operating room (OR)
  - NORA locations

Nonoperating Room Anesthesia

- Historically known as remote anesthesia or out-of-operating room anesthesia
- Nonoperating room anesthesia (NORA) is an anesthesia service provided in a hospital unit, away from ORs.
- Common NORA procedures include the following:
  - Cardiac catheterization
  - Electrophysiology procedures
  - Gastrointestinal endoscopy
  - Interventional radiology procedures
- Challenges of providing anesthesia care in NORA location
  - Patients deemed "too sick" for surgery under general anesthesia
  - Limited physical access to patients during procedure due to room size or large equipment such as fluoroscopy
  - Limited resources including availability of specialized anesthesia equipment, staff, and medications
- NORA patients compared to patients in a general OR
  - Tend to be older
  - More likely to receive monitored anesthesia care instead of general anesthesia

Office-Based Anesthesia

- Involves surgery and other procedures performed at small offices outside of a hospital or ASC setting
- Most common procedures are short-duration elective surgeries associated with minimal blood loss.
  - Examples: cosmetic, dental, podiatric, and certain vascular procedures such as varicose vein treatment
- Office-based facilities are less regulated than ASCs.
  - Patient safety concerns have led to increasing state legislation and professional society guidelines.
  - Some offices are equipped with anesthesia machines; some require anesthesia providers to transport their own equipment and medications.
  - Logistical issues regarding management of Drug Enforcement Administration controlled medications can be a challenge.

- Office-based providers experience a different professional environment than hospital-based providers.
  - Advantages include greater scheduling and financial arrangement flexibility.

PATIENT SELECTION

- Patient selection and optimization are essential for safe outpatient anesthesia.
- Type of facility should be appropriate for procedure and patient comorbidities.
- Preoperative evaluation process should be the same as for inpatient surgery.
- ASA Practice Guidelines for Postanesthetic Care recommend that a responsible individual should accompany a patient home after surgery.

SURGERIES AND PROCEDURES

The most commonly performed ambulatory surgery procedures are listed in the box below.

Ten Most Common Ambulatory Procedures in the United States

1. Lens and cataract procedures
2. Muscle, tendon, and soft tissue operating room procedures (most commonly, rotator cuff repair and trigger finger surgery)
3. Incision or fusion of joint or destruction of joint lesion (most commonly knee and shoulder arthroscopies)
4. Cholecystectomy and common duct exploration
5. Excision of semilunar cartilage of knee
6. Inguinal and femoral hernia repair
7. Repair of diaphragmatic, incisional, and umbilical hernia
8. Tonsillectomy and/or adenoidectomy
9. Decompression of peripheral nerve
10. Operating room procedures of the skin and breast, including plastic procedures of breast

- The spectrum of ambulatory surgeries has been expanding due to several factors.
  - Substantial growth in equipment, techniques, and expertise in minimally invasive surgeries
  - For example, freestanding ASCs have embarked on performing major joint surgeries (e.g., knee and hip arthroplasty) as an outpatient procedure.
  - Successful programs include the following:
    - Strict patient selection criteria
    - Anesthetic regimen facilitating early mobility and adequate pain control
    - Presence of a dedicated team, perioperative care protocol, scheduling, preoperative nutrition, patient education, discharge planning, postoperative pain, and physical therapy management

PREOPERATIVE EVALUATION

- Several conditions can present challenges in providing ambulatory anesthesia.

Obstructive Sleep Apnea

- Obstructive sleep apnea (OSA) is the most common sleep-related breathing disorder.
- Risks of OSA include difficult airway management, intraoperative hypoxemia (potentially life-threatening), need for postoperative tracheal reintubation, and unanticipated hospital admission.
- SAMBA consensus statement on selection of patients with OSA for ambulatory surgery includes the following considerations.
  - Recommended use of STOP-BANG tool for OSA screening
    - STOP-BANG score ≥3 is associated with increased postoperative complications.
  - Screen the patient for common comorbid conditions such as hypertension, arrhythmias, cerebrovascular disease, and metabolic syndrome.
  - Because opioids can exacerbate OSA, consider whether painful surgery that is not amenable to nonopioid analgesia techniques should be performed as inpatient surgery instead of as an ambulatory procedure.
  - Patients with known OSA should continue continuous positive airway pressure (CPAP) or bilevel positive airway pressure (BiPAP) postoperatively.
- ASA has also published practice guidelines for perioperative management of OSA.

Obesity

- Patient obesity has been a much-debated issue in ambulatory anesthesia for many years.
- In patients with BMI >30 undergoing ambulatory surgery, observational studies document an increased likelihood of developing intraoperative and postoperative respiratory events.
- Other perioperative concerns include increased risk of OSA, difficult airway management, use of vasopressors, and risk of unplanned admission or readmission.
- Facility logistics include OR bed capacity, equipment requirements, presence of a lift team, and other resources.
- For patients who also have OSA, a multimodal analgesia approach to reduce opioid use is recommended.
- Most freestanding ASCs have developed their own criteria for accepting patients with obesity.
  - Some use BMI cutoff (most commonly BMI >50).

Chronic Kidney Disease

- Patients with end-stage renal disease (ESRD) on dialysis can safely undergo surgery in an ambulatory setting.
- Preoperative considerations
  - Timing and method of dialysis
  - Comorbidities: hypertension, coronary artery disease, diabetes mellitus, electrolyte abnormalities, altered volume status, and platelet dysfunction
- Anesthetic implications of ESRD
  - Consider using agents with minimal dependence on renal excretion.
  - Succinylcholine causes the same rise in potassium for patients with or without ESRD.
  - Consider use of nondepolarizing muscle relaxants if baseline potassium is not normal.
  - Regional anesthesia is an attractive option, but patients may exhibit uremic platelet dysfunction.

Implanted and Other Medical Devices

- Patients with many implanted medical devices can safely undergo ambulatory surgery.
- Devices safe for ambulatory surgery include pacemaker, implantable cardioverter-defibrillator (ICD), spinal cord or peripheral nerve stimulator, and insulin pump.
  - Devices need to be evaluated preoperatively.
  - Cardiac implantable electrical devices (pacemakers, ICDs) may require reprogramming.
  - Certain devices may require coordination with a specialist not readily available at an ASC.

Difficult Airway Management

- Anticipated or known difficult airway is not an absolute contraindication for ASC care though may be considered a relative contraindication.
- One option is to avoid airway management altogether.
  - Use a carefully executed regional technique as the primary anesthetic.
  - Use caution when administering sedatives that can cause respiratory depression.
- ASC should have equipment to manage an unanticipated difficult airway.

Substance Use Disorders

- Patients with acute intoxication are not suitable for ASC care.
- Patients with substance use disorder may be safely cared for at an ASC.
- Potential issues for patients with opioid use disorder: postoperative pain management, opioid tolerance, use of medication-assisted treatment with buprenorphine
- Multimodal analgesia is recommended to minimize complications.

ANESTHETIC TECHNIQUES

- For outpatient surgeries, the most common risk of general anesthesia that prolongs stay is postoperative nausea and vomiting (PONV).
- Spinal anesthesia can be used for lower extremity surgeries.
  - Advantages
    - No need for airway instrumentation
    - Lower risk of PONV
  - Disadvantage
    - Prolonged motor blockade can delay patient's time to discharge home.
- Peripheral nerve blocks can be used for surgical anesthesia and/or postoperative analgesia.
  - Advantages
    - Nerve blocks can reduce total amount of opioid administered.
    - Risk of PONV is reduced from opioid-sparing or from avoidance of general anesthesia.
- Monitored Anesthesia Care (MAC)
  - Definition: a specific anesthesia service in which an anesthesiologist has been requested to participate in the care of a patient undergoing a diagnostic or therapeutic procedure
  - MAC can encompass a wide range of anesthesia management, including monitoring without administering any medication, actively managing hemodynamics, inducing varying degrees of sedation on the depth-of-sedation continuum, and even general anesthesia.
  - The term MAC is commonly used to describe deep sedation or general anesthesia in a spontaneously breathing patient without an airway device in place.
  - Advantages
    - The absence of inhaled anesthetics translates into a lower risk of PONV.
  - Disadvantages
    - Risks of an unsecured airway (e.g., airway obstruction)
    - Occasional patient discomfort if there is concern for excessive respiratory depression with additional sedative/analgesic administration
  - Closed-claim analysis of patients undergoing MAC suggests that respiratory depression after sedative or opioid administration is the most common mechanism of injury.

POSTOPERATIVE CARE

- Postoperative recovery includes the following three phases.
  - Phase I
    - Early stage of recovery that typically occurs in a postanesthesia care unit (PACU)

        - Patient awakens from the sedative effects of medications, physiologic reflexes return, and pain management and PONV are managed.
    - Phase II
        - Begins when patient is awake and hemodynamically stable with minimal PONV or pain and ends when patient is ready to go home
        - Occurs in the PACU or in a different area of the facility
        - Scoring systems (e.g., the modified Aldrete score) are commonly used to determine PACU discharge readiness.
    - Phase III
        - Occurs at home after PACU discharge
- Fast-tracking is an approach to admit a patient directory from the OR to phase II recovery, bypassing phase I.
    - This is enabled by improvements in surgical techniques and use of short-acting anesthesia drugs.
- Postdischarge nausea and vomiting (PDNV) is an important issue after ambulatory surgery.
    - The incidence of PDNV is 37% in the first 48 hours postdischarge.
    - Independent predictors of PDNV include the following.
        - Female gender
        - Age <50 years old
        - History of PONV
        - Use of opioids in PACU
        - Nausea in PACU

QUALITY IMPROVEMENT

- Minor adverse events are common after ambulatory surgery.
    - Symptoms can include drowsiness, headache, nausea, emesis, myalgia, and sore throat.
- Outcome measures to track include escalation of care, unplanned admission, and readmission.
- Analysis of closed malpractice claims provides insight into anesthesia safety issues in ambulatory surgery.
- Centers for Medicare and Medicaid Services (CMS) developed a payment incentive program to encourage better care and improve quality of service.
- ASA Committee on Performance and Outcome Measures has a Technical Expert Panel for development of quality measures in ambulatory anesthesia.
- Leadership is needed to monitor quality metrics and develop plans to improve patient care.

ADVANCES AND NEW TRENDS IN OUTPATIENT ANESTHESIA

- New medications may facilitate ambulatory anesthesia, including long-acting local anesthetics using microtechnology, sedatives, and antiemetics.
    - Liposomal bupivacaine
        - Bupivacaine encapsulated within multiple nonconcentric lipid bilayers, which allows slow diffusion over an extended period
        - Duration of action may reach 72 hours.
        - Efficacy and cost-effectiveness are unclear.
    - Remimazolam
        - Ultra-short-acting intravenous benzodiazepine that is rapidly metabolized by nonspecific tissue esterase
        - Advantages include rapid onset and predictable recovery.
- Trends of care at ASC vs. hospital-based outpatient setting
    - Financial: ASC procedure costs are lower
    - Access: shorter wait times for surgical case scheduling may translate into improved access for patients.

CONCLUSION

- Demand for ambulatory anesthesia is increasing.
- Anesthesia providers will care for higher-risk patients undergoing more complex procedures.
- Proper selection of patients and facilities is essential to minimizing complications and cost.

Perioperative Pearls for Outpatient Anesthesia

- Patient selection is essential for safe outpatient anesthesia care.
- Appropriate facility and sufficient clinical resources for procedure and patient comorbidities should be considered.
- OSA: recommend STOP-BANG for screening, minimize opioid use, and CPAP/BiPAP postoperatively
- Obesity: BMI often used to determine threshold criteria based on available resources; recommend multimodal analgesia approach to reduce opioid use
- CKD: consider timing and method of dialysis, use agents with minimal dependence on renal clearance, avoid succinylcholine if potassium is elevated.
- Implanted devices: pacemaker, ICD, spinal cord or peripheral nerve stimulator, and insulin pump are safe for outpatient surgery but should be interrogated preoperatively by specialist.
- Difficult airway: may be a relative, but not absolute contraindication to ambulatory surgery. Consider history, available resources, and techniques to avoid airway management altogether.
- Substance use disorder: acute intoxication is not suitable for ASC, but well managed substance use disorder may be appropriate for ASC. Consider multimodal analgesia.
- Anesthetic techniques: MAC and regional anesthesia may be preferred options over general anesthesia in outpatient settings.

QUESTIONS

INTRODUCTION

1. What are the three distinct practice settings of ambulatory anesthesia, and what types of facilities are used for each?
2. Describe the patient flow in ambulatory surgery.
3. What is nonoperating room anesthesia (NORA)?
4. What are some differences between NORA and the main operating room (OR)? What are the challenges of providing anesthesia care in the NORA setting?
5. What are some common procedures done in office-based anesthesia settings?
6. Describe some of the logistical issues with providing anesthesia in an office-based setting.

PATIENT SELECTION

7. What are some considerations for patient selection in outpatient anesthesia?
8. What is the recommended discharge arrangement for sending a patient home after surgery?

SURGERIES AND PROCEDURES

9. List some of the common procedures that are performed in an ambulatory setting >90% of the time.

PREOPERATIVE EVALUATION

10. What are some anesthetic concerns when caring for patients with obstructive sleep apnea (OSA) in the ambulatory setting?
11. Describe some of the Society for Ambulatory Anesthesia (SAMBA) recommendations related to preoperative selection of patients with OSA in the ambulatory setting.
12. According to ASA practice guidelines for the perioperative management of OSA, what are some factors to consider when determining whether inpatient or outpatient care is most appropriate?
13. Why is obesity a concern for outpatient anesthesia?
14. What are some criteria used by freestanding ambulatory surgical centers (ASCs) for accepting patients with obesity?
15. Describe some of the anesthetic concerns for a patient with end-stage renal disease (ESRD) on dialysis undergoing a procedure in an ambulatory setting.
16. What is the effect of succinylcholine on the serum potassium in a patient with ESRD?
17. Is a patient's history of difficult airway management an absolute contraindication for undergoing surgery at a freestanding ASC?
18. What are some of the anesthetic considerations when caring for patients with substance use disorder?

ANESTHETIC TECHNIQUES

19. For outpatient surgeries, what is the most common risk of general anesthesia that results in prolonged stay?
20. What are some of the potential benefits and side effects of spinal anesthesia for ambulatory surgery?

POSTOPERATIVE CARE

21. What does postoperative recovery phase I entail?
22. What attributes does the modified Aldrete score assess for discharge readiness?
23. Name the four risk factors for postoperative nausea and vomiting (PONV) from the simplified Apfel score.

QUALITY IMPROVEMENT

24. In the analysis of closed malpractice claims, how do the claims related to anesthesia care in ASCs compare with hospital ORs?

ADVANCES AND NEW TRENDS IN OUTPATIENT ANESTHESIA

25. What is liposomal bupivacaine, and how long does it last?
26. Why might remimazolam be preferred over other sedatives for short procedures?

ANSWERS

INTRODUCTION

1. Ambulatory anesthesia involves three distinct entities: outpatient anesthesia, office-based anesthesia (OBA), and nonoperating room anesthesia (NORA). The figure below provides examples of different ambulatory surgery facilities. (671-672)

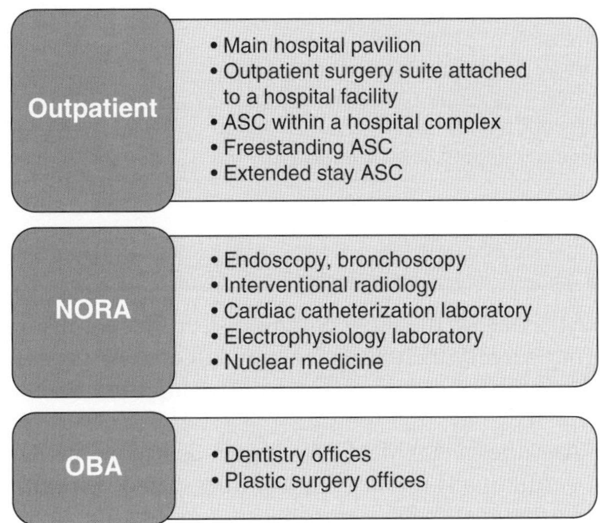

2. In ambulatory surgery, a patient is anticipated to come to the facility on the day of surgery, undergo surgery or an invasive procedure, and be discharged home on the same day or within 23 hours. (671)
3. NORA is an anesthesia service provided in a hospital unit, albeit away from the standard operating rooms (ORs). (672)
4. Compared to the main OR, NORA patients are older, and MAC is the more common anesthesia choice. Some challenges of the NORA setting include (1) patients may be deemed "too sick" for an invasive surgery under general anesthesia and are now offered a minimally invasive alternative; (2) limited physical access to patients because of obstacles such as fluoroscopy equipment; and (3) limited availability of medication, staff, or rescue equipment. (672)
5. Office-based anesthesia is performed outside a hospital or ambulatory surgical center (ASC) setting at small offices. These are generally elective surgeries of short duration with minimal estimated blood loss. Some examples are cosmetic surgery, complex dental procedures, podiatric procedures, and low-risk vascular procedures like varicose vein treatment. (672)
6. When providing office-based anesthesia, the anesthesia providers may need to transport their equipment and medications from one office to another. Further, there may be complicated logistical issues related to managing DEA-controlled medications, especially going from site to site. (672)

PATIENT SELECTION

7. Careful patient selection and optimization are essential for safe outpatient anesthesia. The preoperative evaluation and optimization process should proceed like a patient scheduled for inpatient surgery. In addition, one must consider whether the facility is appropriate for the patient to undergo the scheduled procedure. (673)
8. The ASA Practice Guidelines for Postanesthetic Care recommend that a responsible individual should accompany a patient home after surgery. (673)

SURGERIES AND PROCEDURES

9. The box below lists procedures performed in an ambulatory setting >90% of the time. (673)

Procedures Performed in an Ambulatory Setting >90% of the Time
▪ Operations on the eye ▪ Tympanoplasty; any myringotomy ▪ Excision of semilunar cartilage of knee ▪ Inguinal and femoral hernia repair ▪ Tonsillectomy and/or adenoidectomy ▪ Decompression of peripheral nerve ▪ Lumpectomy or quadrantectomy of breast ▪ Bunionectomy or repair of toe deformities ▪ Plastic procedures on nose ▪ Varicose vein stripping (lower limb)

PREOPERATIVE EVALUATION

10. Obstructive sleep apnea (OSA) is one of the most common sleep-related disorders. Concerns about OSA for patients undergoing ambulatory surgery include the risk of difficult airway management, intraoperative hypoxemia, need for tracheal reintubation, unanticipated hospital admission, and hypoxemic brain injury and death. (673)
11. The Society for Ambulatory Anesthesia (SAMBA) recommends use of the STOP-BANG questionnaire for preoperative OSA screening. Additionally, other comorbidities such as hypertension, arrhythmias, heart failure, cerebrovascular disease, and metabolic syndrome should be evaluated. Since opioids are likely to exacerbate OSA in the perioperative period, painful procedures not amenable to nonopioid analgesia techniques may need to be reconsidered as an inpatient procedure. SAMBA recommends the use of continuous positive airway pressure (CPAP) or bilevel positive airway pressure (BiPAP) postoperatively. (673)
12. The ASA Task Force on Perioperative Management of Patients with OSA recommends the following factors be considered for determining whether inpatient or outpatient care is most appropriate: sleep apnea status, anatomic and physiologic abnormalities, status of coexisting disease, nature of surgery, type of anesthesia, need for postoperative opioids, patient age, adequacy of postdischarge observation, and capabilities of the outpatient facility. (674)
13. Patients with obesity have increased likelihood of developing intraoperative and postoperative respiratory events; they are at increased risk of OSA, difficult airway management, use of vasopressors, and risk of unplanned admission or readmission. (674)
14. Many freestanding ASCs have developed their own criteria for accepting patients with obesity based on BMI cutoffs and other factors, such as the type of obesity (central vs. peripheral), type of procedure, availability of resources, and options for an extended postoperative stay. (674)
15. Patients with end-stage renal disease (ESRD) on dialysis can safely undergo procedures in ambulatory settings. Some issues that a provider should pay close attention to are the timing and method of dialysis and potential difficult intravenous access (due to presence of current or prior dialysis fistula). Patients with ESRD may have comorbidities like hypertension, coronary artery disease, diabetes mellitus, electrolyte abnormalities, altered volume status, and platelet dysfunction. In terms of anesthetic agents, a provider should consider options with minimal dependence on renal excretion. (674)
16. Succinylcholine causes the same rise in potassium for patients with or without ESRD. However, the baseline potassium is more likely to be elevated in a patient with ESRD. Other muscle relaxants can be considered if the baseline potassium is not known to be normal. (674)
17. Patients with a history of (or anticipated) difficult airway management do not represent an absolute contraindication to having the surgery at a freestanding ASC. However, the anesthesia provider must also consider the context of the planned procedure, nature of airway difficulty, availability of specialized airway equipment, skills of the anesthesia provider, and available resources when deciding whether to proceed at the ASC. (674)

18. Patients with substance use disorders may be cared for at ambulatory surgical centers, but patients with acute intoxication are not suitable for ambulatory surgery. Multimodal analgesia may be beneficial to overcome potential issues with postoperative pain management, opioid tolerance, or use of medication-assisted treatment with buprenorphine. (674)

ANESTHETIC TECHNIQUES

19. Postoperative nausea and vomiting (PONV) is the most common risk associated with prolonged stay after general anesthesia. (675)
20. The potential benefits of spinal anesthesia include no need for airway instrumentation and decreased risk of PONV. However, prolonged motor blockade can delay discharge. (675)

POSTOPERATIVE CARE

21. The postoperative recovery period is divided into three phases. The earliest stage of recovery is termed phase I; it typically occurs in the postanesthesia care unit (PACU). During this phase, the patient awakens from the sedative effects of anesthesia medications, physiologic reflexes return, and issues such as pain management and nausea/vomiting are managed. Once the patient is awake, is hemodynamically stable, and has minimal PONV or pain, they can be transferred to phase II of recovery. (675)
22. The modified Aldrete score is a scoring system used to determine PACU discharge readiness. The scoring system consists of activity, respiration, circulation, consciousness, and oxygenation. (675)
23. The four risk factors in the simplified Apfel score to predict PONV are female sex, nonsmoker status, postoperative opioid use, and history of PONV/motion sickness. Each factor adds approximately 20% to the risk of PONV. (675)

QUALITY IMPROVEMENT

24. An approach to study anesthesia-related safety concerns is to analyze closed malpractice claims. When comparing claims against ASCs with hospital operating rooms, ASC claims were more likely to be classified as medium severity than hospital operating room claims and were more likely to involve dental damage or pain. In contrast, ASC claims were less likely to involve death or respiratory or cardiac arrest, and mean indemnity payment was significantly lower for ASC claims. (676)

ADVANCES AND NEW TRENDS IN OUTPATIENT ANESTHESIA

25. Liposomal bupivacaine is bupivacaine hydrochloride encapsulated within multiple nonconcentric lipid bilayers. This allows the medication to diffuse slowly and can last up to 72 hours (compared to approximately 8 hours for plain bupivacaine). (676)
26. Remimazolam is an ultra-short-acting benzodiazepine that can be administered intravenously. It is rapidly metabolized by nonspecific tissue esterases into inactive metabolites. For quick procedures, remimazolam may have an advantage over other sedatives due to its rapid onset and predictable short half-life. (676)

Chapter

38 ANESTHESIA FOR PROCEDURES IN NONOPERATING ROOM LOCATIONS

Chanhung Lee and Wilson Cui

Clinical Pearls for Nonoperating Room Anesthesia

- Clear communication between the anesthesia and intervention teams is crucial.
- Have a detailed plan for communicating with more centrally located anesthesia colleagues in case of needing urgent help.
- Adhere to the same practice standards as those for the operating rooms.
- Ensure all the necessary safety equipment is available.
- Severe reactions to contrast materials necessitate aggressive intervention.
- The level of sedation and/or anesthesia for NORA procedures should be tailored to the mental status of the patient, the severity of their comorbidities, the intraprocedural need, and the risk of complications.
- The most common complications in the endoscopic suite are adverse respiratory events
  - Adverse events can include hypoxemia, hypercapnia, aspiration, loss of airway, and cardiopulmonary arrest.
- Providing anesthesia to patients in the interventional cardiology suite is challenging.
  - A discussion with the cardiologist is essential to understand the complex anatomy, hemodynamic goals, procedural plans, and potential complications.
- The anesthesia provider should be familiar with the basic operation of an external defibrillator/pacemaker.
- The rule of thumb for a patient with cyanotic heart disease is to maintain preanesthetic hemodynamic and oxygenation baseline.
- Many anesthetic agents can affect the effectiveness of induced seizure in ECT.
- Significant postictal swings in the autonomic nervous system can have profound effects on the vital signs.

INTRODUCTION

- Compared with the traditional operating room (OR), nonoperating room anesthesia (NORA) has
  - Higher mean age of patients
  - Higher number of ASA class III and IV patients
  - Slightly higher incidences of death in NORA radiology and cardiology

CHARACTERISTICS OF NORA LOCATIONS

Importance of Communication

- Know the identity and role of personnel participating in the procedure.
- Have a mutual understanding with the procedural team of the specifics and challenges in the procedures.
- Clear communication is prudent for efficient and safe practice.
  - With the entire procedural team
  - With centrally located anesthesia colleagues and technicians in the event of urgent needs

Standard of Care and Equipment

- Adhere to the same practice standards as those for the ORs.
- Follow the same standard and precautions against infectious diseases.
- Hazards for NORA can include the distance of the anesthesia workstation, radiation exposure, loud sound levels, heavy mechanical equipment, and distance to the postanesthesia care unit.

- Personal protective safety equipment should be available.
- Know the location of the nearest defibrillator, fire extinguisher, gas shutoff valves, and exits.

SAFETY AND CONCERNS IN RADIOLOGY SUITES

Radiation Safety Practices

- Radiation intensity and exposure decrease with the inverse square of the distance from the emitting source.
- Clear communication is crucial for limiting radiation exposure.

Monitoring the Radiation Dose

- Radiation exposure can be monitored with one or more film badges.
- Federal guidelines set a limit of 50 mSv for the maximum annual occupational dose.
  - 1 Sv = 100 rem = 1 joule (J) of energy per kilogram of recipient mass

Adverse Reactions to Contrast Materials

Types of Adverse Reactions to Contrast Materials

- Anaphylaxis—IgE-mediated immune response
- Direct mediator release from mast cells and basophils (non–immune-mediated)
- Chemotoxic
- Nephrogenic systemic fibrosis

- Anaphylaxis (IgE-mediated) and non–immune-mediated reactions
  - More common after injection of iodinated agents (used for computed tomography [CT]) rather than gadolinium agents (used for magnetic resonance imaging [MRI])
  - Signs and symptoms can vary.
    - Mild: nausea, pruritus, diaphoresis
    - Moderate: faintness, emesis, urticaria, laryngeal edema, bronchospasm
    - Severe: seizures, hypotensive shock, laryngeal edema, respiratory or cardiac arrest
  - May necessitate aggressive intervention with epinephrine; support with oxygen and IV fluids
  - Premedication (steroids, antihistamines) can be used to inhibit the activation of mast cells and basophils.
  - Adequate hydration is important to prevent aggravation of coexisting hypovolemia or azotemia.
- Chemotoxic reaction is related to contrast osmolarity and ionic strength.
  - Dose and concentration dependent
- Nephrogenic systemic fibrosis (NSF) can occur after exposure to gadolinium-based MRI contrast agents.
  - Occurs in patients with severe renal impairment
  - Results in fibrosis of the skin, connective tissue, and sometimes internal organs
  - Severity ranges from mild to fatal.

MAGNETIC RESONANCE IMAGING

Challenges for MRI Anesthesia

- Scanning sequences can be up to several hours long.
- Motion artifact degrades images.
  - Patients must lie motionless.
- The MRI "bore" is narrow, making patient cooperation difficult.
  - Anesthesia requests are often for children or adults with claustrophobia, severe pain, or critically illness.

MRI Safety Considerations

- Hearing loss from high sound levels
- Electrical burns from incompatible monitoring equipment
- Large magnetic field is always "on" and attracts metal objects with alarming speed and force.
  - Missile injury from ferromagnetic objects
  - Must screen patients for ferromagnetic material, e.g., orthopedic hardware or implanted cardiac devices
- "Quenching" process to turn off magnet releases cryogen into a venting system.
  - Cryogen escape into MRI room can displace oxygen, causing cold injury and asphyxiation.

Monitoring Issues in MRI Suites

- Anesthesia provider stationed outside the magnet room during scans must have access to monitors and see the patient via a window or video monitor.
- Radiofrequency pulse can cause artifact in the pressure transducer and pulse oximeter.
- Non–MRI-compatible equipment may require extensions or stopcocks to lengthen distance from the magnet, increasing the risk of inadvertent disconnection.

Compatible Equipment

- Outside the magnet room: primary workstation for anesthetizing the patient
- Inside the magnet room: the anesthesia machine, fully functioning suction, physiologic monitoring, and ventilator capability should be MRI safe

- Critical intervention needed during the MRI: scan is stopped and the patient is promptly transferred to primary workstation for optimal care

ANESTHESIA FOR NONINVASIVE IMAGING PROCEDURES

- Anxiolysis or moderate sedation may suffice for painless imaging.

Indications for NORA Provider in Noninvasive Imaging
▪ Need for deep sedation on general anesthesia, especially for pediatric patients ▪ Significant comorbidities (e.g., airway compromise, severe cardiopulmonary disease, morbid obesity) ▪ Maintenance of adequate oxygenation and hemodynamic stability ▪ Provide for patient immobilization

Physiologic Monitoring

- ASA Standards for Basic Anesthetic Monitoring
- Ventilation must be continuously assessed by either
  - Sampling CO_2, which can be from an integrated nasal cannula that shows respiratory rate and pattern
  - Visual inspection and/or auscultation

Oxygen Administration

- Supplemental oxygen via a nasal cannula should come from a dedicated flowmeter, preferably humidified for longer duration cases.
- Must have capability to rapidly deploy noninvasive ventilatory support for hypoxemia or hypoventilation/apnea

Pharmacologically Induced Sedation

- Various medication options depending on need, for example
  - Rapid, short-acting medication such as remifentanil for short procedures
  - Benzodiazepines, opioids, or continuous infusions of propofol for longer procedures
  - Dexmedetomidine to minimize respiratory depression or frequently assess mental status

Management of Anesthesia for CT

- Sedation or general anesthesia may be required in children and adults in acute settings, including traumatic injury (head and abdominal), stroke, and altered mental status.

Management of Anesthesia for MRI

- Pediatrics: nasal cannula, laryngeal mask airway, or endotracheal tube may be needed for airway management, based on patient comorbid conditions
- Adults: may need general endotracheal anesthesia to minimize motion artifact which can occur with supraglottic airway and spontaneous ventilation.

INTERVENTIONAL RADIOLOGY

Interventional Neuroradiology

Anesthesia Choice

- General anesthesia: useful for complex procedures, long duration, patient immobility, controlled ventilation, and/or intermittent apnea
- Sedation: allows assessment of neurologic function during the procedure

Access and Monitoring

- C-arm device may require IV tubing with extensions between IV bag and patient.
  - Continuous infusions should be plugged into a port proximal to the IV catheter.
- Fluid and contrast agent may be administered by the interventional team.
  - Monitoring urine output may be useful.

Arterial Blood Pressure Management

- Target blood pressure should be discussed with the interventional team in advance.
- Deliberate hypertension or prevention of arterial hypertension may be requested by the interventional team for specific clinical circumstances.
- Postintervention individual targets may be guided by near-infrared spectroscopy or neuroangiographic findings.

Management of Neurologic and Procedural Crises

- Communication with procedural team will determine next steps (e.g., augmentation of blood pressure for vascular occlusion, or reversal of heparin with protamine for hemorrhage).

Body Interventional Radiology

- Imaging modalities may include CT, MRI, ultrasonography, and radiography.

Anesthesia Evaluation and Management

- The choice of anesthetic technique should be based on patient evaluation and procedural needs.
- The anesthesia provider should be ready to escalate the level of sedation and anesthesia if deemed necessary.

Transjugular Intrahepatic Portosystemic Shunt

- Preanesthesia evaluation should include assessment of other sequelae of cirrhosis, comorbid cardiopulmonary conditions, and coagulopathy.
- General anesthesia is preferred due to the unpredictable duration, risk of aspiration of gastric contents, and the need for internal jugular access.
- Postprocedural complications include encephalopathy, massive hemorrhage, and worsening liver function.

Challenges: Hemostasis and Anticoagulation

- Anticoagulation with heparin or other agents may be requested to prevent thrombosis at access sites.
- Embolization for acute hemorrhage can require transfusions of fluid and blood products, ideally guided by laboratory data along with clinical judgment.

ENDOSCOPY AND ENDOSCOPIC RETROGRADE CHOLANGIOPANCREATOGRAPHY

- Upper endoscopy is used for diagnosis and therapeutic intervention.
- Typically done with the patient in left lateral position and with a bite block

Anesthesia Evaluation and Management

- Anesthesia provider is generally requested if the procedure is expected to be challenging or prolonged.
- Propofol is commonly used in gastrointestinal endoscopy to provide a deeper level of anesthesia, favored for its rapid onset and short duration of action.
- ERCP is a high-risk procedure due to the frequency of hepatobiliary disease and limited access to the airway of the prone patient.
  - ASA class >3, Mallampati airway score of 4, ascites, obesity, sleep apnea, chronic lung disease, and significant alcohol use are risk factors for adverse events, and general anesthesia with endotracheal intubation may be preferred.

Challenges and Complications

- Adverse respiratory events are the most common complications, including hypoxemia, hypercapnia, aspiration, loss of airway, and cardiopulmonary arrest.
  - Effectiveness of ventilation should be continuously assessed and monitored.
  - Hypoxemia is a late sign of hypoventilation.
- Perforation and gas embolism are procedure-related complications that are rare but can be life threatening.
- Acute upper gastrointestinal (GI) bleeding can make tracheal intubation challenging and requires large-bore venous access for resuscitation and correction of coagulopathy.

CATHETER-BASED CARDIOLOGY PROCEDURES

Adult Cardiac Catheterization

- A dedicated anesthesia provider can provide more effective anesthesia, airway management, and hemodynamic support during percutaneous coronary intervention (PCI) such as
  - High-grade stenosis or chronic total occlusion (CTO)
  - In patients with severe anxiety, chronic pain, or inability to lie flat
- General anesthesia in patients with coronary ischemia is high risk but may be needed if
  - The patient is uncooperative or mentally altered
  - There is ongoing need for pulmonary resuscitation
  - Surgical incision is needed for advanced device support

Electrophysiology Studies

Catheter-Based Ablation

- Preanesthesia evaluation: cardiopulmonary reserve, signs and symptoms during offending arrhythmia, airway, comorbid conditions, and relevant medications, especially anticoagulants

Anesthesia Considerations for Electrophysiology Studies

- Possibly prolonged duration
- Potential hemodynamic instability during induced tachyarrhythmia
- Vascular sheaths are continuously flushed, increasing intravascular volume.
- Catheterization of left heart typically requires anticoagulation.
- For patients with chronic atrial fibrillation, the success rate is higher with general anesthesia.
- General anesthesia allows for esophageal temperature monitoring (to avoid left atrial perforation) and detection of phrenic nerve stimulation.

- An anesthetic regimen for an electrophysiology study should ideally provide
  - Patient comfort and immobility
  - Predictable respiratory pattern
  - Unchanged autonomic tone, inducibility of arrhythmia, and intrinsic pacemaker function and conduction

Cardiac Implantable Electronic Devices

- The anesthesia provider should understand the indication for the procedure and the operation of devices for emergency transcutaneous pacing and defibrillation.
- Ventricular fibrillation may be induced to test the device's ability to sense and terminate it.
  - Patients may require sedation prior to and support following fibrillation.

Cardioversion

- Transesophageal echocardiography (TEE) is often performed immediately before cardioversion due to the risk of thromboembolism and stroke in atrial fibrillation.
  - Sedation with a short-acting hypnotic such as propofol is common.
  - Maneuvers to relieve airway obstruction are frequently necessary.

Structural Heart Disease Intervention

- Preprocedural discussion should involve the anesthesia provider, interventional cardiologist, and cardiac surgeon regarding
  - Cardiac anatomy
  - History of previous cardiac surgery or intervention
  - Potential concerns of abnormal physiology or hemodynamic challenges
- General anesthesia is preferred: motionless patient, controlled respiratory movement, safety of continuous TEE examination, and a secure airway in the case of instability or salvage surgery

Pediatric Studies

- Special challenges in neonates, infants, and children with congenital cardiac diseases
  - Typically require general anesthesia
  - Possibility of difficult airway/intubation
  - Respiratory insufficiency can rapidly lead to cardiovascular collapse.
  - Prone to hypothermia
  - Complex cardiac anatomy, shunts, and neonatal/transitional physiology
  - Pulmonary vascular reactivity
- The rule of thumb: keep the cyanotic child at their preanesthetic hemodynamic and oxygenation baseline (easier said than done)

Challenges and Complications

- Most common complications: bleeding, hematoma, pneumothorax, and vascular injury
- Cardiac perforation is a rare but serious complication.
  - Signs: persistent hemodynamic instability refractory to routine measures
  - Diagnosis: echocardiography
  - Management depends on the size and rate of effusion accumulation.
    - "Wait-and-watch" for a small, self-limited effusion
    - Pericardial drain placement
    - Surgical decompression of tamponade for hemodynamic compromise

ELECTROCONVULSIVE THERAPY

- ECT effectively treats severe depression by inducing a generalized seizure to change the patient's neurobiology.
- Efficacy of ECT is influenced by electrode placement, duration of convulsion, and the number of ECT treatments.

Electrically Induced Seizures

- Goal is to trigger a seizure of at least 15 seconds duration.
- Monitored with a single-channel electroencephalogram (motor activity stops before electrical activity)
- Prolonged seizures (>120 seconds) can be harmful and may require intervention.

Anesthesia Evaluation

- There is no absolute contraindication to ECT, but special attention should be given to the presence of coexisting cardiovascular and central nervous system (CNS) diseases.
  - Unstable cardiac disease (malignant hypertension, decompensated heart failure, or arrhythmia) should be evaluated and optimized by a cardiologist.
  - An unstable fracture may be at risk due to motor seizure activity.

Psychotropic Medications

- Medications that may shorten seizure duration should be avoided or tapered, e.g., lithium, anticonvulsants, and benzodiazepines.
- Many psychotropic medications have sympathomimetic, anticholinergic, and CNS effects and can cause drug–drug interactions with common perioperative medications.
  - Monoamine oxidase inhibitors
  - Serotonin reuptake inhibitors
  - Tricyclic antidepressants
  - Lithium

Management of Anesthesia and Seizure

- Cardiac implantable electronic devices (CIEDs) should be reprogrammed to avoid electrical artifact and an abnormal response.
  - Defibrillators should be temporarily deactivated.
  - Pacemakers should be converted to asynchronous mode in patients who are pacemaker dependent.
- Methohexital (most common), etomidate, and ketamine have all been used to induce general anesthesia in ECT.
- A fast-acting neuromuscular blocker (NMB), usually succinylcholine, is used to minimize the side effects from motor convulsion (myalgia).
  - A tourniquet inflated on a distal limb prior to the administration of NMB is used to observe the seizure-related motor activity in that limb.

Physiologic Responses to Seizure and Treatment

- Seizure can have profound effects on the patient's vital signs.
  - First (tonic) phase: parasympathetic discharge, bradycardia, atrioventricular (AV) block, ectopy, arrhythmia, hypotension, or asystole
  - Second (clonic) phase: sympathetic stimulation, tachycardia, and hypertension
  - Treatment may be required for patients at risk for ischemia.

Side Effects

- Review previous records for hemodynamic responses, or post-ECT symptoms such as headache, muscle pain, or nausea.

QUESTIONS

CHARACTERISTICS OF NORA LOCATIONS

1. For nonoperating room anesthesia (NORA), name at least five examples for each of the following: anesthesia-related concerns, special challenges, and safety concerns.
2. What are some fundamental capabilities available in the operating room that must also be available for NORA?

SAFETY AND CONCERNS IN RADIOLOGY SUITES

3. How might anesthesia providers limit their exposure to radiation during diagnostic and therapeutic radiologic procedures?
4. What is the federal guideline limit of annual occupational exposure to radiation in Sievert units? How does this compare to radiation exposure during a chest radiograph or a computed tomography (CT) scan of the head?
5. Which type of contrast agent is most likely to cause an adverse drug reaction? How can it be treated?
6. What prophylaxis may be administered to patients at risk of a serious adverse reaction to an intravenously administered contrast agent?
7. What is the potential serious adverse reaction that can occur in patients with severe renal impairment receiving gadolinium-based magnetic resonance imaging contrast agents?

MAGNETIC RESONANCE IMAGING

8. What is magnetic resonance imaging (MRI)?
9. Complete the following table describing how each factor contributes to challenges for the anesthesia provider that are unique to MRI.

Factor	Challenges Unique to MRI
Magnet	
Patient experience in scanner	
Monitoring	
Accessibility to patient	
Airflow	

ANESTHESIA FOR NONINVASIVE IMAGING PROCEDURES

10. What anesthetic techniques may be used for noninvasive imaging procedures?
11. How does the management of anesthesia for patients undergoing CT compare with the management of anesthesia for patients undergoing MRI?

INTERVENTIONAL RADIOLOGY

12. Is general anesthesia preferred over sedation for procedures in interventional radiology? What are the advantages of each technique?
13. Why is blood pressure management crucial in interventional neuroradiology procedures?
14. What is the concern with the administration of intravenous contrast agents for patients with renal failure who are on metformin therapy?
15. What are some anesthetic concerns related to anesthesia for patients scheduled to undergo transjugular intrahepatic portosystemic shunt (TIPS) placement in interventional radiology?
16. Why might anticoagulation be necessary during interventional radiology procedures?
17. What are some challenges related to anesthetizing patients with acute hemorrhage in interventional radiology?

ENDOSCOPY AND ENDOSCOPIC RETROGRADE CHOLANGIOPANCREATOGRAPHY

18. What complications might occur with endoscopic procedures?
19. What are the anesthetic challenges in caring for a patient with acute upper gastrointestinal bleeding undergoing endoscopy?

CATHETER-BASED CARDIOLOGY PROCEDURES

20. Why might patients require anesthesia for interventional cardiology procedures?
21. What adverse effects might the anesthetic have on cardiac function during interventional cardiology procedures?
22. Why does a patient undergoing elective electrical cardioversion require sedation and amnesia?
23. Describe the steps in the anesthetic management of a patient undergoing elective electrical cardioversion.
24. For catheter-based cardiology procedures, complete the table below by naming some preanesthesia and intraprocedure anesthetic considerations that are specific to the given procedure or patient population.

Catheter-Based Cardiology Procedure	Specific Preanesthesia and Intraprocedural Anesthetic Considerations
Electrophysiology catheter-based ablation	
Cardiac implantable electronic device placement	
Structural heart disease intervention	
Pediatric patients	

25. What are the implications of an intracardiac shunt on the anesthetic management of pediatric patients undergoing interventional cardiology procedures?
26. Name some potential complications the anesthesia provider may encounter in interventional cardiology procedures.
27. How might pericardial effusion or tamponade present during an interventional cardiology procedure? How should it be managed?

ELECTROCONVULSIVE THERAPY (ECT)

28. What are some indications for ECT? What are the absolute and relative contraindications to ECT?
29. How is ECT accomplished, and what monitors are used?
30. Complete the table describing the considerations of each factor for patients undergoing ECT.

Factor	Considerations for ECT
Benzodiazepines	
Esmolol	
Methohexital	
Propofol	
Etomidate	
Ketamine	
Succinylcholine	
Implanted defibrillator	
Pacemaker	

31. How can the airway of the patient undergoing ECT be managed? What equipment should be available to the anesthesia provider?
32. What are the cardiovascular responses to ECT and their consequences?
33. What are some post-ECT manifestations in the patient?

ANSWERS

CHARACTERISTICS OF NORA LOCATIONS

1. The concerns and challenges for providing anesthesia care in a nonoperating room anesthesia (NORA) setting are summarized in the following table. (679–680)

Anesthesia-related concerns	• Patient immobility
	• Patient comfort
	• Patient physiologic stability
	• Readiness for sudden, unexpected complications
	• Perioperative anticoagulation management
	• Sedation at appropriate times during the procedure
	• Smooth and rapid emergence from anesthesia
	• Appropriate postprocedure monitoring for transport
	• Appropriate postprocedure management
Special challenges	• Communication regarding the procedure and expectations
	• Limited access to the patient's airway
	• Poor availability of accessory help
	• Potential difficulty in quickly obtaining emergency equipment
	• Distance to transport the patient before reaching the postanesthesia care unit
	• Need for supplemental oxygen delivery and continuous monitoring with transport
	• Communication regarding the procedure and expectations
Safety concerns	• Possibility of exposure to increased radiation
	• Loud sound levels
	• Heavy mechanical equipment
	• Scavenging of waste anesthetic gases
	• Availability of protective gear: lead aprons, lead thyroid shields, portable lead-glass shields, earplugs
	• Elevator keys for transport if necessary
	• Locations of the nearest defibrillator, fire extinguisher, gas shutoff valves, and exits

2. Anesthesia care provided in NORA must adhere to the same standards that apply to the operating room; the American Society of Anesthesiologists (ASA) has issued a statement regarding minimal guidelines for NORA care. Fundamental capabilities for monitoring, the delivery of supplemental oxygen, noninvasive and mechanical ventilation of the lungs, the availability of suction, the delivery and scavenging of inhaled anesthetics, and an adequate supply of anesthetic drugs and ancillary equipment must all be available for the delivery of anesthesia in remote locations. (680)

SAFETY AND CONCERNS IN RADIOLOGY SUITES

3. Anesthesia providers should attempt to limit their exposure to radiation by wearing a lead apron and thyroid shield, using movable lead-glass screens, and by remaining as far away as possible from the radiation source, preferably at least 1 to 2 meters. A recent study also highlighted the importance of eye protection for anesthesia providers working significant hours in the radiology suite. Finally, clear communication between the radiology and anesthesia teams is crucial for limiting radiation exposure. The radiation exposure can be monitored by wearing radiation exposure badges. (680)
4. Federal guidelines set a limit of 50 mSv (millisieverts) for the maximum annual occupational dose of radiation. By comparison, for patients receiving a chest radiograph the dose is 0.1 mSv, whereas for those receiving a computed tomography (CT) scan of the head the dose is 2 mSv. The average background radiation exposure in the United States is 3 mSv per year. (680)

5. The administration of iodinated contrast agents, as used for x-ray examinations such as CT, is most likely to cause adverse reactions. The signs and symptoms can range from mild to severe, and treatment is relative to the reaction. Treatment may require the administration of oxygen, intravenous fluids, and epinephrine if necessary. The newer nonionic contrast dyes of lower osmolarity are associated with a decreased incidence of allergic reactions. (681)
6. Patients at risk for an adverse reaction to a contrast agent should be pretreated with steroid and antihistamine medications, both the night before and on the morning of the procedure. A typical regimen for a 70-kg adult is 40 mg prednisone, 20 mg famotidine, and 50 mg diphenhydramine. Adequate hydration is necessary to maintain intravascular volume because the intravenous contrast medium also acts as an osmotic load for the patient, inducing diuresis. (681)
7. Nephrogenic systemic fibrosis (NSF) is a serious adverse reaction that can occur in patients with severe renal impairment receiving gadolinium-based magnetic resonance imaging (MRI) contrast agents. In NSF, there is fibrosis of the skin, connective tissue, and sometimes internal organs. The severity of NSF can range from mild to severe and can be fatal. (681)

MAGNETIC RESONANCE IMAGING

8. MRI is a radiologic technology that provides digitalized tomographic images of the body by exposing the body to a very high-strength constant magnetic field and high-frequency alternating electric and magnetic fields. MRI does not produce any ionizing radiation. These studies are useful for the evaluation of neurologic and soft tissues because they can distinguish among fat, vessels, and tumor. (681–682)
9. The following table describes how each factor contributes to challenges for the anesthesia provider that are unique to MRI. (681–682)

Factor	Challenges Unique to MRI
Magnet	Ferromagnetic objects can become missiles when attracted by magnet. Patient must be screened for implanted magnetic objects (e.g., artificial pacemakers, some aneurysm clips, orthopedic hardware, wire-enforced epidural catheters, and some pulmonary artery catheter temperature probes). Magnetic objects can become heated and cause electrical burns. All anesthesia equipment, including gas cylinders, must be MR compatible (plastic, nonmagnetic steel, and aluminum components replace ferromagnetic ones).
Patient experience	MRI table is cold, narrow, and hard. The patient must lie still. MRI scans can last 1 hour or longer. The table moves within a thin tube with walls close to the face, making some patients claustrophobic. The scanner makes loud booming noises (can reach >90–100 decibels).
Monitoring	Blood pressure monitors, pulse oximeter probes, standard electrocardiogram electrodes, and temperature probes must all be MR compatible or risk burning the patient. Arterial lines with long lengths of pressure tubing and the pulse generated from the MRI may generate artificial spikes in the pressure waveform. The anesthesia provider needs to be able to view the monitor and patient from outside or remain inside the magnet room.
Accessibility to patient	The distance to the patient and the movement of the table during imaging require extensions on tubing for IV, capnogram, arterial lines, and other monitors. The patient will need to be promptly transferred out of the scanner room for any critical issues. For example, accidental extubation or life-threatening events will require moving far enough away from the scanner to use metallic resuscitative equipment at an anesthesia workstation.
Airflow	Airflow through the magnet increases patient heat loss, risking hypothermia.

ANESTHESIA FOR NONINVASIVE IMAGING PROCEDURES

10. Anxiolysis, moderate sedation, and general anesthesia are all anesthetic techniques that may be used for noninvasive imaging procedures. For pediatric patients, deep sedation or general anesthesia may be required. In all cases, the ASA Standards of Basic Monitoring apply, capnography may be useful, and supplemental oxygen should be available. (682–683)
11. Anesthesia for a CT scan is similar to that for MRI. That is, access to the patient is limited and monitoring is remote. CT scanning differs from MRI in that the scans are typically shorter, the scanner is an open space making claustrophobia less likely, and the avoidance of ferromagnetic equipment is not necessary. CT scanners emit ionizing radiation, whereas MRI does not. (683)

INTERVENTIONAL RADIOLOGY

12. Anesthetic requirements of patients undergoing interventional radiology procedures vary. Evidence is limited on which technique is superior. General anesthesia ensures airway security, limits movement artifact, and guarantees patient comfort during prolonged cases. The ability to hyperventilate and produce mild hypocapnia may also be beneficial in patients with elevated intracranial pressures. Sedation with spontaneous respiration causes minimal perturbation to hemodynamics and allows faster recovery. The choice depends on the procedural need, the patient's comorbid conditions, and the anesthesia provider's clinical judgment. (683)
13. Blood pressure management and manipulation may be crucial in interventional neuroradiology procedures, making arterial line placement and communication with the interventional radiology team important. Deliberate hypertension may be necessary during occlusive cerebrovascular disease to promote collateral cerebral blood flow, in patients with a subarachnoid hemorrhage in whom vasospasm has developed, or in patients with compromised blood flow to spinal cord, kidneys, or other organs. Conversely, the prevention of arterial hypertension may be critical in patients with recently ruptured intracranial aneurysms or those who have undergone carotid artery angioplasty and stent placement who are susceptible to hyperperfusion injury. Predetermined arterial blood pressure ranges should be established prior to a procedure. (684)
14. Patients with renal failure who are on metformin therapy are at risk for lactic acidosis with the administration of intravenous contrast. (685)
15. Some anesthetic concerns related to anesthesia for patients scheduled to undergo transjugular intrahepatic portosystemic shunt (TIPS) placement in interventional radiology include the effects of liver failure on other organ systems; cardiopulmonary comorbidities, coagulopathy, and thrombocytopenia that may require correction prior to the procedure; the possible need for general endotracheal anesthesia; and the potential for post-TIPS complications, including altered mental status from encephalopathy, massive hemorrhage, and worsening liver failure from decreased portal vein blood flow. (685)
16. Interventional radiology procedures often involve the management of coagulation parameters depending on the anticoagulation status of the patient and the nature of the procedure. Procedures that involve catheters in the arterial tree require anticoagulation, often with heparin, to avoid thromboembolic complications. When the catheters are removed, the anticoagulation effect of heparin is usually reversed with protamine. Unexpected or excessive bleeding during the procedure may also occur and necessitate immediate heparin reversal. (685)
17. Challenges related to anesthetizing patients with acute hemorrhage in interventional radiology include the rapid and safe induction of anesthesia, the establishment of adequate intravenous access with long tubing, and the administration of intravenous fluids and blood products to replace losses and correct potential coagulopathy and thrombocytopenia. (685)

ENDOSCOPY AND ENDOSCOPIC RETROGRADE CHOLANGIOPANCREATOGRAPHY

18. Complications that may occur with endoscopy can be grouped by sedation and airway-related, procedure-related, and patient-related factors. Most complications are adverse respiratory events such as hypoxemia, hypercapnia, aspiration, loss of airway, and even cardiopulmonary arrest. The use of propofol provides faster onset of adequate anesthesia and shorter recovery, but severe respiratory depression can occur and limits its use to anesthesia providers. Procedural complications include laryngospasm, laryngeal injury, esophageal or intestinal perforation, and bleeding. Clinical signs and symptoms associated with perforation can be nonspecific, such as neck, chest, or abdominal pain; tachycardia; tachypnea; hypotension; and abdominal distention. Gas embolism is more common in ERCP than other gastrointestinal endoscopic procedures. (687)
19. The challenges of caring for a patient with acute upper gastrointestinal bleeding undergoing endoscopy include hematemesis making endotracheal intubation difficult, difficult venous access, massive transfusion and volume resuscitation, correction of coagulopathy, and maintaining hemodynamic stability. The patient may have underlying medical issues such as cirrhosis and coagulopathy that require treatment. Anesthetic management of such critically ill patients is further complicated by the location being outside the operating room, where resources and help may not be nearby. (687)

CATHETER-BASED CARDIOLOGY PROCEDURES

20. Patients may undergo interventional cardiology procedures for diagnostic angiography, angioplasty with or without stent placement, electrophysiology study with possible ablation of dysrhythmia, implantation of pacemaker or defibrillators, and percutaneous intervention of valvular defects or other congenital structural

heart diseases. The goal of the anesthesia provider is to ensure patient comfort and safety, to provide hemodynamic monitoring, and to assist in cardiopulmonary resuscitation during an emergency. In a cooperative patient, minimal sedation and analgesia are sufficient when local anesthetic is provided prior to percutaneous vascular access. However, general anesthesia is necessary if surgical exposure is anticipated, there is ongoing need for pulmonary resuscitation, or the patient is uncooperative because of mental status. (688)

21. General anesthesia and positive-pressure ventilation can cause additional myocardial depression and cardiovascular instability in vulnerable patients undergoing interventional cardiology procedures. Coronary ischemia, sometimes induced by angioplasty, as well as dysrhythmia can lead to sudden instability. The use of vasoconstrictors or inotropic agents may be necessary during interventional cardiology procedures. (688)
22. The electrical shock during cardioversion would be painful and can be traumatic to the patient if done without sedation and amnesia. Furthermore, elective electrical cardioversion may be preceded by transesophageal echocardiography (TEE) to examine the left atrium for thrombus, which may increase the length of the procedure. (668)
23. Before undergoing elective electrical cardioversion, the patient should have fasted according to the NPO guidelines. Standard monitors—pulse oximetry, electrocardiogram, blood pressure—are placed. Emergency medication and airway equipment for endotracheal intubation, suction, oxygen supply, and methods of positive-pressure ventilation should be immediately available. Adequate preoxygenation should be achieved prior to the administration of sedative. The upper airway may be topically anesthetized with local anesthetics to suppress the gag reflex during probe insertion, weighing the potential drawback of lingering loss of airway reflex lasting longer than the procedure making it difficult for the patient to handle secretions. With propofol, the anesthesia provider can titrate the level of sedation to allow the passage of the TEE probe, maintain patient cooperation during the TEE examination, and ensure amnesia of the electric shock. During and immediately after sedation, the patient may require manual relief of airway obstruction. Monitoring of the patient is necessary until the recovery of mentation, airway reflexes, and unencumbered respiration. (689)
24. For catheter-based cardiology procedures, the table describes some preanesthesia and intraprocedure anesthetic considerations that are specific to the given procedure or patient population. (689–690)

Catheter-Based Cardiology Procedure	Specific Preanesthesia and Intraprocedural Anesthetic Considerations
Electrophysiology catheter-based ablation	Preanesthesia: Signs and symptoms (eg, syncope, angina) during the offending arrhythmia reflect degree of cardiac compromise during the event. Intraprocedure: Potential hemodynamic instability during induced arrhythmia Autonomic tone and arrhythmia inducibility must be preserved as much as possible and may limit drug choice and dose. Vascular sheaths are continuously flushed, increasing intravascular volume. Anticoagulation is usually required. May need esophageal temperature (to avoid left atrial perforation) and phrenic nerve monitoring
Cardiac implantable electronic device placement	Preanesthesia: Understand the indication for the procedure, the underlying cardiac rhythm, and if the patient is pacemaker dependent. Intraprocedure: Transcutaneous pacing and defibrillation may be necessary. Fibrillation may be intentionally induced to test the newly implanted device, requiring additional sedation and possibly invasive arterial blood pressure monitoring.
Structural heart disease intervention	Preanesthesia: Cardiac anatomy, previous cardiac interventions, and abnormal physiology or hemodynamic challenges should be discussed. Intraprocedure: Patient must remain motionless, preferably with controlled respiratory movement. Continuous transesophageal echocardiography may be required. Acute instability may require emergent salvage cardiac surgery.
Pediatric patients	Typically require general anesthesia Vascular access can be challenging. Syndromic patients may have a difficult airway. May have complex cardiovascular anatomy, shunts, or transitional physiology Respiratory insufficiency can lead to rapid cardiovascular collapse. Prone to hypothermia

25. The presence of a left-to-right shunt has minimal effect on the rate of induction of anesthesia in pediatric patients with either inhaled or intravenous agents. However, hyperoxia and hyperventilation with general anesthesia in these patients may lead to pulmonary vasodilation, increase of shunt fraction, pulmonary congestion, and a decrease in systemic cardiac output. Conversely, the induction of anesthesia with inhaled agents in the

presence of a right-to-left shunt is slowed owing to dilution by shunted blood, whereas the induction of anesthesia with intravenous agents is more rapid. Such patients are cyanotic, have right-sided heart dysfunction, and can be quite ill. In these patients, deep sedation or general anesthesia can pose significant risk. Secondary polycythemia in cyanotic patients also puts them at higher thrombotic risk. The rule of thumb is to have the cyanotic patient remain at preanesthetic hemodynamic and oxygenation baseline, which can be challenging. Hypoxia, hypercapnia, excessive positive airway pressure, metabolic acidosis, hypothermia, and painful stimulation can lead to increases in pulmonary vascular resistance and right-sided heart failure and are best avoided in pediatric patients undergoing interventional cardiology procedures. Judicious de-airing and intravenous fluid are essential to avoid paradoxical embolism regardless of the direction of shunt. (690)

26. Potential complications the anesthesia provider may encounter in interventional cardiology procedures include bleeding, hematoma, pneumothorax, vascular injury, arrhythmias, heart block, and cardiac perforation leading to pericardial effusion and tamponade. (690)
27. A pericardial effusion or tamponade during an interventional cardiology procedure may present as persistent hemodynamic instability unrelated to induced arrhythmias and refractory to medicines. The diagnosis is confirmed with echocardiography. After discussion with the cardiologist, blood products should be ordered, anticoagulation may be reversed, and volume resuscitation should be initiated. If the pericardial effusion is small and self-limiting, the plan may be to do nothing but wait and observe. Otherwise, a pericardial drain may be placed, or rapid mobilization for surgical decompression of tamponade may be necessary. The vascular access placed by the cardiologist may be used for monitoring (arterial line) and/or fluid resuscitation (central venous line). (690)

ELECTROCONVULSIVE THERAPY (ECT)

28. Patients who have severe clinical depression that is refractory to medications, who have become acutely suicidal, who are acutely psychotic or schizophrenic, and with acute mania are all candidates for ECT. The American Psychiatric Association also recommends ECT for maintenance therapy. There is no absolute contraindication to ECT. Relative contraindications include malignant hypertension, severe cardiomyopathy, hemodynamically significant dysrhythmia, recent cerebrovascular accident, and aortic or intracranial aneurysms. Patients with CIEDs and women with low-risk pregnancy can undergo ECT safely. (690–691)
29. ECT is accomplished by administering an electrical stimulus to the patient that is sufficient to induce a generalized seizure of >15 seconds' duration, but no longer than 2 minutes. The mechanism for the short-term benefit derived from ECT is unknown but is thought to be the result of changes in the neurobiology of neurotransmitter levels in the central nervous system and the suppression of hypothalamic–pituitary–adrenal axis hyperactivity. Routine monitors must be used during an ECT procedure, including pulse oximetry, blood pressure monitoring, and a continuous electrocardiogram. A peripheral nerve stimulator may be useful to confirm neuromuscular blockade and the recovery of skeletal muscle from neuromuscular blockade. An electroencephalogram may also be used to confirm generalized seizure activity during ECT. (692)
30. The table below depicts the considerations of each factor for patients undergoing ECT. (690–692)

Factor	Considerations for ECT
Benzodiazepines	Contraindicated because they raise the seizure threshold, shorten seizure duration, and delay awakening
Esmolol	Can be given prophylactically if excessive sympathetic responses have been seen with previous ECT
Methohexital	Decreases the seizure threshold and is the induction agent of choice
Propofol	Increases seizure threshold and shortens seizure duration, but rapidly clears
Etomidate	Decreases the seizure threshold but can induce myoclonus, nausea and vomiting, and adrenal suppression
Ketamine	Increases intracranial pressure and may cause post-ECT confusion, so is least likely choice
Succinylcholine	Can reduce the risk of musculoskeletal injury during the generalized seizure. The motor seizure can be monitored in an isolated limb with the use of a tourniquet prior to injection.
Implanted defibrillator	Defibrillator function should be deactivated prior to the procedure so the device does not misinterpret the ECT stimulus as arrhythmia.
Pacemaker	Patients who are pacemaker dependent may need to have their pacemaker set in asynchronous mode (e.g., with magnet placement) so the ECT stimulus does not lead to pacemaker inhibition and bradycardia.

31. The airway of the patient undergoing ECT can be managed by hand with a mask, provided the patient is not at risk for the aspiration of gastric contents. Before the induction of anesthesia, the patient must be well pre-oxygenated. The anesthesia provider must be prepared to mask ventilate by hand using supplemental oxygen before the onset of seizure activity and in the postictal period, given that apnea may follow seizure activity even after the termination of the effects of succinylcholine. A laryngeal mask airway may be useful to manage the airway of patients in whom bag-mask ventilation is predicted to be difficult or who have obstructive sleep apnea. The anesthesiologist must have all the equipment needed to intubate the trachea of the patient should it become necessary. Suction must also be available in the event that the regurgitation of gastric contents or excessive oral secretions should occur. (692)
32. Cardiovascular responses to ECT occur in two phases. The first (tonic) phase is characterized by profound parasympathetic discharge that can lead to bradycardia, atrioventricular block, atrial arrhythmias, premature atrial or ventricular contractions, and even asystole. Atropine or glycopyrrolate may be necessary treatment during this phase. The second (clonic) phase is characterized by sympathetic nervous system overstimulation. Therefore after ECT bradycardia and hypotension may occur first, followed by tachycardia and hypertension, which may be severe and persistent. Myocardial ischemia and cardiac dysrhythmia can occur and are the most common causes of fatality after ECT. (691)
33. After ECT and the resultant generalized seizure, the patient is likely to be postictal. Headache, confusion, agitation, cognitive impairment, and memory loss may be present after the procedure. (692)

Chapter

39 POSTANESTHESIA RECOVERY

Matthias R. Braehler and Ilan Mizrahi

INTRODUCTION

- Postanesthesia care unit (PACU)
  - Designed and staffed to care for patients who are recovering from anesthesia and surgery
  - Transition from one-on-one monitoring in the operating room to one of the following:
    - Hospital ward (lower level of monitoring)
    - Independent function of the patient at home
  - PACU can be site of care for critically ill patient requiring short-term intensive care unit (ICU) stay.

ADMISSION TO THE POSTANESTHESIA CARE UNIT

- PACU is staffed by specially trained nurses.
  - Skilled in the prompt recognition of postoperative complications
- Handoff from anesthesia provider to PACU nurse
  - Pertinent details of the patient's history, medical condition, anesthesia, and surgery
- PACU monitoring
  - Vital signs recorded as often as necessary but at least every 15 minutes.
  - Oxygenation (pulse oximetry)
  - Ventilation (breathing frequency, airway patency, capnography)
  - Circulation (systemic blood pressure, heart rate, electrocardiogram)
  - Level of consciousness
- Documentation
  - Vital signs and other pertinent information recorded as part of the patient's medical record

EARLY POSTOPERATIVE PHYSIOLOGIC CHANGES

- Emergence from general anesthesia and surgery
  - May be accompanied by physiologic disturbances that affect multiple organ systems

Physiologic Disorders Manifested in the Postanesthesia Care Unit
Neurologic
Delayed awakening
Emergence agitation
Delirium
Nausea and vomiting
Pain
Respiratory
Upper airway obstruction
Arterial hypoxemia
Hypoventilation
Cardiovascular
Hypotension
Hypertension
Cardiac arrhythmias
Renal
Oliguria
Hematologic
Bleeding
Coagulopathy
Metabolic
Decreased body temperature
Electrolyte and acid-base abnormalities

- Most common PACU complications
  - Postoperative nausea and vomiting (PONV)
  - Need for upper airway support
  - Hypotension
- Most serious PACU adverse outcomes
  - Airway/respiratory issues
    - Especially vulnerable to airway obstruction and hypoventilation on transport to PACU
  - Cardiovascular compromise

UPPER AIRWAY OBSTRUCTION

Loss of Pharyngeal Muscle Tone

- The most frequent cause of upper airway obstruction in PACU

- Contributors to loss of pharyngeal tone
  - Persistent medication effects
    - Inhaled and intravenous anesthetics
    - Neuromuscular blocking drugs
    - Opioids
- Upper airway function in an awake patient
  - Pharyngeal muscles contract
  - Diaphragm generates negative inspiratory pressure
  - Tongue and soft palate pulled forward
  - Airway tented open during inspiration
- Upper airway function during sleep
  - Pharyngeal muscle activity depressed during sleep
  - Decrease in muscle tone can promote airway obstruction.
  - Possible vicious cycle promoting obstruction
    - Collapse of compliant pharyngeal tissue during inspiration
    - Reflex compensatory increase in inspiratory effort
    - Negative inspiratory pressure further worsens airway obstruction
- Paradoxical breathing pattern
  - Clinical manifestation of breathing against an obstructed airway
    - Retraction of sternal notch
    - Exaggerated abdominal muscle activity
    - Rocking motion that becomes more prominent with increasing airway obstruction
- Relieving upper airway obstruction from loss of pharyngeal tone—first steps
  - Open the airway with "jaw thrust maneuver"
  - Continuous positive airway pressure (CPAP) applied via a facemask
- Relieving upper airway obstruction—next steps
  - Oropharyngeal or nasopharyngeal airway placement
  - Supraglottic airway placement
  - Endotracheal intubation

Residual Neuromuscular Blockade

- Postoperative residual neuromuscular blockade is very common.
  - Incidence between 20% and 60%
- Evaluation of upper airway obstruction should consider residual neuromuscular blockade.
- Residual neuromuscular blockade may not be evident upon PACU arrival.
  - Diaphragm recovers from neuromuscular blockade before pharyngeal muscles.
    - Prior to extubation, patient may have normal end-tidal CO_2 and minute ventilation.
  - Pharyngeal muscles may have residual neuromuscular blockade.
    - Ability to maintain a patent upper airway and clear upper airway secretions remains compromised.
  - Factors keeping upper airway open before PACU arrival
    - Stimulation associated with tracheal extubation
    - Activity of patient transfer to the gurney
    - Encouragement to breathe deeply may keep the airway open during transport to the PACU.
  - Upper airway obstruction may become evident only after the patient is calmly resting in the PACU.
- Methods to assess recovery from neuromuscular blockade
  - Clinical assessment
  - Nerve stimulator
- Train-of-four (TOF) measurement
  - Measuring TOF ratio by touch or observation is often misleading.
  - Qualitative TOF measurement and 5-second sustained tetanus at 50 Hz do not detect residual paralysis.
  - Quantitative TOF measurement most reliable indicator of adequate reversal
    - Significant clinical weakness persists up to a ratio of 0.7.
    - However, pharyngeal function is not restored until adductor pollicis TOF ratio ≥0.9.
- Clinical evaluation methods
  - Grip strength
  - Tongue protrusion
  - Ability to lift the legs off the bed
  - Ability to lift the head off the bed for a full 5 seconds
- Issues with 5-second sustained head lift
  - Had been considered to be the standard clinical assessment method
  - However, multiple studies document that 5-second head lift is remarkably insensitive.
- Ability to strongly oppose the incisor teeth against a tongue depressor is a more reliable indicator of pharyngeal muscle tone.
  - Correlates with an average TOF ratio of 0.85
- Clinical signs of residual neuromuscular blockade in PACU
  - Respiratory distress
  - Agitation
- Management of suspected residual neuromuscular blockade
  - Prompt review of possible etiologic factors, as noted in the boxes below.

Factors Contributing to Prolonged Nondepolarizing Neuromuscular Blockade

Drugs
- Inhaled anesthetic drugs
- Local anesthetics (lidocaine)
- Cardiac antiarrhythmics (procainamide)
- Antibiotics (polymyxins, aminoglycosides, lincosamides, metronidazole, tetracyclines)
- Corticosteroids

- Calcium channel blockers
- Dantrolene
- Furosemide

Metabolic and physiologic states
- Hypermagnesemia
- Hypocalcemia
- Hypothermia
- Respiratory acidosis
- Hepatic/renal failure
- Myasthenia syndromes

Factors Contributing to Prolonged Depolarizing Neuromuscular Blockade
Excessive dose of succinylcholine
Reduced plasma cholinesterase activity
▪ Decreased levels
▪ Extremes of age (newborn, old age)
▪ Disease states (hepatic disease, uremia, malnutrition, plasmapheresis)
▪ Hormonal changes
▪ Pregnancy
▪ Contraceptives
▪ Glucocorticoids
Inhibited activity
▪ Irreversible (echothiophate)
▪ Reversible (edrophonium, neostigmine, pyridostigmine)
Genetic variant
▪ Atypical plasma cholinesterase

- Simple measures to facilitate recovery from neuromuscular blockade
  - Warming the patient
  - Airway support
  - Correction of electrolyte abnormalities
- Impact of neuromuscular reversal in patients receiving neuromuscular blocking drugs
  - For patients who received neuromuscular blocking drugs, but did not receive reversal agents
    - 2.3 times greater risk of developing postoperative pneumonia compared to those who did receive reversal agents
  - Neostigmine reversal requires a baseline twitch response.
    - Time for TOF ratio to reach ≥0.9 is highly variable.
  - Sugammadex can be administered at any depth of neuromuscular blockade.
    - Full recovery (TOF ratio ≥0.9) typically occurs within several minutes after administration.
  - Use of sugammadex compared to neostigmine significantly lowers the risk of
    - Postoperative pneumonia
    - Respiratory failure
    - Other major complications

Laryngospasm

- Sudden vocal cord spasm that occludes the laryngeal opening
- Timing
  - Most likely to occur during emergence after extubation in OR
  - Can occur in patient still asleep on arrival to PACU
- Triggered by airway irritants (secretions, blood)
- Treatment
  - Suction to remove irritant
  - Jaw thrust with CPAP
  - Muscle relaxation with potential intubation
    - If intubating, do not force ETT through closed glottis.

Airway Edema or Hematoma

- Risk factors for airway edema
  - Long-duration surgery in the prone or Trendelenburg position
  - Airway and neck surgery
  - Large volume resuscitation
  - Repeated airway instrumentation
- Assessment
  - Facial and scleral edema (may not correlate with pharyngeal edema)
  - Leak test before extubating
    - Ability to breathe around the endotracheal tube with cuff deflated
    - Measure intrathoracic pressure required to generate leak around ETT (with cuff deflated).
    - Exhaled tidal volume before and after cuff deflation
- Treatment to facilitate edema resolution
  - Place patient in sitting position to promote venous drainage
  - Diuretics
  - IV dexamethasone
- Hematoma as cause of external airway compression
  - Most often occurs after thyroid, parathyroid, carotid surgery
  - Decompress airway by releasing sutures and evacuating hematoma.
  - Intubation can be difficult, need emergency equipment available
  - Consider awake intubation.

Obstructive Sleep Apnea

- Many patients with obstructive sleep apnea (OSA) undiagnosed at time of surgery
  - Increased risk of airway obstruction
    - Extubate when fully awake.
  - Increased sensitivity to opioids and benzodiazepines
    - Prioritize multimodal analgesia.
- PACU management of patient with OSA
  - CPAP therapy
  - Continuous pulse oximetry postoperatively

DIFFERENTIAL DIAGNOSIS OF ARTERIAL HYPOXEMIA IN THE PACU

Alveolar Hypoventilation

- Hypoventilation leads to hypercapnia, which can cause hypoxemia.
- Treatment
  - Supplemental oxygen
  - Normalize PCO_2 by increasing minute ventilation.
    - Stimulate/awaken the patient.
    - Reverse opioids or benzodiazepines.
    - Mechanical ventilation in severe cases

Decreased Alveolar Partial Pressure of Oxygen

- Diffusion hypoxia
  - Nitrous oxide diffuses rapidly into the alveoli and decreases PaO_2 and $PaCO_2$.
    - Can persist for 5 to 10 minutes after its discontinuation
  - Causes arterial hypoxemia and decreases respiratory drive
  - Treat with supplemental oxygen.

Ventilation-Perfusion Mismatch and Shunt

- Hypoxic pulmonary vasoconstriction
  - Lungs normally vasoconstrict poorly ventilated regions to direct pulmonary blood flow to well-ventilated regions.
  - Inhaled anesthetics and vasodilators inhibit hypoxic pulmonary vasoconstriction.
- True pulmonary shunt
  - Unlike ventilation/perfusion (VQ) mismatch, does not respond to supplemental oxygen
- Causes of postoperative pulmonary shunt
  - Atelectasis (most common cause)
    - Treatment: mobilize patient to sitting position, incentive spirometry, CPAP
  - Pulmonary edema
  - Gastric aspiration
  - Pulmonary emboli
  - Pneumonia

Increased Venous Admixture

- Typically refers to low cardiac output states
  - Normally <5% of cardiac output shunted through the lungs
  - With low cardiac output, blood returns to the heart severely desaturated.
- Decreased alveolar oxygenation is also a cause (e.g., pulmonary edema, atelectasis).
- Mixing of desaturated shunted blood with saturated arterialized blood decreases PaO_2.

Decreased Diffusion Capacity

- Can occur from underlying lung disease
  - Emphysema
  - Interstitial lung disease
  - Pulmonary fibrosis
  - Primary pulmonary hypertension

PULMONARY EDEMA IN THE PACU

- Most often cardiogenic
  - Intravascular volume overload
  - Congestive heart failure
- Noncardiogenic pulmonary edema also possible
  - Postobstructive pulmonary edema
  - Sepsis and acute respiratory distress syndrome (ARDS)
  - Transfusion-related acute lung injury (TRALI)

Postobstructive Pulmonary Edema

- Also called negative pressure pulmonary edema (NPPE)
  - Rare consequence of laryngospasm
  - Can occur after other causes of upper airway obstruction
- Etiology
  - Exaggerated negative intrathoracic pressure during inspiration against closed glottis
  - Augments venous return
  - Promotes fluid movement into alveolar and interstitial spaces
- Timing
  - Develops quickly, usually within 90 minutes of obstruction
- Signs and symptoms
  - Dyspnea
  - Pink frothy sputum
  - Bilateral fluffy infiltrates on chest x-ray (CXR)
- Treatment
  - Supplemental oxygen
  - Diuresis
  - Positive-pressure ventilation
- Resolution
  - Monitoring needed for 2 to 12 hours postoperatively
  - Resolves within 12 to 48 hours when treated immediately

Transfusion-Related Acute Lung Injury

- Consider in patients who develop pulmonary edema in PACU after receiving plasma-containing blood products in OR.
  - Fresh frozen plasma, whole blood, packed red blood cells, platelets

- Timing and presentation
  - Typically, 2 to 4 hours after transfusion (up to 6 hours)
  - Recovery usually in 48 to 96 hours
- Mechanism
  - Recipient neutrophils activated by donor plasma
  - Release of inflammatory mediators
  - Increased pulmonary vascular permeability and pulmonary edema
- Signs and symptoms
  - Fever
  - Cyanosis
  - Systemic hypotension
  - Pulmonary infiltrates on CXR
- Treatment
  - Supplemental oxygen
  - Diuresis
  - Mechanical ventilation for severe hypoxemia
  - Vasopressors for refractory hypotension

MONITORING AND TREATMENT OF HYPOXEMIA

Oxygen Supplementation

- Pulse oximetry is a PACU standard.
  - A significant percentage of patients develop hypoxemia during PACU stay.
- Supplemental oxygen must be available at all times.

Limitations of Pulse Oximetry

- Pulse oximetry does not reflect ventilation.
- Close observation by trained personnel needed in PACU

Oxygen Delivery Systems

- Factors in choosing PACU oxygen delivery system
  - Degree of hypoxemia
  - Surgical procedure
    - Facemasks may be avoided after head and neck surgery to avoid pressure necrosis on incisions and microvascular flaps.
  - Patient compliance
- Oxygen delivery options
  - Use humidified oxygen with all methods of oxygen delivery.
    - Prevents dehydration of nasal and oral mucosa
  - Nasal cannula
    - Flow is usually limited to 6 L/min to minimize discomfort.
    - Each 1 L/min flow increases FiO_2 by 0.04.
    - Thus 6 L/min delivers approximately FiO_2 0.44.
  - Simple facemasks
    - Oxygen flow rate should be at least 5 L/min to prevent rebreathing of exhaled CO_2.
  - High-flow nasal cannula (HFNC)
    - Can deliver oxygen up to FiO_2 1.0 at 60 L/min, 37°C, and 99% relative humidity
    - FiO_2 is equivalent to traditional facemasks.
    - High flow rates generate CPAP effect and decrease work of breathing.

Continuous Positive Airway Pressure

- Mechanism of benefit
  - Decreases hypoxemia from atelectasis by recruiting alveoli
- CPAP after major abdominal surgery
  - May reduce atelectasis, pneumonia, and reintubation
  - Should be used carefully after esophageal or gastric surgery
    - Concern that positive airway pressure may expand stomach and cause anastomotic disruption

Noninvasive Positive-Pressure Ventilation

- An alternative to endotracheal intubation and mechanical ventilation
  - Well described in ICU setting
  - Limited PACU use
- Delivery mechanisms
  - Facemask
    - Via ICU mechanical ventilator in pressure support mode
  - Nasal pillows, nasal mask, or facemask
    - Via dedicated biphasic positive airway pressure machine
- Relative contraindications
  - Hemodynamic instability or life-threatening arrhythmias
  - Altered mental status
  - High risk of aspiration
  - Inability to use nasal or facial mask
  - Refractory hypoxemia
- Patient conditions that may benefit from NIPPV in PACU
  - OSA
  - Chronic obstructive pulmonary disease
  - Cardiogenic pulmonary edema

HEMODYNAMIC INSTABILITY

Systemic Hypertension

- Multiple factors associated with hypertension in PACU, as noted in the box below.

Factors Leading to Postoperative Hypertension
Cardiovascular
■ Preoperative hypertension
■ Hypervolemia
Respiratory
■ Arterial hypoxemia
■ Hypercapnia
Neurologic
■ Pain
■ Emergence agitation
■ Shivering
■ Nausea/vomiting
■ Increased intracranial pressure
■ Increased sympathetic nervous system activity
Drug-related
■ Withdrawal from β-blocker, clonidine
■ Withdrawal from opioids, benzodiazepines
■ Alcohol withdrawal
■ Substance use (e.g., cocaine, methamphetamine, phencyclidine)
Gastrointestinal/genitourinary
■ Bowel distention
■ Urinary retention

- Most common surgical procedures associated with hypertension
  - Carotid endarterectomy
  - Intracranial procedures

Systemic Hypotension

Hypovolemic Shock

- Common causes of hypovolemia (decreased preload) in PACU
  - Ongoing third-space translocation of fluid
  - Inadequate intraoperative fluid replacement
  - Loss of sympathetic nervous system tone from neuraxial blockade
  - Ongoing surgical bleeding
- Clinical signs
  - Tachycardia
    - May be masked by β-blockers
  - Tachypnea
  - Mottled skin
  - Decreased urine output

Distributive Shock

- Possible causes of distributive shock in PACU
  - Sympathectomy from regional/neuraxial anesthesia
    - Blockade at T4 will block cardioaccelerator fibers.
    - Pharmacologic treatment with vasopressors and ephedrine
  - Critically ill patient with decreased vascular tone
    - May rely on increased sympathetic tone to maintain hemodynamics
    - Anesthetics/opioids/sedatives are impactful, even at minimum doses.
  - Allergic reactions (anaphylactic)
    - Symptoms may include rash, bronchospasm, stridor, facial edema.
    - Treatment: stop offending agents, steroids, H1/H2 blockers, fluid, epinephrine
    - Most common causes include neuromuscular blockers, latex, antibiotics.
    - Diagnosis: tryptase obtained within 2 hours may be helpful (results likely not available for days).
  - Sepsis
    - Diagnosis: send blood cultures
    - Treatment: give empiric antibiotics, fluids, vasopressors if needed
- Less common causes of distributive shock
  - Burns
  - Spinal shock (spinal cord injury)
  - Adrenal insufficiency

Cardiogenic Shock

- Mortality rate of patients in cardiogenic shock approaches 70%.
- Cardiogenic causes of postoperative hypotension
  - Myocardial ischemia or infarction
  - Cardiomyopathy
  - Valvular disease
  - Cardiac arrhythmias
  - Drug induced
    - β-Blockers, calcium channel blockers, local anesthetic systemic toxicity
- Diagnosis
  - CVP monitoring
  - Echocardiography
- Treatment
  - Cardiac catheterization/stenting, mechanical support, or cardiac surgery

Extracardiac/Obstructive Shock

- Mechanism is impaired diastolic filling ultimately causing decreased preload.
- Causes of extracardiac/obstructive shock
  - IVC compression
  - Intrathoracic tumor
  - Tension pneumothorax
    - Treatment: needle decompression and chest tube placement
  - Cardiac tamponade
    - Treatment: pericardiocentesis
  - Excessive positive end-expiratory pressure (PEEP)
  - Pulmonary embolus
    - Treatment: thrombolysis, embolectomy
  - Pericardial disease (pericarditis)
- Diagnosis
  - Point-of-care ultrasound

Myocardial Ischemia

- Detection of myocardial ischemia in the PACU can be challenging.
  - Patient's inability to identify or communicate symptoms
  - Only 35% of patients with myocardial infarction complain of typical chest pain.
- Interpreting ECG ST-segment changes in the PACU
  - Consider patient's cardiac history and cardiac risk index

Low-Risk Patients

- In low-risk patients (i.e., patient <45 years of age, no known cardiac disease, only one risk factor)
  - Postoperative ST-segment changes do not usually indicate myocardial ischemia.
  - Relatively benign causes of ST-segment changes in these patients
    - Anxiety
    - Esophageal reflux
    - Hyperventilation
    - Hypokalemia
- Low-risk patients require only routine PACU observation.
  - Unless associated signs and symptoms warrant further clinical evaluation
- More aggressive evaluation if the ECG changes are accompanied by the following:
  - Cardiac rhythm disturbances
  - Hemodynamic instability
  - Angina
  - Associated symptoms

High-Risk Patients

- ST-segment and T-wave changes in high-risk patients can be significant.
  - Even in the absence of typical signs or symptoms of myocardial ischemia
- Any ST-segment, T-wave, or rhythm changes that are compatible with myocardial ischemia should prompt further evaluation.
- Serum troponin levels are indicated when myocardial ischemia or infarction is suspected.
- Once blood samples for measurement of troponin and a 12-lead ECG are completed
  - Appropriate cardiology follow-up
- Value of routine postoperative 12-lead ECG and troponin measurement
  - Insufficient evidence for these tests in asymptomatic patients
  - In unselected patient population, guidelines recommend against routine troponin screening

Cardiac Arrhythmias

- Perioperative cardiac arrhythmias are frequently transient and multifactorial in cause.

Reversible Causes of Perioperative Cardiac Arrhythmias

- Hypoxemia
- Hypoventilation and associated hypercapnia
- Endogenous or exogenous catecholamines
- Electrolyte abnormalities
- Acidemia
- Excessive intravascular fluid
- Anemia
- Substance withdrawal

Tachyarrhythmias

- Sinus tachycardia is the most common PACU tachyarrhythmia.
  - Most common causes in PACU
    - Postoperative pain
    - Agitation
    - Hypoventilation with associated hypoxemia and hypercapnia
    - Hypovolemia (continued postoperative bleeding)
    - Shivering
    - Presence of a tracheal tube causing stimulation
- Atrial arrhythmias
  - Incidence of new postoperative atrial arrhythmias
    - As high as 10% after major noncardiothoracic surgery
    - Incidence even higher after cardiac and thoracic procedures
  - New-onset atrial arrhythmias are not benign.
    - Associated with longer hospital stays and increased mortality rate
- Atrial fibrillation
  - Immediate goal in the treatment of new-onset atrial fibrillation
    - Control of the ventricular response rate
    - May require prompt electrical cardioversion if hemodynamically unstable
  - Pharmacologic treatment
    - Intravenous β-blocker or calcium channel blocker
    - Ventricular rate control with these drugs often chemically cardioverts the patient.
    - If the goal of therapy is chemical cardioversion, amiodarone infusion can be initiated in the PACU.
- Ventricular arrhythmias
  - Premature ventricular contractions (PVCs) and ventricular bigeminy are common.
    - PVCs often reflect increased sympathetic nervous system stimulation (e.g., from tracheal intubation or transient hypercapnia).
  - Ventricular tachycardia is uncommon.
    - True ventricular tachycardia is indicative of underlying cardiac disease.

- For torsades de pointes, QT-interval prolongation on the ECG may be intrinsic or drug related (e.g., from amiodarone, procainamide, methadone, haloperidol, or droperidol).

Bradyarrhythmias

- Bradycardia in the PACU is often iatrogenic.
- Drug-related causes
  - β-adrenergic blocker therapy
  - Neostigmine reversal of neuromuscular blockade
  - Opioid administration
  - Dexmedetomidine
- Procedure- and patient-related causes
  - Bowel distention
  - Increased intracranial or intraocular pressure
  - Spinal anesthesia

Treatment

- Urgency of treatment
  - Depends on the physiologic consequences of the arrhythmia
  - Most concerning is systemic hypotension and/or myocardial ischemia.
- Tachyarrhythmia
  - Decreases diastolic and coronary perfusion time
  - Increases myocardial oxygen consumption
  - Impact depends on the patient's underlying cardiac function.
    - Most harmful in patients with coronary artery disease
- Bradycardia
  - More deleterious in patients with a fixed stroke volume
    - Infants
    - Patients with restrictive pericardial disease
    - Patients with cardiac tamponade

RENAL DYSFUNCTION

- Postoperative renal dysfunction often has multifactorial causes.
  - Intraoperative insult can exacerbate preexisting renal insufficiency.

Differential Diagnosis of Postoperative Renal Dysfunction

Prerenal
- Hypovolemia (bleeding, sepsis, third-space fluid loss, inadequate volume resuscitation)
- Hepatorenal syndrome
- Low cardiac output
- Renal vascular obstruction or disruption
- Intraabdominal hypertension

Renal
- Ischemia (acute tubular necrosis)
- Radiographic contrast dyes
- Rhabdomyolysis
- Tumor lysis
- Hemolysis

Postrenal
- Surgical injury to the ureters
- Obstruction of the ureters with clots or stones
- Mechanical (urinary catheter obstruction or malposition)

- Patient factors in developing acute kidney injury (AKI)
  - Preexisting renal insufficiency, diabetes, hypertension, obesity, male sex, old age
- Surgical factors
  - Cardiac, vascular, transplant, thoracic, and emergency surgery
- Fluid management during surgery
  - Balanced crystalloid (lactated Ringer, Plasma-Lyte) may decrease AKI compared to saline.
  - Hydroxyethyl starch (HES) should be avoided.
- Blood pressure and postoperative AKI
  - Risk of AKI increased when MAP <60 mmHg for 20 minutes or MAP <55 mmHg for 10 minutes.

Oliguria

Intravascular Volume Depletion

- Intravascular volume depletion is the most common cause of oliguria in PACU
  - Fluid challenge with 500 to 1000 mL should restore urine output.
  - Patients with hypertension may require higher MAP for renal perfusion.
- Assessment of possible hypovolemia
  - Fractional excretion of sodium (FeNa)
  - Central venous pressure monitoring
  - Echocardiography

Postoperative Urinary Retention

- Ultrasonography can measure bladder volume.
  - Urinary retention defined as bladder volume >600 mL
- ASA PACU guidelines do not require voiding prior to PACU discharge.

Contrast Nephropathy

- IV contrast is increasingly required for procedures.
  - Angiography for coronary, aortic, vascular, cerebral procedures
- Timing
  - Creatinine increases within 24 to 48 hours after contrast.
  - Returns to baseline within a week
- Management
  - Intravascular volume expansion with isotonic saline is most effective protection.

- No role for acetylcysteine or urine alkalinization with bicarbonate in preventing AKI after contrast

Intraabdominal Hypertension

- Consider in patients with oliguria and tense abdomen after abdominal surgery.
- Adverse effects of intraabdominal hypertension (IAH)
  - Increased intrabdominal pressure (IAP) impedes renal perfusion and venous drainage
    - Normal IAP 5 mmHg
    - IAH: IAP sustained >12 mmHg
  - Oliguria typically when IAP >15 mmHg
  - Anuria typically when IAP >30 mmHg
- Abdominal compartment syndrome (ACS)
  - Diagnosis requires sustained IAP >20 mmHg with new organ dysfunction/failure
- IAP measurement
  - Bladder pressure indirectly assesses IAP
- Management
  - Medical management
    - Improve abdominal wall compliance
    - Decompress GI contents
    - Correct fluid overload
  - Surgical management
    - For primary ACS, surgical decompression may be required.

Rhabdomyolysis

- Patients at risk for rhabdomyolysis
  - After major crush or thermal injury
  - Morbidly obese patients having bariatric surgery
  - Increased BMI and length of surgery pose increased risk.
- Clinical manifestations
  - Myalgias, abdominal pain, nausea, weakness
  - Myoglobinuria, elevated creatine kinase (CK) levels
- Treatment
  - Maintain urine output.
    - Aggressive hydration, loop diuretics
  - Correct electrolytes.
    - Hyperkalemia, hyperphosphatemia, hypocalcemia
  - Management of renal tubular toxic effect of myoglobin
    - Mannitol and bicarbonate are of unclear benefit.

POSTOPERATIVE HYPOTHERMIA AND SHIVERING

- Postoperative hypothermia
  - Defined as core temperature <36 °C
  - Can occur after general and neuraxial anesthesia
- Temperature goal
  - Core temperature should be at least 36°C within 15 minutes after anesthesia ends
- Impact of mild to moderate hypothermia (33°C to 35°C)
  - Exacerbates postoperative bleeding
    - Inhibits platelet function
    - Inhibits coagulation factor activity
  - Inhibits drug metabolism
    - Prolongs neuromuscular blockade
  - May delay awakening
  - Long-term deleterious effects of hypothermia
    - Increased incidence of myocardial ischemia and myocardial infarction
    - Delayed wound healing
- Postoperative shivering
  - Often occurs after general and neuraxial anesthesia
  - Incidence as high as 66% after general anesthesia
  - Independent risk factors for shivering
    - Young age
    - Joint replacement surgery
    - Core hypothermia

Mechanism

- Heat loss and heat redistribution during surgery
- Shivering in hypothermic patient
  - Due to thermoregulatory mechanisms
- Shivering in normothermic patient
  - More rapid recovery of spinal cord function compared to brain function
  - Uninhibited spinal reflexes may manifest as clonic activity.

Treatment

- Actively warm patient using forced air warmer or warm blankets.
- Accurate core body temperature measurement
  - Tympanic membrane (may be technically challenging)
  - Oral and axillary temperature are usually close to core temperature.
- Treatment of shivering
  - Opioids and α_2-adrenergic agonists effective
    - Most used agent in adults: meperidine (12.5 to 25 mg IV)

POSTOPERATIVE NAUSEA AND VOMITING

- Incidence
  - Without prophylaxis, one third of patients who undergo inhalational anesthesia develop postoperative nausea and vomiting (PONV).
- Consequences of PONV
  - Delayed discharge from the PACU
  - Unanticipated hospital admission
  - Increased incidence of pulmonary aspiration
  - Significant postoperative discomfort

- Benefits of identifying high-risk patients for prophylactic intervention
  - Improved quality of patient care
  - Greater patient satisfaction in the PACU

Prevention and Treatment

- Patient-related risk factors
  - Female sex
  - Nonsmoking status
  - History of PONV and/or motion sickness
  - Need for postoperative opioids
  - Young age (<50 years)
- Anesthesia-related risk factors
  - Use of volatile anesthetics and nitrous oxide
  - Higher doses of perioperative opioids
  - Neostigmine for reversal of neuromuscular blockade
- Surgery-related risk factors
  - Length of surgery
  - Certain surgical procedures
    - Cholecystectomy
    - Laparoscopy
    - Gynecological surgery
- Prophylactic measures to prevent PONV
  - Pharmacologic intervention
    - Multiple drugs available for prophylaxis and treatment of PONV (see box below)
  - Modification of anesthetic technique
    - Use of regional anesthesia technique
    - Minimize the use of volatile anesthetics and nitrous oxide.
    - Use of multimodal analgesia to reduce postoperative opioid requirement
- Antiemetic therapy—guidelines for prevention
  - Administer two antiemetic agents to all patients with one or two risk factors.
  - Administer three or four antiemetic agents to all patients with more than two risk factors.
  - Drug class
    - Do not redose any medication of the same class within 6 hours after the initial dose.
    - If a patient requires PONV treatment in PACU, choose a drug from another class that has not previously been administered.

Commonly Used Antiemetics, With Adult Doses

Anticholinergics
Scopolamine: transdermal patch, 1.5 mg
Apply to a hairless area behind the ear before surgery; remove 24 hours postoperatively.

Antihistamines
Hydroxyzine: 12.5 to 25 mg IM

Phenothiazines
Promethazine: 12.5 to 25 mg IV/IM
Prochlorperazine: 2.5 to 10 mg IV/IM

Butyrophenones
Droperidol: 0.625 to 1.25 mg IV
See black box warning regarding torsades de pointes: monitor the ECG for prolongation of the QT interval for 2 to 3 hours after administration—preoperative 12-lead ECG recommended
Haloperidol: 0.5 to <2 mg IM/IV
Use with caution if prolonged QT interval present in ECG

Nk-1 Receptor Antagonists
Aprepitant: 40 mg PO prior to induction of anesthesia
Casopitant: 150 mg PO prior to induction of anesthesia

Prokinetic
Metoclopramide: 10 to 20 mg IV
Minimal antiemetic properties, avoid in patients with any possibility of gastrointestinal obstruction

Serotonin Receptor Antagonists
Ondansetron: 4 mg IV 30 minutes before conclusion of surgery
Granisetron: 0.35 to 3 mg IV near the conclusion of surgery
Tropisetron: 2 mg IV near the conclusion of surgery
Ramosetron: 0.3 mg IV near the conclusion of surgery
Palonsetron: 0.075 mg IV with induction of anesthesia
Dolasetron: 12.5 mg IV 15 to 30 minutes before conclusion of surgery (no longer marketed in the United States due to risk of QTc prolongation and torsades de pointes)

Corticosteroids
Dexamethasone: 4 to 8 mg IV with induction of anesthesia
Methylprednisolone: 40 mg IV with induction of anesthesia

ECG, Electrocardiogram; *IM,* intramuscularly; *IV,* intravenously; *PO,* by mouth.

DELIRIUM

- Postoperative delirium (POD) definition
  - Acute and fluctuating alteration of mental state with reduced awareness and disturbance of attention
- POD timing
  - Often starts in the recovery room
  - Can occur up to 5 days after surgery
- Incidence of POD
  - Depends on peri- and intraoperative risk factors and is highly variable
  - Reported incidence between 4% and 75%
- POD and patient outcomes
  - Worse surgical outcomes
  - Increased hospital length of stay
  - Functional decline
  - Higher rates of institutionalization
  - Higher mortality
  - Higher cost and resource utilization
- Subtypes of delirium
  - Hyperactive
  - Hypoactive
    - May easily go unnoticed and therefore go untreated
    - Potentially linked to a worse outcome

Risk Factors

- Postoperative delirium has been linked to multiple risk factors as noted in the box below:
- Types of risk factors
  - Predisposing factors (inherent to the patient)
  - Precipitating factors (triggering the onset of delirium)

Risk Factors for Delirium

Predisposing (baseline)
- Cognitive impairment (e.g., dementia)
- Age >65 years
- Sensory impairment (vision, hearing)
- Severe illness (e.g., requiring ICU admission)
- Presence of infection
- Poor functional status (e.g., frailty, limited mobility)
- Alcohol abuse
- Malnutrition

Precipitating
- Medications or medication withdrawal: psychotropic medications (antidepressants, antiepileptics, antipsychotics, benzodiazepines), anticholinergics, muscle relaxants, antihistamines, GI antispasmodics, opioid analgesics, antiarrhythmics, corticosteroids, more than six total medications, more than three new inpatient medications
- Pain
- Hypoxemia
- Hypoglycemia
- Electrolyte abnormalities
- Malnutrition
- Dehydration
- Environmental change (e.g., ICU admission)
- Sleep/wake cycle disturbances
- Urinary catheter use
- Restraint use
- Infection

GI, **Gastrointestinal;** *ICU*, **intensive care unit.**

- Highest-risk procedures include cardiac, vascular, and hip fracture surgeries.

Prophylaxis and Management

- Patients at high risk should be identified prior to surgery
  - Delirium risk screening tools, e.g., AWOL-S tool
- Patients who screen high risk should be placed on a delirium reduction pathway.
  - Pathway should include recommendations for the pre-, intra-, and postoperative care of the patient.
- Avoid deliriogenic medications in PACU.
  - Anticholinergics
  - Sedative-hypnotics
  - Meperidine
  - Unless the specific needs for any of these medications outweigh their potential risks (e.g., benzodiazepines for seizures or for benzodiazepine/alcohol withdrawal)
- Simple measures to decrease the incidence of developing postoperative delirium
  - Frequent reorientation
  - Sensory enhancement
    - Glasses
    - Hearing aids
    - Listening amplifiers
  - Pain control
  - Cognitive stimulation
  - Simple communication approaches to prevent behavior escalation
  - Keeping the patients in their circadian rhythm
- Screening for delirium in the PACU
  - Should be performed before the patient leaves the unit
    - NuDESC (Nursing Delirium Screening Scale)
    - CAM (Confusion Assessment Method) score
- For patients screening positive for delirium in PACU
  - Evaluate for possible precipitating factors.
    - Uncontrolled pain
    - Hypoxia
    - Pneumonia
    - Infection (pneumonia, wound, catheter, bloodstream, urinary tract, sepsis)
    - Electrolyte abnormalities
    - Urinary retention
    - Fecal impaction
    - Medications
    - Hypoglycemia
  - Treat symptoms and causative factors immediately.
  - Multicomponent nonpharmacological interventions described above should be used.
  - Pharmacological interventions
    - Only use in the lowest effective dose
    - Primarily for agitated delirious patients when other interventions have failed
    - Patients who pose a substantial harm to themselves or others
    - Medication of choice: haloperidol starting at 0.5 to 1 mg IM/IV

Emergence Agitation

- Definition
  - Transient confusional state that is associated with emergence from general anesthesia
- Incidence
  - Common in children
    - Peak age is between 2 and 4 years.
    - More than 30% experience agitation or delirium during their PACU stay.
  - Incidence in adults is 3% to 5%.
- Timing
  - Usually occurs within the first 10 minutes of recovery
    - Most frequently associated with rapid emergence from inhalational anesthesia

- Can occur later in children who are brought to the recovery room asleep
- Typically resolves quickly and is followed by uneventful recovery
- Other possible etiologic factors
  - Intrinsic characteristics of the anesthetic
  - Postoperative pain
  - Type of surgery
  - Age
  - Preoperative anxiety
  - Underlying temperament
  - Adjunct medications

DELAYED AWAKENING

- A response to stimulation should occur within 60 to 90 minutes after surgery.
- If emergence has not taken place at that point, consider the following:
  - Residual anesthetic drug effect (most frequent cause)
    - Benzodiazepines
    - Opioids
    - Neuromuscular blocking drugs
    - Propofol and volatile anesthetics (after prolonged anesthetic)
  - Acute alcohol or illicit drug intoxication
  - Central anticholinergic syndrome
  - Metabolic disturbances
    - Hypothermia (<33°C)
    - Electrolyte imbalances (e.g., hyponatremia, hypercalcemia, hypermagnesemia)
    - Hypo- or hyperglycemia
    - Underlying metabolic diseases (e.g., liver, kidney, or thyroid)
  - Neurologic complications
    - Cerebral hypoxia
    - Seizures (with consequent postictal state)
    - Elevated ICP
    - Intracerebral event (hemorrhage, thrombosis, embolus)

Treatment

- Management of patient who presents with delayed emergence
  - Assess airway, breathing, and circulation.
  - Confirm that all anesthetic agents are discontinued.
  - Rewarm patient actively if hypothermia is present.
  - Perform cardiopulmonary and neurological examinations.
  - Use neuromuscular transmission monitor to detect residual neuromuscular blockade.
  - If residual opioid effect is suspected
    - Give naloxone in small increments.
  - If a residual benzodiazepine effect is suspected
    - Titrate flumazenil to effect.
  - Treat hypoglycemia with dextrose.
  - Treat hyperglycemia with insulin.
  - Obtain an ABG and electrolyte panel.
    - Treat carbon dioxide narcosis with hyperventilation (and potentially intubation).
    - Correct electrolyte disturbances.
  - Consider central anticholinergic syndrome (CAS) as a diagnosis of exclusion and administer physostigmine.
  - If concern for acute stroke
    - Consult neurology (e.g., as "code stroke" activation).
    - Obtain a stat head CT.
  - Admit to the ICU for neurologic monitoring if patient still not emerging after above steps.

DISCHARGE CRITERIA

- Specific PACU discharge criteria may vary by institution.
- General principles that are universally applicable
  - Patients routinely required to have a responsible person accompany them home
  - Requiring patients to urinate before discharge may be necessary only in selected patients.
  - Demonstrated ability to drink and retain clear fluids may be appropriate for selected patients.
  - A minimum mandatory stay in the unit should not be required.
  - Patients should no longer be at increased risk for cardiorespiratory depression.
  - Mental status is clear or has returned to baseline.

POSTANESTHESIA SCORING SYSTEMS

- To standardize and facilitate discharge from PACU, different scoring systems have been developed.
- The Modified Aldrete score is most commonly used.
  - Assigns 0, 1, or 2 points to five variables: activity, respiration, circulation, consciousness, oxygen saturation
- Other scores designed to determine readiness for discharge home after outpatient surgery
  - E.g., Postanesthesia Discharge Scoring System (PADS)
- ASA PACU Standards of Care require that a physician accept responsibility for the discharge of patients from the unit
  - Even when the decision to discharge the patient is made by the PACU nurse in accordance with hospital-sanctioned discharge criteria or scoring systems
  - If discharge criteria are to be used, they must first be approved by the department of anesthesia and the hospital medical staff.
  - A responsible physician's name must be noted in the medical record.

QUESTIONS

ADMISSION TO THE POSTANESTHESIA CARE UNIT

1. What are the standards of postoperative care outlined in the ASA Standards for Postanesthesia Care?
2. Which vital signs need to be monitored and recorded in the PACU and how frequently should this be done?

EARLY POSTOPERATIVE PHYSIOLOGIC CHANGES

3. Name physiologic disorders that can manifest while the patient is in the PACU.

UPPER AIRWAY OBSTRUCTION

4. What is the most frequent cause of upper airway obstruction?
5. What is the clinical presentation of upper airway obstruction?
6. What interventions are used to treat upper airway obstruction?
7. Why may residual neuromuscular blockade not immediately be evident upon arrival in the PACU?
8. How is residual neuromuscular blockade assessed in an awake patient?
9. What is laryngospasm, and when is it likely to occur?
10. How should laryngospasm be treated?
11. What operative factors may result in airway edema in the immediate postoperative period?
12. What tests can be performed to evaluate airway patency in patients at risk for airway edema prior to extubation?
13. What measures can facilitate resolution of airway edema that precludes extubation?
14. How can upper airway obstruction in the PACU due to hematoma after thyroid or carotid surgery be treated?
15. What are some special considerations for patients with obstructive sleep apnea (OSA) for postanesthesia care?

DIFFERENTIAL DIAGNOSIS OF ARTERIAL HYPOXEMIA IN THE PACU

16. What are some potential causes of hypoxemia in the PACU? Which of these is most common?
17. What are some potential causes of postoperative hypoventilation?
18. In a patient with a normal A-a gradient, what would be the resulting PaO_2 of a patient breathing room air if the patient's $PaCO_2$ increased from 40 to 80 mmHg?
19. In the PACU, how can arterial hypoxemia secondary to hypercapnia be reversed?
20. What is diffusion hypoxia?
21. Describe the hypoxic pulmonary vasoconstriction (HPV) response, and name some medications that may inhibit it.
22. What are some causes of a true shunt that may present as arterial hypoxemia in the PACU? What is the response to supplemental oxygen in these patients?
23. What is the most common cause of pulmonary shunting presenting as arterial hypoxemia in the PACU? How can it be treated?
24. What is the significance of an increased venous admixture in the PACU?
25. What coexisting lung diseases may result in a decreased diffusion capacity and subsequent arterial hypoxemia in the PACU?

PULMONARY EDEMA IN THE PACU

26. What are the typical causes of cardiogenic and noncardiogenic pulmonary edema in the PACU?
27. What is postobstructive pulmonary edema? How might postobstructive pulmonary edema present in the PACU?
28. How is postobstructive pulmonary edema diagnosed and treated?
29. What is transfusion-related acute lung injury (TRALI)? When is it likely to present?

MONITORING AND TREATMENT OF HYPOXEMIA

30. What is the FiO_2 that can be delivered through a simple nasal cannula? What are some other options for oxygen delivery in the PACU?

31. What is a high-flow nasal cannula (HFNC)? What are its advantages?
32. Is there a role for continuous positive airway pressure (CPAP) and noninvasive positive-pressure ventilation (NIPPV) in the PACU?

HEMODYNAMIC INSTABILITY

33. What are some factors associated with hypertension in the PACU?
34. What are some causes of hypotension in the PACU?
35. What are the most common causes of allergic reactions leading to hypotension in the perioperative setting?
36. What are specific considerations for detecting myocardial ischemia in the postoperative patient?
37. What are common causes of sinus tachycardia in the PACU?
38. What are some reversible causes of cardiac arrhythmias in the postoperative patient?
39. Describe the management of new-onset atrial fibrillation in the PACU.
40. What drugs may contribute to ventricular tachycardia and torsades de pointes in the PACU?
41. What are some possible causes of bradycardia in the PACU?

RENAL DYSFUNCTION

42. What is the differential diagnosis of postoperative renal dysfunction?
43. How is oliguria defined? What is the most common cause of oliguria in the PACU?
44. How should oliguria due to decreased intravascular volume be managed in the PACU?
45. What are the risk factors for postoperative urinary retention?
46. Which patients are at risk for acute renal dysfunction due to contrast nephropathy? How should it be managed?
47. How does intraabdominal hypertension (IAH) lead to oliguria and postoperative renal dysfunction? How can IAH be managed?
48. Which patients are at risk for acute renal dysfunction due to rhabdomyolysis? How should they be managed?

POSTOPERATIVE HYPOTHERMIA AND SHIVERING

49. How is postoperative hypothermia defined, and what are its detrimental effects?
50. How high can the incidence of postoperative shivering be, and what are independent risk factors of this entity?
51. What is the appropriate treatment of postoperative hypothermia and shivering?

POSTOPERATIVE NAUSEA AND VOMITING

52. What are risk factors for postoperative nausea and vomiting (PONV)?
53. How does the number of PONV risk factors influence the approach to PONV prophylaxis?
54. What are the different classes of antiemetic drugs available for prophylaxis and treatment of PONV?

DELIRIUM

55. How is postoperative delirium defined, and how frequently does it occur?
56. What are the predisposing and precipitating risk factors for postoperative delirium?
57. What measures can be taken to reduce the likelihood of postoperative delirium?
58. How do you treat a patient with suspected postoperative delirium?
59. How is emergence agitation defined?

DELAYED AWAKENING

60. A patient in the PACU has delayed awakening 60 minutes after all general anesthesia medications have been stopped? What is the differential diagnosis?
61. What is the workup and treatment of a patient who presents with delayed awakening?

DISCHARGE CRITERIA

62. What are general principles that are universally applicable to determine readiness for discharge from the PACU?

POSTANESTHESIA SCORING SYSTEMS

63. What are the five criteria to determine readiness for discharge used in the Modified Aldrete score? What criteria need to be met for a score of 10?

ANSWERS

ADMISSION TO THE POSTANESTHESIA CARE UNIT

1. The ASA Standards for Postanesthesia Care outline the care for all patients who have received general anesthesia, regional/neuraxial anesthesia, or monitored anesthesia care. These patients need to be recovered in a dedicated postanesthesia care unit, which should have appropriate design, staffing, and equipment. The patients should be transported to the PACU by an anesthesia provider with continuous monitoring, evaluation, and treatment, as necessary. The care will be transferred from the anesthesia provider to the PACU nurse after the patient has been reevaluated and verbal report has been given. During the stay in the PACU, the patient will be continually evaluated, and an accurate written record will be maintained. Finally, the patient will be discharged from the unit under the responsibility of a physician. (698)
2. During the stay in the PACU, the following vital signs should be monitored and recorded: oxygenation (pulse oximetry), ventilation (breathing frequency, airway patency, capnography), and circulation (systemic blood pressure, heart rate, electrocardiogram [ECG]). Vital signs are recorded as often as necessary but at least every 15 minutes while the patient is in the unit. (698)

EARLY POSTOPERATIVE PHYSIOLOGIC CHANGES

3. While a patient is in the recovery room, the following physiologic disorders can occur: upper airway obstruction, arterial hypoxemia, hypoventilation, hypotension, hypertension, cardiac dysrhythmias, oliguria, bleeding, decreased body temperature, delirium (or emergence agitation), delayed awakening, nausea and vomiting, and pain. Prompt recognition and treatment are required to prevent further harm to the patient. (698)

UPPER AIRWAY OBSTRUCTION

4. The most frequent cause of upper airway obstruction in the immediate postoperative period is the loss of pharyngeal muscle tone in a sedated or obtunded patient. The persistent effects of inhaled and intravenous anesthetics, neuromuscular blocking drugs, and opioids all contribute to the loss of pharyngeal tone in the PACU patient. (698)
5. The effort to breathe against an obstructed airway is characterized by a paradoxical breathing pattern consisting of retraction of the sternal notch and exaggerated abdominal muscle activity. Collapse of the chest wall and protrusion of the abdomen with inspiratory effort produces a rocking motion that becomes more prominent with increasing airway obstruction. (698)
6. Obstruction secondary to loss of pharyngeal tone can be relieved by simply opening the airway with the "jaw thrust maneuver" or continuous positive airway pressure (CPAP) applied via a facemask (or both). Support of the airway is needed until the patient has adequately recovered from the effects of drugs administered during anesthesia. If the airway obstruction cannot be overcome by the steps described above, placement of an oropharyngeal or nasopharyngeal airway, a supraglottic airway device, or an endotracheal tube may be required. (698–699)
7. Residual neuromuscular blockade may not be evident upon arrival in the PACU because diaphragm function recovers from neuromuscular blockade more rapidly than pharyngeal muscle function. With an endotracheal tube in place prior to extubation, end-tidal carbon dioxide concentrations and tidal volumes may indicate adequate ventilation while the ability to maintain a patent upper airway and clear upper airway secretions remains compromised. The stimulation associated with tracheal extubation, followed by the activity of patient transfer to the gurney and subsequent encouragement to breathe deeply may keep the airway open during PACU transport. Upper airway obstruction may become evident only after the patient is calmly resting in the PACU. (699)
8. In an awake patient, clinical assessment of reversal of neuromuscular blockade is preferred to the application of painful TOF monitoring. Clinical evaluation includes grip strength, tongue protrusion, the ability to lift the legs off the bed, and the ability to lift the head off the bed for a full 5 seconds. For many years, the 5-second sustained head lift had been considered the standard, reflecting not only generalized motor strength but, more importantly, the patient's ability to maintain and protect the airway. However, studies document the insensitivity of the 5-second head lift as a marker of neuromuscular blockade reversal, and this maneuver should not routinely be used to assess recovery from neuromuscular blockade. A more reliable clinical assessment is the ability to strongly oppose the incisor teeth against a tongue depressor. This maneuver correlates with an average TOF ratio of 0.85. If there is any doubt about residual neuromuscular blockade in the PACU, a quantitative TOF measurement should be used to rule out this condition. (699)

9. Laryngospasm is bilateral vocal cord spasm that completely occludes the laryngeal opening. Laryngospasm usually occurs during emergence from anesthesia immediately after extubation in the operating room, but can occur when patients are awakening after general anesthesia in the PACU. (700)
10. Laryngospasm can be treated initially with jaw thrust and continuous positive airway pressure (CPAP) up to 40 cm H_2O. This typically is sufficient, but if laryngospasm persists, succinylcholine can be administered (0.1 to 1 mg/kg IV or 4 mg/kg IM) to relax the vocal cords. For persistent laryngospasm, a full intubating dose of muscle relaxant and induction agent should be administered to facilitate emergent tracheal intubation. (700)
11. Operative factors that may result in airway edema in the immediate postoperative period include prolonged procedures in the prone or Trendelenburg position; large-volume fluid resuscitation; surgical procedures involving the airway and neck (thyroidectomy, carotid endarterectomy, and cervical spine procedures); and hematoma at the surgical site (again, commonly thyroidectomy and carotid endarterectomy). Visible external signs (e.g., facial or scleral edema, noticeable hematoma) may not accompany life threatening edema or airway compression. (700)
12. Leak tests can be performed to evaluate airway patency in patients at risk for airway edema prior to extubation. One leak test evaluates the patient's ability to breathe around an occluded endotracheal tube (ETT) with the cuff deflated. An alternative leak test measures the intrathoracic pressure required to produce an audible leak around the ETT with the cuff deflated. Another method is to measure the exhaled tidal volume before and after the ETT cuff is deflated during volume control ventilation. (700)
13. Three interventions can help resolve airway edema: (1) sitting the patient upright to ensure venous drainage and reduce any component of dependent edema, (2) diuretic administration, and (3) IV dexamethasone to decrease airway swelling. (700)
14. Upper airway obstruction due to hematoma after thyroid or carotid surgery can be treated by decompressing the airway by releasing the clips or sutures on the wound and evacuating the hematoma. This temporizing measure may be required because mask ventilation and endotracheal intubation by direct laryngoscopy can be difficult secondary to airway displacement. (700)
15. Patients with OSA should not be extubated until they are fully awake and following commands. Because of their increased risk for airway obstruction, opioids and benzodiazepines should be minimized, along with any other medications that depress respiratory drive. To this end, regional anesthesia and multimodal opioid-sparing analgesic techniques should be used whenever possible. CPAP should be available to use postoperatively. Patients' home CPAP devices should be available for use upon arrival in the PACU. If they do not use CPAP at home or do not have their machines with them, a respiratory therapist may need to ensure the proper fit of a CPAP device and titrate the pressure to relieve the airway obstruction. Patients with known or suspected OSA should have continuous pulse oximetry monitoring in the postoperative period. (700–701)

DIFFERENTIAL DIAGNOSIS OF ARTERIAL HYPOXEMIA IN THE PACU

16. There are multiple potential causes of hypoxemia in the PACU. The physiologic mechanisms include alveolar hypoventilation, decreased alveolar partial pressure of oxygen, ventilation-perfusion mismatch and shunt, increased venous admixture, and decreased diffusion capacity. Disease processes include congestive heart failure, pulmonary edema, respiratory depression from anesthetic medication effects, diffusion hypoxia, aspiration of gastric contents, pulmonary embolus, pneumothorax, increased oxygen consumption (from shivering), advanced age, and obesity. Of these, atelectasis (shunt) and alveolar hypoventilation from medications are the most common causes of postoperative hypoxemia in the PACU. (701)
17. Among the potential causes of postoperative hypoventilation are drug-induced central nervous system depression (e.g., from volatile anesthetics, opioids), residual effects of neuromuscular blocking drugs, increased carbon dioxide production, and coexisting pulmonary disease. Each of these causes of alveolar hypoventilation leads to a corresponding increase in arterial partial pressure of carbon dioxide ($PaCO_2$). (701)
18. In a patient breathing room air at sea level, hypoventilation to a $PaCO_2$ of 80 mmHg will result in hypoxemia, even when the patient has normal lungs without a significant A-a gradient. This is demonstrated through the alveolar gas equation. Alveolar oxygen pressure (P_AO_2) in this scenario is 50 mmHg. Supplemental oxygen can mask alveolar hypoventilation by maintaining normal oxygen saturation on pulse oximetry. (701)
19. Arterial hypoxemia secondary to hypercapnia can be reversed by the following interventions: administering supplemental oxygen; external stimulation to awaken the patient; the pharmacologic reversal of the effects of opioids, benzodiazepines, and muscle relaxants; or in some patients controlling respiration with mechanical ventilation. (701)

20. Diffusion hypoxia refers to the rapid diffusion of nitrous oxide into the alveoli at the end of a nitrous oxide anesthetic. Nitrous oxide dilutes the alveolar gas, producing a transient decrease in alveolar oxygen pressure that can persist for up to 5 to 10 minutes after discontinuation of nitrous oxide. In the absence of supplemental oxygen, arterial hypoxemia may ensue and contribute to hypoxemia in the PACU. (702)
21. The hypoxic pulmonary vasoconstriction (HPV) response is the attempt of normal lungs to optimally match ventilation and perfusion by constricting vessels that perfuse poorly ventilated alveoli. This vasoconstrictive response shifts blood flow to well-ventilated regions of the lung. When the HPV response is inhibited, arterial hypoxemia may result. Agents that produce pulmonary vasodilation and thus inhibit the HPV response include inhaled anesthetics, nitroprusside, and dobutamine. (702)
22. Some causes of a true shunt that may present as arterial hypoxemia in the PACU include atelectasis, pulmonary edema, gastric aspiration, pulmonary emboli, and pneumonia. Patients with arterial hypoxemia secondary to a true shunt will not respond to supplemental oxygen. (702)
23. The most common cause of pulmonary shunting presenting as arterial hypoxemia in the PACU is atelectasis. It can be treated by sitting the patient up right, incentive spirometry, and if necessary, positive airway pressure via a facemask. (702)
24. Increased venous admixture refers to the contribution of mixed venous blood to arterial hypoxemia. This effect is typically significant only in cases of low cardiac output when blood returns to the heart in a severely desaturated state. Normally, only 2% to 5% of the cardiac output is shunted through the lungs, but conditions that increase shunt fraction may significantly increase the effect of venous admixture on arterial oxygenation. (702)
25. Coexisting lung diseases such as emphysema, interstitial lung disease, pulmonary fibrosis, or primary pulmonary hypertension may result in a decreased diffusion capacity and subsequent arterial hypoxemia in the PACU. (702)

PULMONARY EDEMA IN THE PACU

26. Pulmonary edema in the immediate postoperative period is most often due to cardiogenic causes, typically from intravascular volume overload or congestive heart failure. Noncardiogenic causes of pulmonary edema in the PACU include postobstructive pulmonary edema, sepsis with acute respiratory distress syndrome, or transfusion-related acute lung injury (TRALI). (702)
27. Postobstructive pulmonary edema (also called negative-pressure pulmonary edema) is a potential consequence of laryngospasm. It is a transudative edema that results from exaggerated negative intrathoracic pressure during inspiration against a closed glottis, which increases venous return, afterload, and pulmonary venous pressures. These conditions promote transudation of fluid into the alveoli. Young, muscular, patients are at increased risk owing to their ability to generate significant inspiratory force. Postobstructive pulmonary edema presents as arterial hypoxemia and respiratory distress within 90 minutes of relief of the obstruction. (702)
28. Clinical manifestations of postobstructive pulmonary edema include hypoxemia and bilateral fluffy infiltrates on chest radiograph. Treatment is supportive with supplemental oxygen, diuresis, and if necessary, positive-pressure ventilation with CPAP or intubation and mechanical ventilation. (702)
29. TRALI refers to pulmonary edema associated with fever and hypotension after the transfusion of plasma-containing blood products. Although fresh frozen plasma and whole blood are the most common culprits, packed red blood cells and platelets can also trigger TRALI. Typically, TRALI manifests within 2 to 4 hours but can occur up to 6 hours after transfusion. The diagnosis is made by an increased alveolar-to-arterial oxygen gradient, bilateral pulmonary infiltrates on a chest radiograph, and systemic hypotension. (702)

MONITORING AND TREATMENT OF HYPOXEMIA

30. As a general rule, each liter per minute of oxygen flow through a simple nasal cannula will increase the FiO_2 by 0.04. The delivery of oxygen by this method is limited by lack of humidification and temperature correction of the gas. The maximum rate of 6 L/min results in approximately 0.44 FiO_2. Other options for oxygen delivery in the PACU include a simple face mask, nonrebreather face mask, and high-flow nasal cannula. Other than the high-flow nasal cannula, each of these oxygen delivery methods is limited in the FiO_2 they can provide secondary to the entrainment of room air when the patient inhales. (703)
31. High-flow nasal cannula can deliver oxygen at rates as high as 60 L/min. Patients tolerate such high flows because the inspired gas is humidified and warmed to 99.9% relative humidity and 37°C. These devices deliver oxygen directly to the nasopharynx throughout the respiratory cycle, and the high flow may enhance the FiO_2 and decrease the work of breathing by a CPAP effect. (703)

32. The decision to use noninvasive modes of ventilation in the PACU must be guided by careful consideration of both patient and surgical factors. Hemodynamic instability, refractory hypoxemia, and the inability to protect the airway due to altered mental status are standard contraindications to noninvasive positive-pressure ventilation (NIPPV). Additional contraindications to consider in this setting include an increased risk of aspiration due to the surgical procedure (e.g., esophagectomy), inability to properly apply the nasal or face mask delivery apparatus because of facial surgery (e.g., sinus surgery), or the need to avoid oropharyngeal and gastric distention by positive-pressure ventilation (e.g., esophageal and abdominal operations). With the previous considerations in mind, home settings of CPAP are recommended routinely for patients with obstructive sleep apnea in the PACU. In the appropriate patient population, application of CPAP or NIPPV in the PACU can help prevent pneumonia, acute respiratory failure, and reintubation. (703–704)

HEMODYNAMIC INSTABILITY

33. Patients with essential hypertension are at greatest risk for postoperative hypertension in the immediate postoperative period. Additional factors to consider include pain, arterial hypoxemia, hypoventilation, hypercapnia, increased intracranial pressure, urinary retention, bowel distention, drug or alcohol withdrawal, emergence agitation, and shivering. Surgical procedures that predispose the patient to hypertension include craniotomy and carotid endarterectomy. (704)
34. A combination of one or more of the following physiologic derangements may account for hypotension in the PACU: a decrease in preload (hypovolemia), intrinsic pump failure (cardiogenic), a decrease in afterload (distributive), or an extracardiac/obstructive cause. Decreased preload may be due to inadequate volume resuscitation in patients who undergo preoperative bowel preparation or after surgery with ongoing translocation of fluid (e.g., major intraabdominal procedures), unrecognized or ongoing blood loss, or loss of sympathetic tone because of neuraxial blockade (spinal or epidural). Intrinsic pump failure often results from exacerbation of preexisting cardiac conditions (e.g., cardiomyopathy, valvular disease, arrhythmias, or coronary artery disease). Decreased afterload can be attributed to iatrogenic sympathectomy (e.g., high neuraxial blockade), blunting of sympathetic drive by narcotics and residual intravenous anesthetics, sepsis, burns, spinal shock, and anaphylaxis. Obstructive causes of hypotension (e.g., cardiac tamponade, pulmonary embolus, and tension pneumothorax) should be ruled out in at-risk patients, such as those who undergo intraoperative central-line placement, intrathoracic or mediastinal procedures, or total hip arthroplasty. (704–706)
35. The most common causes of allergic reaction leading to hypotension in the perioperative setting are neuromuscular blocking drugs, followed by latex and antibiotics. (705)
36. Detection of myocardial ischemia in the PACU can be challenging because of the patient's inability to identify or communicate symptoms related to cardiac ischemia. One study found that only 35% of postoperative patients with myocardial infarction complained of typical chest pain. ST-segment changes on the ECG in the PACU should be interpreted based on the patient's cardiac history and risk index. In low-risk patients (<45 years of age, no known cardiac disease, only one risk factor), postoperative ST-segment changes on the ECG do not usually indicate myocardial ischemia. Relatively benign causes of ST-segment changes in these low-risk patients include anxiety, esophageal reflux, hyperventilation, and hypokalemia. In general, low-risk patients require only routine PACU observation unless associated signs and symptoms warrant further clinical evaluation. A more aggressive evaluation is indicated if the changes are accompanied by cardiac rhythm disturbances, hemodynamic instability, angina, or associated symptoms.

    In high-risk patients, ST-segment and T-wave changes on the ECG can be significant even in the absence of typical signs or symptoms of myocardial ischemia. In this patient population, any ECG changes that are compatible with myocardial ischemia should prompt further evaluation. Determination of serum troponin levels is indicated when myocardial ischemia or infarction is suspected in the PACU. Once blood samples for measurement of troponin and a 12-lead ECG are completed, arrangements must be made for the appropriate cardiology follow-up. (706)
37. Common causes of sinus tachycardia in the PACU include postoperative pain, agitation, hypoventilation with associated hypoxemia and hypercapnia, hypovolemia (e.g., from continued postoperative bleeding), shivering, and the presence of an endotracheal tube. (706)
38. Reversible causes of cardiac arrhythmias in the postoperative period include hypoxemia, hypoventilation and associated hypercapnia, endogenous or exogenous catecholamines, electrolyte abnormalities, acidemia, excessive intravascular fluid, anemia, and substance withdrawal. (706–707)
39. Control of the ventricular response rate is the immediate goal in the treatment of new-onset atrial fibrillation in the postoperative patient. Hemodynamically unstable patients may require prompt electrical cardioversion,

but most patients can be treated pharmacologically with an intravenous β-blocker or calcium channel blocker. Ventricular rate control with these drugs is often enough to chemically cardiovert the postoperative patient whose arrhythmia may be catecholamine driven. If the goal of therapy is chemical cardioversion, an amiodarone infusion can be initiated in the PACU. (707)

40. Ventricular tachycardia is uncommon, whereas premature ventricular contractions (PVCs) and ventricular bigeminy are common. PVCs often reflect increased sympathetic nervous system stimulation, as may accompany tracheal intubation and transient hypercapnia. True ventricular tachycardia is indicative of underlying cardiac disease, and in the case of torsades de pointes, QT-interval prolongation on the ECG may be intrinsic or drug related (e.g., amiodarone, procainamide, methadone, haloperidol, or droperidol). (707)
41. Bradycardia in the PACU is often iatrogenic. Drug-related causes include β-adrenergic blocker therapy, neostigmine reversal of neuromuscular blockade, opioid administration, and treatment with dexmedetomidine. Procedure- and patient-related causes include bowel distention, increased intracranial or intraocular pressure, and spinal anesthesia. A high spinal block of cardioaccelerator fibers originating from T1 through T4 can produce severe bradycardia. The resulting sympathectomy, and possible intravascular volume depletion and associated decreased venous return can result in sudden cardiac arrest, even in young healthy patients. (707)

RENAL DYSFUNCTION

42. The differential diagnosis of postoperative renal dysfunction includes prerenal, renal, and postrenal causes. Prerenal causes include hypovolemia (bleeding, sepsis, third space fluid losses, and inadequate volume resuscitation), hepatorenal syndrome, low cardiac output, renal vascular obstruction, or intraabdominal hypertension. Intrarenal causes include acute tubular necrosis, radiographic contrast dyes, rhabdomyolysis, tumor lysis, and hemolysis. Postrenal causes include urinary retention, surgical injury or obstruction to the ureters, or mechanical obstruction to the urinary catheter. Frequently the cause is multifactorial, and a preexisting renal insufficiency may be exacerbated by an intraoperative insult. For example, preoperative infection and perioperative or intraoperative contrast radiologic studies may put patients at risk for acute renal dysfunction. In the PACU, diagnostic efforts should focus on the identification and treatment of readily reversible causes of oliguria. (707–708)
43. Oliguria is defined as a urine output of <0.5 mL/kg/h. The most common cause of oliguria in the PACU is intravascular volume depletion. (708)
44. Oliguria due to decreased intravascular volume is usually responsive to a 500- to 1000-mL bolus of intravenous crystalloid. Intravenous fluids should be continued as necessary to maintain renal perfusion and prevent further ischemic injury and development of acute tubular necrosis. If a fluid challenge is contraindicated or oliguria persists, central venous monitoring or echocardiography may facilitate diagnosis of volume depletion. (708)
45. Postoperative urinary retention refers to the inability to void despite a bladder volume of more than 600 mL. Risk factors include age >50 and intraoperative fluid >750 mL. (708)
46. Contrast nephropathy should be considered in patients who have undergone angiography for aortic, peripheral vascular, cerebral vascular, or coronary artery disease. These patients often have chronic renal insufficiency and are at increased risk of developing renal failure secondary to an intravenous contrast load. Intravascular volume expansion with isotonic saline is the only effective means to prevent contrast nephropathy. Unfortunately, acetylcysteine or urine alkalinization with sodium bicarbonate infusions have shown no benefit and are not recommended. (708–709)
47. Persistently elevated intraabdominal pressure impedes renal perfusion and leads to renal ischemia. Intraabdominal hypertension is defined as a sustained intraabdominal pressure (IAP) higher than 12 mmHg, and abdominal compartment syndrome is defined as a sustained IAP greater than 20 mmHg that is associated with new organ dysfunction. Oliguria does not develop until IAP reaches 15 mmHg. Intraabdominal hypertension should be ruled out by measuring the bladder pressure in any patient with a tense abdomen and oliguria postoperatively. Prompt intervention is necessary to restore renal perfusion. Medical management includes measures to improve abdominal wall compliance, evacuation of gastrointestinal contents, correction of positive fluid balance, and (if necessary) surgical decompression of the abdomen. (709)
48. Rhabdomyolysis should be suspected in oliguric patients who have suffered a major crush or thermal injury. The incidence is also increased in morbidly obese patients undergoing bariatric surgery. A creatine kinase (CK) level should be measured in suspected patients. It is treated by early aggressive hydration to maintain urine output. In addition, electrolyte abnormalities must be corrected. Mannitol and bicarbonate infusion to prevent renal tubular myoglobin toxicity is commonly practiced but may not provide any further benefit. (709)

POSTOPERATIVE HYPOTHERMIA AND SHIVERING

49. Postoperative hypothermia is defined as a core temperature <36°C. Besides being unpleasant for the patient, it can inhibit platelet function, coagulation factor activity, and drug metabolism. Furthermore, it exacerbates postoperative bleeding, prolongs neuromuscular blockade, and may delay awakening. Finally, long-term deleterious effects include an increased incidence of myocardial ischemia and myocardial infarction, and delayed wound healing. (709)
50. The incidence of postoperative shivering may be as high as 66% after general anesthesia. Independent risk factors include young age, joint replacement surgery, and core hypothermia. (709)
51. Patients who arrive hypothermic in the PACU should be actively warmed by using a forced air warmer or warm blankets. Accurate core body temperature should be obtained, with oral or axillary measurement being feasible locations. Several opioids as well as α_2-adrenergic agonists have been shown to abolish shivering; the most commonly used agent in adults is meperidine (12.5 to 25 mg IV). (709)

POSTOPERATIVE NAUSEA AND VOMITING

52. There are several risk factors for PONV, and the likelihood of PONV increases with the number of these risk factors. These factors can be divided into patient-related, anesthesia-related, and surgery-related risk factors. Patient-related risk factors include female gender, nonsmoking status, history of PONV and/or motion sickness, the need for postoperative opioids, and young age (<50 years). Anesthesia-related risk factors include the use of volatile anesthetics and nitrous oxide as well as the administration of higher doses of perioperative opioids and neostigmine for reversal of neuromuscular blockade. Surgery-related risk factors include the length of surgery as well as certain surgical procedures (cholecystectomy, laparoscopy, gynecological surgery.) (710)
53. The expert guidelines "Fourth Consensus Guidelines for the Management of Postoperative Nausea and Vomiting" advocate a liberal approach to prophylaxis based on number of PONV risk factors. The guidelines recommend giving two antiemetic agents to all patients with one or two risk factors, and giving three or four antiemetic agents to all patients with three or more risk factors. If an adequate number and dose of antiemetic drugs given at the appropriate time is ineffective, simply giving more of the same class of drug in the PACU is unlikely to produce any significant benefit. Therefore it is recommended not to redose any medication of the same class within 6 hours after the initial dose. Instead, a drug from another class that has not previously been administered should be chosen for the treatment of PONV in the PACU. (710)
54. There are drugs from several different pharmacological classes available for prophylaxis and treatment of PONV. These groups are anticholinergics, antihistamines, phenothiazines, butyrophenones, Nk-1 receptor antagonists, prokinetics, serotonin receptor antagonists, and corticosteroids. A combination of drugs from different groups is recommended, and the number of drugs should be chosen based on the number of PONV risk factors. (710–711)

DELIRIUM

55. Postoperative delirium (POD) is defined as an acute and fluctuating alteration of mental state with reduced awareness and disturbance of attention. POD often starts in the recovery room but can occur up to 5 days after surgery. The incidence of POD depends on peri- and intraoperative risk factors and is highly variable, with incidences between 4% and 75% reported in the literature. (710)
56. Risk factors for postoperative delirium are commonly divided between predisposing factors (inherent to the patient) and precipitating factors (triggering the onset of delirium). Major predisposing risk factors are reduced cognitive reserve (e.g., dementia, depression, advanced age), reduced physical reserve (e.g., atherosclerotic disease, renal impairment, pulmonary disease, advanced age, preoperative β-blockade), sensory impairment (e.g., vision, hearing), alcohol use disorder, malnutrition, dehydration, and presence of infection. Major precipitating risk factors include the performed surgical procedure (physiologic stressor) and medications or medication withdrawal such as psychotropic medications (antidepressants, antiepileptics, antipsychotics, benzodiazepines), anticholinergics, muscle relaxants, antihistamines, GI antispasmodics, opioid analgesics, antiarrhythmics, corticosteroids, more than six total medications, more than three new inpatient medications. Additional major precipitating factors include pain, hypoxemia, electrolyte abnormalities, malnutrition, dehydration, environmental change (e.g., ICU admission), sleep/wake cycle disturbances, urinary catheter use, restraint use and infection. (711)

57. Patients at high risk of postoperative delirium should be identified prior to entering the operating room by using a delirium risk screening tool. Patients who are screened as high risk for developing delirium should ideally be placed on a delirium reduction pathway to decrease their likelihood of developing delirium in the postoperative phase of care. Such a pathway should include recommendations for the pre-, intra-, and postoperative care of the patient. Once the patient is in the recovery room, any deliriogenic medications should be avoided, unless the specific needs for any of these medications outweighs their potential risks (e.g., benzodiazepines for seizures or for benzodiazepine/alcohol withdrawal). Simple measures, such as frequent reorientation, sensory enhancement (ensuring glasses, hearing aids, or listening amplifiers are available upon arrival in the PACU), pain control, cognitive stimulation, simple communication standards and approaches to prevent the escalation of behaviors, and keeping the patients in their circadian rhythm can decrease the incidence of developing postoperative delirium by 30% to 40%. (711)
58. If a patient develops postoperative delirium, prompt evaluation of possible precipitating factors should occur. These include uncontrolled pain, hypoxia, pneumonia, infection (wound, indwelling catheter, and bloodstream, urinary tract, sepsis), electrolyte abnormalities, urinary retention, fecal impaction, medications, and hypoglycemia. Treatment of causative factors and symptoms has a major impact on reducing the duration of delirium and should be initiated immediately. Generally, multicomponent nonpharmacological interventions should be used for all patients with delirium (e.g., frequent reorientation, calm environment, eliminating restraint use, familiar objects in the room, bringing glasses and hearing aids to the patient). Pharmacologic interventions should be reserved and only used in the lowest effective dose for agitated delirious patients when other interventions have failed and when patients pose a substantial harm to themselves or others. The medication of choice is haloperidol starting at 0.5 to 1 mg IM/IV. (711)
59. Emergence agitation is a transient confusional state that is associated with emergence from general anesthesia. Emergence agitation is common in children, with more than 30% experiencing agitation or delirium at some period during their PACU stay. It usually occurs within the first 10 minutes of recovery but can have onset later in children who are brought to the recovery room asleep. The peak age of emergence agitation in children is between 2 and 4 years. Unlike delirium, emergence agitation typically resolves quickly and is followed by uneventful recovery. In children, emergence agitation is most frequently associated with rapid emergence from inhalational anesthesia. Other possible etiologic factors include intrinsic characteristics of the anesthetic, postoperative pain, type of surgery, age, preoperative anxiety, underlying temperament, and adjunct medications. Awareness of these contributors allows one to identify and treat children who are at increased risk. In contrast to children, the incidence of emergence agitation in adults is estimated to only be between 3% and 5%. (711)

DELAYED AWAKENING

60. Residual drug effects are the most frequent cause of delayed emergence after general anesthesia. The most common drugs to consider are benzodiazepines, opioids, and neuromuscular blocking drugs. However, after a long-duration anesthetic, propofol and volatile anesthetics can also cause a delay in emergence. Furthermore, acute alcohol or illicit drug intoxication can be other culprits. Another often overlooked drug effect is the central anticholinergic syndrome, as several drugs used during anesthesia can block the central cholinergic neurotransmission and therefore delay the wakeup. Metabolic disturbances such as hypothermia (<33°C), electrolyte imbalances (e.g., hyponatremia, hypercalcemia, hypermagnesemia), hypo- or hyperglycemia, as well as underlying metabolic diseases (e.g., liver, kidney, or thyroid abnormalities) can delay emergence after anesthesia. Finally, neurologic complications such as cerebral hypoxia, seizures (with postictal state), elevated ICP, as well as any intracerebral event (hemorrhage, thrombosis, embolus) should be considered. (712)
61. In any patient who presents with a delayed emergence, the initial assessment should begin with the airway, breathing, and circulation. It is important to confirm that all anesthetic agents are discontinued. The patient's body temperature should be checked upon arrival in the PACU, and if hypothermia is present, the patient should be actively rewarmed. A cardiopulmonary and neurologic exam should be performed. The use of a neuromuscular transmission monitor is instrumental in detecting residual neuromuscular blockade, which should be reversed if present. If a residual opioid effect is suspected, naloxone in small increments can be titrated to effect. Similarly, if a residual benzodiazepine effect is suspected, flumazenil can be titrated to effect. A blood glucose level should be checked, and hypoglycemia should be treated with dextrose; hyperglycemia can be treated with insulin as needed. An ABG and electrolyte panel should be obtained. Carbon dioxide narcosis can be treated with assisted ventilation (and potentially intubation). Electrolyte disturbances should be corrected. If the cause of delayed awakening remains elusive, central anticholinergic syndrome (CAS) should

be considered, for which physostigmine IV could be administered. An acute cerebrovascular event should also be considered. Additional steps could include obtaining a stat head CT and consulting a neurologist. If the patient remains minimally responsive, admission to the ICU for further monitoring and serial exams should be initiated. (712)

DISCHARGE CRITERIA

62. For a patient to be determined ready for discharge from the PACU, the following general principles are applied. All outpatients are routinely required to have a responsible person accompany them home. The requirement to urinate before discharge may only be necessary in selected patients. Similarly, the ability to drink and retain clear fluids may only be appropriate for selected patients. A minimum mandatory stay in the unit should not be required. At the time of PACU discharge, the patient should no longer be at an increased risk of cardiac or respiratory depression and their mental status should be clear or should have returned to baseline. (713)

POSTANESTHESIA SCORING SYSTEMS

63. The Modified Aldrete score assesses activity (ability to move extremities), breathing, circulation (systemic blood pressure), consciousness, and oxygen saturation (pulse oximetry). In each category a patient can get 0, 1, or 2 points, as noted in the table below. Readiness for discharge is indicated by a score of ≥9, as noted in the table below. (713)

Criteria for Determining Release From the Postanesthesia Care Unit: The Modified Aldrete Score

Variable Evaluated	*Score*
Activity	
Able to move four extremities on command	2
Able to move two extremities on command	1
Able to move no extremities on command	0
Breathing	
Able to breathe deeply and cough freely	2
Dyspnea	1
Apnea	0
Circulation (systemic blood pressure)	
Within 20% of the preanesthetic level	2
20%–49% of the preanesthetic level	1
≥50% of the preanesthetic level	0
Consciousness	
Fully awake	2
Arousable	1
Not responding	0
Oxygen saturation (pulse oximetry)	
>92% while breathing room air	2
Needs supplemental oxygen to maintain saturation >90%	1
<90% even with supplemental oxygen	0

Adapted from Aldrete JA. The post anaesthesia recovery score revisited. *J Clin Anesth*. 1995;7:89–91.
Score ≥9 required for discharge.

Chapter

40 PERIOPERATIVE PAIN MANAGEMENT

Carolyn Kloepping and Sarah Greene

INTRODUCTION

- Postoperative pain
  - Complex reaction to tissue injury
  - Can result in adverse effects in multiple organ systems
  - Leads to significant morbidity, patient discomfort
  - Increased healthcare costs (e.g., longer postanesthesia care unit [PACU], intensive care unit [ICU], or hospital stay)
- Chronic postsurgical pain (CPSP)
  - Defined as postsurgical pain lasting longer than the normal recuperative healing time
  - Affects 10% to 65% of patients
  - Most common after the following procedures
    - Limb amputation (30% to 83%)
    - Thoracotomy (22% to 67%)
    - Sternotomy (27%)
    - Breast surgery (11% to 57%)
    - Gallbladder surgery (up to 56%)

COMMON TERMINOLOGY

- Pain
  - An unpleasant sensory and emotional experience caused by actual or potential tissue damage or described in terms of such damage
- Acute pain
  - Follows injury to the body and generally recedes when the bodily injury heals
- Chronic (persistent) pain
  - Pain that has persisted beyond the time of healing
  - Duration of persistent pain is determined by the nature of the injury.
  - Usually considered chronic when the duration exceeds 3 months' duration
- Pain management
  - Clinical practice of relieving acute, subacute, and chronic (persistent) pain
  - Achieved through the implementation of psychological, physical, therapeutic, pharmacologic, and interventional methods

In-Hospital (Inpatient) Pain Service

- Types of inpatient pain medicine services
  - Perioperative (acute) pain medicine
  - Chronic (persistent) pain medicine
- Many institutions do not have separate pain services.

NEUROBIOLOGY OF PAIN

Nociception

- Process of recognition and transmission of painful stimuli from the periphery to the sensory cortex
- Nociceptors
  - Free afferent nerve endings of myelinated Aδ and unmyelinated C fibers
  - Present in peripheral visceral and somatic sites
  - Activated by inflammatory mediators released in response to painful stimuli
    - Thermal, mechanical, or chemical tissue damage

Afferent Sensory Pathway

- First-order neurons: periphery to dorsal horn of spinal cord
  - Integration with inhibitory input
  - Some impulses pass to ventral horn and initiate spinal reflexes.
- Second-order neurons: dorsal horn of spinal cord to thalamus
  - Crosses to contralateral side of spinal cord before ascending
  - Divides and sends projections to reticular activating system and periaqueductal gray matter
- Third-order neurons: thalamus to sensory cortex
  - Produces cortical responses and the perception of pain

Modulation of Nociception

- Spinal cord modulation
  - Via excitatory or inhibitory neurotransmitters at the dorsal horn of spinal cord
  - Via descending inhibitory pathways that originate from the brainstem

- Peripheral sensitization
  - Caused by continuous release of inflammatory mediators in periphery
  - Results in
    - Activation of dormant nociceptors
    - Decreased threshold for activation
    - Increased discharge rate with activation
    - Increased rate of spontaneous discharge
- Central sensitization
  - Pain hypersensitivity resulting from persistent central nervous system postinjury changes
- Hyperexcitability
  - Condition that can occur after tissue damage
  - Neurons with exaggerated and prolonged responsiveness to normal afferent input
  - Key receptors: *N*-methyl-D-aspartate (NMDA)
  - Neurotransmitters or second messengers involved include:
    - Substance P
    - Protein kinase C-γ

Preventive Analgesia

- Rationale
  - Central or peripheral sensitization after injury or surgical incision can amplify postoperative pain.
  - Therefore attempt to block pain transmission throughout
    - Before injury or incision
    - During noxious stimuli
    - After (postoperative/postinjury)
- Potential benefits of preventive analgesia
  - May prevent development of central sensitization
  - May reduce acute postprocedural pain/hyperalgesia and chronic pain after surgery

Multimodal Approach to Perioperative Recovery

- Multimodal approach may include a combination of the following:
  - Interventional analgesic techniques
    - Neuraxial analgesia
    - Peripheral nerve catheter or peripheral nerve block
  - Systemic pharmacologic therapies
    - E.g., nonsteroidal anti-inflammatory drugs (NSAIDs), α-adrenergic agonists, NMDA receptor antagonists, membrane stabilizers, and opioids
- Requires multidisciplinary collaboration
- Potential benefits
  - May decrease perioperative morbidity
  - Decrease length of hospital stay
  - Improve patient satisfaction without compromising safety

Multimodal Analgesia: Goals and Approach

- Goals
  - Sufficient diminution of the patient's pain to instill a sense of control over the pain
  - Enable early mobilization
  - Allow early enteral nutrition
  - Attenuate the perioperative stress response
  - Maximize the benefit (analgesia) while minimizing the risk (side effects of the medications)
- Approach
  - Local anesthesia
  - Regional techniques
    - Single shot vs catheter
  - Nonopioid analgesics
    - E.g., acetaminophen, NSAIDs, or cyclooxygenase (COX)-2–specific inhibitors
  - Other analgesic adjuncts
    - Ketamine, lidocaine, magnesium

Opioid-Induced Hyperalgesia

- Paradoxical effect after postoperative short-term administration of opioids
  - Increase in patient's pain severity
  - Decrease in pain tolerance
- Involves activation of NMDA receptors

Opioid-Sparing Versus Opioid-Free Techniques

- Growing concern of persistent postoperative opioid use following surgery
- No significant difference has been shown between opioid-sparing and opioid-free techniques.

ANALGESIC DELIVERY SYSTEMS

- Traditional delivery systems for perioperative pain management
  - Oral and parenteral on-demand analgesics
- Newer approaches
  - IV infusions of analgesics
  - Patient-controlled analgesia (PCA)
  - Other routes: subcutaneous, neuraxial, peripheral nerve

Patient-Controlled Analgesia

- PCA advantages over intermittent intravenous (IV) or intramuscular (IM) opioids
  - Better analgesia
  - Greater safety
  - Less sedation
  - Less total drug use
  - Fewer sleep disturbances
  - More rapid return to physical activity
- PCA parameters
  - PCA dose limit per unit time

- Lockout interval (minimum time between doses)
- Option for continuous basal infusion if needed
- Monitors
  - Pulse oximetry may not detect respiratory depression when supplemental oxygen is used.
  - Capnography should be considered in patients with substantial comorbidities.

SYSTEMIC THERAPY

Oral Administration

- Oral analgesics not optimal in immediate postoperative period due to NPO status
- Perioperative oral medication options
  - NSAIDs
  - Acetaminophen
  - Opioids
  - Amine reuptake inhibitors (tricyclic antidepressants [TCAs], serotonin, and norepinephrine reuptake inhibitors [SNRIs])
  - Vitamin C (preoperative and postoperative)
  - Gabapentinoids
    - Risk of respiratory depression, particularly when combined with opioids
    - Not recommended for routine use

Intravenous Administration

- Use
  - Common in PACU or ICU to treat acute or severe pain
  - Continuous nursing care and monitoring provide safety.
- Characteristics of IV compared to oral administration
  - Quicker onset
  - Less variability in plasma concentration
  - Rapid redistribution
  - Shorter duration of analgesia
- Opioids
  - The table below lists commonly used parenteral and oral analgesics

Oral and Parenteral Analgesics for Treatment of Perioperative Pain

Agent	Route of Administration	Dose (mg)	Half-life (hr)	Onset (hr)	Analgesic Action (hr)	Peak Duration (hr)
Opioids and Opioid Derivatives						
Morphine	Intravenous	2.5–15	2–3.5	0.25	0.125	2–3
	Intramuscular	10–15	3	0.3	0.5–1.5	3–4
	Oral	30–60	3	0.5–1	1–2	4
Codeine	Oral	15–60	4	0.25–1	0.5–2	3–4
Hydromorphone	Intravenous	0.2–1.0	2–3	0.2–0.25	0.25	2–3
	Intramuscular	1–4	2–3	0.3–0.5	1	2–3
	Oral	1–4	2–3	0.5–1	1	3–4
Fentanyl	Intravenous	20–50 (μg)	0.5–1	5–10 min	5 min	1–1.5
	Transmucosal*	200–1600 (μg)	2–12	0.1–0.25	0.5–1	0.25–0.5
	Transdermal	12.5–100 (μg)	20–27	12–24	20–72	72
Oxymorphone	Oral	5–10	3.3–4.5	0.5	1	2–6
	Intravenous	0.5–1	3–5	0.15	0.25	3–6
	Subcutaneous	1–1.5	3–5	0.15	0.25	3–6
	Intramuscular	1–1.5	3–5	0.15	0.25	3–6
Hydrocodone	Oral	5–7.5	2–3	30	90	3–4
Oxycodone	Oral	5	3–5	0.5	1–2	4–6
Methadone	Oral	2.5–10	3–4	0.5–1	1.5–2	4–8
Other						
Tramadol†	Oral	50–100	5–6	0.5–1	1–2	4–6

*Transmucosal fentanyl is most appropriately reserved for breakthrough malignant (cancer) pain.
†Not classified by the U.S. Food and Drug Administration as an opioid; however, tramadol possesses naloxone partial-reversal analgesia.

- Ketamine
  - Subanesthetic doses for postoperative analgesia
    - Does not cause cognitive impairment or hallucinations
  - Reduces opioid-induced hyperalgesia
    - May suppress central sensitization
  - Preoperative and intraoperative infusions reduce CPSP risk.
- Lidocaine
  - Continuous infusion for intraoperative and postoperative analgesia
  - Reduced pain scores, nausea, ileus duration, opioid requirements, and length of hospitalization
  - Effect can persist for hours or days after terminating the infusion.
  - Mechanism
    - Involved in inflammatory signaling
    - Blocks excitatory responses of glycine in wide-dynamic range neurons
  - Toxicity at low doses is rare.
    - Monitor postoperatively for symptoms of perioral numbness, tinnitus, or cardiac dysrhythmias.
- Acetaminophen
  - No difference in efficacy compared to oral administration
  - IV dose is useful for patients who are NPO.
- Dexamethasone
  - Preoperative administration decreases acute postoperative pain scores and opioid consumption.
  - Increased efficacy at dose >10 mg
- Clonidine
  - Modest analgesic effect of decreased postoperative pain
  - Limited by side effects of bradycardia and hypotension
- Magnesium
  - Given intraoperatively reduces postoperative pain and opioid requirements
  - Blocks NMDA receptors

Subcutaneous Administration

- For patients without IV access or in palliative care

Transmucosal Administration

- Provides rapid onset of drug effect
- Rarely used for postoperative pain

Perioperative Management of Buprenorphine

- Food and Drug Administration (FDA)-approved medication for opioid dependence
  - Other medications include methadone and naloxone
- Partial mu agonist, kappa antagonist
  - Duration of action is unpredictable.
  - Risk for respiratory depression when combined with full opioid agonist
- Perioperative management of patient receiving buprenorphine
  - Ideal to discontinue 3–5 days before surgery
  - If unable to taper/discontinue before surgery
    - Administer baseline buprenorphine dose.
    - Multimodal analgesia
  - Alternatively, preoperative transition from buprenorphine to methadone
    - Methadone is a long-acting opioid.
    - May be useful if surgery is major or severe pain is expected
- Challenges
  - Discontinuation can precipitate withdrawal symptoms.
  - Time course to surgery may limit planning with patient's buprenorphine prescriber.

NEURAXIAL ANALGESIA

- Neuraxial and peripheral regional techniques
  - Generally provide superior analgesia compared with systemic opioids
  - May decrease morbidity and mortality

Intrathecal Administration

- Onset of intrathecal opioid is proportional to lipid solubility of the drug.
  - Duration of effect longer if opioid is hydrophilic.
- Advantages
  - Can place drug near the site of action
  - Short to intermediate duration of postoperative analgesia after single dose
- Disadvantage
  - Single-shot lacks flexibility for duration of effect.
  - Intrathecal catheter placement controversial due to reports of cauda equina syndrome

Epidural Administration

- Continuous local anesthetic only
  - Significant failure rate
  - Frequently causes motor block and hypotension
  - Effect determined by total dose (not volume or concentration)
- Continuous opioid only
  - No motor block or hypotension
  - Hydrophilic opioids have a spinal mechanism of action.
  - Lipophilic opioids have a systemic site of action.
- Local anesthetic plus opioid combination
  - Generally more effective analgesia than single class of medication

Side Effects of Neuraxial Analgesic Drugs

- Many medication-related side effects can occur.
- Standing orders and nursing protocols for analgesic regimens
  - Neurologic monitoring
  - Treatment of side effects
  - Physician notification about critical variables

Most Common Side Effects

- The most common side effects are noted in the box below.

Most Common Side Effects of Neuraxial Analgesia for Perioperative Pain Management

- **Urinary retention** (10%–30%): Epidural administration of local anesthetics and/or opioids is associated with urinary retention.
- **Nausea, vomiting, and pruritus** (15%–18%): Pruritus is one of the most common side effects of epidural or intrathecal administration of opioids, with an incidence of approximately 60% compared with about 15%–18% for local epidural anesthetic administration or systemic opioids.
- **Motor block** (2%–3%): In most cases motor block resolves within 2 hr after discontinuing the epidural infusion. Persistent or increasing motor block should be promptly evaluated, and spinal hematoma, spinal abscess, and intrathecal catheter migration should be considered as part of the differential diagnosis.
- **Hypotension** (0.3%–7%): Local anesthetics used in an epidural analgesic regimen may block sympathetic fibers and contribute to postoperative hypotension.
- **Respiratory depression** (0.1%–0.9%): Neuraxial opioids administered in appropriate doses are not associated with a more frequent incidence of respiratory depression than that seen with systemic administration of opioids. Risk factors for respiratory depression with neuraxial opioids include larger dose, geriatric age group, concomitant administration of systemic opioids or sedatives, the possibility of prolonged or extensive surgery, the presence of comorbidities, and thoracic surgery.

Anticoagulants

- Increased risk of spinal hematoma in patients receiving anticoagulants
- ASRA consensus statements
  - Recommends timing for neuraxial needle/catheter placement and removal in relation to specific anticoagulants to minimize risk of spinal hematoma

Infection

- Meningitis and spinal abscess are rare (<1 in 10,000).
- Increased risk
  - Longer duration of epidural analgesia
  - Immunocompromised patient
  - Malignancy or trauma

SURGICAL SITE (INCISION) INFILTRATION

- Local anesthetic infiltration before incision and/or before closure is recommended to reduce postoperative pain.

INTRAARTICULAR ADMINISTRATION

- Intraarticular opioids
  - Analgesia up to 24 hours postoperatively
    - Effect may not be superior to that of systemic opioids.
  - May prevent CPSP
  - Opioid receptors at peripheral terminals of primary afferent nerves
- Local anesthetics
  - Glenohumeral continuous catheters with bupivacaine are associated with chondrolysis.
  - Extended-release bupivacaine may not be more effective than traditional local anesthesia combined with opioid.

PARAVERTEBRAL BLOCKS

- Beneficial effects for patients undergoing breast surgery
  - Effective acute pain control
  - Demonstrated to decrease development of CPSP
- Can be performed as single-shot or continuous catheter
- Thoracic, cardiac, and pediatric applications

PERIPHERAL NERVE BLOCK

- Single-shot injections for intraoperative analgesia
  - Adding an adjuvant drug provides intermediate (<24 hours) relief.
- Continuous perineural catheters for longer duration of analgesia

Techniques

- Anatomic landmarks
- Nerve stimulation
- Ultrasound-guided

Adjuvant Drugs

- Epinephrine
  - Increased duration of block due to vasoconstriction

- Clonidine
  - α_2-Adrenergic receptor mechanism
  - Dose-dependent extension of duration of block up to 2 hours
- Dexmedetomidine
  - Improves analgesia duration and opioid reduction

REGIONAL ANALGESIA

- Regional analgesia can be an effective technique for perioperative pain.
- Can be part of multimodal analgesic plan
- Can increase pain relief, patient satisfaction, and sleep quality

Catheter Versus Single-Shot Techniques

Upper Extremity

- Example: continuous interscalene block for shoulder surgeries

Lower Extremity

- Example: perineural catheters for joint surgery of hip, knee, ankle, and foot
- Alternate approaches include epidural or lumbar plexus catheter.

TRANSVERSUS ABDOMINIS PLANE BLOCK

- Potential advantages of transversus abdominis plane (TAP) block
  - Increased analgesia
  - Decreased urinary retention
  - Decreased systemic medication requirement and systemic side effects
- Procedures for which TAP block may be appropriate
  - Hysterectomy
  - Cesarean section
  - Laparoscopic cholecystectomy

QUESTIONS

COMMON TERMINOLOGY

1. Fill in the table below describing the potential adverse effects of postoperative pain on each of the listed physiologic systems.

	Adverse Effect(s) of Postoperative Pain
Pulmonary System	
Cardiovascular System	
Endocrine System	
Immune System	
Coagulation System	
Gastrointestinal System	
Genitourinary System	

2. What factors correlate with the severity of postoperative pain?
3. How are in-hospital pain management services structured?

NEUROBIOLOGY OF PAIN

4. List examples of endogenous inflammatory mediators.
5. What is the neurologic pathway of afferent pain impulses?
6. Where along the pathway of afferent pain impulses can modulation occur?
7. Name excitatory and inhibitory neurotransmitters that have a role in pain modulation.
8. What is the difference between preemptive analgesia and preventive analgesia?
9. What is multimodal perioperative analgesia?
10. What is opioid-induced hyperalgesia (OIH)?

ANALGESIC DELIVERY SYSTEMS

11. Describe patient-controlled analgesia (PCA), including settings, advantages, and risks associated with use.

SYSTEMIC THERAPY

12. What limitations exist in using oral opioids in the perioperative period?
13. What role does ketamine have in the perioperative period? What are the side effects?
14. How do the efficacy and potency of acetaminophen compare between oral and intravenous administration?
15. What are some side effects of intravenous clonidine that limit its analgesic use?
16. What is buprenorphine? How should a patient taking oral buprenorphine be managed preoperatively, intraoperatively, and postoperatively?

NEURAXIAL ANALGESIA

17. Why might a local anesthetic be added to an opioid for administration in the epidural space for the management of postoperative pain?
18. What are the potential adverse effects of neuraxial opioids for postoperative analgesia?
19. Which patients may be most at risk for respiratory depression from neuraxial opioids?
20. What concerns exist regarding the concurrent use of anticoagulants and neuraxial analgesia?
21. What factors increase the risk of epidural abscess associated with epidural analgesia?

SURGICAL SITE INFILTRATION

22. What is the benefit of surgical site infiltration with liposomal bupivacaine?

INTRAARTICULAR ADMINISTRATION

23. What are the advantages and disadvantages of intraarticular analgesics?

PERIPHERAL NERVE BLOCK

24. What are some adjuvant drugs that can be used for peripheral nerve blockade?

REGIONAL ANALGESIA

25. What are some advantages of perioperative continuous perineural catheters in upper extremity surgeries?
26. What are some advantages of perioperative continuous perineural catheters in lower extremity surgeries?

TRANSVERSUS ABDOMINIS PLANE BLOCK

27. What are the indications for a transversus abdominis plane block?

ANSWERS

COMMON TERMINOLOGY

1. The following table describes the potential adverse physiologic effects of postoperative pain. (716–717)

	Adverse Effects of Postoperative Pain
Pulmonary System	Atelectasis
	Decreased lung volume
	Ventilation-to-perfusion mismatching
	Arterial hypoxemia
	Hypercapnia
	Pneumonia
Cardiovascular System	Sympathetic nervous system stimulation
	Systemic hypertension
	Tachycardia
	Myocardial ischemia
	Cardiac dysrhythmias
Endocrine System	Hyperglycemia
	Sodium and water retention
	Protein catabolism
Immune System	Decreased immune function
Coagulation System	Increased platelet adhesiveness
	Decreased fibrinolysis
	Hypercoagulation
	Deep venous thrombosis
Gastrointestinal System	Ileus
Genitourinary System	Urinary retention

2. Factors that positively correlate with the severity of postoperative pain include preoperative opioid intake, increased body mass index, anxiety, depression, pain intensity level, characteristics of fibromyalgia, and the duration of surgery. Factors that are negatively correlated include the patient's age and the level of the surgeon's operative experience. (716)
3. The goals of an in-hospital acute pain management service are to reduce postsurgical pain, decrease the period of recuperation, and inhibit the development of chronic persistent pain via early pain management intervention. A chronic pain medicine service can additionally help manage patients with preexisting chronic/persistent pain and cancer-related pain using a multidisciplinary team and diverse treatment modalities, with the goal of transitioning the patient to outpatient care. Inpatient pain service groups may be staffed by regional anesthesiologists, pain physicians, and advanced practice clinicians. (718)

NEUROBIOLOGY OF PAIN

4. Endogenous mediators of inflammation include prostaglandins (PGE_1 and PGE_2), histamine, bradykinin, serotonin, acetylcholine, lactic acid, hydrogen ions, and potassium ions. (719)
5. Nociceptors are free afferent nerve endings activated by thermal, mechanical, or chemical tissue damage. Nociceptors send axonal projections to the dorsal horn of the spinal cord where they synapse with second-order neurons. The axonal projections of the second-order neurons cross to the contralateral half of the spinal cord

and ascend the spinothalamic tract to the thalamus in the brain. In the thalamus, these second-order neurons synapse with third-order neurons that send axonal projections to the sensory cortex. Before reaching the thalamus, the second-order neurons divide and send axonal branches to the reticular formation and periaqueductal gray matter. (718)

6. Modulation of a painful stimulus can occur at almost every level along the afferent neurologic pain pathway. In the periphery, modulation can occur by decreasing or eliminating the endogenous mediators of inflammation in the vicinity of the nociceptor. Pharmacologic agents useful for the modulation of painful stimuli in the periphery include aspirin and nonsteroidal anti-inflammatory drugs (NSAIDs), which decrease the synthesis of prostaglandins. At the level of the spinal cord, modulation of painful stimuli can occur through the effects of excitatory or inhibitory neurotransmitters in the dorsal horn. Above the level of the spinal cord, modulation of painful stimuli can occur through the effects of a descending inhibitory pathway that originates in the brainstem. (718–719)
7. Examples of excitatory pain-modulating neurotransmitters include glutamate, aspartate, vasoactive intestinal polypeptide, cholecystokinin, gastrin-releasing peptide, angiotensin, and substance P. Examples of inhibitory neurotransmitters that are believed to modulate painful stimuli include enkephalins, endorphins, and somatostatin. (718–719)
8. Preemptive analgesia is defined as an analgesic intervention initiated before the noxious stimulus develops to block peripheral and central pain transmission at the time of initial stimulation. Preventive analgesia is functionally defined as an attempt to block pain transmission prior to the injury (surgical incision), during the noxious insult (surgery itself), and after the injury throughout the recovery period. Limiting analgesia to the immediate preoperative or early intraoperative period may not be clinically appropriate because the inflammatory response can last into the postoperative period and continue to maintain peripheral sensitization. (719)
9. Multimodal perioperative analgesia is a broad definition that refers to managing postprocedural pain through multiple approaches. For example, postoperative pain can be managed through a combination of interventional analgesic techniques (epidural or peripheral nerve catheters) and systemic pharmacologic therapies (NSAIDs, α-adrenergic agonists, NMDA receptor antagonists, membrane stabilizers, and opioids). The goals of multimodal perioperative analgesia include sufficient diminution of the patient's pain to instill a sense of control over the pain, enable early mobilization, allow early enteral nutrition, and attenuate the perioperative stress response. The secondary goal of this approach is to maximize the benefit (analgesia) while minimizing the risk (side effects of the medications being used). (720)
10. Opioid-induced hyperalgesia (OIH) describes the paradoxical increase in pain severity and decrease in pain tolerance after a patient receives perioperative short-term opioids. This effect is known to occur after patients received an intraoperative opioid infusion for operative analgesia and has also been demonstrated in human and animal experimental models. (720)

ANALGESIC DELIVERY SYSTEMS

11. Patient-controlled analgesia (PCA) is a method of delivering medication that a patient controls. Medication delivery can be oral, intravenous, subcutaneous, neuraxial, or via peripheral nerve catheter. The most common is the intravenous route, in which a patient controls the administration of an opioid by pressing a button connected to a pump. The pump is programmed to deliver a preset small intravenous dose of opioid when triggered. The lockout interval is the interval of time that must pass after the last self-administered dose before the patient can deliver another small dose of opioid to themselves.

    Advantages of PCA include improved titration of drug and subsequent patient comfort with less total drug administered, less sedation, improved sleep at night, and a more rapid return to physical activity after surgery. The major risk of PCA use is respiratory depression. Respiratory depression is best monitored by continuous capnography and respiratory rate monitoring, but these are not readily available and not sufficiently sensitive and specific. Continuous pulse oximetry is better than no monitor, but it may not reveal respiratory depression, particularly in patients receiving supplemental oxygen. (721-722)

SYSTEMIC THERAPY

12. The limitation of the oral administration of opioids for the management of acute postoperative pain is the lack of ability to titrate it effectively to pain and the prolonged amount of time it takes to reach its peak effect. Patients are also limited by their perioperative NPO status. The oral route of opioid administration is appropriate when the patient's pain is decreased and there is no longer a need for rapid adjustments in the level of analgesia. (722)

13. Ketamine can be effective in small doses for postoperative analgesia partly due to its NMDA antagonistic properties, which can attenuate central sensitization and opioid tolerance. A preoperative bolus of 0.5 mg/kg followed by an infusion of 4–5 μg/kg/min can reduce pain and CPSP. Low-dose ketamine infusions have a low incidence of hallucinations or cognitive impairment. Ketamine is comparable to opioids with regard to side effects of dizziness, itching, nausea, or vomiting. The use of ketamine in patients at high risk for the development of chronic postsurgical pain or who have opioid use disorders or significant opioid tolerance should be considered. (723)
14. No clinical trial has demonstrated a difference in efficacy or potency between oral and intravenous acetaminophen. There is a difference in bioavailability, and the time to onset of analgesia is shorter with intravenous administration. (724)
15. Side effects of bradycardia and hypotension associated with intravenous clonidine may limit its analgesic use in the treatment of postoperative pain. (724)
16. Buprenorphine is a long-acting partial agonist at the mu-opioid receptor, but when used with a full mu-opioid agonist, functions as an antagonist. Therefore the analgesia the patient experiences is less than what the patient would normally experience for a given dose of an opioid. Buprenorphine is commonly used for detoxification or maintenance therapy for patients with opioid use disorders (addiction), and is now also prescribed for the treatment of pain in those without opioid use disorders as well.

    The pharmacokinetics of buprenorphine are somewhat unpredictable, making it hard to predict when its partial agonist properties will have worn off after the last dose of buprenorphine taken prior to surgery. This uncertainty leads to the risk of unexpected respiratory depression from the full opioid agonist as the buprenorphine unbinds from the opioid receptor. In addition, its antagonist properties can make opioid pain medications ineffective, leading to poor postoperative pain control.

    If there is no ability to wean the patient from buprenorphine preoperatively (at least 72 hours prior to surgery), the best approach is to maintain the buprenorphine therapy throughout the perioperative setting, either as an IV formulation, or transdermal/sublingual. Any additional analgesic needs can be addressed with an additional full agonist opioid as well as through a multimodal approach. (724–725)

NEURAXIAL ANALGESIA

17. Local anesthetic added to the opioid solution for administration in the epidural space results in a synergistic analgesic effect. This is believed to occur because of the blockade of painful stimuli at two different sites in the spinal cord. The opioid administered acts by binding to opioid receptors. The local anesthetic administered acts at the nerve roots and in the dorsal root ganglia by blocking the transmission of afferent impulses. The synergistic effect of these two classes of drugs allows for a decreased dose of each to be administered to the patient. This has the added benefit of a decreased risk of the potential side effects of both drugs. (726)
18. Potential adverse effects of the neuraxial administration of opioids for postoperative analgesia include pruritus, urinary retention, nausea and vomiting, sedation, and early and delayed depression of ventilation. Local anesthetic infusions are more likely to cause hypotension and motor block than opioid infusions. (726–727)
19. Factors that increase the risk for respiratory depression from neuraxial opioids include larger doses, geriatric age group, concomitant administration of systemic opioids or sedatives, the possibility of prolonged or extensive surgery, the presence of comorbid conditions, and thoracic surgery. (726–727)
20. The concern regarding the concurrent use of neuraxial analgesia and anticoagulants is the development of a spinal or epidural hematoma. The incidence of spinal or epidural hematoma related to neuraxial analgesia is rare, but it can be catastrophic and requires immediate surgical attention. General concepts for the management of neuraxial analgesia with anticoagulation include (1) the timing of neuraxial needle or catheter insertion or removal should reflect the pharmacokinetic properties of the specific anticoagulant, (2) frequent neurologic monitoring is essential, (3) concurrent administration of multiple anticoagulants may increase the risk of bleeding, and (4) the analgesic regimen should be tailored to facilitate neurologic monitoring, which may be continued in some cases for 24 hours after epidural catheter removal. The American Society of Regional Anesthesia and Pain Medicine has created consensus statements on the management of anticoagulants in relation to neuraxial anesthesia and administration (insertion/removal) of neuraxial techniques in the presence of various anticoagulants. (726–727)
21. Factors that increase the risk of postoperative epidural abscess associated with epidural analgesia include longer duration of anesthesia and the presence of coexisting immunocompromising or complicating diseases (e.g., malignancy, trauma). The overall incidence of postoperative epidural abscess associated with epidural analgesia is extremely rare. A trial of postoperative epidural analgesia with a mean catheter duration of 6.3 days in 4000 surgical cancer patients did not reveal the occurrence of epidural abscess. (727)

SURGICAL SITE INFILTRATION

22. Liposomal bupivacaine has been approved for surgical site infiltration by the FDA. It is an extended-release formulation that is designed to provide analgesia for over 96 hours after injection, but it has only been found to be superior to placebo for the first 24 hours after administration. (727)

INTRAARTICULAR ADMINISTRATION

23. Intraarticular injection of opioids may provide analgesia for up to 24 hours postoperatively and prevent the development of chronic postsurgical pain. However, the superiority of this delivery method over systemic administration has not been demonstrated. Of note, continuous intraarticular administration of bupivacaine has been associated with chondrolysis in the glenohumeral joint. (728)

PERIPHERAL NERVE BLOCK

24. Adjuvant drugs that can be used for peripheral nerve blockade include epinephrine, clonidine, opioids, and dexmedetomidine. Epinephrine significantly increases the duration of blockade with minimal side effects. Clonidine is beneficial in extending the duration of preoperative blockade by about 2 hours but has less utility with perineural catheters. Clonidine is a better preemptive analgesic when added to a local anesthetic block than when used as a single drug. Side effects, including hypotension, bradycardia, and sedation, are less likely to occur with lower doses. (728)

REGIONAL ANALGESIA

25. Continuous perineural catheters for upper extremity procedures have been associated with increased pain relief with minimal need for opioid supplementation. Patients also have increased satisfaction and sleep quality. An example is continuous interscalene blockade for shoulder surgery. (728)
26. Continuous perineural catheters for lower extremity surgery (e.g., hip, knee, ankle, foot) are associated with an earlier discharge from the postanesthesia care unit. Lumbar plexus catheters can be used as part of a multimodal regimen with better pain scores at rest and during physical therapy. The advantage over epidural anesthesia is that there is unilateral blockade rather than unnecessary bilateral blockade. (729)

TRANSVERSUS ABDOMINIS PLANE BLOCK

27. The transversus abdominis plane block has been used for many abdominal procedures, including abdominal hysterectomy, cesarean section, and laparoscopic cholecystectomy. Theoretical advantages of this technique include avoidance of both neuraxial involvement and lower extremity blockade, decreased urinary retention, and decreased systemic side effects. Ultrasound guidance has made this a safer and more reliably achieved peripheral blockade. (729)

Chapter

41 CRITICAL CARE MEDICINE

Anne L. Donovan and Ashish Agrawal

INTENSIVE CARE UNIT DEFINITIONS, INTERPROFESSIONAL CARE, AND PHYSICIAN STAFFING

- Intensive care unit (ICU)
  - Geographically separated nursing care area
  - Critically ill patients for intense observation, diagnosis, and therapeutic procedures
- Interprofessional care
  - Expertise from many healthcare professionals working toward a common goal
  - Improves outcomes in the ICU

ORGAN FAILURE AND SUPPORT

- Single or multiple organ dysfunction is common in critically ill patients.
- Severity scores can predict mortality.

Neurologic: Encephalopathy and Delirium

- Encephalopathy
  - Neurologic process that causes altered levels of consciousness or sensorium
- ICU delirium
  - Specific type of encephalopathy diagnosed based on the following presentation
    - Waxing/waning mental status
    - Inattention
    - Disorganized thinking
    - Altered level of consciousness
  - Affects >30% of ICU patients and >80% of mechanically ventilated patients
  - Confusion Assessment Method for the ICU (CAM-ICU): most used delirium screening tool

Prevention and Treatment of ICU Delirium

Nonpharmacologic strategies
- Frequent reorientation
- Restore day/night and sleep cycles.
- Presence of family members
- Physical therapy and and mobilize out of bed
- Sensory aids (e.g., glasses, hearing aids)
- Avoid triggering medications (e.g., benzodiazepines).

Pharmacologic agents
- May help control symptoms
- Do not prevent delirium or shorten course
- Examples
  - Melatonin
  - Haloperidol
  - Atypical antipsychotics

Cardiovascular: Shock

- Shock
  - Insufficient delivery of oxygen to critical organs and tissues to maintain normal function
  - Categorized by underlying cause

Hypovolemic Shock

- Decreased circulatory volume often from bleeding, dehydration, or fluid loss

Compensatory Responses to Hypovolemia

- Translocation of interstitial fluid into circulating volume
- Activation of the renin-angiotensin-aldosterone system
  - Sodium conservation by kidneys
- Baroreceptor reflex
  - Increases heart rate
- Catecholamine release and sympathetic nervous system stimulation
  - Vasoconstriction diverts blood from skin, skeletal muscle, and splanchnic circulation.
  - Maintains perfusion to vital organs

- Clinical manifestations
  - Hypotension
  - Tachycardia
  - Vasoconstriction
  - Dry mucous membranes
  - Cold and clammy skin
- Treatment
  - Volume resuscitation with blood (for bleeding)
    - Treat coagulopathies.

    - Consider administration of tranexamic acid to reduce fibrinolysis (if within 3 hours of traumatic injury).
    - Replace calcium.
    - Maintain normothermia.
    - Allow permissive hypotension until bleeding is controlled.
  - Volume resuscitation with fluid (for dehydration)
    - Isotonic, balanced crystalloid
  - Vasopressors should only be used to temporize.

Cardiogenic Shock

- Left or right ventricle is unable to fill with volume or contract effectively to generate effective stroke volume.
- Clinical manifestations depend on ventricle involved.
  - Left ventricular (LV) failure: pulmonary edema
  - Right ventricular (RV) failure: distended neck veins, peripheral edema, hepatic congestion
  - Cold and poorly perfused extremities in both RV and LV failure
- Treatment is tailored to particular cardiac physiology.
  - Treatment goals
    - Improve cardiac output
    - Normalize cardiac filling pressure
    - Restore balance between myocardial oxygen supply and demand
  - Pharmacologic therapy can include the following:
    - Vasopressors
    - Inotropes
    - Diuretics
    - Systemic vasodilators
    - Pulmonary vasodilators
  - Mechanical circulatory support devices
    - Intraaortic balloon pump
    - Extracorporeal membrane oxygenation
    - Ventricular assist devices
    - Impella
  - Treat specific underlying cause if possible.
    - Cardiac revascularization for shock related to myocardial infarction

Obstructive Shock

- Physical obstruction to flow either within the heart or the large vessels of the pulmonary or systemic circulation
  - Results in decrease in LV filling
- Causes
  - Pulmonary embolism, pericardial tamponade, tension pneumothorax
- Treatment
  - Relieve cause of obstruction by thrombolysis, pericardiocentesis, or chest tube placement.

Distributive Shock

- Also called vasodilatory shock
- Profound dilation of the arterial vascular system leading to decreased systemic vascular resistance (SVR)
  - Only type of shock with warm, well-perfused extremities on exam
- Three types
  - Septic
  - Anaphylactic
  - Neurogenic
- Septic shock
  - Life-threatening organ dysfunction resulting from dysregulated host response to infection
    - Organ dysfunction is emphasized as the major contributor to mortality.
    - Mortality rate in septic shock is 40%.
  - Diagnosis
    - The Quick Sequential Organ Failure Assessment (qSOFA) score identifies patients at high risk of death or ICU admission.
  - Treatment
    - Early recognition, prompt antibiotics, rapid fluid resuscitation, treatment of infectious source
    - Frequent assessment of composite clinical endpoints (e.g., clinical exam, fluid responsiveness, lactate clearance)
    - Vasopressors (e.g., norepinephrine) to support organ perfusion after intravascular volume repletion
    - Avoid excess fluid after the acute phase of sepsis treatment.
- Anaphylactic shock
  - Systemic, immediate hypersensitivity reaction mediated by IgE results in basophil and mast cell degranulation
  - Diagnosis
    - Mucocutaneous: urticaria, pruritus, flushing, angioedema
    - Respiratory: wheezing, stridor, upper airway obstruction
    - Gastrointestinal: nausea/vomiting
    - Cardiovascular: hypotension, shock
  - Treatment
    - Epinephrine, intravenous fluids, corticosteroids, antihistamines, bronchodilators
- Neurogenic shock
  - Interruption of sympathetic outflow to the periphery leading to unopposed parasympathetic tone
    - Often due to traumatic spinal cord injury
    - Injury above the fourth thoracic level can be associated with bradycardia.
  - Treatment
    - Early neurosurgical intervention

- Prevention of secondary injury by maintaining perfusion to brain and spinal cord (fluids, elevated mean arterial pressure [MAP] goals)

Hemodynamic Monitoring

- Complex physiology of patients in shock
- Advanced monitoring tools may be appropriate.
  - Arterial catheter
  - Central venous catheter
  - Pulmonary artery catheter
  - Noninvasive cardiac output monitors
  - Point-of-care ultrasonography

Pulmonary: Respiratory Failure

- Categorized based on two aspects
  - Acuity (acute vs. chronic)
  - Pathophysiology (hypoxemic vs. hypercapnic)

Hypoxemic Respiratory Failure

- Pathophysiology
  - Alveolar to arterial (A-a) gradient often present
    - Problem with diffusion between the alveolus and arterial capillary, ventilation-perfusion mismatch, or shunting
  - Absence of A-a gradient
    - Indicates hypoventilation or inhalation of hypoxic gas mixture (rare)
- ARDS (acute respiratory distress syndrome)
  - Diffuse, inflammatory injury of the lung
  - Diagnosis
    - Based on the Berlin definition, summarized in the box below.

Berlin Definition of Acute Respiratory Distress Syndrome

Timing	Within 1 week of a known clinical insult or new or worsening respiratory symptoms
Oxygenation	Mild: PaO_2/FiO_2 >200 ≤300 mmHg with PEEP or CPAP ≥5 cmH_2O Moderate: PaO_2/FiO_2 >100 ≤200 mmHg with PEEP ≥5 cmH_2O Severe: PaO_2/FiO_2 ≤100 mmHg with PEEP ≥5 cmH_2O
Chest Radiograph	Bilateral opacities not fully explained by effusions, lobar/lung collapse, or nodules
Edema	Respiratory failure not fully explained by cardiac failure or fluid overload
Risk Factor	If no risk factor for lung injury identified, then need objective assessment such as echocardiography to exclude hydrostatic edema

ARDS, Acute respiratory distress syndrome; *CPAP,* continuous positive airway pressure; *FiO_2,* fraction of inspired oxygen; *PaO_2,* arterial partial pressure of oxygen; *PEEP,* positive end-expiratory pressure.
Adapted from Acute respiratory distress syndrome: The Berlin definition. *JAMA.* 2012;307(23).
Modified from Liu LL, Gropper MA: Critical care anesthesiology. Ch 101. In Miller RD (ed): Miller's Anesthesia, 8th ed. Philadelphia: Elsevier, 2015.

  - Treatment
    - Treat underlying cause of ARDS.
    - Use lung protective ventilation strategy, described below.

Lung Protective Ventilation

- Tidal volume—6 cc/kg ideal body weight
  - Ideal body weight is based on height and gender, not actual weight.
- Limit plateau pressure <30 cm H_2O.
  - Lower tidal volume if plateau pressure is higher.
- Use higher positive end-expiratory pressure (PEEP)
- Accept lower PaO_2 and higher $PaCO_2$ goals (permissive hypoxemia and hypercapnia)
  - PaO_2 >55 mmHg
  - pH >7.25

    - Restrictive fluid management and prone positioning
    - Unclear mortality benefit of inhaled pulmonary vasodilators or extracorporeal membrane oxygenation (ECMO)

Hypercapnic Respiratory Failure

- Causes
  - Hypoventilation (e.g., from drug intoxication, neuromuscular weakness)
  - Increased dead space (e.g., severe COPD or asthma)

Respiratory Support

- Used in both hypoxemic and hypercapnic respiratory failure
- Supplemental oxygen
  - Low-flow
    - Nasal cannula
    - Simple facemask
    - Nonrebreather mask
  - High-flow
    - Heated and humidified high-flow nasal cannula
- Noninvasive positive pressure ventilation
  - Types
    - Continuous positive airway pressure (CPAP)
    - Bilevel positive airway pressure (BiPAP)
  - Indications
    - COPD with acute hypercapnic respiratory failure (can reduce mortality and intubation rate)
    - Acute cardiogenic pulmonary edema
    - Postoperative respiratory failure
    - Hypoxemic respiratory failure in immunocompromised patients
  - Drawbacks
    - Potential for aspiration
    - Inability to control tidal volume and airway pressure
    - Potential delays in endotracheal intubation

- Mechanical ventilation
  - So-called "invasive" mechanical ventilation is delivered via endotracheal tube or tracheotomy.
  - Goals
    - Decrease work of breathing
    - Improve oxygen delivery
    - Facilitate CO_2 removal
    - Minimize ventilator-associated lung injury
  - Modes of ventilation
    - Continuous mandatory ventilation (volume control, pressure control)
    - Intermittent mandatory ventilation (synchronized, or SIMV, is most common)
    - Spontaneous ventilation (pressure support is most common)

Lung Compliance and Mechanical Ventilation

- Compliance = ΔVolume/ΔPressure
- Volume-controlled ventilation
  - Tidal volume is specified.
  - To attain the targeted tidal volume, airway pressure will vary according to the lung compliance.
- Pressure-controlled ventilation
  - Airway pressure is specified.
  - At the targeted airway pressure, tidal volume will vary according to the lung compliance and airway resistance.

- Weaning from mechanical ventilation
  - Weaning process should be initiated after patient recovers from cause of respiratory failure.
  - Risk of ventilator-associated pneumonia (VAP) increases with the duration of mechanical ventilation.
  - Protocol-based weaning by respiratory therapist and/or nurses facilitates more rapid weaning.

Considerations for Weaning from Mechanical Ventilation

- Oxygenation
- Ventilation
- Respiratory mechanics
  - Rapid shallow breathing index
  - Maximum inspiratory force
- Secretions
- Upper airway patency
  - Cuff leak test
- Mental status
- Hemodynamic stability
- Clinical course

- Tracheotomies
  - May facilitate rehabilitation for patients requiring prolonged mechanical ventilation
  - Timing of tracheotomy remains controversial.
    - Mean airway pressure and alveolar derecruitment can result from placement.
    - Should be deferred in patients who are unstable or with high PEEP or oxygen requirements
  - Inadvertent dislodgement within 7 days of placement
    - Blind replacement can result in false subcutaneous passage.
    - Replace under direct visualization via orotracheal intubation (if possible) or with use of a pediatric laryngoscope/fiberoptic scope in tracheal stoma.

Gastrointestinal: Nutrition

- Goal of ICU nutrition
  - Preserve lean body mass.
  - Avoid malnourishment.
    - Associated with increased mortality rate, prolonged hospital stay, poor wound healing, increased infection risk
- Diagnosis of malnutrition
  - History and targeted physical exam
- Route of nutrition
  - Enteral nutrition is preferred over parenteral nutrition
    - Helps maintain gut integrity
    - Reduced risk of gastrointestinal (GI) bleeding
- Timing of ICU nutrition
  - Early achievement of feeding at goal rate (within the first week) not shown to have significant benefit in previously well-nourished patients

Perioperative Considerations for Enteral Feedings

- Continuing enteral feeds for patients undergoing frequent surgeries may prevent malnutrition.
  - Avoids multihour nutritional holds starting at midnight
- Institutional preferences can vary.
  - For fasting intervals
    - May be influenced by gastric feeds versus postpyloric or jejunal feeds
  - For acceptable gastric residuals
    - Volumes of up to 500 mL can be accepted.
  - For aspiration of residual volume prior to surgery
- Procedures involving manipulation of endotracheal tubes
  - General recommendation is to hold enteral feeds for 6 to 8 hours.

Renal: Acute Kidney Injury

- Epidemiology
  - Incidence of acute kidney injury (AKI) is 35% in ICU patients.
  - New requirement for dialysis associated with in-hospital mortality of 50%

- Diagnosis
  - Multiple criteria can be used, e.g., RIFLE criteria (risk, injury, failure, loss, end-stage renal disease)
- Causes of acute renal failure
  - Categorized by cause, as noted in the box below.

Causes of Acute Renal Failure
Prerenal
▪ Hypovolemia
▪ Low effective circulating volume (e.g., from decompensated heart failure or liver disease)
Renal
▪ Glomerulonephritis
▪ Toxins (e.g., NSAIDs, cisplatin, aminoglycosides, contrast agent, myoglobin, hemoglobin)
▪ Vasculitis (e.g., TTP/HUS)
▪ AIN (e.g., from PCN, cephalosporins, cimetidine, SLE, sarcoidosis)
▪ Tubular disease (e.g., ATN, tumor lysis syndrome)
Postrenal
▪ Obstructive nephropathy

AIN, Acute interstitial nephritis; *ATN,* acute tubular necrosis; *NSAIDs,* nonsteroidal antiinflammatory drugs; *PCN,* penicillin; *SLE,* systemic lupus erythematosus; *TTP/HUS,* thrombotic thrombocytopenic purpura/hemolytic uremic syndrome.

- Treatment
  - Supportive care including maintenance of euvolemia
  - Avoid nephrotoxins (e.g., contrast, nonsteroidal antiinflammatory drugs).
  - Dialysis for excessive intravascular volume or electrolyte disturbances
    - Can be offered as intermittent hemodialysis (IHD)
    - Continuous renal replacement therapy also possible (associated with better hemodynamics compared to IHD)

Infectious Disease: Hospital-Acquired Infections

- Prevention of hospital-acquired infections can help improve outcomes in the ICU.
- Prevention strategies
  - Catheter-associated urinary tract infection (CAUTI)
    - Aseptic technique during placement
    - Limit duration of urinary catheters.
  - Ventilator-associated pneumonia (VAP)
    - Use VAP bundles (elevate head of bed to 30 degrees, subglottic suction, daily spontaneous awakening trials, and SBTs)
    - Avoid excessive use of stress ulcer prophylaxis.
  - Catheter-related blood stream infection (CRBSI)
    - Sterile placement of vascular access
    - Prompt removal when not needed

Endocrine: Glucose Management

- Intensive insulin therapy to achieve blood glucose 80–110 mg/dL does not improve survival.
  - Increases risk of hypoglycemia and mortality
- Goals of ICU glucose management
  - Avoid severe hypoglycemia (<40 mg/dL).
  - Avoid hyperglycemia (>200 mg/dL).
  - Target moderate glucose ranges of 140–180 mg/dL.

Prophylaxis

- Venous thromboembolism (VTE)
  - Increased risk in ICU patients
  - Unfractionated heparin or low molecular weight heparin reduces the risk of VTE.
  - Mechanical thromboprophylaxis
    - Less effective than chemoprophylaxis
    - May reduce risk in patients with increased risk of bleeding complications
- GI
  - Stress ulcers more likely in ICU patients.
    - Increased gastric acid production
    - Functionally impaired mucosal barrier
  - Proton pump inhibitors or H_2 blockers can reduce rates of stress ulcer–related GI bleeding.
    - May increase risk of hospital-associated pneumonia or *C. difficile*.

A-F BUNDLE

- Postintensive care syndrome (PICS)
  - A constellation of physical, cognitive, or psychological symptoms that persist in critically ill patients (or their family members) after an ICU stay
- A-F bundle
  - A care strategy developed to prevent or ameliorate impairments related to PICS

A: Assess, Prevent, and Manage Pain

- Pain affects nearly all ICU patients.
- Use pain assessment tools that are validated in ICU.
  - Numerical Rating Scale
  - Behavioral Pain Scale
  - Critical Care Pain Observation Tool
- Treat pain with opioid and nonopioid medications.
- Nonpharmacologic techniques (e.g., relaxation, music) can be considered.

B: Both SAT and SBT

- Goal is to reduce time patient receives mechanical ventilation.
- SAT
  - Spontaneous awakening trial

        - Pause continuous sedatives.
        - Assess pain and sedation levels.
    - Do not perform SAT in certain patients.
        - Neuromuscular blockade
        - Seizures
        - Elevated ICP
- SBT
    - Spontaneous breathing trial
        - Ventilator mode changed to partial support mode (e.g., pressure support)
- Daily SAT and SBTs at the same time can decrease time to extubation.

C: Choice of Sedation and Analgesia

- Follow stepwise process
    - Treat pain aggressively (e.g., intermittent IV opioids).
    - Once pain is controlled, address agitation or delirium.
- If continuous sedation needed, target light sedation (RASS 0 or –1).
    - Preferentially use propofol or dexmedetomidine.
    - Avoid benzodiazepines for continuous sedation.
        - Increased mortality
        - Increased duration of mechanical ventilation

D: Delirium: Assess, Prevent, and Manage

- Affects up to 80% of mechanically ventilated patients in the ICU
- Strategies in the ICU
    - Assess regularly using delirium screening tool.
    - Prevent with nonpharmacologic strategies.
    - Manage aggressively when delirium is present.

E: Early Mobility

- ICU patients experience rapid deterioration of muscle strength and function.
- Benefits of early mobility
    - Improved outcomes
        - Increased ventilator-free days
        - Reduced duration of delirium
        - Improved functional status at discharge
- Safe in mechanically ventilated patients

F: Family Engagement and Empowerment

- Providing patient- and family-centered care is an important quality focus in the ICU.
- Structures to facilitate shared decision-making and family inclusion
    - Patient and family inclusion on rounds
    - Extended visiting hours
    - Family inclusion on rounds
    - Family presence during procedures

QUESTIONS

ICU DEFINITIONS, INTERPROFESSIONAL CARE, AND PHYSICIAN STAFFING

1. What does interprofessional care mean, and how does interprofessional care contribute to better outcomes for critically ill patients?

ORGAN FAILURE AND SUPPORT

2. What are common causes of encephalopathy in the ICU?
3. How is delirium defined? What are the subtypes commonly encountered in the ICU?
4. What is the most commonly used screening tool for delirium in the ICU? How is the tool administered?
5. How does ICU delirium impact patient outcomes?
6. How is shock defined and categorized?
7. The following table lists different shock types and several important physiologic parameters. In each cell, enter an up or down arrow to indicate the direction of change of each parameter for the different shock types.

Shock Type	Cardiac Output	Systemic Vascular Resistance	Central Venous Pressure	Pulmonary Capillary Wedge Pressure	Mixed Venous Oxygen Saturation
Hypovolemic					
Cardiogenic					
Obstructive					
Distributive					

8. In the table below, list the common causes, clinical findings, and treatment for the four types of shock.

Type of Shock	Common Causes	Clinical Findings	Treatment
Hypovolemic			
Cardiogenic			
Obstructive			
Distributive			

9. What are the components of the qSOFA tool used to identify patients with infections who are at high risk of death? What is its clinical utility for patients not in an ICU setting?
10. Describe the current approach to management of patients with septic shock.
11. List three types of invasive hemodynamic monitors which may be helpful in predicting fluid responsiveness in critically ill patients. Which is most accurate?
12. List three indications for bedside cardiac ultrasonography in the ICU.
13. How can respiratory failure be categorized?
14. What are some common causes of acute hypoxemic respiratory failure?
15. What are some common causes of acute hypercapnic respiratory failure?
16. What are the key differences between low-flow and high-flow oxygen delivery systems?
17. What are the indications and contraindications for noninvasive positive pressure ventilation (NIPPV)?
18. What are the goals of mechanical ventilation?
19. List three modes of mechanical ventilation, and describe how spontaneous patient respiratory effort is supported in each mode.
20. Describe parameters that are set versus variable in volume control ventilation, pressure control ventilation, and pressure support ventilation.
21. How does the set inspiratory flow rate influence inspiratory and expiratory times?
22. How does a ventilator switch between inspiration and expiration in the following ventilator modes: volume control, pressure control, and pressure support ventilation?

23. What is PEEP? How does it improve oxygenation?
24. What are some patient characteristics that indicate readiness for a trial of weaning from mechanical ventilation? What are the criteria for extubation?
25. What is the rapid shallow breathing index? What value predicts successful weaning from mechanical ventilation?
26. What are basic principles for mechanical ventilation in patients with ARDS? What are some other therapies that could be considered for patients with severe refractory hypoxemia?
27. What is the most accurate way of determining a patient's nutritional status in critically ill patients?
28. In nonmalnourished patients, what are the general recommendations for timing of nutrition and for route of delivery (enteral vs. parenteral)?
29. What are the RIFLE criteria that are used to describe the spectrum of acute kidney injury (AKI)?
30. Describe prerenal, intrarenal, and postrenal causes of AKI.
31. What are the treatment options for AKI?
32. Is continuous renal replacement therapy or intermittent hemodialysis the more appropriate renal replacement therapy in critically ill patients?
33. What are some common hospital-acquired infections, and how can their risk be minimized?
34. What is the most appropriate glucose target for critically ill patients? Why?
35. What are some risk factors for venous thromboembolism in critically ill patients? What are pharmacologic and nonpharmacologic methods for prevention?
36. When should medication be used for prevention of stress ulcers in critically ill patients? Which medications are available?

A-F BUNDLE

37. What are some common symptoms experienced by survivors of critical illness? What is the name for this condition?
38. What is the A-F bundle? Complete the table below to describe what each letter stands for and the corresponding outcome that can be addressed through the use of this bundle.

A	
B	
C	
D	
E	
F	

39. What are commonly used assessment tools for pain, agitation, and delirium in the ICU? Why is protocolized screening important?
40. How do spontaneous awakening and breathing trials impact patient outcomes in mechanically ventilated patients?
41. What is the most appropriate target for sedation? If continuous sedative medications are necessary, which medications are preferred? Which medications should be avoided?
42. How can early mobility improve patient outcomes? What can be done to facilitate early mobility?

ANSWERS

ICU DEFINITIONS, INTERPROFESSIONAL CARE, AND PHYSICIAN STAFFING

1. Interprofessional care is healthcare that is provided by a team of professionals from multiple different training backgrounds. Examples include physicians, nurses, and respiratory care practitioners. The collective expertise from these individuals is necessary to provide modern critical care to patients of ever-increasing complexity. (735)

ORGAN FAILURE AND SUPPORT

2. Encephalopathy is a neurologic process that causes altered levels of consciousness or sensorium. It can be caused by primary neurological causes (e.g., stroke, seizure, tumor) or secondary causes. Common secondary causes include toxic (e.g., illicit drug use or exposure to certain medications), metabolic (e.g., electrolyte disturbances, hypoxia, acid-base disturbances, hyperammonemia), or infectious (e.g., sepsis) etiologies. Delirium is a specific subtype of encephalopathy that can be triggered by any of the above causes. (736)
3. Delirium is the acute onset of a disturbance in attention, awareness, and cognition that is a direct consequence of a medical condition and is not explained by a preexisting neurocognitive disorder. Delirium develops over a short period of time (i.e., hours to days) and tends to fluctuate throughout the day. Patients with delirium can display hyperactive (e.g., agitation and restlessness), hypoactive, or mixed phenotypes. Hypoactive delirium is the most common subtype even though it is likely underdiagnosed and has been associated with worse outcomes in critically ill patients. (736)
4. The Confusion Assessment Method for the ICU (CAM-ICU) is the most commonly used screening tool for delirium in the ICU. To perform CAM-ICU, the clinician first determines whether there has been an acute change in mental status from baseline or a fluctuating mental status in the past 24 hours. If so, the patient is assessed for inattention by asking him or her to squeeze the clinician's hand each time a letter is repeated in the spelling of a phrase (e.g., squeeze each time you hear the letter "A" in the phrase "SAVE-A-HAART"). If more than two errors are detected, the patient's consciousness is assessed using the Richmond Agitation Sedation Scale (RASS). If RASS is anything other than zero (i.e., calm, cooperative), the patient is considered CAM-positive (i.e., delirium is present). If RASS is zero, the patient is assessed for disorganized thinking using questions or commands that require abstract thinking. If the patient is unable to complete the task, he or she is considered CAM-positive. (736)
5. ICU delirium has been associated with numerous poor outcomes in ICU patients, including longer hospital and ICU lengths of stay, fewer mechanical ventilator-free days, more frequent discharge to an institution, increased cost, long-term cognitive impairment, and increased mortality. Since delirium is preventable in some cases, it is an important target for quality improvement in the ICU. (736)
6. Shock is a state where there is insufficient delivery of oxygen to the body's critical organs and tissues to maintain normal function. Shock can be categorized based on its underlying cause: hypovolemic (e.g., bleeding, dehydration), cardiogenic (e.g., left or right ventricular failure), obstructive (e.g., pulmonary embolism, pericardial tamponade), and distributive (e.g., septic, neurogenic, anaphylactic). (736)
7. Shock types and key physiologic parameters are summarized in the table below. (736)

Characteristics of Various Shock States

Shock Type	Cardiac Output	Systemic Vascular Resistance	Central Venous Pressure	Pulmonary Capillary Wedge Pressure	Mixed Venous Oxygen Saturation
Hypovolemic	↓	↑	↓	↓	↓
Cardiogenic	↓	↑	↑	↑ *	↓
Obstructive	↓	↑	↑	↓ **	↓
Distributive	↑ or even	↓	↓	↓	↑ or even

*Pulmonary capillary wedge pressure is normal to low in right ventricular failure.
**Pulmonary capillary wedge pressure is elevated in cardiac tamponade.

8. A summary of the common causes, clinical findings, and treatment for the four types of shock are described in the table below. (737–741)

Type of Shock	Common Causes	Clinical Findings	Treatment
Hypovolemic	Bleeding (e.g., trauma, surgery, gastrointestinal hemorrhage). Dehydration (e.g., diarrhea, vomiting, sweating)	Dry mucous membranes, decreased skin turgor, and cold/clammy skin	Resuscitation with the appropriate fluid lost; hemorrhagic patient may require blood components in a 1:1:1 ratio. Dehydrated patient may require an isotonic, balanced crystalloid such as Plasmalyte or Lactated Ringer's solution
Cardiogenic	Myocardial infarction, cardiomyopathy, myocarditis, arrhythmia, valvular rupture, or ventricular septal defect	Cold and poorly perfused extremities; LV failure—often have pulmonary edema; RV failure—often have distended neck veins, peripheral edema, and hepatic congestion	Optimizing preload with fluid or diuresis; maintaining cardiac output with inotropy; decreasing afterload to improve cardiac output; treat reversible causes of cardiogenic shock (e.g., thrombolytics for acute myocardial infarction, treating tachyarrhythmias)
Obstructive	Massive pulmonary embolism, pericardial tamponade, and tension pneumothorax	Distended neck veins and venous congestion	Relieving the etiology of obstruction, such as pericardial effusion drainage, thrombolytics for pulmonary embolism, or needle thoracostomy for tension pneumothorax
Distributive	Three main types: septic, anaphylactic, and neurogenic shock	Warm extremities	Targeted toward the etiology, such as antibiotics for septic shock, epinephrine and steroids for anaphylactic shock, and vasopressors and neurosurgical intervention for neurogenic shock

9. The quick SOFA (qSOFA) score is a simplified tool which identifies high-risk patients who are at 3- to 14-fold increased risk of mortality. To be identified as high risk, patients have a suspected infection plus two out of three of the following criteria: altered mental status (GCS <15), respiratory rate ≥ 22, systolic blood pressure ≤ 100. The qSOFA score may be used in the non-ICU setting such as hospital ward or step-down unit to help inform a decision whether to transfer to the ICU. (740)
10. The modern treatment of sepsis includes early recognition of septic shock, rapid fluid resuscitation, prompt antibiotic administration, treatment of the infectious source, and support of organ perfusion with vasopressors. While in the past specific fluid targets were used (i.e., 30 cc/kg), fluid resuscitation is now guided by the clinical exam, dynamic fluid responsiveness, and lactate clearance. (740)
11. Invasive hemodynamic monitors in the ICU include arterial lines, central venous catheters, and pulmonary artery catheters. Arterial lines and monitoring of systolic pressure variation (SPV) and pulse pressure variation (PPV) have been shown to be more accurate in a mechanically ventilated patient than monitoring central venous pressure (CVP) with a central venous catheter or pulmonary artery occlusion pressure (PAOP) with a pulmonary artery catheter. (741)
12. Bedside cardiac ultrasonography in the ICU can be an important tool to diagnose the etiology of undifferentiated shock. It can quickly evaluate for hypovolemic shock by examination of the IVC in a spontaneously ventilating patient, for obstructive shock by evaluation for a pericardial effusion or tamponade, and for cardiogenic shock by evaluation of right or left ventricular systolic function. (741)
13. Respiratory failure is often categorized based on acuity (i.e., acute vs. chronic) and whether the problem lies with oxygenation (i.e., hypoxemic respiratory failure) or ventilation (i.e., hypercarbic respiratory failure). It is common for more than one process to exist at the same time; for example, a person with chronic hypoxemia may develop acute-on-chronic hypoxemic respiratory failure with or without acute hypercarbic respiratory failure. (741–742)
14. Common causes of acute hypoxemic respiratory failure, including those that injure the lung directly and those causing indirect lung injury, are noted in the table below. (742)

Triggers of Acute Respiratory Distress Syndrome

Causes of Direct Lung Injury	Causes of Indirect Lung Injury
Pneumonia	Sepsis
Aspiration of gastric contents	Severe trauma
Pulmonary contusion	Cardiopulmonary bypass
Reperfusion pulmonary edema	Drug overdose
Amniotic fluid embolus	Acute pancreatitis
Inhalational injury	Near-drowning
	Transfusion-related acute lung injury

Data from Ware LB, Matthay MA. The acute respiratory distress syndrome. *N Engl J Med.* 2000;342:1334–1349.

15. Acute hypercapnic (hypercarbic) respiratory failure is commonly caused by obstructive lung disease (e.g., asthma, COPD), neuromuscular weakness (e.g., critical illness neuromyopathy, myasthenia gravis, amyotrophic lateral sclerosis), sleep disordered breathing (e.g., obstructive sleep apnea, obesity hypoventilation syndrome), other problems with respiratory mechanics (e.g., diaphragmatic weakness), or medications that depress respiratory drive (e.g., opioids, benzodiazepines). Any process that interferes with gas exchange across the alveolar capillary membrane, such as ARDS, can also cause hypercarbia. (743)
16. Low-flow oxygen delivery systems, which deliver up to 15 L of oxygen per minute, include nasal cannula, simple face mask, and nonrebreather mask. High-flow nasal cannula is the most common type of high-flow oxygen delivery system (20–60 liters per minute). Key differences include maximum FiO_2 delivery, PEEP delivery, and circuit requirements. In any supplemental oxygen delivery system, the inspired FiO_2 depends on how much room air is entrained with each breath. This, in turn, depends on how much of the patient's anatomic nasopharyngeal reservoir has been filled with oxygen between breaths. Quiet breathing with a normal respiratory rate allows more time between breaths for the nasopharyngeal reservoir to fill with oxygen, and therefore each breath will have a higher inspired FiO_2 when compared with breathing at a higher respiratory rate and a higher peak inspiratory flow (e.g., the patient with respiratory distress and tachypnea). Therefore high-flow systems can deliver a higher FiO_2 than low-flow systems, and FiO_2 is less dependent on patient respiratory effort. High-flow systems may deliver a small amount of PEEP and help with CO_2 elimination at very high flows. High-flow oxygen must be delivered through a heated and humidified circuit to promote patient comfort and prevent complications such as nosebleeds. (743)
17. The most widely accepted indications for NIPPV use include treatment of COPD exacerbations and cardiogenic pulmonary edema. Notably, these conditions can resolve or improve quickly with appropriate treatment such as inhaled bronchodilators (COPD) and diuretics (pulmonary edema). Other supported uses of NIPPV include respiratory failure in postoperative patients or in immunocompromised patients. The contraindications to NIPPV are listed in the box below.

Contraindications for Noninvasive Positive-Pressure Ventilation
Impaired neurologic state (coma, seizures, encephalopathy) Respiratory arrest or upper airway obstruction Shock or severe cardiovascular instability Severe upper gastrointestinal bleeding Recent gastroesophageal surgery Vomiting Excessive airway secretions Facial lesions that prevent proper fit of nasal or facial masks

NIPPV should be used with caution (if at all) in patients with ARDS, because tidal volume and pressure cannot be adequately controlled. Appropriate judgment must always be used to avoid delays in necessary intubation, which could make the intubation procedure higher risk and increase patient mortality. (743)

18. The goals of mechanical ventilation may include any or all of the following: 1) to decrease work of breathing, 2) to improve oxygen delivery, and/or 3) to facilitate carbon dioxide removal. Whenever mechanical ventilation is used, minimizing ventilator-induced lung injury (i.e., barotrauma, volutrauma, atelectrauma, and biotrauma) using a lung-protective strategy is an important goal. (743)
19. The three modes of mechanical ventilation are continuous mandatory ventilation (CMV), intermittent mandatory ventilation (IMV), and spontaneous. In CMV, every breath is fully supported by the ventilator. Assist control (AC) is a commonly used subtype of CMV, where the ventilator provides a fully supported breath regardless of whether the breath is initiated by the ventilator (i.e., the "set" or "controlled" breaths) or by the patient (i.e., the "spontaneous" breaths). In IMV, in particular synchronized IMV (SIMV), the ventilator delivers fully supported breaths at a set rate, but also allows breaths to be initiated by the patient. The degree of support provided for spontaneous breaths depends on both timing of the spontaneous breath and what is programmed by providers. If a patient-initiated breath occurs within a prespecified window of time before a controlled breath, the ventilator will provide a fully supported (i.e., "synchronized") breath. If, however, a patient-initiated breath occurs outside of that window of time, the ventilator delivers whatever degree of support providers have specified. For example, providers may specify that spontaneous breaths receive pressure or volume support, or no ventilator support. In spontaneous mode, all breaths are initiated by the patient and are supported (most commonly by pressure support). Spontaneous modes have a back-up mode (e.g., CMV) which is activated in case the patient becomes apneic or does not trigger an adequate number of breaths. (744)
20. The table below indicates parameters that are ordered in each ventilator mode, as well as additional settings that can be ordered. In volume control ventilation (VCV), a minimum minute ventilation is guaranteed. Peak inspiratory pressure will vary from patient to patient depending on the individual patient's lung compliance. In pressure control ventilation (PCV), tidal volume will vary from patient to patient depending on an individual patient's lung compliance. Because of the variance in tidal volume, a minimum minute ventilation is not guaranteed in PCV. In pressure support ventilation (PSV), respiratory rate will vary between patients depending on an individual patient's respiratory drive, and tidal volume will vary from patient to patient depending on individual patient factors including lung compliance and respiratory drive. (744–745)

Mechanical Ventilator Orders

Example	Ventilator Orders Written	Additional Settings That Can Be Ordered	Explanation
Example 1: Assist control–volume control (AC/VC)	Mode AC/VC Rate 10 V_T 500 mL PEEP 5 cmH_2O FiO_2 1.0	Flow rate: typically 60 L/min Trigger: flow or pressure	Ventilator will deliver the preset tidal volume of 500 mL 10 times a minute; if the patient's respiratory rate is greater than 10, each breath will also be 500 mL
Example 2: Assist control–pressure control (AC/PC)	Mode AC/PC Rate 10 PIP 20 cmH_2O PEEP 5 cmH_2O FiO_2 1.0	I:E ratio: typically 1:2 Inspiratory time Trigger: flow or pressure	Ventilator will deliver 10 breaths per minute; each breath will reach a peak pressure of 20 cmH_2O; if the patient's respiratory rate is greater than 10, each breath will also reach a peak pressure of 20 cmH_2O
Example 3: Synchronized intermittent mandatory ventilation–volume control (SIMV-VC)	Mode SIMV-VC Rate 10 V_T 500 mL Pressure support 5 cmH_2O PEEP 5 cmH_2O FiO_2 0.5	Flow rate: typically 60 L/min Trigger: flow or pressure (this applies to all the breaths, SIMV, or pressure support)	Ventilator will deliver 10 breaths per minute with tidal volume 500 mL; if the patient's respiratory rate is greater than 10, those non-mandatory breaths will receive inspiratory pressure support to peak pressure 5 cmH_2O above the PEEP of 5 cmH_2O
Example 4: Pressure support ventilation (PSV)	Mode PSV Driving pressure 8 cmH_2O PEEP 5 cmH_2O FiO_2 0.5	Trigger: flow or pressure	Patient must be breathing spontaneously; each breath will receive inspiratory pressure support to peak pressure 8 cmH_2O above the PEEP of 5 cmH_2O

FiO_2, Fraction of inspired oxygen; *I:E,* inspiratory:expiratory ratio; *PEEP,* positive end-expiratory pressure; *PIP,* peak inspiratory pressure; *VT,* tidal volume.

21. Inspiratory flow rate is set by providers in VCV (typically at 60 L/min) and is determined by the patient (i.e., "demand flow") in PCV and PSV. In VCV, higher inspiratory flow rate results in a shorter inspiratory (I) time and a longer expiratory (E) time, because it takes less time to provide the pre-set tidal volume at a higher flow rate. Increasing inspiratory flow rate in VCV is one technique that can be used to improve ventilator synchrony for patients experiencing air hunger (usually patients with ARDS). In PCV, patients determine their own inspiratory flow rate, a concept known as "demand flow." Because I time or I:E ratio is set in PCV, the peak inspiratory flow rate does not affect I or E time; rather, higher flow rates result in higher tidal volume and increased mean airway pressure because PCV is a time cycled mode. (745)
22. Switching between inspiration and expiration is a concept known as "cycling." In VCV, inspiration stops and expiration begins when the set tidal volume is delivered. Thus VCV is a volume-cycled mode. PCV is a time-cycled mode. The ventilator stops delivering inspiratory flow after a set amount of time, determined by either the set I time or I:E ratio and respiratory rate, regardless of the tidal volume delivered to that point. PSV is flow-cycled. Inspiration stops once inspiratory flow rate, which is determined by the patient, drops to a specified threshold (e.g., 25% of peak inspiratory flow). (745)
23. PEEP is positive end-expiratory pressure, or the pressure that is delivered by the ventilator throughout expiration. PEEP increases mean airway pressure, which may recruit collapsed alveoli, and increases functional residual capacity, which prevents collapse of small airways during expiration. Therefore usual application of PEEP improves ventilation-perfusion matching and decreases shunt, which serves to improve oxygenation. Application of excessive amounts of PEEP can have deleterious consequences, such as overdistension of alveoli, increased dead space, and decrease in venous return. (744)
24. There are many potential strategies to wean patients from mechanical ventilation. Prior to extubation, patients should have indicators of successful breathing without ventilator support. These include adequate oxygenation (PaO_2/FiO_2 >150 cmH_2O with <8 cmH_2O PEEP), ventilation (tidal volume 5–6 cc/kg with minimal ventilatory support and/or minute ventilation <10 L/min with appropriate respiratory mechanics), secretions that can be cleared by the patient both in terms of quantity and quality, a patent upper airway (i.e., free of anatomic obstruction and without significant upper airway edema), and appropriate mental status to protect their airway. In addition, hemodynamic stability and resolution of the process that resulted in intubation should also be considered. (745)
25. The rapid shallow breathing index (RSBI) is a quick measure of a patient's respiratory mechanics, calculated as the ratio between respiratory rate (breaths/min) and tidal volume in liters. RSBI >105 is an indicator that the patient will fail an attempt at extubation, whereas RSBI <105 is only somewhat associated with extubation success. (745–746)
26. Management of ARDS is largely supportive, using lung-protective (ARDSnet) ventilation, which is aimed at minimizing ventilator-associated lung injury. The important features of this ventilation strategy include: 1) lower tidal volumes (~6 cc/kg ideal body weight), 2) plateau pressure <30 cmH_2O, 3) higher PEEP, 4) permissive hypercapnia (pH >7.25) and hypoxemia (PaO_2 >55 mmHg). Other therapies that are evidence-based and can be considered on a case-by-case basis include neuromuscular blockade, prone positioning, and restrictive fluid management. Inhaled pulmonary vasodilators and extracorporeal life support are sometimes used to support patients with refractory hypoxemia; however, evidence for a mortality benefit for these therapies in a broad population is lacking. (742–743)
27. Laboratory tests such as albumin and prealbumin are not reliable markers of nutritional status due to fluctuating volume status and impaired protein synthesis in the critically ill. Measurements such as body mass index (BMI) similarly are not reflective of nutritional status. A thorough nutrition assessment should include a careful history and a targeted nutritional physical exam. (747)
28. For patients who are not malnourished, enteral nutrition is generally preferred over parenteral nutrition to maintain gut integrity and reduce the risk of gastrointestinal bleeding. While meeting reasonable caloric and protein goals are important for long-term recovery in all critically ill patients, initiating early goal enteral feeds in the first week has not been shown to be superior to initiating low volume tube feeds in the first week or goal tube feeds in the second week of critical illness. (747)
29. The RIFLE criteria stands for risk, injury, failure, loss, and end-stage renal disease. For each increase in RIFLE criteria, there is a stepwise increase in mortality. The criteria are shown in the table below. (747–748)

The RIFLE Criteria

RIFLE Category	GFR Criteria	UO Criteria	OR Hospital Mortality
Risk	Cr increased × 1.5 or GFR decreased >25%	< 0.5 mL/kg/hr × 6 hr	2.2 (95% CI 2.17–2.3)
Injury	Cr increased × 2 or GFR decreased >50%	< 0.5 mL/kg/hr × 12 hr	6.1 (95% CI 5.74–6.44)
Failure	Cr increased × 3 or GFR decreased >75% or Cr >4 mg/dL	< 0.3 mL/kg/hr × 24 hr or anuria × 12 hr	8.6 (95% CI 8.07–9.15)
Loss	Complete loss of renal function for >4 weeks		
ESRD	End-stage renal disease		

Cr, Creatinine; *ESRD,* end-stage renal disease; *GFR,* glomerular filtration rate; *OR,* odds ratio; *UO,* urine output.
Data modified from KDI Global, OKAKIW Group. Kidney Disease Improving Global Outcomes (KDIGO) clinical practice guideline for acute kidney injury. *Kidney Int.* 2012;(Suppl 2):1–138.

30. Prerenal causes of AKI include hypovolemia or other causes of low effective circulating volume such as decompensated heart failure and liver disease. Intrarenal causes include glomerulonephritis, toxins (e.g., NSAIDs, contrast), vasculitis, acute interstitial nephritis (AIN), or tubular disease (ATN). Postrenal causes include any cause of obstructive nephropathy such as bladder tumors or kidney stones. (747–748)
31. Supportive care for AKI includes optimizing volume status, avoiding nephrotoxic agents (e.g., NSAIDS, contrast), dose adjustment for medications to match creatinine clearance, and electrolyte and acid-base monitoring. Should AKI progress to failure, loss, or ESRD, hemodialysis is ultimately required. (748)
32. While there are reasons to choose one renal replacement modality over another in some critically ill patients, no single renal replacement therapy is appropriate for all critically ill patients. Patients who are hemodynamically unstable or who are susceptible to osmotic or fluid shifts (e.g., acute liver failure, traumatic brain injury) are more likely to benefit from continuous renal replacement, while those who require urgent clearance of toxins or electrolytes, or who are receiving ongoing chronic outpatient dialysis, may benefit from intermittent hemodialysis. (748)
33. Common hospital-acquired infections include catheter-associated urinary tract infections (CAUTI), ventilator-associated pneumonia (VAP), and catheter-related bloodstream infections (CRBSI). In general, risk for these hospital-acquired infections can be minimized by following evidence-based bundles, which generally include optimal sterile technique for placing sterile devices (urinary catheters and central venous catheters), proper care of these devices when placed, and prompt removal when these devices are no longer needed. (748–749)
34. A moderate glucose range of 140–180 mg/dL is the most appropriate glucose target for critically ill patients. Severe hypoglycemia (<40 mg/dL) is associated with increased mortality, so the moderate glucose range is designed to reduce the risk of severe hypoglycemia while also preventing significant hyperglycemia (>200 mg/dL). (749)
35. Risk factors for venous thromboembolism in critically ill patients include immobility, mechanical ventilation, presence of a central venous catheter, and use of vasopressors. Prevention includes both pharmacologic methods such as unfractionated heparin (UFH) and low-molecular-weight heparin (LMWH) as well as nonpharmacologic methods such as compression stockings and pneumatic compression devices. (749)
36. Patients at risk for stress ulcers should be treated with an H_2 blocker or proton pump inhibitor. Indications for stress ulcer prophylaxis are shown in the box below. (749)

Indications for Stress Ulcer Prophylaxis
History of GI bleed within last year
Mechanical ventilation >48 hours
Coagulopathy not from pharmacologic anticoagulation (platelet count <50 × 10^9/L, INR >1.5, or PTT > 2 × control)
Trauma
Spinal cord injury
Severe traumatic brain injury
Extensive thermal injury or burns
High-dose steroids in patients with severe sepsis or septic shock

GI, Gastrointestinal; *INR,* international normalized ratio; *PTT,* partial thromboplastin time.

A-F BUNDLE

37. Survivors of critical illness or their family members commonly experience impairment in cognitive and physical function that can be long-lasting. They may also develop a variety of psychological symptoms such as anxiety, depression, and post-traumatic stress disorder that may persist beyond their ICU stay. This syndrome is called post-intensive care syndrome (PICS), or for family members, PICS-family. (749–750)
38. The A-F bundle is a strategy developed to help with implementation of the Pain, Agitation, Delirium, Immobility, Sleep (PADIS) guidelines, which outline best practices for management of these important issues in the ICU. The overall goal is to help prevent or lessen the symptoms experienced by survivors of critical illness. The table below describes what each letter stands for and the corresponding outcome that is addressed through the use of this bundle. (750–751)

A	**Assess**, prevent, and manage pain
B	**Both** spontaneous awakening trial (SAT) and spontaneous breathing trial (SBT)
C	**Choice** for sedation and analgesia
D	**Delirium**: assess, prevent, and manage
E	**Early** mobility
F	**Family** engagement and empowerment

39. When a patient is able to communicate, pain is preferably measured with a scale that relies on self-reporting, such as the Numeric Rating Scale (NRS). If a patient is unable to communicate, the Critical Care Pain Observation Tool (CPOT) or Behavioral Pain Scale (BPS) are two well-validated tools for measuring pain. Agitation is most commonly assessed using the Richmond Agitation-Sedation Scale (RASS) or Sedation-Agitation Scale (SAS). CAM-ICU is the most well-validated delirium assessment tool in ICU patients. It is important to screen for pain, agitation, and delirium proactively and at regular intervals so that signs and symptoms can be detected early and appropriate treatment targeted to the cause can be implemented. For example, in an agitated patient, pain should be adequately treated prior to providing continuous sedation, since pain may be the underlying trigger for the patient's agitation. (750–751)
40. Performance of daily spontaneous awakening trial (SAT) and spontaneous breathing trial (SBT) has been shown to decrease the duration of mechanical ventilation. Some studies also show reduction in hospital length of stay and mortality using this approach. SAT and SBT should be performed together to increase the likelihood of successful SBT and to reduce continuous sedation to the lightest plane necessary. (750)
41. Targeting a light plane of sedation (RASS 0 or –1) in mechanically ventilated patients is considered best practice in the ICU. Prior to starting continuous sedation, pain should be adequately treated with intermittent boluses of an opioid such as fentanyl. If, after achieving adequate pain control, continuous sedation is needed to control patient agitation, propofol or dexmedetomidine are the preferred agents. Continuous infusions of benzodiazepines have been associated with increased duration of mechanical ventilation and increased mortality, so should be avoided whenever possible. (750)
42. Early mobility can help prevent the rapid decline in muscle strength and deterioration in functional status experienced by critically ill patients. Early mobility practices have been associated with increased ventilator-free days, reduced duration of delirium, and improved functional status at the time of ICU discharge. Performing all elements of the A-F bundle is important to ensuring that a patient is able to participate in early mobilization. To facilitate patient participation, pain must be well controlled, sedation must be kept at a light plane, and agitation and delirium must be minimized. Family can be empowered and engaged to participate in mobilization practices. Early mobilization is an excellent example of how the entire A-F bundle must be implemented together to achieve the best outcomes. (749–751)

Chapter

42 PERIOPERATIVE MEDICINE

Emilee Borgmeier, Matthew D. McEvoy, and Jeanna D. Blitz

INTRODUCTION

- Practice of anesthesiology
  - Historically focused on care of the individual patient during surgery
  - Track record of improving quality and safety
- Concept of perioperative medicine
  - Focus on nonoperative care of patients undergoing major surgery
  - An evolving specialty with anesthesiology as most appropriate path
  - Promote value-based, patient-centered care
  - Focus on improvement in overall surgical outcomes

THE PERIOPERATIVE MEDICINE CONSULTANT

- Perioperative medicine
  - A natural expansion of the specialty of anesthesiology
  - Expands focus to optimization of patient care for long-term outcome improvement

Distinct Skillset of the Perioperative Medicine Consultant
Knowledge ▪ Medicine ▪ Surgery ▪ Anesthesiology ▪ Geriatrics ▪ Psychology ▪ Psychometrics **Proficiency** ▪ Care coordination ▪ Business management ▪ Clinical quality principles

- Key aspects of perioperative medicine
  - Preoperative medical, psychological, and physical fitness optimization
  - Goal-directed, evidence-based anesthetic management
  - Optimization of the recovery process

IMPROVING PERIOPERATIVE OUTCOMES AND OPERATIONALIZING PERIOPERATIVE MEDICINE

- Historical focus
  - Safety of the intraoperative and immediate postoperative periods
- Current focus on outcomes is broadening.
  - In-hospital complications
  - 30-day complications
  - 1-year complications and disability-free survival
- Enhance focus on holistic patient-centered care.
  - Functional capacity
  - Social interactions
  - Pain interference
  - Sleep disturbances
- Expanded focus includes three distinct phases of care.
  - Preoperative prehabilitation
  - Immediate postoperative care and in-hospital recovery
  - Postdischarge recovery/rehabilitation

VALUE-ADDED PREOPERATIVE SCREENING AND TESTING

- Evolving indications for preoperative testing
  - Shift away from routine preoperative testing
  - Use of value-based, patient-specific, and evidence-driven testing
    - Target modifiable patient problems that could affect perioperative outcomes
- Enhance history and physical with targeted use of screening tools
- Rationale for commonly used screening labs
  - Direct further tests.
  - Provide referrals to medical specialties.
  - Overall aim is to improve patient's perioperative outcomes.

Commonly Used Preoperative Screening Tools
Revised Cardiac Risk Index (RCRI) ▪ Risk of major adverse cardiac events **STOP-BANG** ▪ Likelihood of obstructive sleep apnea **PONS (Perioperative Nutrition Screening)** ▪ Risk of malnutrition **CFS (Clinical Frailty Scale)** ▪ Summarize overall level of fitness or frailty in elderly patient **American College of Surgeons (ACS) National Surgical Quality Improvement Project (NSQIP) risk calculator** ▪ Evaluates domains from many areas of health ▪ Provides holistic and specific calculations of risk for many postoperative outcomes

- Examples of screening labs
  - Cardiac biomarkers
    - Suspect undiagnosed cardiac disease and screening echocardiography not readily available
  - Hemoglobin A_{1c}
    - Suspect uncontrolled or undiagnosed diabetes mellitus type 2
  - Complete blood count (CBC)
    - If anemia is suspected based on history
    - For known anemia (additional labs discussed below)
  - Vitamins C and D, folate, and/or albumin levels
    - Suspected malnutrition

MEDICAL MANAGEMENT OF THE MOST COMMON COMORBIDITIES

Anemia

- Preoperative anemia is common.
  - May affect up to 50% of surgical patients
  - Most common in patients scheduled for orthopedic, gynecologic, or colorectal surgery
- Increased perioperative risks for patients with anemia
  - 16-fold increase in perioperative mortality
  - Double the risk of perioperative acute kidney injury (AKI), major adverse cardiac events (MACE), and increased length of stay
- Iron deficiency is most common cause of perioperative anemia.
  - Vitamin B_{12} and folate deficiencies must also be considered.
- Patients more likely to develop anemia
  - Rapidly growing oncologic mass
  - Hematuria or gastrointestinal bleeding
  - Significant inflammatory states
- Diagnosis
  - Patient symptoms include fatigue, dyspnea.
  - Physical exam with pallor in severe anemia
- Workup
  - CBC plus iron level and total iron-binding capacity (TIBC), as noted in the box below

Diagnosis and Workup of Iron Deficiency Anemia
▪ Hemoglobin <12 g/dL in females, <13 g/dL in males ▪ Ferritin <100 μg/L and/or – Transferrin saturation (Tsat) <30% and/or – Reticulocyte hemoglobin content <30% ▪ Supported by mean corpuscular volume <80 fL ▪ Must also evaluate folate and B_{12} levels.

- Treatment with either oral or parenteral (IV) iron depending on timing of surgery and underlying mechanism of anemia
  - Oral iron
    - Limited effectiveness in perioperative patients due to poor absorption, intolerance to side effects
    - 4–8 weeks required to see results
    - Consider trial of therapy for patients with mild anemia and planned surgery >4 weeks in advance.
  - IV iron
    - Bypasses limitations posed by poor absorption of oral iron
    - Response typically seen within 1 week
    - Maximum response takes 3–4 weeks after IV infusion.
    - Some patients are not candidates for iron therapy.
- Erythropoiesis-stimulating agents (ESAs)
  - Consider when therapy with iron, B_{12}, or folate is ineffective.
    - One example may be anemia of chronic disease.
  - May be prothrombotic, use caution in patients predisposed to DVT/PE
  - Contraindicated in patients with active malignancy

Nutritional Optimization

- Malnutrition may affect 50%–70% of surgical patients.
  - Only detected and treated in 10% of patients
  - Highest incidence of malnutrition
    - Patients requiring gastrointestinal surgery
    - Patients with frailty syndrome
- Risks of malnutrition
  - Higher rates of wound infection, prolonged hospitalization, and mortality
- Diagnosis of malnutrition
  - GLIM criteria
    - Subnormal BMI, weight loss, reduced muscle mass, decreased food intake, and presence of disease burden
    - These criteria can be subjective to assess.
- Screening tools are essential for detection.
  - Perioperative Nutrition Screening (PONS)

- Malnutrition Screening Tool (MST)
- Vitamins C and D levels
- Consider serum albumin (included in PONS screening tool).

- Treatment approach
  - Preoperative oral nutritional supplementation that is high in protein, with or without immunonutrition (IMN)
    - Protein supplementation goal is >1.5 g/kg/day.
    - IMN typically contains arginine, glutamine, omega-3 fatty acids.
  - Total parenteral nutrition (TPN) for those unable to take PO
  - Duration of 2–4 weeks of preoperative nutrition supplements is currently recommended.
    - Benefits may begin in as few as 3 days.
    - Postoperatively—continue TPN, protein supplementation, or IMN in hospital and after discharge, if needed
- Vitamin D
  - Plays several key intracellular roles
  - Deficiency associated with worse mortality after hospital admission
  - Improvement in mortality if supplementation provided to patients who are deficient
- Vitamin C
  - Vitamin C treatment may improve outcomes in the critically ill.
  - Low vitamin C levels are associated with worse outcomes in the general surgical patient.
  - No improvement has been shown in perioperative period with vitamin C supplementation.

Smoking Cessation

- Approximately 14% of US adults currently smoke cigarettes.
- Current smokers are at significantly higher risk for perioperative complications.
  - 20% increase in perioperative mortality compared to nonsmokers
  - 40% increased risk for wound infections, postoperative pulmonary complications (PPCs), stroke, pulmonary embolism, septic shock, myocardial infarction, and cardiac arrest
  - Patient-reported outcomes are worse in those who continue to smoke.
- Physiologic benefits of smoking cessation depend on the duration of abstinence.
  - Reduced carbon monoxide levels—within 4 hours
  - Improvement in immune system function—4 weeks
  - Decreased rate of PPCs—4 weeks, with greatest benefit after 8 weeks
  - Improved wound healing—3 months
  - Smoking cessation of any duration provides tremendous overall health benefit.
    - Encourage at any perioperative timepoint.

Approach to Smoking Cessation–The 5 A's Approach

Discussion with the patient in the preoperative clinic; plan for surgery is a major life event creating a "teachable moment."

Ask to identify all tobacco users at every visit.
Advise tobacco users to quit.
- Offer cessation assistance via a quitline/hotline.

Assess their willingness to attempt quitting.
Assist tobacco users.
- Refer to quitline-delivered counseling and provide numbers.
- Provide prescription for nicotine replacement therapy (e.g., gum, lozenges, patches).

Arrange for a follow-up meeting.
- Beginning first week after quit date

Glycemic Control

- Perioperative hyperglycemia is associated with poor perioperative outcomes
  - Increased mortality risk, higher risk of wound infection, poor wound healing
  - Likely the result of impaired immune function, direct cellular damage, vascular dysfunction
- Screening by lab evaluation
  - Hemoglobin A_{1c} or fasting/nonfasting blood glucose

Diagnosis of Diabetes Mellitus Type 2

Any one of the below fulfills criteria for diagnosis
- Hemoglobin A_{1c} ≥6.5%
- Random blood glucose ≥200 mg/dL
- Fasting blood glucose ≥126 mg/dL

- Screening in the perioperative context is more nuanced than screening in primary care.
  - Consider testing prior to major inpatient surgery for the following patients.
    - Age >45 years, BMI >25 kg/m^2, history of gestational diabetes, or higher-risk ethnic group (Hispanic, African American), family history of diabetes
  - Consider preoperative hemoglobin A_{1c} for patients with known diabetes mellitus (either type) without A_{1c} in the past 3 months.
    - Higher risk for perioperative complications if A_{1c} ≥8%
    - Corresponds to average glucose ~180 mg/dL
  - Diagnosis in patients with moderate to severe anemia
    - Serum fructosamine level can replace hemoglobin A_{1c}.
    - Fructosamine level can also assess response to therapy in a shorter time frame (2–3 weeks) compared to A_{1c} (months).

- Management of patients with elevated preoperative hemoglobin A_{1c}
  - If A_{1c} ≥8%, discuss with surgical team.
    - Delay of elective procedures allows for referral to endocrinology or return to primary care, with goal to improve glycemic control.
  - If A_{1c} ≥6.5% but <8%, elective surgery may proceed.
    - Consult a glucose-management service postoperatively.
  - Regardless of A_{1c} level, give enough time prior to surgery to improve management.
    - Consider referral to endocrinology or primary care, especially for a new diagnosis.
- Perioperative treatment of hyperglycemia
  - Intraoperative: goal is modest reduction in blood glucose levels
    - Typically target blood glucose <180 mg/dL
    - Most often treated with IV insulin infusion
  - Postoperative: treatment usually with subcutaneous insulin protocols
  - Avoidance of severe hypoglycemia is a strong consideration.
    - Severe hypoglycemia can be life-threatening.
    - Typical symptoms (e.g., nausea, dizziness, tremors) will not be evident during general anesthesia.
    - Must check glucose frequently enough to detect.
    - Glucose goal of <180 mg/dL (not lower) may help reduce hypoglycemia risk.

Obstructive Sleep Apnea and Chronic Obstructive Pulmonary Disease

- Postoperative pulmonary complications
  - Dangerous to patient, costly to health systems (average of $25,000 per episode)
  - Risk factors for PPCs
    - Untreated pulmonary disease (e.g., COPD, asthma)
    - Untreated obstructive sleep apnea (OSA)
    - Current smokers
  - Detection and treatment of modifiable risk factors may improve outcomes.
- COPD
  - Risk factors
    - ≥20 years smoking history, age ≥45 years and/or ≥20–40 pack years
  - Symptoms to assess
    - Self-reported chronic cough, sputum production, wheezing, and significant dyspnea with activity
  - Formally diagnosed with pulmonary function tests (PFTs)
    - Spirometry findings include $FEV_1/FVC < 0.7$
  - Treatment
    - Approach to medical management described in box below
    - Continue inhaled medications on the day of surgery, with the exception of theophylline.

Treatment of Newly Diagnosed COPD

- First line: monotherapy with inhaled bronchodilator (short (SABA) or long acting (LABA))
- Additional medications for symptom control
- Consider preoperative initiation of combination therapy (LAMA + LABA) for patients with moderate to severe disease (GOLD III/IV or groups B, C, D), and time to surgery <1 month

- OSA
  - Moderate to severe OSA may be undiagnosed and untreated.
  - Increases perioperative risk
    - Cardiac and respiratory outcomes (e.g., hypoxemia, respiratory failure)
    - Postoperative opioid-related adverse events
  - Screening for OSA is important.
    - Patients with STOP-BANG score ≥5 or STOP-BANG ≥3 and serum bicarbonate ≥28 mEq/L should be referred for formal evaluation (>75% chance of moderate to severe OSA)
    - Formal diagnosis made by polysomnography (PSG) or home sleep study (HSS)
  - Patients with known OSA
    - If using home CPAP, bring device to be used perioperatively.
    - If not using CPAP, consider postoperative respiratory-monitoring ward for 24–48 hours after surgery.
  - High-risk patients for OSA who are not currently treated
    - Consider respiratory-monitored ward for 24–48 hours postoperatively.
    - Be prepared to start perioperative CPAP for hypoxemia or witnessed apnea.

Prehabilitation

- A specific combination implemented prior to elective surgery incorporating three elements
  - Physical exercise
  - Nutritional optimization (e.g., supplementation)
  - Psychological preparation (e.g., anxiety reduction)
- Goal is to improve physiologic and psychological stamina to withstand high levels of stress in the perioperative period.
- Prehabilitation approaches increasingly used for multidimensional syndromes such as frailty
- Challenges of prehabilitation
  - Resource- and time-intensive

- Large heterogeneity in approaches to interventions makes definitive recommendations difficult.
- Potential benefits of prehabilitation
  - Some evidence-based support for improved outcomes in colorectal, esophageal, prostate, and some orthopedic surgeries

Physical Exercise Regimen

- Assessment of physical status may be done in clinic with simple tests of ability.
  - Timed Up and Go (TUG)
    - Measures time required to stand from a seated position and walk 10 feet away, then return
    - Time >12 seconds on the TUG reveals increased risk for impaired mobility/falls
  - 6-Minute Walk Test (6MWT)
    - Measures amount of distance covered by patient walking at a tiring pace
    - Normal values vary by age range and gender.
    - Correlates most closely with cardiopulmonary exercise testing (CPET)
  - 1 Minute Sit-to-Stand Test
    - Measures number of times a patient can rise from seated position and return to seated position in 1 minute
    - May reveal instability or poor functional reserve
- A "one-size-fits all" approach to physical exercise regimen may be impractical.
- Components of prehabilitation-focused exercise regimen
  - Aerobic exercise for 30 minutes daily
  - Lightweight strength training
  - Exercises to promote balance and flexibility
  - Patient-specific considerations
    - Functionally limited patient—start with improving core strength (e.g., sit-to-stand exercises, arm movements); may require physical and/or occupational therapy
    - Patient at high risk of PPCs—inspiratory muscle training
- Physical exercise and outcomes
  - Studied interventions have significant heterogeneity.
  - No definitive evidence that improved aerobic capacity and strength improve perioperative outcomes.

PSYCHOLOGICAL STATE: ASSESSMENT AND INTERVENTIONS

- Anxiety and depression are common in patients preparing for surgery.
  - Prevalent and undertreated in the general population, especially the elderly
  - If untreated, these conditions may represent barriers to preoperative optimization.
- Perioperative risks of anxiety, depression, PTSD, and other psychiatric illnesses
  - Associated with prolonged pain and opioid use, longer hospitalization, and increased risk of in-hospital mortality
- Screening for anxiety and depression
  - Can occur in the preoperative clinic to assist in patient preparation
  - Hospital Anxiety and Depression Score (HADS)
  - Patient Health Questionnaire (PHQ)
    - Screens for depression alone
- Interventions
  - Individually tailored, nonpharmacologic low-cost interventions
  - Psychological preparation
    - Strategies to modify patient's thoughts and perceptions
    - Provide detailed procedural and sensory information
    - Procedural: what, how, when certain events will occur
    - Perceptions: expected sensations, sounds and smells
  - Relaxation-based interventions
    - Perioperative music therapy can be very effective at reducing anxiety.
    - Music activates limbic system and can decrease sympathetic output by modification of endogenous opioids, oxytocin, cortisol, and catecholamines.
  - Cognitive behavioral therapy (CBT)
    - Time-intensive approach that requires specially trained providers
    - 4–8 weeks of CBT prior to surgery associated with faster recovery and improved perioperative pain control

COGNITIVE SCREENING AND INTERVENTIONS

- Screening for cognitive dysfunction should be done preoperatively.
- Primary goal is to identify patients at highest risk for perioperative delirium.
- Most used screening tool is the Mini-Cog.
  - Fast, easy-to-implement, reliable results
  - Three-word recall (1 point each) and a clock drawing test (2 points for normal)
  - Scores ≤2 are considered at risk for postoperative delirium
- Approach to patients at high risk of delirium
  - Preoperative interventions addressed in box below
  - Strategies can be implemented pre-, intra-, and postoperatively.
  - Up to 40% of perioperative delirium cases may be preventable.

Preoperative Interventions for High-Risk Delirium

Educate patient and family about signs and symptoms of delirium.

Educate family about mitigation strategies.
- Return of sensory aids
- Frequent reminders by family of location and reason
- Assistance with recovery of natural sleep/wake cycles

Consultation with a geriatrician and/or PCP to wean deliriogenic medications
- E.g., benzodiazepines, anticholinergics, sleep aids, opioids, multiple psychotropic medications

HEALTH LITERACY AND SHARED DECISION MAKING

- Goal of health literacy
  - Health information and services provided for the patient match the patient's ability to understand and use those services
- Patients with low health literacy
  - Poorly understand their own health
  - Overestimate their ability to manage their health
- Risk of poor health literacy
  - Higher risk for surgical complications
  - Longer hospital stay after major surgery
- Approach to patient with low health literacy
  - Face-to-face discussions
  - Repeated verbal instructions with video or infographic instructions as well
  - Goal is for patient to be able to participate in shared decision-making.
- Goals of shared decision-making
  - Patient fully understands risks/benefits of proposed surgery/anesthetic.
  - Patient understands alternatives to proposed therapy, including foregoing treatment.
- Facilitating shared decision making
  - "Teach-back method" can enhance retention, identify gaps in understanding
  - Consider standardized discussion template as described in box below.

Keys to Shared Decision-Making

- Asking permission to introduce a topic
- Ascertaining patient's understanding of their illness
- Exploring goals of their care
- Exploring fears related to their care
- Identification of an alternate decision-maker

OTHER OPPORTUNITIES TO IMPROVE PERIOPERATIVE OUTCOMES

- Other comorbidities should be assessed perioperatively.
- E.g., cardiac, thyroid, renal dysfunction

FUTURE DIRECTIONS IN PERIOPERATIVE MEDICINE: SOCIAL DETERMINANTS OF HEALTH

- Social and economic factors contribute to poor outcomes.
- Health disparities arise from multifactorial causes.
- Further research is needed to identify perioperative interventions related to social, economic, and physical environmental issues.

QUESTIONS

IMPROVING PERIOPERATIVE OUTCOMES AND OPERATIONALIZING PERIOPERATIVE MEDICINE

1. Describe how perioperative medicine reflects an expanded focus on anesthesia patient care and safety.

VALUE-ADDED PREOPERATIVE SCREENING AND TESTING

2. Describe some specific screening tools that are useful in perioperative medicine when used in conjunction with the history and physical.
3. What is the role of routine screening in the preoperative evaluation? List three examples of inappropriate preoperative testing.

MEDICAL MANAGEMENT OF THE MOST COMMON COMORBIDITIES

4. What are the risks of preoperative anemia? What type of anemia is most common in patients presenting for surgery?
5. What labs are required to evaluate for iron deficiency anemia? What results will confirm that diagnosis?
6. What are the goals of iron repletion therapy? Describe two methods of delivering iron therapy to patients and the advantages/disadvantages of each method.
7. What is an erythropoiesis-stimulating agent (ESA)? What are the contraindications for the use of an ESA in the treatment of anemia?
8. Which patients are at greatest risk for nutritional deficiencies? What are the risks of malnutrition for a patient undergoing surgery?
9. What are the criteria used by the nutrition screening tools PONS (Perioperative Nutrition Screen) and MST (Malnutrition Screening Tool)? What scores are necessary in each to be considered "at risk" for nutritional deficiencies?
10. What is the recommended minimum intake of protein for a perioperative patient?
11. What is the optimal timing of smoking cessation prior to surgery? Is there any risk to patients who quit smoking prior to surgery?
12. What are the goals for glycemic management in the preoperative, intraoperative, and postoperative phases of care? What is the perioperative risk of pursuing normoglycemia in a patient with diabetes?
13. What are some examples of a postoperative pulmonary complication (PPC)? What types of pulmonary disease may lead to increased risk of PPCs if left untreated?
14. For patients with COPD, how can the severity of airflow limitation be assessed using the GOLD criteria?
15. What are the three key components of the concept of prehabilitation?
16. The cardiopulmonary exercise test (CPET) measures parameters such as oxygen consumption during exercise in a pulmonary laboratory setting. What screening tool that can be used in a preoperative clinic best reflects the findings on CPET?
17. Is there a universally effective preoperative exercise regimen that improves outcomes? What are some general targets for physical activity?
18. What cautions should be used when prescribing preoperative exercise therapy? Under what circumstances might physical therapy/occupational therapy (PT/OT) be helpful?

PSYCHOLOGICAL STATE: ASSESSMENT AND INTERVENTIONS

19. What are the perioperative risks of psychological disorders such as anxiety and depression? What preoperative interventions may improve those risks and increase patient satisfaction?

COGNITIVE SCREENING AND INTERVENTIONS

20. What is the goal of perioperative cognitive screening? What screening tool is most used, and what score represents the highest risk for delirium?

21. For a patient identified as high risk for delirium, what are the highest-yield preoperative interventions to prevent delirium after surgery?

HEALTH LITERACY AND SHARED DECISION MAKING

22. What are the implications of a patient's poor understanding of their health with respect to perioperative complications? Describe some high-yield teaching methods that may help patients with poor health literacy.

ANSWERS

IMPROVING PERIOPERATIVE OUTCOMES AND OPERATIONALIZING PERIOPERATIVE MEDICINE

1. Traditionally, anesthesia care has been described in three phases: preoperative, intraoperative, and postoperative. Perioperative medicine can be described as having an expanded focus on anesthesia patient care that includes prehabilitation, immediate perioperative care, and recovery/rehabilitation. This more holistic patient perspective includes attention to functional capacity, social interactions, pain interference, sleep disturbances, and other issues that could affect outcomes. As perioperative care and safety have improved, the focus on outcomes has broadened to include in-hospital, 30-day, and even 1-year intervals after surgery. (754)

VALUE-ADDED PREOPERATIVE SCREENING AND TESTING

2. There are many screening tools designed to supplement the traditional history and physical. This chapter discusses the STOP-BANG (screening for OSA), PONS (screening for malnutrition), and the clinical frailty scale. Other tools include the Mini-Cog to screen for susceptibility to perioperative delirium, as well as the DASI (Duke Activity Status Index) to identify patients who may have poor physiologic reserve. (744–754)
3. Preoperative testing should be based on patient risk factors and the stress of the proposed surgery. In the absence of a clinical indication, routine screening tests should not be performed. For example, in an otherwise healthy, asymptomatic patient, ECG, routine blood tests (e.g., complete blood count and chemistry panel), and chest radiograph should not be ordered. (754)

MEDICAL MANAGEMENT OF THE MOST COMMON COMORBIDITIES

4. Anemia increases overall perioperative risk, including 16-fold greater mortality risk and 2-fold greater risk of acute kidney injury, major adverse cardiac events, and increased length of hospital stay. Iron deficiency is the most common cause of preoperative anemia. (755)
5. The table below summarizes the lab tests and results that are consistent with the diagnosis of iron deficiency anemia. (755–756)

Test	Result
Transferrin saturation	<30%
Ferritin	<100 μg/L
Reticulocyte hemoglobin content	<30%

6. The goal of iron repletion therapy is to correct preoperative anemia, which should improve postoperative outcomes. There are two routes of therapy: oral or intravenous. Oral therapy is inexpensive and readily accessible; however, 4–8 weeks of therapy are required, and many patients develop gastrointestinal side effects. IV iron has a more rapid onset of effect (within 1 week) with maximum response in 3–4 weeks. IV iron has the potential for more serious adverse effects, including anaphylaxis with earlier formulations. (756)
7. Erythropoiesis-stimulating agents (ESAs) are medications that stimulate bone marrow to produce red blood cells, thus increasing hemoglobin. Most guidelines consider active malignancy to be a contraindication, but use may be considered if the malignancy is being treated with chemotherapy or if the goals of care are palliative only. For patients without a contraindication, ESAs may be combined with iron therapy to increase the rate and magnitude of response when correcting preoperative anemia. (756)
8. Patients scheduled for gastrointestinal surgery and patients who meet criteria for frailty syndrome have the greatest risk for nutritional deficiencies. Untreated malnutrition is associated with wound infection, prolonged hospitalization, and increased mortality. (756–757)
9. The following tables contain the components of the PONS and MST screening tools. Those considered "at risk" for nutritional deficiencies will have a score of >1 on the PONS or ≥2 on the MST. (757)

PONS (Perioperative Nutrition Screen) Questions	Points: yes = 1, no = 0
Have you lost ≥10% of body weight in past 6 months without trying?	
Have you been eating <50% of your normal diet in the last week?	
Is the patient's BMI <18.5, or if age >65, is their BMI <20?	
Is albumin <3 g/dL?	

MST (Malnutrition Screening Tool) Questions	Points
Have you lost weight recently without trying?	
No Unsure	0 2
If yes, how much weight (kilograms) have you lost?	
1–5 6–10 11–15 >15 Unsure	1 2 3 4 2
Have you been eating poorly because of a decreased appetite?	
No Yes	0 1

10. For a patient undergoing surgery, protein intake >1.5 g/kg/day is considered adequate for oral nutritional supplementation. For example, in a 60-kg patient, this would equal 90 g of daily protein. High protein supplementation is most effective when it is initiated at least 2–4 weeks prior to surgery. (757)
11. While there is no consensus on optimal timing for smoking cessation prior to surgery, a duration greater than 4 weeks is when most benefit is seen. After 4 weeks, evidence shows a reduction in respiratory complications, as well as improved wound healing. However, the half-lives of nicotine and carbon monoxide are <24 hours, so cessation even 24 hours prior to surgery will improve tissue oxygen delivery and reduce sympathetic output during surgery. There is no significant risk associated with short-term smoking cessation prior to surgery. Two observational studies from the 1980s suggested that secretions and complications might increase with shorter periods of smoking cessation, but this has not been borne out in subsequent larger analyses. (758–759)
12. Preoperatively, reduction of hemoglobin A_{1c} to <8% before surgery likely reduces the risk of perioperative complications such as poor wound healing and greater risk for infections. Both the intraoperative and postoperative goals for glycemic management target a modest reduction in blood glucose levels of <180 mg/dL. Intraoperatively, this is most commonly pursued with an IV insulin infusion and postoperatively with subcutaneous sliding scale insulin protocols. Large studies have shown that pursuing normoglycemia, or "tight" glucose management (e.g., glucose 80–110 mg/dL) leads to significantly increased risk of hypoglycemia, which can be life-threatening. (759)
13. Postoperative pneumonia, unplanned reintubation, and prolonged mechanical ventilation are considered true PPCs. Patients with pulmonary diseases such as COPD, asthma, OSA, and current cigarette smoking, are considered at increased risk of PPCs. Appropriate medical management may modify the risk of these conditions. Other pulmonary pathologies that likely increase risk of PPCs include interstitial and restrictive lung disease, but these may have a less modifiable impact on outcomes. Management with a pulmonologist is recommended. (758–760)
14. The Global Initiative for Obstructive Lung Disease (GOLD) classification of airflow limitation severity in COPD is based on pulmonary function test spirometry values, specifically the FEV_1. The specific spirometry cut-points in the box below are assessed after at least one short-acting bronchodilator. Airflow limitation is only one aspect of COPD. There is also a GOLD ABCD assessment tool that incorporates patient symptoms, health status impairment, and outcomes such as requirement for hospital admission. (760)

	FEV_1 (% of predicted)
GOLD 1	≥80
GOLD 2	50–79
GOLD 3	30–49
GOLD 4	<30

15. Prehabilitation refers to the specific combination of nutritional optimization, improvement of physical stamina, and psychological preparation. The major goal of prehabilitation is to improve the patient's ability to tolerate the perioperative stress associated with surgery. (760)
16. The 6-Minute Walk Test (6MWT) requires a patient to ambulate a 30-meter stretch of level ground for 6 minutes, with the goal to walk as far as possible without jogging or running. The total distance traveled, compared with averages for the patient's age and sex, correlates well with CPET oxygen consumption values. (761)
17. Unfortunately, there is no universally effective preoperative exercise regimen as a patient's functional status may differ with respect to issues such as balance, gait speed, and physical strength. Understanding a patient's current activity level, access to equipment, and assistance with balance are key to developing an individual plan. In general, physical exercise regimens include 30 minutes of daily aerobic exercise with lightweight strength training (8–15 repetitions with various muscle groups) if possible. Exercises that promote balance and flexibility may be helpful as well. (761)
18. Caution should be used when discussing preoperative exercise in patients with known or suspected severe cardiac disease, high oxygen requirements, or who are at high risk for falls without assistance. For patients with these issues, PT/OT referral is highly recommended. (761, 763)

PSYCHOLOGICAL STATE: ASSESSMENT AND INTERVENTIONS

19. Patients with untreated anxiety and depression are at risk for prolonged pain and opioid use, longer hospitalization, and increased risk of in-hospital mortality. In addition, patients with these disorders may avoid seeking care, especially if they have had prior negative experiences in the healthcare setting. Anxiety and depression may also limit successful engagement in preoperative optimization. If enough time is available prior to surgery, cognitive behavioral therapy (CBT) may be a helpful intervention. This is typically resource intensive and requires 4–6 weeks to see improvement in outcomes. Other interventions could include in-depth discussion of procedural/anesthetic care, as well as expectations for sensations perioperatively. Music therapy may also help reduce perioperative stress and anxiety, especially when the patient selects the playlist. (761–762)

COGNITIVE SCREENING AND INTERVENTIONS

20. Perioperative cognitive screening is primarily used to identify patients who are at high risk for postoperative delirium. The Mini-Cog is the most used test in the preoperative setting because it is easy to administer and interpretation is reliable. A score of ≤2 places the patient at greater perioperative risk for delirium. (762)
21. Referral to geriatrician or primary care provider (PCP) may facilitate controlled weaning of medications that may place a patient at higher risk for delirium, such as benzodiazepines, muscle relaxants, sleep aids, opioids, and psychotropic medications. Education of the patient and family regarding symptoms of delirium and ways that the family can assist in reorientation, along with visual aids as needed, are also high-yield interventions. (762)

HEALTH LITERACY AND SHARED DECISION MAKING

22. Patients with low health literacy level are at greater risk for surgical complications and in-hospital mortality after major surgery. Having face-to-face discussions with the patient, including repeated verbal instructions supplemented with video or infographic instructions can all improve their understanding of current plans for intervention. The "teach-back method" is a particularly useful way for the provider to assess the patient's comprehension and identify gaps in understanding that can be further addressed. (762)

Chapter

43 TRAUMA

Benn Morrie Lancman, Katrina Gabriel-Ramos, and Marc P. Steurer

INTRODUCTION

Physiology in Trauma

- Causes of hypotension
  - Hemorrhagic shock (most common cause)
  - Obstructive shock (e.g., tension pneumothorax or cardiac tamponade)
  - Cardiogenic shock
  - Neurogenic shock
- Phases of hemorrhagic shock
  - Compensatory
    - Up to 10% to 15% of blood volume lost
    - Degree of hemorrhage can be masked.
    - Systemic perfusion may be maintained without intervention.
  - Progressive
    - Ongoing hemorrhage leads to a sequence of events.
    - Inadequate perfusion, tissue ischemia, local hypoxia, cardiac dysfunction, metabolic acidosis, and multiorgan failure

Compensatory Mechanisms in Hemorrhagic Shock

- Reflex pathways
  - Sympathetic nervous system
  - Carotid sinus and aortic arch baroreceptors
  - Renin-angiotensin system and vasopressin secretion
- Physiologic response
  - Increased total peripheral resistance
  - Increased venous return
  - Increased heart rate

- Trauma-induced coagulopathy
  - Endogenous causes (direct result of injury)
    - Inflammatory factors and cellular dysfunction
    - Factor deficiency, hyperfibrinolysis, platelet dysfunction
  - Iatrogenic causes (resuscitation-associated)
    - Hemodilution, hypocalcemia, hypothermia, acidosis
- Lethal triad: hypothermia, coagulopathy, and acidosis

INITIAL MANAGEMENT

- Standardized initial assessment and management processes
- Processes run swiftly and in parallel

Prearrival Preparation

- Universal organization and deployment of multiple resources
- Essential, succinct information about the patient
- Prearrival briefing can include introductions and roles.

Trauma Bay

Primary Survey

- Advanced Trauma Life Support (ATLS) approach to assess the patient
- Identify and treat immediate life-threatening injuries (ABCDE).
  - **A**irway
    - If time allows, optimize patient and perform neurologic assessment.
    - Preoxygenation may be difficult, which reduces apneic time.
    - Assume a full-stomach, rapid sequence induction is standard.
  - **B**reathing and oxygenation
  - **C**irculation and hemorrhage control
    - Stop bleeding (e.g., direct pressure, sutures).
    - Damage control resuscitation (DCR) to prevent end-organ damage
  - **D**isability
    - Rapid assessment of neurologic status (e.g., pupils, gross limb function)
    - Glasgow Coma Scale (GCS) score
  - **E**xposure
    - Check for other injuries, entire body
- Special groups
  - Suspected cervical spine injury
    - Manual in-line stabilization if suspected spine injury

- Can remove front of hard collar during the time of laryngoscopy
- May need to be relaxed slightly if failed intubation, hypoxia are risks
- Airway burns
  - Need expedited airway management
  - Can rapidly progress to an occluded airway from expanding edema
  - Signs include facial burn, soot in upper airway, carbonaceous sputum, stridor, explosive injuries
- Oral trauma
  - Blood may obscure videolaryngoscope or fiberoptic view.
  - Surgical airway team available
- Direct airway injury
  - Tracheal trauma can cause stridor, subcutaneous emphysema
  - Endotracheal tube cuff should be advanced past injury.

Managing the Trauma Airway

- Induction of anesthesia can result in hypotension.
  - Intravascular volume loss from bleeding
  - Abolishes the sympathetic nervous system response
  - Consider peri-induction resuscitation to reduce the likelihood of hypovolemic arrest.
- Anesthetic drug choices
  - In general, decreased doses are needed.
  - Have vasopressors immediately available.
- Anticipate difficulty.
  - Explicit team briefing of airway management plan and backup
- For the soiled airway (e.g., blood)
  - Have two suctions available in case of blockage.
- Primary use of a videolaryngoscope
  - May reduce pressure applied to the immobilized cervical spine
  - Consider as first-line approach.
- For the unstable patient post initiation of positive pressure ventilation
  - Consider evolving tension pneumothorax.

INTRAOPERATIVE MANAGEMENT

- Massive hemorrhage is a cause of hemodynamic shock in trauma patients.
  - Management is divided into three phases.
  - Other causes should be considered.

Differential Diagnosis of Hemodynamic Shock in Trauma Patient

- Massive hemorrhage
- Tension pneumothorax
- Cardiac tamponade
- Cardiac contusion
- Neurogenic shock

Phase 1: Uncontrolled Hemorrhage

- Basic principles
  - Massive transfusion protocol
  - Management of additional personnel
  - Ventilation with 100% FiO_2
  - Direct-to–operating room (OR) improves outcomes.
- Damage control resuscitation
  - Permissive hypotension (systolic blood pressure <100 mmHg, mean arterial pressure 50 to 60 mmHg)
  - Caveats: traumatic brain or spinal cord injury, coronary artery disease, carotid stenosis, pediatrics, obstetrics
  - Limit crystalloids and colloids.
  - Early and empiric 1:1:1 transfusion (packed red blood cells [PRBCs]:fresh-frozen plasma [FFP]:platelets)
- Consider procoagulants (e.g., tranexamic acid); balance thromboembolic risk.
- Avoid vasopressors to prevent extreme vasoconstriction in hypovolemia.
- Minimum of two large-bore peripheral intravenous (PIV) lines; consider central access if significant/prolonged
- Rapid infuser system for delivery of large amounts of warmed blood products

Phase 2: Controlled Hemorrhage (with partial surgical control)

- Mainstay: point-of-care testing (POCT) to guide the resuscitation
- Viscoelastic tests: thromboelastography (TEG) and rotational thromboelastometry (ROTEM) to tailor transfusion/coagulation requirements
- Invasive monitoring and possible transesophageal echocardiogram (TEE)
- Arterial blood gases (ABGs), lactate/base deficit to guide fluid therapy

Phase 3: Restoration of Physiology (surgical hemostasis is complete)

- Deepening of anesthesia gradually
- Replenish intravascular volume.
- Consider use of low-dose vasoactive infusions.
- Indicator is normalization of serum lactate and base deficit.

Intraoperative Management of the Trauma Patient

- Principles of damage control surgery and resuscitation are paramount.
  - Stop the bleeding/contamination and prevent coagulopathy.

Intraoperative Management of the Trauma Patient—Continued

- Maintain high-frequency, two-way communication with surgeons.
  - Hemodynamic stability, blood loss, etc.
- In the patient with shock, start with very low-dose anesthesia and uptitrate as patient physiology allows.
  - Normal anesthetic doses imply adequate resuscitation.
- Do not forget to increase OR temperature.
- Consider unrecognized injury (different body compartment) if ongoing instability despite apparent surgical control.

SPECIAL CONSIDERATIONS

Traumatic Brain Injury

- Primary neurologic injury
  - Irreversible neuronal damage that occurs at the moment of injury
  - Includes skull fractures, diffuse axonal injuries, hematomas
- Secondary neurologic injury
  - Subsequent injury to the brain
  - Causes: intracranial hypertension, systemic hypotension, hypoxia, hyperthermia, coagulopathy, hyper/hypoglycemia, acidosis
- Management goals
  - Optimize patient physiology and limit secondary injury.
- Airway considerations
  - Early intubation and airway control (e.g., GCS score <8, intracranial hypertension)
  - Avoid nasal airways/tubes in facial/head trauma.
  - Concurrent airway or cervical spine injuries
- Anesthetic goals and emergent neurosurgical management
  - Hemodynamic stability to maintain cerebral perfusion pressure (CPP)
    - Maintain CPP between 50 and 70 mmHg.
  - Propofol and etomidate
    - Reduce cerebral blood flow (CBF).
    - "Coupled" reduction of cerebral metabolic rate of oxygen ($CMRO_2$)
  - Ketamine and succinylcholine
    - No significant clinical effect on intracranial pressure (ICP) and CBF
  - Volatile anesthetics
    - Increase CBF while decreasing $CMRO_2$ ("uncoupling").
    - Keep <0.5 MAC (or <1 MAC for sevoflurane) to minimize increased CBF.
  - Total intravenous anesthesia (TIVA)
    - Decreases ICP but is less titratable
  - Volatile vs. TIVA
    - There is no definitive study demonstrating superiority of either.
  - Cushing reflex in patients with high ICP
    - Causes catecholamine release and arteriolar vasoconstriction
    - Can mask intravascular volume depletion
    - Profound hypotension can occur after ICP normalizes.
  - Before dural opening
    - Achieve/maintain euvolemia.
    - Have vasopressors and inotropes available.
    - Gradually decrease anesthetics.
  - Postoperative airway management
    - Discuss plan with surgeons.
    - Controlled ventilation avoids hypoxia, hypoventilation.
    - Neuromuscular blocking drug (small dose) prevents coughing, bucking with transport.

Managing Traumatic Brain Injury

- For surgically amenable lesions (e.g., subdural hematoma [SDH]), surgical decompression is a priority.
  - Time is brain.
- Hypovolemia is significantly exacerbated by mannitol.
  - Make sure the patient has had adequate fluid replacement before the dura is opened.
- A good choice for large-bore venous access is the saphenous vein.
  - Place while facilitating rapid cranial decompression.
- Get an ABG early to assess for $ETCO_2$ to $PaCO_2$ gradient.
  - Gradient can be large in concomitant pulmonary injury (e.g., contusion, aspiration, hemorrhage).

Spinal Cord Injury

- Disruption of sensory, motor, or autonomic function due to acute trauma
  - Complete: no motor or sensory function below level of injury
  - Incomplete: varying degrees of sensory or motor function below injury
- Spinal cord precautions for suspected spinal injury
  - Cervical collar placement and strict logroll precautions
- Cervical spine injuries
  - May have diaphragm impairment and weakness
  - Can have decreased vital capacity and inability to cough/clear secretions
- Thoracic and high lumbar injuries
  - Intercostal or abdominal muscle weakness
  - Increased work of breathing, paradoxical abdominal movement
- Endotracheal intubation
  - Succinylcholine use is safe within first 24 hours of injury.
    - Avoid after 48 hours due to risk of severe hyperkalemia.
  - Severe bradycardia and hypotension possible with high injury levels

- Neurogenic shock
  - Cervical and high thoracic (T4 and above) injuries
  - Disruption of sympathetic cardiac accelerators
    - Exaggerated bradycardia and systemic vasodilation (severe hypotension)
  - Treat with vasopressors and volume.
- Anesthetic management
  - Maintain mean arterial pressure (around 85 to 90 mmHg) for adequate spinal cord perfusion.

Burns

- Assessment of burns
  - Burn surface area (BSA) estimated commonly by the "rule of nines."
  - Severity as superficial, partial-thickness, or full-thickness.
  - Types are thermal, chemical, or electrical.
    - Initial treatment is dependent on the type of burn.
- Fluid management
  - Cornerstone of burn management
  - Most common is the modified Parkland formula (4 mL/kg/% BSA) over initial 24 hours after injury.
  - First 24 hours, use crystalloid only due to protein leak (colloids ineffective).
  - Tailor resuscitation using vital signs, urine output, and labs.
  - Excessive fluids can cause acute respiratory distress 3 to 5 days after injury.
- Airway management
  - Rapid-onset edema can result in total airway obstruction.
  - Early intubation with slightly smaller-diameter endotracheal tube.
- Carbon monoxide (CO) toxicity
  - Not detectable on standard monitors
  - High binding affinity to hemoglobin can result in tissue hypoxia.
  - High FiO_2 for patients suspected of CO inhalation
- Pain management
  - Severe and prolonged pain can require pain specialist consultation.
- Infection
  - Major cause of morbidity and death
  - Use antibiotics and sterile dressing to cover burns.
  - Avoid overresuscitation of fluids, which increases risk.

Extremes of Age

Pediatric Trauma

- Most common cause of morbidity and fatality in pediatrics
- Nonaccidental injury should always be considered.
- Pediatric physiology
  - Significant blood loss can be masked initially.
  - Rapid deterioration occurs once a compensatory threshold is reached.
- Vascular access
  - Can be difficult, early IO advocated (if >2 attempts at a PIV line)
- Weight
  - For drug dosing, fluid administration, equipment, and estimated blood loss
  - Blood administration: PRBCs increase Hb by 2 to 2.5 g/dL for every 10 mL/kg administered.
  - Broselow Pediatric Emergency Tape useful to estimate weight

Geriatric Trauma

- Preexisting illness and declining physiologic reserve
  - Minimal trauma can result in significant injuries (e.g., fractures, subdural bleed).
  - Affects survival
- Medications
  - Can exacerbate or mask hemodynamic changes (e.g., β-blockers)
- Elder abuse is a consideration.
- End-of-life and goals of care may influence the appropriateness of an intervention.

Trauma in Pregnancy

- Gestational age affects injury patterns.
  - First trimester: uterus is intrapelvic, well protected
  - Second trimester: uterus is extrapelvic; increased risk of fetal injury
  - Third trimester: maternal organs relatively protected by the uterus
- Maternal physiology
  - Blood changes
    - Increased volume can mask significant blood loss.
    - Increased clotting factors or hypercoagulable state near term
  - Compensated respiratory alkalosis
    - Normal PCO_2 of about 30 mmHg
  - Aortocaval compression starting around 20 weeks' gestational age
    - Use left uterine displacement.
  - Increased risk of difficult intubation
    - Airway edema
    - Increased breast size affecting laryngoscopy
    - Reduced functional residual capacity and apnea time
    - Higher aspiration risk
- Anti-D immunoglobulin
  - Given to Rh-negative mothers with major trauma within 72 hours
- Fetal monitoring
  - Usually for >24 weeks gestational age

  - Consider once maternal stability is achieved.
  - Perfusion to the uteroplacental unit is *not* autoregulated.
  - Fetal deterioration should prompt reassessment of maternal hemodynamics.
- Delivery
  - May be necessary to optimize maternal or fetal survival
  - Consider cesarean section if >5 minutes of maternal cardiac arrest.
- Unique differential diagnoses
  - Amniotic fluid embolism
  - Placental abruption
  - Uterine rupture
  - Eclampsia

Care for Trauma Patients in Non-OR Settings

- Locations of care can include computed tomography (CT) scanner, interventional radiology suite, magnetic resonance imaging (MRI) scanner, intensive care unit (ICU).
  - Patients often evaluated in CT scanner before other triage.
- Equipment considerations
  - Anesthesia machine, emergency airway equipment, anesthetic medications, hemodynamic medications
- Anesthesia provider must be ready for cardiopulmonary resuscitation, massive transfusion.

QUESTIONS

INTRODUCTION

1. What types of shock can cause hypotension after a trauma-induced injury?
2. What are some compensatory reflexes in the hypotensive trauma patient? What is the result when these mechanisms fail?
3. Describe the features of acute traumatic coagulopathy.

INITIAL MANAGEMENT

4. How is the ATLS approach used during the initial management of a trauma patient?
5. What are some special considerations when managing the airway of a trauma patient?

INTRAOPERATIVE MANAGEMENT

6. Intraoperative resuscitation of massively hemorrhaging trauma patients can be divided into three phases. Complete the following chart listing the strategies and special considerations for each phase.

	Phase 1	Phase 2	Phase 3
Clinical Status	**Life-Threatening Uncontrolled Hemorrhage**	**Ongoing Hemorrhage With Partial Surgical Control**	**Controlled Hemorrhage**
Clinical priorities			
Blood products			
Crystalloids and colloids			
Special points			

7. Describe the principles of damage control resuscitation.
8. The graphical readout of the thromboelastograph (TEG) and rotational thromboelastometry (ROTEM) coagulation tests include three phases. In the chart below, indicate which procoagulant interventions are most appropriate to administer for a deficiency in each of these three phases.

Phase	Procoagulant Intervention Guided by Deficiency
Preclot formation • Coagulation cascade is triggered. • Platelets are activated.	
Clot formation • Beginning of clot formation to maximum clot formation	
Clot stability • Detects and quantifies fibrinolysis	

SPECIAL CONSIDERATIONS

9. What are some common causes for secondary injury in patients with traumatic brain injury (TBI)?
10. What are some considerations for the endotracheal intubation of patients with TBI?
11. What are the main principles for the intraoperative management of patients with TBI?
12. What is the Cushing reflex and its clinical significance?
13. What are specific considerations when caring for patients with acute spinal cord injury?
14. What is spinal shock and specific considerations in the management of patients with spinal shock?
15. What are specific considerations in the management of patients with acute burn injury?
16. What are some specific considerations in the acute management of the pediatric trauma patient?
17. What are some specific considerations in the acute management of the elderly trauma patient?
18. What are some specific considerations in assessing and managing pregnant trauma patients?

ANSWERS

INTRODUCTION

1. Hemorrhagic shock is the most common cause of hypotension in trauma, though other causes must also be considered during the evaluation. Other causes include cardiogenic shock, neurogenic shock, and obstructive shock, as in the cases of tension pneumothorax or cardiac tamponade. (769)
2. Compensatory reflexes via the sympathetic nervous system, carotid sinus, aortic arch baroreceptors, and other low-pressure receptors may mask early hemorrhage and result in normotension (compensated shock). Progressive shock occurs as these mechanisms fail to provide adequate end-organ perfusion. If uncorrected, this can lead to tissue and cellular necrosis, metabolic acidosis, cardiac dysfunction, and, ultimately, death. (769)
3. Acute traumatic coagulopathy is characterized by factor deficiency, hyperfibrinolysis, and platelet dysfunction. It results from tissue hypoperfusion, which leads to a complex interaction among inflammatory factors, cellular dysfunction, and intrinsic anticoagulants. This is separate from other causes of coagulopathy and can be present on arrival to the emergency department. Acute traumatic coagulopathy can be exacerbated by iatrogenic resuscitation factors, including hemodilution, hypocalcemia, hypothermia, and acidosis. These processes lead to a positive feedback loop that can result in death if not corrected. (769)

INITIAL MANAGEMENT

4. ATLS is Advanced Trauma Life Support, an approach to the trauma patient developed by the American College of Surgeons. It provides a shared and consistent approach to a major trauma patient. It is based on a Primary Survey (to identify and treat immediately life-threatening injuries), a Secondary Survey (to identify serious but not immediately life-threatening injuries), and a Tertiary Survey (to assess for any additional injuries). The Primary survey is organized into the ABCDE mnemonic: (A) Airway and cervical spine control, (B) Breathing and oxygenation, (C) Circulation and hemorrhage control, (D) Disability, and (E) Exposure. Disability is a neurologic assessment to identify potentially catastrophic injuries requiring prompt management. Exposure refers to inspecting the patient on all sides for other injuries while simultaneously avoiding hypothermia. Control Catastrophic Bleeding is often added to the start of the ABCDE mnemonic to address the most common cause of early preventable death from exsanguinating hemorrhage. (770)
5. Challenges in the airway management of trauma patients may involve airway anatomy (e.g., maxillofacial trauma), baseline hemodynamic instability, trauma-induced organ dysfunction (e.g., hypoxemia, head injury, altered mental status, burns), or need for transport immediately afterward. Preoxygenation may be difficult due to direct pulmonary injury, patient noncompliance, or preexisting illness. The assumption of a "full stomach" during induction requires consideration of rapid sequence induction of anesthesia. Additionally, acute intravascular volume loss from bleeding can be masked by sympathetic overstimulation caused by pain and distress, resulting in exaggerated hemodynamic effects of induction agents. Trauma patients with suspected cervical spine injury should have a hard collar placed to stabilize their spine. During laryngoscopy, the front of the collar should be loosened, and an additional provider should manually stabilize the head and neck to minimize cervical spine movement. Video laryngoscopy can reduce the force required for intubation and improve first-attempt visualization. (770–773)

INTRAOPERATIVE MANAGEMENT

6. The following chart lists the strategies and special considerations for each phase of care of the massively hemorrhaging trauma patient. (776–783)

	Phase 1	Phase 2	Phase 3
Clinical Status	**Life-Threatening Uncontrolled Hemorrhage**	**Ongoing Hemorrhage With Partial Surgical Control**	**Controlled Hemorrhage**
Clinical priorities	• Stop the bleeding • Control the airway • Ventilate with 100% FiO_2 • Damage control resuscitation	• Tailored resuscitation • Insertion of arterial and central lines • Prevent hypothermia with warmed fluid/blankets	• Restore physiology • Rapid intravascular filling • Stepwise deepening of anesthesia

	Phase 1	Phase 2	Phase 3
Clinical Status	**Life-Threatening Uncontrolled Hemorrhage**	**Ongoing Hemorrhage With Partial Surgical Control**	**Controlled Hemorrhage**
Blood products	• Activate massive transfusion protocol • Consider emergency (un-matched) blood products • Empiric 1:1:1 transfusion ratio	• TEG/ROTEM to guide coagulation products • ABG to guide red blood cell transfusion	• Only as required on testing • Deactivate massive transfusion protocol when appropriate
Crystalloids and colloids	• Cautious use only	• Use to treat hypovolemia with normal coagulation and hemoglobin	• Attempt to normalize lactate and base deficit
Special points	• Consider $CaCl_2$ 1 g for every three blood products • Large bore IV access • Rapid infusing system (e.g., Belmont) • Avoid vasoconstrictors	• Ventilatory adjustments • Consider cell salvage • Aim to repeat TEG/ROTEM/ ABG every 30 min • Consider TEE for difficult cases	• Consider vasoactive infusions if necessary

7. Damage control resuscitation (DCR) principles are permissive hypotension, rapidly achieving hemostasis, early use of hemostatic and blood products, and minimal crystalloid and colloid use. Permissive hypotension temporarily targets a lower-than-normal blood pressure (systolic blood pressure 80 to 90 mmHg) in an actively hemorrhaging patient until hemostasis is achieved or until the patient's condition further deteriorates, with adjustment of the tolerable systolic blood pressure in the elderly, those with preexisting cardiac disease or hypertension, and special populations (including TBI, spinal cord injury, obstetric and pediatric patients). Massive transfusion initially focuses on a ratio of 1:1:1 of packed red blood cells, fresh-frozen plasma, and platelets. With ongoing life-threatening uncontrolled hemorrhage, adding cryoprecipitate to provide fibrinogen and tranexamic acid (an antifibrinolytic) to prevent coagulopathy may be helpful. Crystalloid administration should be avoided because of hemodilution and increased rate of bleeding (due to higher blood pressure). Synthetic colloid administration in the acutely bleeding patient increases coagulopathy by impairing fibrinogen polymerization and platelet function. (777–778)
8. Viscoelastic testing (TEG/ROTEM) can be used to rapidly assess the magnitude and nature of a patient's individual coagulopathy and help tailor the resuscitation as indicated by the following chart. (780–782)

Phase	Procoagulant Intervention Guided by Deficiency
Preclot formation • Coagulation cascade is triggered. • Platelets are activated.	• Prothrombin complex concentrate • Fresh-frozen plasma
Clot formation • Beginning of clot formation to maximum clot formation	• Cryoprecipitate • Fibrinogen concentrate • Platelet concentrates
Clot stability • Detects and quantifies fibrinolysis	• Antifibrinolytic

SPECIAL GROUPS

9. The most common causes of secondary injury in TBI patients include intracranial hypertension, arterial hypotension, hypoxia, hyperthermia, coagulopathy, hyperglycemia, hypoglycemia, and acidosis. TBI management focuses on limiting secondary injury by avoiding and treating these potential causes. (783)
10. A secured airway should be established in TBI patients if they cannot maintain a patent airway (owing to loss of reflexes) or cannot adequately oxygenate or ventilate, have signs of intracranial hypertension, uncontrollable seizure activity, or progressively worsening mental status. These factors often correlate with a deteriorating GCS score, usually eight or less, or another concurrent injury. Special attention must also be paid to cervical spine immobilization during airway manipulation because TBI patients are at higher risk of having concurrent

cervical spine injuries. The effect of induction agents on the TBI patient's hemodynamics and cerebral perfusion pressure must be cautiously considered. (783–784)

11. The goal of managing TBI patients intraoperatively is to reduce ICP and maintain a cerebral perfusion pressure of 50 to 70 mmHg. This involves arterial line monitoring to ensure sufficient systolic blood pressure and to promptly treat systemic hypotension, administering mannitol and antiseizure medications, maintaining euvolemia, facilitating venous drainage through reverse Trendelenburg positioning, and the avoidance of high peak inspiratory pressures and positive end-expiratory pressure. Generally, hyperventilation is not recommended within the first 24 hours of injury unless treating impending herniation. Another factor pertinent to management is the availability of blood products to treat bleeding and coagulopathy. (784)
12. The Cushing reflex is the intense sympathetic nervous system response to a high ICP to maintain cerebral perfusion. The reflex is characterized by systemic hypertension and may mask intravascular fluid volume depletion. Profound intraoperative hypotension may occur after decompression and normalization of the ICP due to a sudden decrease in systemic sympathetic activity. Before decompression, the patient's intravascular fluid volume should be repleted, anesthetic agents should be decreased, and vasopressors and inotropes should be available for administration. Blood should also be available in case of abrupt bleeding. (784)
13. Spinal cord precautions must be undertaken immediately in patients with acute spinal cord injury, including cervical collar placement and strict logroll precautions when moving. The adequacy of ventilation and oxygenation should be evaluated. Patients with cervical or thoracic spinal cord injuries, especially those with complete injuries, may have diaphragmatic, intercostal, and abdominal weakness, leading to decreased vital capacity and the inability to cough and clear secretions. Succinylcholine can safely be used for neuromuscular blockade for endotracheal intubation within the first 24 hours of injury in acute spinal cord injury patients. (785)
14. Spinal shock describes the acute cardiovascular effects of high thoracic or cervical injury (usually T4 and above) due to disruption of the sympathetic cardioaccelerator fibers causing sympathetic blockade. This results in significant bradyarrhythmias, atrioventricular block, systemic vasodilation, hypotension, and motor and sensory findings below the level of the lesion. Spinal shock treatment is supportive with isotonic fluid, vasopressors, and inotropes as necessary, with care not to overresuscitate the patient with IV fluids. The mean arterial blood pressure should be maintained at 85 to 90 mmHg to maintain adequate spinal cord perfusion, unless contraindicated by concurrent injuries. The American Association of Neurological Surgeons no longer recommends the administration of large-dose steroids, which have been associated with adverse effects, including death. (785–786)
15. Considerations in the management of patients with acute burn injury include intravascular volume resuscitation, the potential for airway edema and total airway obstruction, providing adequate analgesia, the risk of inhalation injury and carbon monoxide poisoning, the potential for infection, the potential for compartment syndrome due to reduced compliance of circumferentially burned tissues, and the potential need for transfer to a tertiary care center. Intravascular volume resuscitation happens commonly with a balanced salt solution and can be guided by multiple available formulas. There is increasing recognition of the risk of precipitating acute respiratory distress syndrome (ARDS) 3 to 5 days after burn injury with excessive volume administration. Supplemental high-concentration oxygen is essential for treating inhalational injuries if carbon monoxide poisoning is suspected. Standard pulse oximetry monitors can read an erroneously normal value despite tissue hypoxemia in patients with carbon monoxide poisoning. The administration of high-concentration oxygen significantly decreases the half-life of carbon monoxide in the blood. It should be used as an initial measure until carbon monoxide poisoning has been excluded through laboratory analysis. Physicians should also consider the risk of cyanide toxicity or other inhalational toxidromes based on the location of the burn/inhalational injury. For example, a house fire would expose a patient to significant burnt plastics and synthetic fibers. (786–787)
16. Special considerations in the acute management of the pediatric trauma patient include late physiologic decompensation because pediatric patients can mask significant hemodynamic compromise due to their robust underlying physiology, potentially difficult IV access and the need for potential interosseous access, achieving patient compliance with radiologic testing, and dosing drugs and blood transfusions based on weight. In pediatric patients, any blood loss can be significant. There should also be an awareness of the potential for nonaccidental injury. Some indications of nonaccidental injury include injuries inconsistent with developmental milestones, multiple injuries (especially if over a prolonged period), frequent presentations, and inconsistent history of the incident. (788–789)
17. Special considerations in the acute management of the elderly trauma patient include preexisting illness and reduced physiologic reserve, medications the patient may have taken or missed, the potential for the masking of blood loss by the lack of tachycardia as a result of the β-adrenergic blockade, the increased risk of trauma from

minimal impact including fractures and subdural hematoma, an awareness of the potential for elder abuse, and the consideration of end-of-life care and the patient's wishes concerning interventions that would be acceptable to the patient. When providing damage control resuscitation to elderly trauma patients, higher blood pressure targets should be considered due to the reduced tolerance for end-organ relative hypoperfusion. (790)

18. Special considerations in the acute management of the pregnant trauma patient include the fact that typical signs of blood loss may occur late, that fetal distress may be the first sign of maternal compromise, left uterine displacement reduces aortocaval compression, a reduced functional residual capacity can lead to rapid oxygen desaturation, improper seatbelt use can affect the injury pattern, and the awareness that intimate partner violence increases during pregnancy. Other considerations include the changes in maternal physiology (e.g., hypercoagulable state), the higher likelihood of having difficult intubation, the need for anti-D immunoglobulin in Rh-negative mothers with major trauma (ideally within 72 hours of the trauma), reducing radiation exposure (without delaying diagnosis), the potential need for fetal heart rate monitoring, and the potential need for delivery of the fetus to control massive uterine bleeding or to optimize maternal and/or fetal survival. In addition, the nature of maternal and fetal injury changes as the fetus develops during the pregnancy. Starting in the second trimester, the uterus moves to an extra-pelvic position, and there is a progressively increased risk of direct injury to the fetus until term. At the same time, the maternal organs become more shielded. In the third trimester, there is an increased risk of injury to the bladder and an increased likelihood of precipitating early labor. (790–791)

Chapter

44 CHRONIC PAIN MANAGEMENT

Christopher R. Abrecht

INTRODUCTION

- Pain medicine is inherently multidisciplinary.
- Multiple certification pathways exist for training in pain management, with the most established and comprehensive being ACGME-accredited fellowships in pain medicine.
- While the board certification examination is administered by the American Board of Anesthesiology (ABA), several specialties may become board certified in pain medicine, including neurology, physical medicine and rehabilitation, family medicine, and more.

CHRONIC PAIN FOUNDATIONS

Terminology

- Pain is defined as "an unpleasant sensory and emotional experience associated with, or resembling that associated with, actual or potential tissue damage."
- Pain is possible even without evidence of tissue damage.
- Pain is a biological, psychological, and social experience (biopsychosocial model of pain).

Epidemiology

- According to a 2016 study from the Centers for Disease Control and Prevention, up to 8% of adults in the United States have high-impact chronic pain, wherein pain limits activities of daily living.
  - This pain is more common in females, older adults, unemployed adults who were previously employed, and adults in lower socioeconomic groups.

Pathophysiology

- Three neurons are part of a simplified pain transmission framework.
  - First order: nociceptive afferent with cell body in dorsal root ganglion which synapses in the spinal cord
  - Second order: cell body in the spinal cord which synapses in the thalamus
  - Third order: cell body in the thalamus which synapses in the cortex
- The thalamus is a key center for pain processing.
- Sensitization, a phenomenon in which neurons sense pain with inputs that were not previously associated with pain, is implicated in chronic pain states.
  - Peripheral sensitization is from increased sensitivity to nociceptive input at the terminal ends of the first-order neurons.
    - Inflammatory molecules such as substance P mediate these changes.
  - Central sensitization is from changes at the level of the spinal cord and brain.
    - *N*-Methyl-D-aspartate (NMDA) receptor upregulation mediates some of these changes.
- Neuropathic pain is caused by damage to nerve tissue. It can be thought of as a pathological "gain-of-function" process.

PAINFUL CONDITIONS: SPINE

Lower Back Pain: An Overview

- Lower back pain is the top global cause of disability.
- A functional spinal unit includes the following:
  - Two adjacent vertebrae
  - The intervertebral disc
  - Facet joints
  - Spinal ligaments
- Degenerative changes, perhaps better described as age-related changes, are very common but are usually nonspecific.
  - Most older adults will have "degenerative changes," but these are not necessarily pain generators.
- Understanding basic terminology for spinal pathology is key for a pain physician.
  - Spondylosis: arthritis of the spine
  - Spondylolysis: fracture in the pars interarticularis
  - Anterolisthesis: anterior displacement of a vertebral body to the one below

- Spondylolisthesis: anterolisthesis from spondylolysis
- Back pain with "red flag" symptoms should prompt advanced imaging such as lumbar spine MRI.
  - Bowel and/or bladder incontinence
  - Saddle anesthesia
  - New weakness or numbness (concerning for cauda equina syndrome)
  - Unintended weight loss in patient with a history of cancer
  - Fever, especially in patients with immunosuppression or substance use disorder (concerning for spinal infection)

Lumbosacral Spine Pain: Axial Pain Generators

- Myofascial pain is characterized by the presence of taut bands of skeletal muscle and fascia, called trigger points.
- Facet joint pain is characterized by axial pain, worse with maneuvers that increase load on the joint (e.g., lumbar extension and lateral rotation).
  - Radiation may occur with facet joint pain, but it is not in a dermatomal distribution.
- Sacroiliac joint (SIJ) pain is characterized by pain in the lower back, buttocks, or hip area, worse with sitting and with a higher incidence in women.
  - Tenderness at the posterior superior iliac spine (Fortin finger test) and pain with femoral abduction and external rotation (FABER or Patrick's test) are suggestive of SIJ-mediated pain.
- Discogenic pain is characterized by axial lumbosacral pain that is worse with coughing, sneezing, and lumbar flexion.
  - This condition is more common in younger patients and may also be associated with radiculopathy related to nerve root irritation.

Lumbosacral Radiculopathy

- Lumbar or sacral radiculopathy is characterized by paresthesia, sensory deficit, or pain in a dermatomal distribution.
  - Weakness may also be present in a myotomal distribution.
  - In the straight leg raise maneuver, reproduction of pain with elevation of the leg between 30 and 70 degrees is a positive result.
- Acute radiculopathy of less than 6 weeks' duration is usually treated conservatively with NSAIDs and physical therapy.
- Chronic radiculopathy of >6 weeks duration and unresponsive to conservative management may be treated with epidural steroid injections or surgical intervention.
  - There is ongoing debate about when surgical intervention is appropriate, so a patient-specific approach should be pursued.
  - In most cases, the presence of a neurological deficit will prompt surgical intervention.

Lumbar Spinal Stenosis

- Lumbar spinal stenosis is a reduction in the cross-sectional area of the spinal canal from disc herniation, facet arthropathy, ligamentum flavum hypertrophy, and other causes.
- Patients with this condition are usually older and report pain in the lower back, buttocks, and legs.
- Symptoms are improved with sitting and forward flexion of the lumbar spine ("shopping cart sign") and worse while standing and walking upright.
- The pathophysiology of this condition is direct mechanical compression of neural components as well as downstream epidural venous congestion causing a transient compartment syndrome of the cauda equina.

PAINFUL CONDITIONS: NEUROPATHIC PAIN

Peripheral Neuropathy

- Peripheral neuropathy is often used synonymously with polyneuropathy, a disorder affecting multiple peripheral nerves.
- The distal ends are usually affected, with a "glove and stocking" distribution of symptoms.
- Top causes are diabetic peripheral neuropathy, chemotherapy-induced peripheral neuropathy, and alcohol-induced peripheral neuropathy.

Complex Regional Pain Syndrome

- Neuropathic pain in which the sympathetic nervous system (SNS) amplifies pain is known as sympathetically mediated pain.
- Anxiety, stress, and other types of emotional stress activate the SNS and therefore worsen this subtype of neuropathic pain.
  - It is therefore paramount that treatment of these conditions include attention to a patient's psychological state.
- Complex regional pain syndrome (CRPS) is characterized by pain in a distal extremity disproportionate to any inciting event.
  - Hyperalgesia, allodynia, skin color changes, temperature changes, edema, sudomotor, and motor changes are characteristic and delineated in the Budapest Criteria for this condition.
- A common scenario for CRPS is onset after orthopedic trauma or prolonged immobilization, such as from a cast.

- Females are more commonly affected, and patients are usually younger.
- In CRPS 1 ("reflex sympathetic dystrophy"), representing 90% of all cases, there is no clear peripheral nerve injury.
- In CRPS 2 ("causalgia"), injury to a peripheral nerve is identified.
- Treatments serve to reduce pain so that a patient can participate in physical therapy.
  - Desensitization techniques, neuropathic medications, ketamine infusions, sympathetic blocks, and psychological treatment are part of the care plan.

PAINFUL CONDITIONS: CHRONIC POSTSURGICAL PAIN

- Chronic postsurgical pain (CPSP) is pain that develops after a surgery and persists beyond the usual healing process, usually at least 3 months postoperatively.
- CPSP is particularly common after thoracotomy, mastectomy, inguinal herniorrhaphy, knee arthroplasty, and limb amputation.
- Risk factors include young age, female gender, preoperative chronic pain, preoperative opioid use, and poorly controlled postoperative pain.
- Increasingly, there is a movement toward the development of a transitional pain service, with the following elements.
  - A physician board certified in pain medicine overseeing a multidisciplinary team
  - Team goals include optimizing modifiable factors preoperatively, overseeing perioperative pain plans, and ensuring continued high-level pain care posthospital discharge.

PAIN CONDITIONS: ADDITIONAL GENERATORS

- Central pain syndromes include poststroke pain, multiple sclerosis pain, and postherpetic neuralgia.
- Headache conditions include migraine and trigeminal neuralgia.
- Fibromyalgia is marked by widespread pain in multiple points throughout the body, associated with fatigue and impaired sleep.
- Chronic pelvic pain may relate to endometriosis, pelvic floor dysfunction, or other etiologies.

PSYCHOLOGICAL TREATMENT PILLAR: CATASTROPHIZING

- Pain catastrophizing is a dysfunctional cognitive approach to pain, wherein a patient experiences a lack of confidence and control and anticipates negative outcomes regarding pain.
- The Pain Catastrophizing Scale is a validated instrument used to quantify the extent of pain catastrophizing.
- Cognitive-behavioral therapy (CBT) is a structured, active form of therapy wherein patients learn how cognition (distorted thoughts not based on reality) affects behaviors (actions). CBT is helpful for patients with pain catastrophizing.

PHYSICAL MEDICINE TREATMENT PILLAR

- Physical therapy (PT) is an essential part of most painful conditions. It is a treatment in its own right for musculoskeletal and mixed neuropathic conditions such as fibromyalgia.
- A structured PT program also addresses fear avoidance, wherein a concern that movement will result in worsening pain – can in turn lead to deconditioning and worse pain.
- Many patients also benefit from integrative and complementary and alternative medicine (CAM).
  - CAM examples include acupuncture, transcutaneous electrical nerve stimulation, biofeedback, meditation, and dietary changes.

PHARMACOLOGIC TREATMENT PILLAR

Nonopioid Analgesics

- Nonsteroidal antiinflammatory drugs (NSAIDs) are often used for predominantly nociceptive pain, as from osteoarthritis.
  - NSAIDs inhibit the enzyme cyclooxygenase, thereby reducing prostaglandins, which mediate inflammation and pain.
- Muscle relaxants are sometimes used for long-term management of chronic pain syndromes, although the data for long-term use are not robust.
  - In the presence of spasticity, as from multiple sclerosis or cerebral palsy, muscle relaxants are indicated for long-term use.
- First-line neuropathic pain therapy: antiepileptics, antidepressant serotonin-norepinephrine reuptake inhibitor (SNRI), and tricyclic antidepressants (TCA)
  - Gabapentin: effective dose usually 1200 to 3600 mg/day, number needed to treat (NNT) of 6.3; side effects include dizziness, CNS depression, weight gain, and respiratory depression
  - Pregabalin: effective dose usually 300 to 600 mg/day, NNT of 7.7, with similar, although perhaps less prominent, side effects compared with gabapentin

  - SNRI duloxetine: effective dose of 60 mg; side effects include nausea, insomnia, mood changes
  - SNRI venlafaxine: effective dose of 75 to 225 mg/day, NNT of 6.4; side effects include sweating, headache, dizziness, and others similar to duloxetine.
  - TCA nortriptyline: effective dose 25 to 100 mg/day; side effects include anticholinergic dry mouth, constipation, urinary retention, dizziness, NNT 3.6 but often not well tolerated

Opioid Analgesics

- There are no robust studies showing that opioids are effective in the management of chronic, noncancer pain, but there is a wealth of data showing opioid therapy results in myriad problems.
- The Centers for Disease Control and Prevention (CDC) published a landmark guideline for the prescription of opioids for noncancer pain. Suggestions include the following:
  - Short-acting instead of long-acting formulations were recommended.
  - Coprescription of an opioid and a benzodiazepine should be avoided, if possible.
  - For patients with opioid use disorder, medication-assisted treatment with buprenorphine or methadone should be offered.
- In the wake of these guidelines, some patients were rapidly weaned off their opioids, with severe destabilization being the result.
  - In response, another CDC guideline noted that opioid therapy should not be abruptly discontinued.
    - Tapering should be initiated when risks outweigh benefits and should be done very slowly, as little as 10% per month.
    - If tapering becomes problematic, conversion to buprenorphine may be indicated.
- Currently, there is no hard limit on what dose a patient should be prescribed. At higher doses, pain specialist consultation may be sought.
- Safe prescribing includes ongoing assessment for continued analgesia, improved activities of daily living, lack of adverse side effects, lack of aberrant drug behaviors, adherence, a signed opioid agreement, and assessment of misuse and potential for adverse reaction.

PROCEDURAL TREATMENT PILLAR

Epidural Steroid Injections

- Interlaminar: a needle is directed between the lamina and through the ligamentum flavum, using a loss of resistance approach and fluoroscopic guidance.
- Transforaminal: a needle is directed in an oblique trajectory into the foramen, using fluoroscopic guidance. This approach may also be diagnostic, used in surgical planning.
- Risks, in particular in the cervical spine, include epidural hematoma, direct vascular damage, or steroid embolism. One technique to minimize this risk is to avoid use of particulate steroids for cervical (and lumbar) transforaminal injections.

Facet Injections

- The facet joint is the articulation between adjacent vertebral bodies and gets input from two medial branch nerves from corresponding dorsal rami, one from the spinal nerve above and one from the spinal nerve below the joint.
  - To treat facet joint pain, one approach is to block the nerves innervating a joint and then, if diagnostically positive, at a future date perform a radiofrequency ablation (RFA) of these nerves.
  - Another approach is to administer local anesthetic and steroids directly into the joint.

Sympathetic Blockade

- Stellate or cervicothoracic ganglion
  - Blockade is at the anterior tubercle of C6 (Chassaignac's tubercle) or C7.
  - Technique may be fluoroscopic or ultrasound, with the latter increasingly favored to ensure medication is administered superficial to the longus colli muscle.
  - Indications include CRPS, Raynaud's, vascular disease, PTSD, and more.
  - Successful block results in a Horner syndrome: miosis, ptosis, enophthalmos, and anhidrosis.
    - Other signs include unilateral nasal congestion, venodilation, and increase in temperature in the affected limb of at least 1°C.
  - Complications include vascular injury causing hematoma or stroke and seizure from intravascular injection.
- Celiac plexus
  - Blockade is at the anterolateral surface of the aorta at T12-L1
  - Technique by pain physicians is fluoroscopic, with other specialists doing CT- or endoscopy-guided approaches and no technique being uniformly better than another.
  - Transcrural approach administers medication directly onto the celiac ganglion and may involve passage of the needle through the aorta.
  - Splanchnic approach administers medication posterior to the crura, targeting the splanchnic nerves before they coalesce into the plexus.

  - Indications include pain affecting stomach to transverse colon as well as pancreas, liver, and kidneys.
  - Note: Abdominal visceral nociceptive *afferents* accompany sympathetic *efferents*, and thus the celiac ganglion allows blockade of painful nociceptive input.
  - Neurolytic approaches may involve alcohol or phenol.
  - Expected outcomes include relatively increased parasympathetic tone with orthostatic hypotension and diarrhea.
  - Rare but devastating complications include paraplegia from spread of neurolytic medication toward the spinal segmental arteries or the artery of Adamkiewicz.

Celiac Plexus Block

- Sympathetic blockade of the celiac plexus will result in unopposed parasympathetic tone.
- Acute hypotension may result after this procedure from the sympathectomy
  - Other causes of hypotension could include an intraabdominal hematoma, in particular if a transaortic approach is used; another possibility is a pneumothorax.
- Increased GI motility may also result, causing diarrhea; the procedure should not be performed in patients with a bowel obstruction.

- Lumbar sympathetic
  - Blockade is at anterolateral surface of L2-L4 vertebral bodies.
  - Indications include CRPS of the lower extremities.
- Superior hypogastric plexus
  - Blockade is at the anterior surface of the L5 vertebral body and sacral promontory.
  - Indications include pain in the pelvic region.
- Ganglion impar
  - Blockade is anterior to the sacrococcygeal junction.
  - Indications include tailbone or perineal pain.

NEUROMODULATION: ADVANCED INTERVENTIONAL PAIN MEDICINE

- Advanced interventional pain techniques (also known as "surgical pain" interventions) should be performed by physicians who have completed a fellowship with a robust neuromodulation program and start their practice working closely with an experienced colleague.
- Complications of implanted devices are not uncommon and may be biological (e.g., surgical site infection, hematoma, seroma, wound dehiscence) or device related (e.g., lead migration or break, catheter leak, device failure).
- Spinal cord stimulation (SCS) is in essence the administration of electrical impulses at the dorsal column in lieu of pharmacology in the management of pain.
  - Implantation of the electrodes along with an implantable pulse generator (IPG) is typically preceded by a trial, in which electrodes alone are inserted for several days, to determine whether pain relief occurs.
  - The most common indications for SCS are failed back surgery syndrome (postlaminectomy pain syndrome) or CRPS.
- Dorsal root ganglion (DRG) and peripheral nerve stimulation (PNS) target a single nerve root or peripheral nerve, respectively.
- Intrathecal pumps (ITPs) allow the administration of analgesics from an implanted reservoir directly into the cerebral spinal fluid.
  - This therapy is usually reserved for patients who note benefit from systemic analgesics but are limited by side effects.
  - Failed back surgery syndrome and cancer pain are common indications.
  - The three FDA-approved medications for intrathecal use are baclofen, morphine, and ziconidine.
  - In practice, a combination of medications is often administered concurrently; the additional medications include bupivacaine, hydromorphone, clonidine, and others.

SUMMARY

- Pain care is not truly pain care unless it is comprehensive and multidisciplinary.
- Pain specialists are not really pain specialists unless they understand the neurobiology of pain, biopsychological model of pain, and the spectrum of pharmacologic, rehabilitative, integrative, and procedural modalities available.

QUESTIONS

CHRONIC PAIN FOUNDATIONS

1. In the table below, describe a simplified three-neuron pathway of nociceptive pain transmission from the periphery to the brain.

	Neuron Pathway
First-order neuron	
Second-order neuron	
Third-order neuron	

PAINFUL CONDITIONS: SPINE

2. Describe the differences among the following spinal imaging terms: spondylosis, spondylolysis, anterolisthesis, and spondylolisthesis.
3. A patient presents with 5 weeks of lower back pain radiating along the outer aspect of the leg and ending in the dorsal aspect of the foot. What nerve root is most likely involved, and what motor deficit would be expected? What is the best treatment plan for this patient?

PAINFUL CONDITIONS: NEUROPATHIC PAIN

4. A 39-year-old female patient with a known tibial stress fracture and right leg pain is referred for a sympathetic block to treat presumed CRPS. Clinical findings include hyperalgesia throughout the leg, swelling, color changes, diffuse paresthesias, and limited movement of the leg. What management plan would you recommend for this patient?

PSYCHOLOGICAL TREATMENT PILLAR: CATASTROPHIZING

5. A patient with chronic lower back pain states he worries that his pain will get worse, he cannot keep his pain out of his mind, he wonders if something serious is going to happen to him, and he feels that there is nothing he can do to reduce the intensity of his pain. What psychological condition might be present? What are your recommendations for management?

PHARMACOLOGIC TREATMENT PILLAR

6. Describe the pharmacologic treatment options for a patient with neuropathic pain.
7. What are the definitions of the following terms: *opioid tolerance*, *opioid hyperalgesia*, and *opioid use disorder*?

PROCEDURAL TREATMENT PILLAR

8. What are the common pain conditions for which epidural steroid injections are administered?
9. A few minutes after a patient receives a stellate ganglion blockade, he develops a hoarse voice, repeatedly clears his throat, and reports anxiety. What is the differential diagnosis?

NEUROMODULATION: ADVANCED INTERVENTIONAL PAIN MEDICINE

10. What is spinal cord stimulation (SCS)? What are the most common indications?

ANSWERS

CHRONIC PAIN FOUNDATIONS

1. The table below summarizes a three-neuron pathway of nociceptive pain transmission from the periphery to the brain. (795)

	Neuron Pathway
First-order neuron	Input from nociceptive neuron with cell body in dorsal root ganglion, synapsing in spinal cord
Second-order neuron	Input from spinal cord neuron, synapsing in the thalamus (spinothalamic tract)
Third-order neuron	Input from thalamus, synapsing in the sensory cortex, creating pain perception

PAINFUL CONDITIONS: SPINE

2. The table below defines several common radiologic spine findings. (797)

Term	Definition
Spondylosis	General term for arthritis of the spine
Spondylolysis	Fracture in the pars interarticularis (junction of vertebral body and posterior elements)
Anterolisthesis	Anterior displacement of vertebral body relative to the one below
Spondylolisthesis	Anterolisthesis secondary to spondylolysis

3. The most common lumbosacral radiculopathies involve L4, L5, and S1. L5 dermatome involvement manifests as pain in the outer aspect of the hip area, lateral aspect of the leg, and dorsal aspect of the foot. The L5 myotome includes dorsiflexion of the great toe and the foot. Walking on heels would be impaired in a motor L5 radiculopathy. Since the patient's lumbar radiculopathy is acute (less than 6 weeks' duration) – and if his motor deficit is not prominent – nonsurgical management is likely the best option. If the duration of the lumbar radiculopathy exceeds 6 weeks, there is debate whether a surgical management plan would offer benefits such as faster resolution. However, 1-year outcomes for surgical versus nonsurgical management of lumbar radiculopathy appear similar. (799)

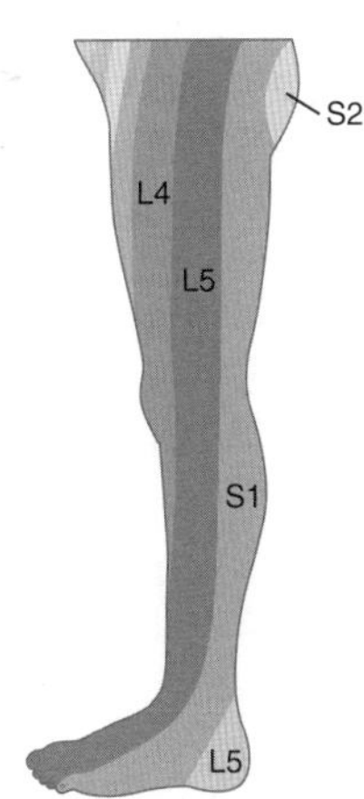

PAINFUL CONDITIONS: NEUROPATHIC PAIN

4. CRPS is a diagnosis of exclusion. While it is important that patients who potentially have this condition are seen in a timely manner by a pain specialist, it is equally important that other conditions are ruled out. This patient, for example, should be seen by an orthopedist. A compartment syndrome, deep vein thrombosis, or vascular insufficiency could explain some of the symptoms the patient reports. Once these other conditions have been ruled out, then a diagnosis of CRPS can be made using the Budapest Criteria. Treatment for lower extremity CRPS includes lumbar sympathetic block as well as desensitization techniques, physical therapy, psychological care, and medication management. (800–801)

PSYCHOLOGICAL TREATMENT PILLAR: CATASTROPHIZING

5. Pain catastrophizing is likely present in this patient. The Pain Catastrophizing Scale may be administered to confirm the diagnosis. In this condition, there is an unhealthy preoccupation about pain and an anticipation of

negative outcomes. Treatment includes engagement with a psychologist for cognitive-behavioral therapy (CBT). In CBT, a patient is taught to identify disordered thoughts and learn how these thoughts affect behaviors in an unproductive way. An action plan is also developed to address these thoughts and behaviors. Patients who undergo treatment in pain catastrophizing are much more likely to enjoy a higher level of functionality and be more responsive to other pain treatments. (802)

PHARMACOLOGIC TREATMENT PILLAR

6. First-line therapy for neuropathic pain includes antiepileptic gabapentinoids (e.g., gabapentin, pregabalin); antidepressant serotonin-norepinephrine reuptake inhibitors (SNRIs) such as duloxetine and venlafaxine; and tricyclic antidepressants (TCAs) such as nortriptyline or amitriptyline. Second-line medications include topical lidocaine and capsaicin. Further therapies for neuropathic pain include opioids, such as tramadol. (802)
7. Opioid tolerance occurs when with repeated exposure to opioids, a decreased therapeutic effect is noted. In other words, a higher dose is needed to achieve the same effect. Opioid-induced hyperalgesia occurs when with repeated exposure to opioids, a paradoxical increase in pain is noted. Opioid use disorder is a neurobiologic condition wherein patients take opioids in larger amounts and over a longer period than intended, resulting in a persistent desire or unsuccessful attempt to decrease their opioid use. (803)

PROCEDURAL TREATMENT PILLAR

8. Epidural steroid injections are administered for a variety of painful conditions, although there is not always robust data to support their use. Arguably the most established condition is lumbar radiculopathy, such as from a herniated disc. Benefit is less likely the longer a radiculopathy is present and if multiple prior epidural steroid injections have already been performed. Another condition is discogenic pain, wherein disc pathology is thought to cause axial pain as well as nerve root irritation. A third condition is lumbar spinal stenosis, wherein a decreased cross-sectional area of the spinal canal causes transient mechanical and venous congestion-mediated neural impingement. In cases of severe lumbar spinal stenosis, epidural steroid injections often do not result in sustained relief. In all cases, epidural steroid injections are meant to transiently decrease neural inflammation and reduce pain, so that a patient is better able to engage in physical therapy and hopefully not need further interventions to treat their painful condition. (803–804)
9. The recurrent laryngeal nerve may be blocked during a stellate ganglion block. The result may be a hoarse voice or coughing. The phrenic nerve can also be blocked, resulting in shortness of breath. Both conditions may also induce anxiety. A pneumothorax is also possible, especially if the procedure was performed at C7, closer to the apex of the lungs, but it is less likely. Ideally, a patient should be counseled before performing the block about a Horner syndrome and recurrent laryngeal and phrenic nerve palsies. (805–806)

NEUROMODULATION: ADVANCED INTERVENTIONAL PAIN MEDICINE

10. Spinal cord stimulation (SCS) is the administration of electrical impulses in the management of pain. Conventional SCS involves placement of electrodes in the dorsal epidural space. First, a patient will undergo a psychological evaluation to rule out suboptimally treated psychiatric conditions, which should be addressed before pursuing neuromodulation. Next, a patient will undergo a trial, wherein temporary electrodes are placed in the epidural space to determine if sufficient pain relief and functionality result from this treatment modality. After 3 to 7 days, these electrodes are removed. Last, if the trial was successful, a patient will undergo permanent implantation of epidural electrodes attached to an implantable pulse generator. The most common indications for SCS include failed back surgery syndrome or CRPS. (807)

Chapter

45 CARDIOPULMONARY RESUSCITATION

Albert Yen and David Shimabukuro

INTRODUCTION

- Cardiopulmonary resuscitation (CPR) is Basic Life Support (BLS).
- Advanced Cardiac Life Support (ACLS) and Pediatric Advanced Life Support (PALS) incorporate advanced and invasive techniques into BLS.
- Outcomes from in-hospital cardiac arrest (IHCA) have improved but are still poor.

EVIDENCE BASED

- Guidelines for CPR and Emergency Cardiovascular Care (ECC)
  - Published by the American Heart Association (AHA) in conjunction with the International Liaison Committee on Resuscitation (ILCOR)
- Guidelines are continually reviewed and updated online.

PRINCIPLES OF MANAGEMENT

Basic Life Support

- Four major components of BLS
  - Recognition of cardiac arrest
  - Activation of the emergency medical services (EMS) system
  - Early administration of cardiopulmonary resuscitation (CPR)
  - Early defibrillation
- The AHA algorithm for the inpatient setting includes
  - Verify scene safety.
  - Check the patient for responsiveness.
  - Activate the resuscitation team.
  - Retrieve resuscitation equipment.
  - Check for adequate breathing and pulse.
  - Begin CPR.
  - Use defibrillator as soon as possible.

Recognition of Cardiac Arrest by Health Care Providers

- Rapid recognition is essential.
- Simultaneously check for pulse and adequate ventilation.
  - Pulse check at carotid or femoral artery.
  - Avoid mistaking agonal gasps as breathing.
- Time elapsed for assessment should not exceed 10 seconds.

Cardiopulmonary Resuscitation

- Compression, airway, breathing (CAB) and defibrillation
  - Early initiation of chest compressions improves the likelihood of return of spontaneous circulation (ROSC).
  - Studies have demonstrated noninferiority to compression-only CPR in out-of-hospital settings.
  - For in-hospital cardiac arrests, providers are still required to provide assisted ventilation.
- Compressions
  - Performed on a firm surface when possible
  - Depth of approximately 2 to 2.5 inches (5 to 6 cm)
  - Rate of 100 to 120 compressions per minute
  - Complete chest recoil is essential to allow blood to fill the heart.
    - Allows for adequate cardiac output
  - Cycle at a ratio of 30 compressions to 2 breaths (30:2).
    - Five cycles are performed in 2 minutes.
  - Minimizing compression interruptions increases the likelihood of ROSC.
- Airway
  - Airway maneuvers should be attempted quickly and efficiently.
    - Airway attempts should minimally interrupt compressions.
  - Definitive airway management is preferred.
  - Alternative options to open the airway if advanced airway not achieved
    - Head tilt-chin lift maneuver
    - Jaw thrust only when cervical spine injury is suspected
    - Properly sized nasal or oral airway

- Breathing
  - Administer maximum oxygen concentration.
  - Tidal volume of approximately 400 to 600 mL, or visible chest rise.
  - Rate of 1 breath every 6 seconds
  - Avoid excessive positive pressure and hyperventilation.
    - Can reduce preload/cardiac output and increase gastric insufflation

Defibrillation

- Defibrillation pads should be attached to the patient as soon as possible.
  - Time to defibrillation is critical for ROSC and survival.
  - Optimal position and alternative locations are available in diagrams.
- Energy to terminate ventricular fibrillation (VF)/ ventricular tachycardia (VT)
  - Monophasic (unidirectional) devices: 360 Joules (J)
  - Biphasic (bidirectional) devices: 120 to 200 J
- CPR should resume for 2 minutes immediately after defibrillation.

Alternative Techniques and Ancillary Devices

- Alternative devices are not supported by the evidence.
- Extracorporeal membrane oxygenation (ECMO) can be considered.
  - Patients with IHCAs with reversible causes
  - When expeditiously available and with available support

Adult Advanced Cardiovascular Life Support

- Builds on the basics of BLS by adding in interventions

Interventions in Advanced Cardiac Life Support

- Airway manipulation
- Medication administration
- Arrhythmia management
- Transition to post-cardiac arrest care

Resuscitation Team Management

- Adapts principles of crisis resource management (CRM) from the aviation industry
- Team leader
  - Delegates tasks and clearly assigns roles
  - Taps into the collective knowledge of the team
- Communication
  - Clear messaging and assignment of tasks
  - Closed loop communication
  - Team leader is the single point of all communication.

Principles of Crisis Resource Management

- Anesthesiology was the first specialty to incorporate CRM principles into the training of its clinicians.
- Team-based approach to averting and mitigating medical crises
- Focuses on behaviors such as team leadership, dynamic decision-making, interpersonal communication, situational awareness, and resource utilization

Monitoring Cardiopulmonary Resuscitation

- Continuous end-tidal carbon dioxide (P_{ETCO2}) monitoring with capnogram waveform
  - Can be used to confirm airway placement
  - Guides adequacy of chest compressions
  - For quality resuscitation target a P_{ETCO2} of 10 mmHg or greater
- Arterial relaxation diastolic pressure
  - Guides adequacy of chest compressions
  - For quality resuscitation target a diastolic pressure of 20 mmHg or greater
- Arterial blood pressure monitoring
- Central venous oxygen saturation
- Cardiac ultrasound

Airway Management

- There is no formal recommendation on timing of placement of an advanced airway.
- Advanced airways include an endotracheal tube (ETT) or a supraglottic airway.
  - Placement should be by an experienced provider.
  - Interruption of chest compressions should be less than 10 seconds.
  - Continuous waveform capnography is recommended for confirmation.
  - Alternative clinical confirmations should also be used.
    - Auscultation, bilateral chest rise, nonwaveform capnography

Management of Specific Arrhythmias

- Bradycardia
  - Clinically significant generally when the heart rate is less than 50
  - Signs and symptoms
    - Hypotension, altered mental status, ischemic chest discomfort, or signs of acute heart failure
  - Treatment
    - Atropine 1 mg intravenous (IV), repeat every 3 to 5 minutes, maximum dose 3 mg
    - If atropine is ineffective, dopamine or epinephrine infusions
    - Consider transcutaneous pacing (TCP).

Adult Bradycardia Algorithm

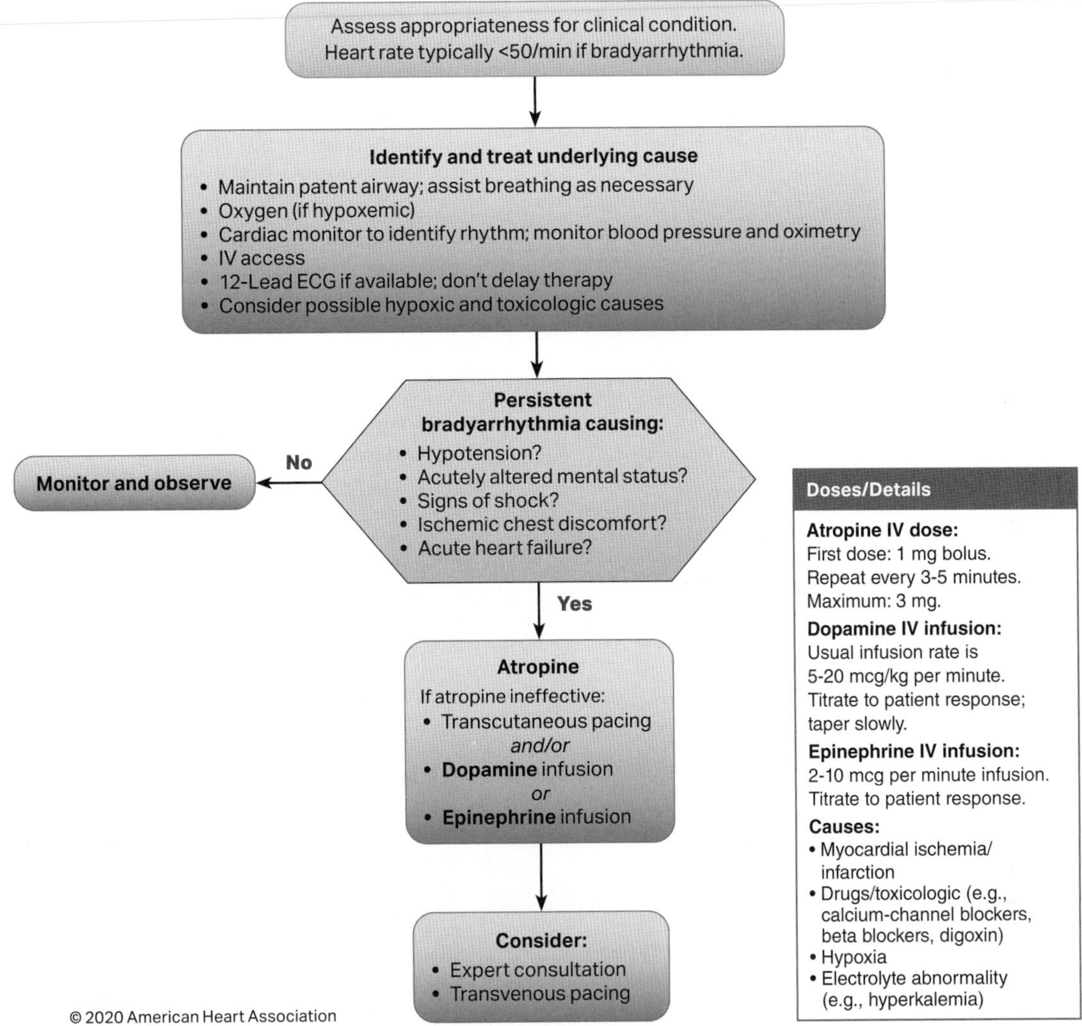

Adult Bradycardia Algorithm (with permission from the AHA). Figure depicts the resuscitation algorithm for bradycardia with a pulse—2020 update. (From 2020 AHA Guidelines for CPR and ECC: Adult Basic & Advanced Life Support. © 2020 American Heart Association.)

- Common causes
  - Excess medication (i.e., β-blockers, calcium channel blockers), hypoxia, myocardial ischemia, and electrolyte abnormalities
- See figure above.

- Tachycardia
  - Clinically significant generally when the heart rate is above 120 to 150
  - Signs and symptoms
    - Hypotension, altered mental status, ischemic chest discomfort, or signs of acute heart failure
  - Treatment depends on risk of hemodynamic compromise
    - If yes, immediate synchronized cardioversion is indicated; repeat if necessary and/or add antiarrhythmic medications.
    - If not, rate control or antiarrhythmic therapy is indicated.
  - Medications
    - Narrow-complex: β-blocker, calcium channel blocker, amiodarone
    - Wide-complex: amiodarone, procainamide, or sotalol
  - See figure on p. 528.
- Pulseless arrest
  - Dysrhythmias that produce pulseless arrest
    - VT (shockable)
    - VF (shockable)
    - Pulseless electrical activity (not shockable)
    - Asystole (not shockable)
  - Treatment
    - Immediate effective chest compressions and rapid defibrillation (for VT/VF)

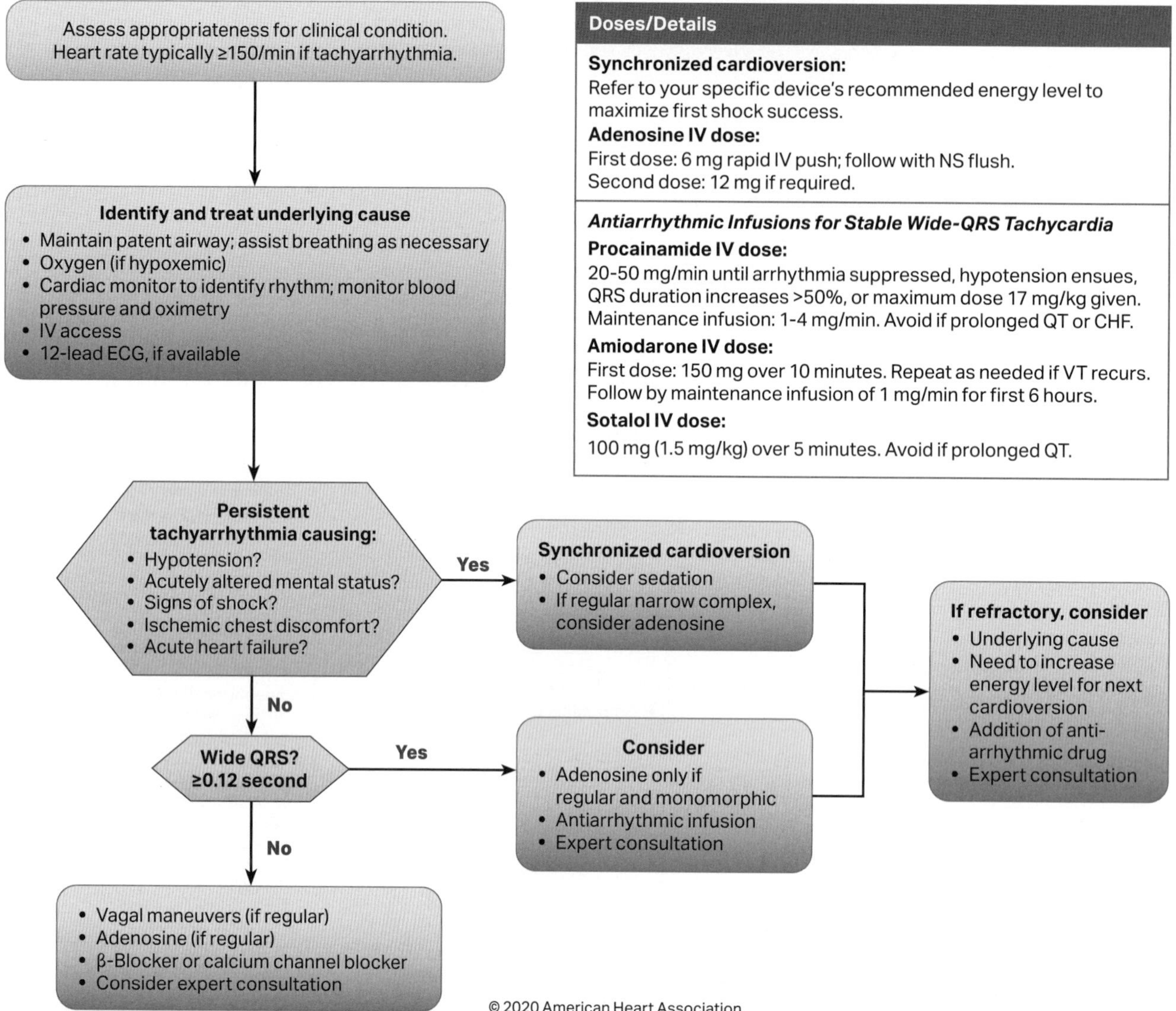

Adult Tachycardia with a Pulse Algorithm (with permission from the AHA). Figure depicts the resuscitation algorithm for tachycardia with a pulse—2020 update. (From 2020 AHA Guidelines for CPR and ECC: Adult Basic & Advanced Life Support. © 2020 American Heart Association.)

    - IV access, definitive airway, and drug therapy follow compressions.
    - Consider possible causes of pulseless arrest.
- Ventricular Fibrillation/Ventricular Tachycardia
  - Defibrillate
  - Immediately resume CPR after every shock.
  - Check pulse every 2 minutes (5 cycles of CPR).
    - No pulse + shockable rhythm: defibrillate and resume CPR
    - No pulse + nonshockable rhythm: move to the asystole/pulseless electrical activity (PEA) algorithm
    - ROSC: move to post-cardiac arrest algorithm
  - Administer epinephrine 1 mg every 3 to 5 minutes.
  - Consider amiodarone or lidocaine administration (not both).
  - Consider advanced airway/capnography.
  - See figure on p. 529.
- Asystole/Pulseless Electrical Activity
  - Needs excellent CPR because these are nonperfusing rhythms.
  - Administer epinephrine 1 mg IV ASAP and every 3 to 5 minutes.
  - Check pulse every 2 minutes (5 cycles of CPR).
    - No pulse + nonshockable rhythm: resume CPR
    - No pulse + shockable rhythm: move to the VF/VT algorithm
    - ROSC: move to post-cardiac arrest algorithm

Adult Cardiac Arrest Algorithm

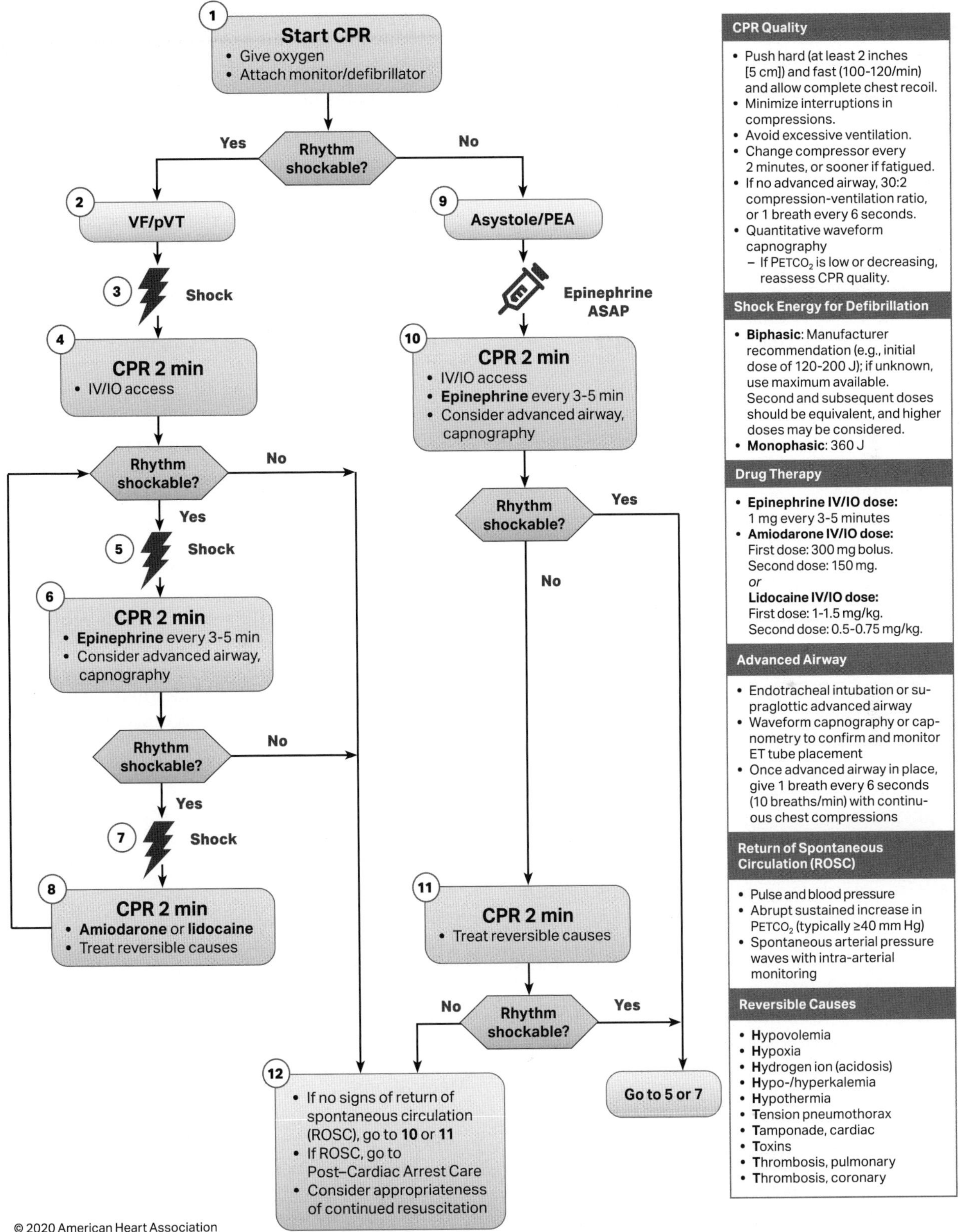

Adult Cardiac Arrest Algorithm (with permission from the AHA). Figure depicts the adult cardiac arrest algorithm—2020 update. (From 2020 AHA Guidelines for CPR and ECC: Adult Basic & Advanced Life Support. © 2020 American Heart Association.)

- Identify and treat reversible causes.
  - Cardiac ultrasound may be useful.
- Establish an advanced airway/capnography.

Medication Administration

- Routes of administration
  - IV
    - A single, large catheter preferred over multiple small catheters
    - Insertion should not interrupt CPR.
  - Intraosseous (IO)
  - ETT
    - Only certain medications (e.g., epinephrine, lidocaine, atropine)
    - Dose is 2 to 10 times the recommended IV dose.
    - Dilute in 5 to 10 mL of sterile water.
- Epinephrine
  - Randomized trials showed increased survival to ROSC and hospital discharge.
  - Can increase diastolic blood pressure and therefore coronary perfusion
  - Disadvantage
    - Increases myocardial demand by increasing heart rate and afterload
- Amiodarone
  - Improves survival in adults with out-of-hospital VF/VT arrest (compared with placebo)
  - Initial dose for VF/VT is 300 mg IV.
    - Additional dose of 150 mg IV for persistent pulseless VF/VT
  - Disadvantages
    - Can interact with volatile anesthetics to produce heart block, profound vasodilation, myocardial depression, and severe hypotension
    - Can prolong the effects of oral anticoagulants, phenytoin, digoxin, and diltiazem.
    - Can exacerbate or induce arrhythmias, especially torsade de pointes
- Other medications
  - Lidocaine was removed, then reinstated to algorithm for refractory VF/VT.
  - Vasopressin was removed due to lack of demonstrable benefit over epinephrine.
  - Naloxone should be considered for cardiac arrest due to opioid overdose.

Pediatric Advanced Life Support

- Most pediatric cardiac arrests are caused by respiratory deterioration.
  - Airway and ventilation management are critical for successful pediatric resuscitation.
- Adult resuscitation algorithms can be used for adolescent children.
- The elements of CAB and high-quality CPR in pediatric patients are same as in adults.
- Differences between CPR in pediatrics compared to adults
  - CPR depth and compression ratios
  - Shock energy for defibrillation
  - Drug therapy dosing is weight based.
  - See figure on p. 531.

Circulation

- Depth one third to one half the anteroposterior diameter of the chest
  - For infants 4 cm, for children 5 cm
- Compression to ventilation ratio
  - 30:2 for one rescuer and no advanced airway
  - 15:2 for two rescuers and no advanced airway (for children)
- Rate of 100 to 120 compressions per minute
- Pulse checks
  - For infants, check the brachial or the femoral artery.
  - For children, check the carotid or femoral artery.
- ECMO can be considered for all pediatric patients, especially for IHCA.

Airway and Ventilation Management

- Advanced airway
  - Pediatric airway differences include proportionally larger tongue and head compared to adult.
  - Straight laryngoscope blades may be preferred.
  - One breath every 2 to 3 seconds once there is an advanced airway
- Head tilt-chin lift is the technique of choice to open the airway.
- Conventional CPR is preferred over compression-only resuscitation.

Defibrillation

- First shock at 2 J/kg
- Second shock at 4 J/kg
- Subsequent shocks >4 J/kg, to a maximum of 10 J/kg or adult dose
- Biphasic AEDs can be used in children older than 1 year outside hospital setting.

Medications

- Epinephrine is associated with an increased rate of ROSC.
  - Dosage is 0.01 mg/kg up to a maximum dose of 1 mg.
  - Repeat every 3 to 5 minutes per ACLS protocols.
- Amiodarone or lidocaine for refractory VT or pulseless VT
  - Amiodarone dosing is 5 mg/kg bolus; repeat up to 3 times for VF/VT.
  - Lidocaine dosing is 1 mg/kg.

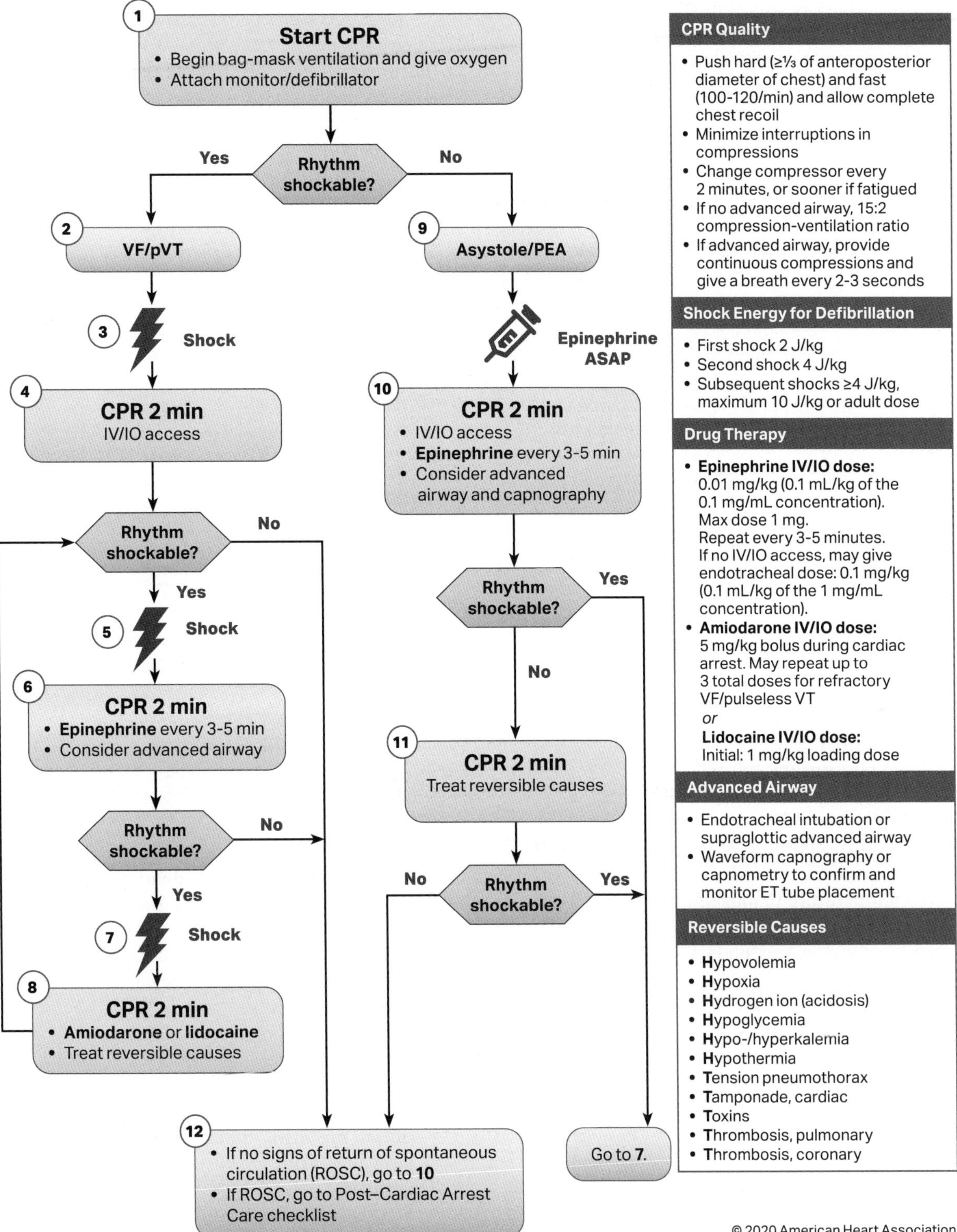

Pediatric Cardiac Arrest Algorithm (with permission from the AHA).Figure depicts the pediatric cardiac arrest algorithm—2020 update. (From 2020 AHA Guidelines for CPR and ECC: Adult Basic & Advanced Life Support. © 2020 American Heart Association.)

Postresuscitation Care and Neuroprognostication

- Transfer to intensive care unit (ICU).
- Optimization of cardiopulmonary function
  - Ensure adequate oxygen delivery and tissue perfusion.
  - Vasopressors and inotropes may be needed for support.
  - See figure on p. 533.

Pulmonary and Hemodynamic Postresuscitation Goals

- Pulmonary
  - Advanced airway placement (if not already done)
  - Pulse oximetry saturation 92% to 98%
  - Ventilate to $PaCO_2$ of 35 to 45 mmHg
- Cardiac/hemodynamic
  - Aggressively treat hypotension (systolic blood pressure [SBP] <90 mmHg, mean aterial blood pressure [MAP] <65 mmHg).
  - Electrocardiogram, echocardiogram, and serial cardiac enzymes
  - Monitor central or mixed-venous oxygen saturation.
  - Check lactate when applicable.
  - Check for reversible causes.

- Acute coronary syndrome
  - Electrocardiogram as soon as possible after ROSC
  - ST-segment elevation indicates need for emergent cardiac angiography.
- Neurologic monitoring
  - Neuroprognostication has a multimodal approach.
  - Evaluation should be >72 hours after return to normothermia.
- Targeted temperature management (TTM)
  - For patients who are not following commands
  - AHA strongly recommends TTM of 32°C to 36°C for 24 hours.
  - Hyperthermia can worsen ischemic brain injury and should be avoided.
  - Complications of lower targeted temperature can include impaired coagulation, hypokalemia, hyperglycemia, worsening of arrhythmias, and an increased risk of infection.
- Blood glucose control
  - Avoid significant hypoglycemia and hyperglycemia.
  - Increased blood glucose is associated with poor neurologic outcome.

Special Perioperative Considerations

- Incidence of intraoperative cardiac arrest (ICA) approximately 7.22 in 10,000 surgeries
- Predictors of ICA
  - Intraoperative blood loss (amount of transfusions received)
  - Anaphylaxis
- Perioperative cardiac arrests compared to other IHCAs
  - Anesthetic medication–related alterations to physiology
  - Usually witnessed and frequently anticipated
  - Are associated with a higher survival rate and better neurologic outcomes

Response to Intraoperative Arrest

- Initiate CPR.
- Call for help.
- Discontinue anesthetic.
- Discontinue surgery and check the field for bleeding, if possible.
- Retrieve emergency equipment.
- Increase FiO_2 to 100%.
- Manually ventilate the lungs.
- Open all intravenous lines.
- Use capnography to assess adequacy of CPR.
- Attach defibrillator (if applicable).

Anaphylaxis

- Agents at highest risk
  - Latex, β-lactam antibiotics, succinylcholine, nondepolarizing neuromuscular blockers, IV contrast material
- Treatment
  - Administer epinephrine.
  - Remove or discontinue offending agent, if possible.
  - Administer steroids and antihistamines.
  - IV fluid administration
  - Consider early, definitive airway support.
  - Proceed to CPR and ACLS if cardiovascular collapse occurs.

Gas Embolism

- Surgeries at risk
  - Laparoscopic surgical procedures, sitting craniotomies, posterior spine surgery, and endobronchial laser procedures
- Treatment
  - Stop insufflation or offending cause.
  - Occlude open veins if possible.
  - Flood the surgical field with saline.
  - Place the patient in Trendelenburg with left side down.
  - Proceed to CPR and ACLS If cardiovascular collapse occurs.

ACLS Health Care Provider Post–Cardiac Arrest Care Algorithm

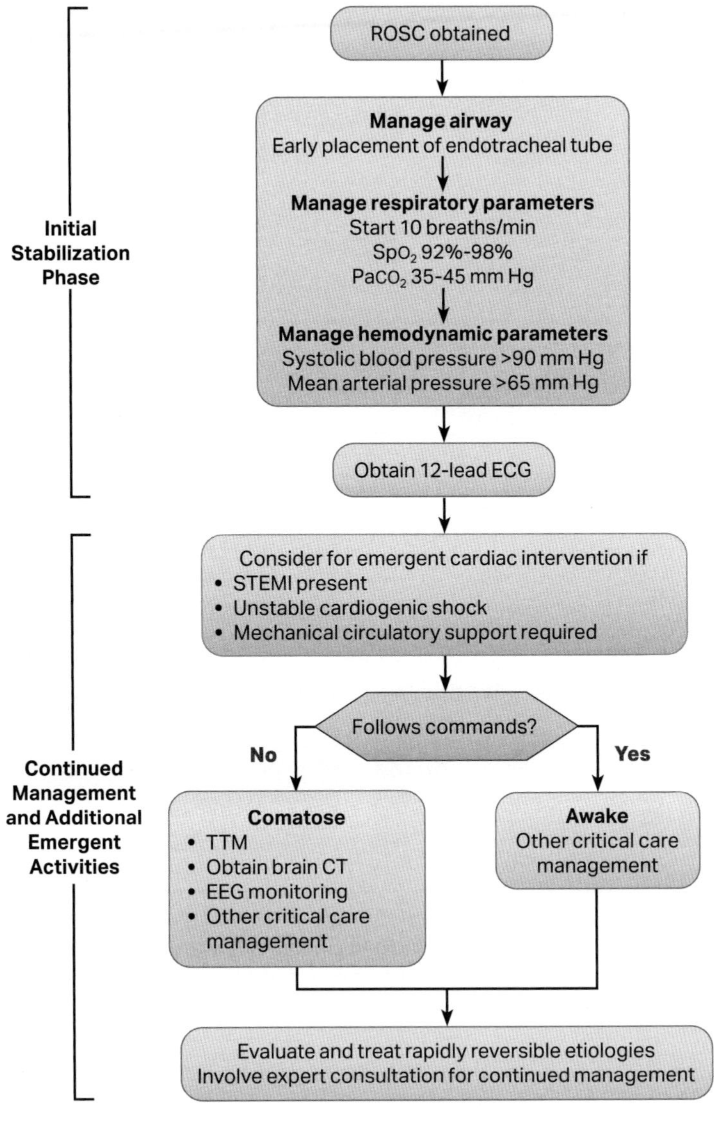

Initial Stabilization Phase

Resuscitation is ongoing during the post-ROSC phase, and many of these activities can occur concurrently. However, if prioritization is necessary, follow these steps:

- Airway management: Waveform capnography or capnometry to confirm and monitor endotracheal tube placement
- Manage respiratory parameters: Titrate FIO_2 for SpO_2 92%-98%; start at 10 breaths/min; titrate to $PaCO_2$ of 35-45 mm Hg
- Manage hemodynamic parameters: Administer crystalloid and/or vasopressor or inotrope for goal systolic blood pressure >90 mm Hg or mean arterial pressure >65 mm Hg

Continued Management and Additional Emergent Activities

These evaluations should be done concurrently so that decisions on targeted temperature management (TTM) receive high priority as cardiac interventions.

- Emergent cardiac intervention: Early evaluation of 12-lead electrocardiogram (ECG); consider hemodynamics for decision on cardiac intervention
- TTM: If patient is not following commands, start TTM as soon as possible; begin at 32-36°C for 24 hours by using a cooling device with feedback loop
- Other critical care management
  - Continuously monitor core temperature (esophageal, rectal, bladder)
  - Maintain normoxia, normocapnia, euglycemia
  - Provide continuous or intermittent electroencephalogram (EEG) monitoring
  - Provide lung-protective ventilation

H's and T's

Hypovolemia
Hypoxia
Hydrogen ion (acidosis)
Hypokalemia/**h**yperkalemia
Hypothermia
Tension pneumothorax
Tamponade, cardiac
Toxins
Thrombosis, pulmonary
Thrombosis, coronary

Post-Cardiac Arrest Care Algorithm (with permission from the AHA). Figure depicts the post–cardiac arrest algorithm—2020 update. (From 2020 AHA Guidelines for CPR and ECC: Adult Basic & Advanced Life Support. © 2020 American Heart Association.)

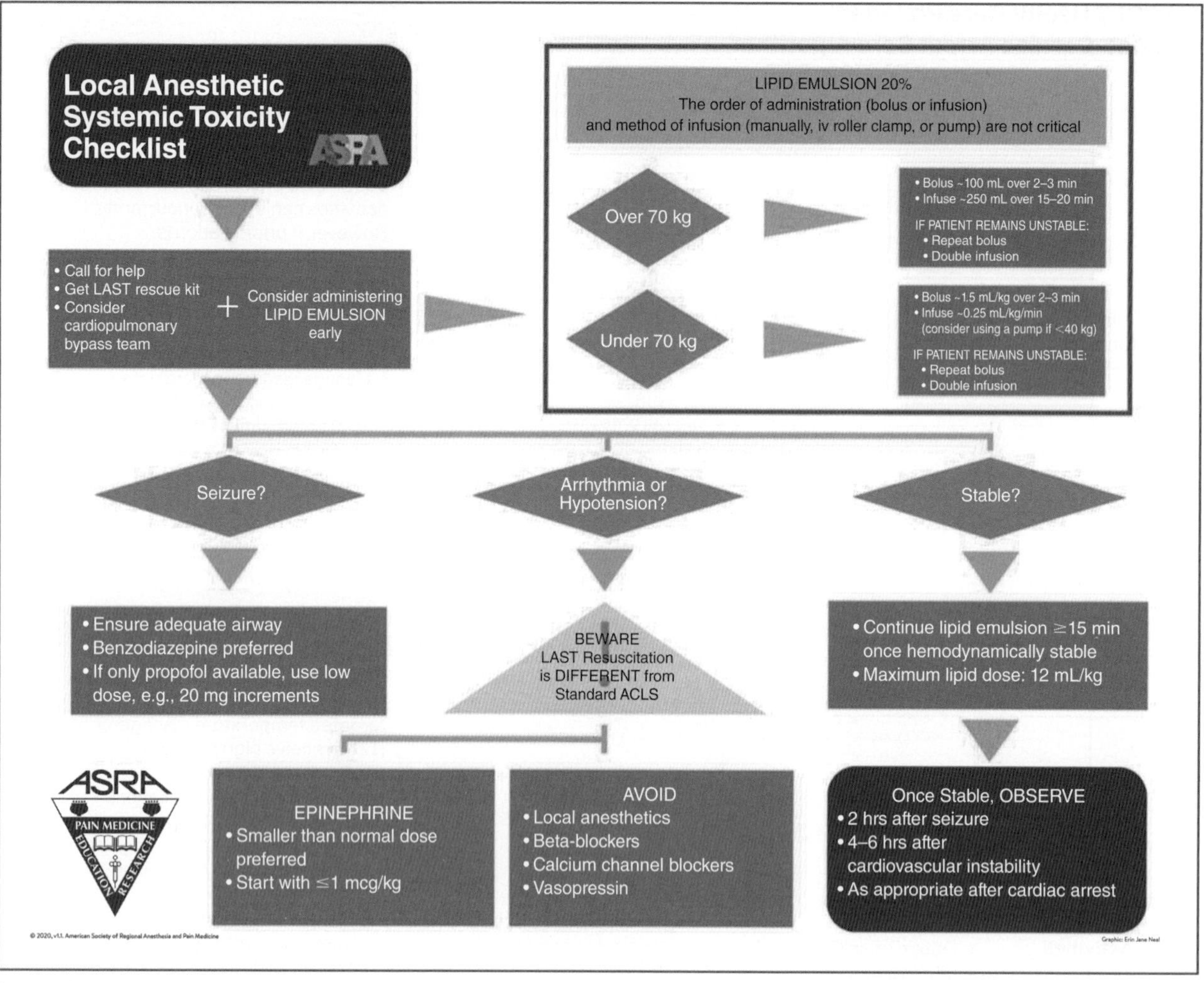

Local Anesthetic Systemic Toxicity Algorithm (with permission from the American Society of Regional Anesthesia and Pain Medicine). Figure depicts the American Society of Regional Anesthesia and Pain Medicine Local Anesthetic Systemic Toxicity Checklist: 2020 version. (Copyright 2020 by the American Society of Regional Anesthesia and Pain Medicine.)

Local Anesthetic Systemic Toxicity

- Cause and effect
  - Dose-dependent toxicity of sodium channels
  - In awake patients, neurologic symptoms precede cardiac signs.
  - Cardiac rhythm ranges from premature ventricular contractions to asystole.
- Treatment
  - Stop the local anesthetic, if possible.
  - Proceed with ACLS if pulseless.
  - Intralipid 20% load of 1.5 mL/kg bolus, then infuse 0.25 mL/kg/hr.
  - Sodium bicarbonate to maintain a pH >7.25
  - Consider transcutaneous or transvenous pacing for bradycardic rhythms.
  - Epinephrine dosing should be decreased to ≤1 μg/kg.
- Cautions
  - Avoid local anesthetics, β-blockers, calcium channel blockers, vasopressin
  - Propofol should not be used as a substitute for intralipid.
  - Cardiopulmonary bypass and/or mechanical circulatory support should be considered if intralipid is ineffective.
  - See figure above.

Cardiovascular Collapse From Neuraxial Anesthesia

- Causes and pathophysiology
  - A high level of spinal anesthesia appears to be most common cause.
  - Seems to occur in young, otherwise healthy patients
  - Autonomic balance shifts toward the parasympathetic system.
  - Venous return decreases from pooling in the splanchnic circulation.
  - Baroreceptor activation stimulates a paradoxical Bezold–Jarisch response.
- Treatment
  - Initiate CPR and ACLS protocols, and immediate epinephrine

Cardiac Arrest in Pregnancy

- Best outcome is successful maternal resuscitation.
- Treatment
  - Initiate high-quality CPR and ACLS.
  - Relieve aortocaval compression with left uterine displacement.
    - Manual displacement if fundal height above diaphragm and no ROSC
  - Perform advanced airway management and administer 100% oxygen.
  - Place IV line above the diaphragm.
  - Discontinue IV magnesium for preeclampsia, and administer calcium chloride.
  - Perimortem cesarean section (PMCD, also called resuscitative hysterotomy) recommended if ROSC is not achieved within 5 minutes.
- Postresuscitation care
  - TTM is recommended.
  - Continuous fetal monitoring if a PMCD is not performed

Debriefing

- Anxiety and posttraumatic stress can occur in rescuers.
- Debriefing and referral for emotional support may be beneficial.
- May allow for review of team performance and subsequent improvement

Systems of Care

- AHA guidelines made recommendations to improve outcomes in IHCA.
- Dependent on appropriate surveillance, prevention, and early recognition
  - Establishment of rapid response teams to reduce the incidence of cardiac arrest
  - Transfer to higher-acuity setting for patients at risk.
- Discussions about patient preferences for resuscitation before an actual event (if possible)
- CRM techniques should be used in order to optimize team dynamics.

QUESTIONS

BASIC LIFE SUPPORT

1. What are some differences between laypersons and health care providers' responses in Basic Life Support (BLS)?
2. What are the components of high-quality CPR?
3. What is the head tilt-chin lift maneuver, and when should it be modified?
4. What locations on the chest represent the most appropriate sites for the placement of defibrillator pads?
5. How many joules (J) of electricity should be delivered during an attempt at external defibrillation?

ADULT ADVANCED CARDIAC LIFE SUPPORT

6. What are some physiologic variables that can be used to monitor CPR?
7. Complete the following table listing the possible causes of pulseless arrest referred to as the 8 "H's" and 8 "T's".

	"H's"	"T's"
1.		
2.		
3.		
4.		
5.		
6.		
7.		
8.		

8. What is the appropriate treatment for ventricular fibrillation/ventricular tachycardia?
9. What is the appropriate treatment for pulseless electrical activity and asystole?

PEDIATRIC ADVANCED LIFE SUPPORT

10. How does the algorithm for CPR compare between children and adults?
11. Complete the following table comparing and contrasting adult and pediatric resuscitation algorithms.

	Adults	Children >1 year old	Infants <1 year old
Artery to check pulse			
Compression rate			
Compression depth			
Breath rate with advanced airway			
Energy for initial shock			
Energy for subsequent shocks			
Epinephrine dose			

12. What is proper rescuer hand placement for chest compressions in infants and in children?
13. Can standard biphasic automated external defibrillators (AEDs) be used in pediatric patients?

POSTRESUSCITATION CARE AND NEUROPROGNOSTICATION

14. How should a cardiac arrest patient be managed after the return of spontaneous circulation?

15. Complete the following table outlining the goals for postresuscitation care.

	Goal
Hemodynamic (targeted blood pressure parameters)	
Oxygenation (targeted oxygen saturation)	
Ventilation (targeted $PaCO_2$)	

16. What is the goal for temperature management in postresuscitation care?
17. Describe the components of the multimodal approach to neuroprognostication.

SPECIAL PERIOPERATIVE CONSIDERATIONS

18. Complete the following table of common causes of perioperative cardiac arrest in the categories listed in the first column.

	Causes of Perioperative Cardiac Arrest
Medications	
Respiratory	
Cardiovascular	

19. What are some exposures or drugs used in the operating room that can precipitate an anaphylactic reaction?
20. What is the treatment for intraoperative anaphylaxis?
21. What is the treatment for an intraoperative gas embolism?
22. What is the treatment for local anesthetic systemic toxicity (LAST)? What drugs should be avoided in the treatment of LAST?
23. How should cardiovascular collapse be managed in a patient who has just received neuraxial anesthesia?

ANSWERS

BASIC LIFE SUPPORT

1. For both laypersons and health care providers, the most essential aspect of Basic Life Support (BLS) is the rapid recognition of cardiac arrest and the initiation of high-quality CPR. For laypersons, there is some flexibility in activation of EMS before breathing and pulse assessment. The initiation of independent or dispatcher-assisted CPR for presumed (versus confirmed) arrest is acceptable for laypersons, as the risk of harm to the patient is low if the patient is not in cardiac arrest. Additionally, compression-only CPR is acceptable for laypersons, whereas health care providers are expected to provide assisted ventilation. Finally, health care providers should check for a pulse while simultaneously evaluating ventilation to reduce the time needed for assessment. (811)
2. Components of high-quality CPR include adequate depth, appropriate rate, and appropriate cycle ratio of compressions. It is important to allow adequate time for chest recoil for the heart to maximally fill with blood. Ideally, compressions should be on a firm surface, interruptions for airway management and to check for a pulse should be less than 10 seconds, and care should be taken not to ventilate with excessive positive pressure. (811)
3. Unconscious patients can have upper airway obstruction due to the tongue falling against the posterior pharynx. The head tilt-chin lift maneuver involves extension of the head and displacement of the mandible to an anterior position, thereby moving the tongue forward away from the posterior pharynx. For many individuals, this is adequate to provide a patent airway. For patients with suspected neck trauma, the rescuer needs to modify the maneuver by excluding the head tilt to avoid exacerbating a potential spinal cord injury. This can be achieved with the jaw thrust maneuver where two fingers are placed behind the angle of the mandible on both sides, the thumb is placed on the cheekbones, and the jaw is thrust forward. (811, 813)
4. The defibrillator pads should be applied to the chest on dry, bare skin, with firm pressure ensuring good skin contact in a position that will maximize the flow of electrical current through the myocardium. The standard placement is with one pad centrally on the chest, and one diametrically opposite this pad on the back of the patient to create a clear line through the heart between the two pads. Alternatively, if rolling the patient is unable to be achieved, the pads can be placed with one below the right clavicle and to the right of the upper sternum and the second pad at the level of the apex of the heart in the midaxillary line. (813)
5. The amount of energy (joules [J]) delivered for external defibrillation depends on whether the defibrillator is monophasic (360 J) or biphasic (120 to 200 J). Though no waveform has been demonstrated to improve ROSC or survival in external defibrillation, biphasic defibrillators (which deliver two pulses of opposite polarity) are thought to be more successful at terminating atrial and ventricular tachyarrhythmias, including ventricular fibrillation (VF) and ventricular tachycardia (VT). They also require less energy and may therefore cause less myocardial damage. (813)

ADULT ADVANCED CARDIAC LIFE SUPPORT

6. Continuous monitoring of end-tidal carbon dioxide (P_{ETCO2}) with quantitative and qualitative waveform capnography can be beneficial during resuscitation as confirmation of advanced airway placement and also as a guide for the adequacy of chest compressions. A P_{ETCO2} of at least 10 mmHg is associated with a greater chance of ROSC while a P_{ETCO2} of less than 10 mmHg is associated with poor outcomes. When ROSC is achieved, the P_{ETCO2} will typically increase significantly and maintain at this increased level. An alternative physiologic measure is arterial pressure monitoring, paying close attention to the diastolic pressure to assess the adequacy of CPR. A diastolic pressure of at least 20 mmHg is associated with adequate chest compressions. Other less commonly used monitors include central venous oxygen saturation and bedside cardiac ultrasound by an experienced sonographer. (814)
7. The following table lists the possible causes of pulseless arrest categorized as the 8 "H's" and 8 "T's". (819)

	"H's"	"T's"
1.	Hypovolemia	Toxins (anaphylaxis/anesthesia)
2.	Hypoxia	Tamponade
3.	Hydrogen ions (acidosis)	Tension pneumothorax (hemothorax)
4.	Hyperkalemia/hypokalemia	Thrombosis of coronary artery

	"H's"	"T's"
5.	Hypoglycemia	Thrombosis of pulmonary artery
6.	Hypothermia	Trauma
7.	Hyperthermia (malignant hyperthermia)	QT interval prolongation
8.	Hypervagal response	Pulmonary hypertension

8. Patients in ventricular fibrillation/ventricular tachycardia (VF/VT) should receive immediate defibrillation of 120 to 200 J with a biphasic (360 J with a monophasic) defibrillator. Good quality CPR should also be immediately instituted and maintained throughout the resuscitation, including prior to defibrillation while equipment is being obtained. Epinephrine 1 mg intravenously may be administered every 3 to 5 minutes if VF or VT persists after one to two sets of CPR-defibrillation cycles. Amiodarone or lidocaine, antiarrhythmic agents of different classes, can be considered for persistent VF/VT as well. Do not use both drugs in the same resuscitation episode. (817–819)
9. Pulseless electrical activity (PEA) and asystole are managed similarly to VF/VT, with the exception that defibrillation provides no benefit for patients in PEA or asystole. PEA, asystole, and VF/VT are all treated with effective CPR with minimal interruptions, identifying and treating reversible causes, the administration of epinephrine, and establishment of an advanced airway. The cardiac rhythm should be checked after every 5 cycles or 2 minutes of CPR. (817, 819)

PEDIATRIC ADVANCED LIFE SUPPORT

10. The algorithm for CPR in pediatric patients is basically the same as that for adults, which is that chest compressions are initiated before airway management and breathing. One distinct difference is the compression:ventilation ratio. In pediatric patients, the pattern should be 30 compressions to 2 breaths for one rescuer, but 15 compressions to 2 breaths for two rescuers. (820)
11. The following table compares and contrasts adult and pediatric resuscitation algorithms. (811–821)

	Adults	Children >1 year old	Infants <1 year old
Artery to check pulse	Femoral or carotid	Femoral or carotid	Femoral or brachial
Compression rate	100–120	100–120	100–120
Compression depth	5–6 cm	5 cm	4 cm
Breath rate with advanced airway	Every 6 seconds	Every 2–3 seconds	Every 2–3 seconds
Energy for initial shock	Biphasic 120–200 J Monophasic 360 J	2 J/kg	2 J/kg
Energy for subsequent shocks	Equivalent to or higher than the initial shock	4 J/kg for second shock 4–10 J/kg for 3+ shocks	4 J/kg for second shock 4–10 J/kg for 3+ shocks
Epinephrine dose	1 mg	0.01 mg/kg	0.01 mg/kg

12. Hand placement during chest compressions in infants is with the rescuer's one hand to support the back while compressions are performed with two fingers of the other hand. An alternative approach is the two thumb encircling hand technique, where the infant is encircled by the hands with both thumbs lying over the sternum. This is the preferred technique if multiple rescuers are present. In children, cardiac compressions can be accomplished with the heel of one hand directly over the lower half of the sternum, between the nipples and above the xiphoid process. (820, 822)
13. Standard biphasic automated external defibrillators (AEDs) can be used in children older than 1 year outside the hospital setting. For AED use on infants or children under 8 years of age, a pediatric dose attenuator system is recommended if available. If this is not available, a standard external defibrillator can be used in pediatric patients. (820)

POSTRESUSCITATION/CARE AND NEUROPROGNOSTICATION

14. The management of the cardiac arrest patient after the return of spontaneous circulation should include transfer to the ICU for close monitoring and optimization of hemodynamics, oxygenation, and ventilation.

Vasopressors, inotropes, and volume expansion with crystalloid may be necessary depending on the clinical scenario. An invasive arterial catheter is recommended. A 12-lead ECG, cardiac enzymes, and an echocardiogram should be immediately obtained as well, and evaluation for utility of cardiac interventions should be determined such as coronary angiography with or without interventions and mechanical circulatory support. In addition, electrolyte, glucose, and metabolic derangements should be corrected as best able. A neurological evaluation should be obtained; if neurological baseline has not been achieved, targeted temperature management should be initiated. (822–824)

15. Patient specifics should drive hemodynamic management. As a general guideline, the following are targeted for patients who are postresuscitation. (823–824)

	Goal
Hemodynamic	MAP >65 mmHg or SBP >90 mmHg
Oxygenation	Pulse oximetry saturation between 92% and 98%
Ventilation	$PaCO_2$ between 35 to 45 mmHg

16. Targeted temperature management (TTM) is indicated in patients who do not follow commands after ROSC. A goal temperature between 32°C and 36°C is recommended, and once achieved it should be maintained for at least 24 hours. Hyperthermia should be avoided in the post-cardiac arrest period as this has been shown to be detrimental. Patient factors should be accounted for when choosing the temperature, as therapeutic hypothermia has several side effects. For example, hypothermia can cause impaired coagulation and increased risk of infection, which may contraindicate its implementation. (824)
17. Neuroprognostication following cardiac arrest has a multimodal approach per AHA guidelines. Factors used within 24 hours include TTM (as soon as possible) and imaging (e.g., head CT). From 24 hours to 48 hours additional factors are electrophysiology (e.g., EEG), clinical examination, and serum biomarkers. Neuroprognistication is delayed until at least 72 hours following achievement of normothermia after targeted temperature management. (822–824)

SPECIAL PERIOPERATIVE CONSIDERATIONS

18. The following are common causes of perioperative cardiac arrest. (824)

	Causes of Perioperative Cardiac Arrest
Medications	Anesthetics High neuraxial blockade Local anesthetic toxicity Drug administration errors
Respiratory	Hypoxemia Auto-positive end-expiratory pressure (PEEP) Acute bronchospasm
Cardiovascular	Vasovagal Hypovolemic/hemorrhagic Distributive shock Obstructive shock Left ventricular failure Right ventricular failure Arrhythmia Acute coronary syndrome

19. Exposures or drugs used in the operating room that can precipitate an anaphylactic reaction include latex, β-lactam antibiotics, succinylcholine, all muscle relaxants, and intravenous contrast material. (825)
20. The main treatment for anaphylaxis is epinephrine. The causative drug should be discontinued or removed if possible. A continuous infusion of epinephrine should be considered, as this has been shown to have improved treatment of anaphylactic shock when compared to bolus dosing of epinephrine. Intravenous fluids may be necessary, and steroids and antihistamines are often administered. Early definitive airway support should be considered if not already in place given the potential for rapid development of oropharyngeal and

laryngeal edema, which can occlude the natural airway. In the event of complete cardiovascular collapse, CPR and ACLS should be started. Of note, larger doses of epinephrine may be required. (825)

21. The treatment of an intraoperative gas embolism is to stop insufflation, occlude open veins, and flood the surgical field with saline. The patient should also be placed in a Trendelenburg position with the left side down. In the case of complete cardiovascular collapse, CPR and ACLS should be started. (825–826)
22. Local anesthetic systemic toxicity (LAST) is characterized by neurologic symptoms prior to cardiac manifestations in the awake patient. Cardiac manifestations can range from premature ventricular contractions to asystole. In the event of cardiovascular toxicity, intralipid 20% IV load of 1.5 mL/kg followed by an infusion of 0.25 mL/kg/hr should be administered. Of note, despite propofol's suspension in a lipid solution, this is not recommended as a treatment for LAST given the profound hemodynamic effects it can have in an already hemodynamically compromised patient. In the event of cardiovascular collapse, CPR and ACLS should be immediately instituted. In this specific scenario, cardiopulmonary bypass or mechanical circulatory support would be warranted. Prolonged resuscitation can result in good neurologic recovery in these patients. Drugs that should be avoided in the treatment of LAST include local anesthetics, β-blockers, calcium-channel blockers, vasopressin. Epinephrine doses should be limited to <1 μg/kg. (826–827)
23. Cardiac arrest from neuraxial anesthesia should be managed with standard CPR and ACLS. (826)

Chapter

46 QUALITY AND PATIENT SAFETY

Meng-Chen Vanessa Lin and Linda L. Liu

INTRODUCTION

- Clinical anesthesia practice is a model for quality and safety in medicine.

DEFINITIONS: QUALITY VERSUS SAFETY

- Safety: the focus is on lack of harm and avoidance of adverse events.
- Quality: the optimal performance of a task, which can be measured by outcome, efficiency, cost, satisfaction, and/or value
  - Strategies often improve both safety and quality.
  - Higher quality may not always signify better safety and vice versa.

SPECIFIC APPROACHES TO ANESTHESIA SAFETY

Learning From Experience

- A large component of anesthesia safety has been based on a history of reporting observations.

Empiric Observation for Patient Safety
▪ Identify and describe an adverse event. ▪ Determine how it may occur in clinical practice. ▪ Develop and test countermeasures. ▪ Disseminate the results. – Technical improvements – Education

- Human interactions with anesthesia delivery systems have also been studied and implemented to optimize the human-anesthesia machine interface for patient safety.
  - For example, "linking" of oxygen and nitrous oxide flowmeters to prevent delivery of hypoxic gas mixtures

Adoption of Specialty-Wide Standards

- Monitoring standards proposed by the American Society of Anesthesiologists in 1986 were the first specialty-wide standards of any medical specialty.

Anesthesia Monitoring Standards Proposed in 1986
▪ An anesthesiologist should be present in the operating room. ▪ Arterial blood pressure and heart rate should be monitored at least every 5 minutes where not clinically impractical. ▪ Electrocardiogram shall be continuously displayed during anesthesia. ▪ Ventilation and circulation shall be continuously monitored during anesthesia. ▪ A method for monitoring breathing system disconnect shall be used in every general anesthetic. ▪ The oxygen concentration in the breathing circuit should be measured with an oxygen analyzer. ▪ During every administration of general anesthesia, temperature should be measured.

From Eichhorn JH, Cooper JB, Cullen DJ, et al. Standards for patient monitoring during anesthesia at Harvard Medical School. *JAMA*. 1986;256:1017–1020.

  - Standards are developed, implemented, and universally applied.
  - Developed from databases of adverse events and not evidence-based because anesthesia-attributable adverse events are rare
- Retrospective observations and clinical experience allude to improved safety, though conclusive benefit has been difficult to establish.

Patient Safety-Focused Programs

- Societies help identify and disseminate quality and safety in anesthetic care.

Examples of Anesthesia Patient-Safety Focused Programs
Anesthesia Patient Safety Foundation (APSF) ▪ Independent nonprofit dedicated to identify areas of anesthesia practice with potential for adverse events ▪ Members include anesthesiologists, nurse anesthetists, manufacturers of equipment and drugs, engineers, and insurers ▪ Worldwide circulation of newsletters, instructional videos, research grants, and conferences
ASA Closed Claims Project ▪ Reviews data from settled anesthesia lawsuits ▪ Identifies patient safety concerns, patterns of injury, and develops prevention strategies
Anesthesia Quality Institute (AQI) ▪ Sponsored by the ASA ▪ Oversees the Anesthesia Incident Reporting System (AIRS) and National Anesthesia Clinical Outcomes Registry (NACOR) ▪ Collects clinical data, provides learning opportunities based on incident reports, benchmarks amongst peers, and performance gap analyses
Multicenter Perioperative Outcomes Group (MPOG) ▪ Receives and analyzes data from multiple institutions ▪ Generates feedback to providers based on quality process and outcome metrics

FROM SAFETY TO QUALITY: MAKING ANESTHESIA BOTH SAFER AND BETTER

- Anesthesia quality includes optimizing safety, efficiency, cost, and patient satisfaction.
- The multidisciplinary nature of perioperative care makes measuring improvements difficult.
  - Attributions isolated to anesthesia are difficult to discern from surgery and nursing.
- Quality measures can usually be divided into three types: process, structure, and outcome.
  - Each method has its limitations.
  - None can lead to improved quality without sustainability.

Process Measures

- Track how a clinical care task should be delivered (e.g., measuring intraoperative glucose, administering antibiotics)
- Determining how the patient's clinical course or outcome is affected by a specific process of anesthesia care is challenging given the multiple aspects of perioperative care.

Structural Measures

- Track organizational elements possibly relevant to the quality of care (e.g., presence of physicians on-call for emergencies in the ICU, availability of diagnostic laboratory and radiologic testing)
- However, the link between structural measures and improved outcomes is difficult to discern.

Outcome Measures

- Measured through large databases from programs like NACOR and MPOG
- Accurate comparison of outcomes between individuals and institutions must adjust for patient comorbidities.
  - Risk adjustment can be difficult to define and implement.
- Outcome measurement alone has limited effectiveness if not properly contextualized.

TOOLS FOR IMPROVING LOCAL OUTCOMES

Structured Quality Improvement Approaches

- Multiple approaches for initiating and executing quality improvement projects exist.
  - FADE: **F**ocus on problem, **A**nalyze baseline performance/root cause, **D**evelop action plan, **E**xecute plan/**E**valuate results
  - PDSA: **P**lan, **D**o, **S**tudy, **A**ct
  - DMAIC: **D**efine, **M**easure, **A**nalyze, **I**mprove, **C**ontrol
- The common approach in these models is to evaluate, implement, and measure.

A Structured Approach for a Quality Improvement Project
Evaluate: the problem that needs improving ▪ Determine the metric that you will be measuring (process, structural, outcome). ▪ Obtain baseline data for the current state. ▪ Set the target goal. **Implement**: the action plan ▪ Define the causal factors that need improvement. ▪ Decide on the action plan. ▪ Disseminate the plan. **Measure**: assess the outcome by measuring the predefined metric **Repeat**: continue to evaluate ▪ Implement new action plans. ▪ Measure for improvement.

- Run chart: tracks performance over time to identify patterns and trends and to determine if interventions are successful

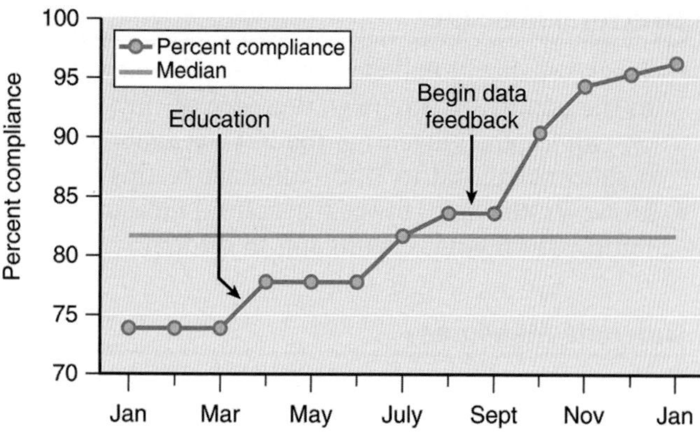

Example of a run chart. The performance measure on the Y axis is compliance with timing of preoperative antibiotics. The X axis represents time in months. Arrows indicate the time of two interventions that were performed. (Figure from Varughese AM, Buck DW, Lane-Fall MB, et al. Quality improvement in anesthesia practice and patient safety. In Gropper M, ed. Miller's anesthesia, 9th ed. Elsevier, 2020: Figure 5.2, Amsterdam, NL.)

- Control chart: a run chart that includes upper and lower performance limits/targets

Multidisciplinary Process Improvement: Root Cause Analysis, "Never Events," and Failure Mode Effects Analysis

- Root cause analysis (RCA) is a **retrospective** analysis using a multidisciplinary group to evaluate every step resulting in an adverse event.
  - Focus is on system processes and not individual provider behavior.
  - A causal factor chart is created detailing the event and all the contributing (causal) factors.

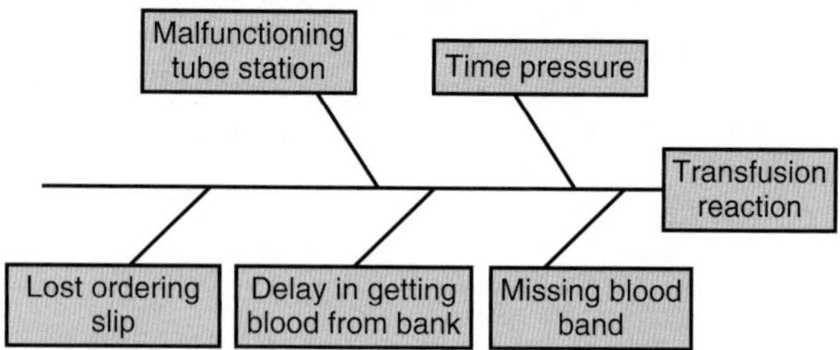

Sample causal factor chart. (From Tung A. Sentinel events and how to learn from them. Int Anesthesiol Clin. 2014;52:53–68.)

  - RCAs and the resultant action plans are mandated by The Joint Commission (TJC) whenever a "sentinel event" occurs.
- Failure mode effects analysis is a **prospective** analysis of a specific process, which aims to identify all the potential ways that it can fail.
  - Can be time-consuming even for straightforward processes
  - Often difficult to implement effective change because the adverse event has not yet occurred
  - Best reserved for large-volume, high-risk processes for which the risk of catastrophic failure is clear

QUESTIONS

DEFINITIONS: QUALITY VERSUS SAFETY

1. What are the key differences between the terms "safety" and "quality"?
2. In the table below, indicate whether the listed intervention represents an improvement in quality, safety, or both.

Intervention	Quality, Safety, or Both
Shorter hospital length of stay	
Ultrasound guidance for central line placement	
The presence of an additional anesthesia provider for patients with known difficult endotracheal intubation	

SPECIFIC APPROACHES TO ANESTHESIA SAFETY

3. Describe how anesthesia safety protocols can be developed from using past experiences.
4. Describe how implementation of specialty-wide standards can play a role in patient safety.

FROM SAFETY TO QUALITY: MAKING ANESTHESIA BOTH SAFER AND BETTER

5. Describe the three main quality measures of process, structure, and outcome, and the limitations of each.
6. Describe whether the task measured in the table below reflects process, structure, or outcome.

Task	Process, Structure, or Outcome
Availability of diagnostic laboratory and radiologic testing	
Mandating perioperative administration of ß-adrenergic blockers in myocardial infarction	
Postoperative acute kidney injury	
An active hospital-based quality improvement program	
Surgical site infections	
Perioperative glucose measures	
Electronic medical record	

TOOLS FOR IMPROVING LOCAL OUTCOMES

7. What are the three main principles that comprise the framework for quality improvement projects?
8. Describe the process of conducting a root cause analysis (RCA). What are some drawbacks to the RCA process?
9. What are sentinel events, and how does The Joint Commission (TJC) mandate they be managed?
10. Describe the process of conducting a failure mode effects analysis.

ANSWERS

DEFINITIONS: QUALITY VERSUS SAFETY

1. Safety refers to the lack of harm and avoidance of adverse events. Quality refers to the optimal performance of a task, which is multidimensional. In addition to avoiding injury (safety), it can refer to outcome, efficiency, cost, satisfaction, or some other metric of performance. (829)
2. The table below describes whether the intervention is an improvement in quality, safety, or both. (829–830)

Intervention	Quality, Safety, or Both
Shorter hospital length of stay	Quality
Ultrasound guidance for central line placement	Both
The presence of an additional anesthesia provider for patients with known difficult endotracheal intubation	Safety

SPECIFIC APPROACHES TO ANESTHESIA SAFETY

3. Collecting information of past adverse events, identifying a pattern, and developing countermeasures to mitigate against those adverse events is the mainstay of developing many anesthesia safety protocols. For example, some institutions developed transfusion goals for prone spinal fusion cases when risk factors associated with ischemic optic neuropathy were identified. (830)
4. Implementation of specialty-wide standards appear to confer improved outcomes in patient safety, although it may be difficult to establish a clear benefit from formal studies. An example of such is the adoption of monitoring standards in anesthesiology, which upon universal application has shown a reduction in reported adverse events. The ASA now endorses three practice standards: anesthetic monitoring, preoperative care, and postoperative care. (831)

FROM SAFETY TO QUALITY: MAKING ANESTHESIA BOTH SAFER AND BETTER

5. There are three main quality measures, and each has its limitations. (832–835)
   a. Process measures analyze the performance of certain tasks. While process measures are easy to measure, the success or failure of implementing a process does not necessarily improve outcome since a patient's clinical course is multifactorial. For example, one large study evaluating the initiation of preoperative β-adrenergic blockers did not clearly improve patient outcomes (fewer myocardial infarctions, but risks of stroke and death were increased).
   b. Structural measures refer to whether certain organizational features are in place to provide for high-quality care. Like process measures, structural measures are easy to measure, but the link to outcomes is difficult to assess. For example, the availability of in-house critical care attendings has not clearly shown an improvement in outcomes.
   c. Outcome measures refer to measuring the quality of medical care by the results, such as postoperative acute kidney injury. Outcome measures can provide information about daily clinical work as data gathering capabilities continue to improve. However, outcome measures require risk adjustment to account for patient-related comorbidities, and variability of this risk adjustment between different healthcare systems can limit the significance of the results.

6. The table below describes whether the task measured reflects process, structure, or outcome. (832–835)

Task	Process, Structure, or Outcome
Availability of diagnostic laboratory and radiologic testing	Structure
Mandating perioperative administration of ß-adrenergic blockers in myocardial infarction	Process
Postoperative acute kidney injury	Outcome
An active hospital-based quality improvement program	Structure
Surgical site infections	Outcome
Perioperative glucose measures	Process
Electronic medical record	Structure

TOOLS FOR IMPROVING LOCAL OUTCOMES

7. Several tools exist to serve as a framework for quality improvement. All of these follow the general model of evaluation, implementation, and measurement. (835)
8. A root cause analysis (RCA) retrospectively evaluates every step resulting in an adverse event using a multidisciplinary group. The goal is to focus on system processes (not individuals) to identify the root cause of the problem under analysis. This is mandated by The Joint Commission (TJC) for certain adverse events but can be used for any incident that a healthcare system would like to analyze. This is often done with a causal factor chart, which details an adverse event and all the contributing factors leading up to the event, or vice versa; the causal factor chart can start with the event, and work backward using logic and time information. A drawback of RCAs is that they are performed after an adverse event has already occurred. (835–837)
9. Sentinel events are events that reveal dangerous gaps in patient care and signal the need for immediate investigation and response. Examples of sentinel events include hemolytic transfusion reactions, wrong site procedures, and any intrapartum maternal death. Within 45 days of a sentinel event, it must be reported to TJC, an RCA performed, and a strategic action plan developed for implementation to reduce the risk of a recurrence. Reporting to TJC is voluntary but also a key element of accreditation visits. (836–837)
10. A failure mode effects analysis (FMEA) prospectively analyses a certain process and aims to anticipate all the potential failures and problems that may occur and lead to an adverse event. A drawback of performing an FMEA is that it can be time-consuming and difficult to implement effective change because it considers all possible adverse events that could result from a process. (837)

Chapter

47 PALLIATIVE CARE

Sarah Gebauer

INTRODUCTION

Definitions
■ **Hospice**: an insurance benefit for patients with a life expectancy of <6 months ■ **Palliative care**: a more inclusive term for care provided to patients with serious illnesses that is appropriate at any age and any stage of illness – Can be provided along with curative, even aggressive, treatment – Approach may be more nuanced, before transitioning to hospice

- Palliative care teams evaluate and manage physical and emotional pain and symptoms.
  - Physical and psychosocial contributing factors are considered, and appropriate expertise solicited (e.g., chaplain, social workers, art therapists)
  - Shared decision making: incorporating the patients' and families' values and goals in making medical recommendations and decisions
- Palliative care teams reduce hospital costs and do not increase the mortality rate.

What Is Hospice?

- Refers to a set of benefits used to decrease patients' symptoms, increase patient and family satisfaction, and reduce costs
- Most hospice services are provided at home, with hospice staff teaching the family how to care for a seriously ill, dying patient.

Medicare Hospice Benefits
Personnel ■ Physician of patient's choice ■ Nurse ■ Social worker ■ Spiritual counselor ■ Volunteers

Medicare Hospice Benefits—Continued
Goods and Services ■ Nursing support available on-call 24/7 ■ Access to short-term inpatient or continuous in-home care ■ Bereavement support for 1 year after the patient's death ■ Medical equipment (bed, walker, etc.) ■ Medical supplies (bandages, catheters, etc.)

Hospice and Palliative Medicine Subspecialty

- Hospice and palliative medicine is a board-certified subspecialty.
  - 1-year fellowship for >10 medical specialties
  - Perioperative advance directives and goals-of-care conversations apply to all anesthesia providers.

Anesthesiologists' Contribution to Palliative Care

- Anesthesiologists have specific skills in symptom management (e.g., pain, nausea) and insight into the risks of a perioperative course.

WHAT DO PALLIATIVE CARE TEAMS DO?

- Palliative care is an interdisciplinary field.
  - Physicians, nurses, social workers, chaplains, and anesthesia providers all contribute to palliative care.
- *Goals-of-care consults:* shared treatment plan that incorporates meaningful goals for the patient and family
- *Symptom management consults:* treatment plans require understanding of the patient's underlying pathophysiology
  - Common symptoms: insomnia, dyspnea, fatigue, pain, anxiety, depression, nausea and vomiting, and constipation

Palliative Care in the Intensive Care Unit

- *Palliative care consultation:* patients in the ICU for >7 days or with an expected mortality of >35%
- Palliative care consults in the ICU decrease time in the ICU and hospital length of stay, with no increase in mortality.
  - Improves communication between patient, family, and providers

Withdrawal of Life Support

- Distinction between withdrawal of life support and withdrawal of care should be discussed.
- Withdrawal of ventilator support requires preparing family on what to expect and having suction and medications available to titrate to patient comfort.

Spirituality in Serious Illness

- The role spirituality or religion plays in the patient and family's lives
- How the family requests the body be treated after death

PALLIATIVE CARE AND PAIN

Use of Opioids at the End of Life

- Opioids should be titrated to patient symptoms, not increased arbitrarily.

The Ethical Principle of Double Effect

A physician can treat symptoms that may hasten death as a secondary effect, provided the doctor's intention is to have a good outcome, like decreased pain and distress, rather than a bad outcome, like death.

Cancer Pain

- The cause of cancer pain is often complex and can be caused by the tumor itself; edema around a tumor; metastases in tissue, nerve, or bone; or the cancer treatment itself, such as chemotherapy- or radiation-induced neuropathies.
- Chemotherapy, radiation therapy, and/or surgery may be appropriate to alleviate cancer pain even when there is no anticipated increase in life expectancy.

Noncancer Pain

- Noncancer pain in seriously ill patients is often undertreated, though treatment is warranted.
  - Patients with dementia may have pain but are unable to communicate its source.
  - Patients with COPD with pain may not receive opioids due to concern about worsening the respiratory symptoms.

CHALLENGES IN THE PALLIATIVE CARE PATIENT

Identifying Palliative Care and Hospice Patients

Who Should Get a Palliative Care Consultation?

- Seriously ill patients without clear treatment preferences or decision-makers
- Patients whose care causes a conflict among staff members
- Patients with refractory symptoms

Inpatient Palliative Care Consults

- Patients with any of the following should be considered for a palliative care consultation.
  - Life-threatening diseases like metastatic cancer or liver failure
  - Illnesses with a high possibility of death such as multiorgan failure, severe trauma, or sepsis
  - Patients likely to die in the next year
  - Patients with complex psychosocial or symptom needs

Hospice Consults

- Hospice consultations should be considered for patients with a life expectancy of ≤6 months who are interested in treating symptoms, rather than a curative intent.

Prognosis

- Prognosis estimate helps make appropriate medical decisions.

Physician Estimate

- Physicians tend to be inaccurate at determining patient prognosis.
  - ICU physicians generally underestimate survival.
  - Physicians who know the patient well overestimate survival.
- Asking "Would I be surprised if this patient died in the next 12 months?" is a relatively good tool to assess prognosis broadly.

Disease Trajectories

- Disease-specific trajectories may help patients know what to expect.

Prognostic Tools

- Can be helpful in framing the patient's likely course
  - Limited in accounting for comorbid conditions or assessing life expectancy

Functional Status

- Functional status correlates well with prognosis.

Communication

- Ensure patient and family understand the medical issues.
- Determine how much detail they would like to know.

Goals-of-Care Conversations

- Gather family members, multidisciplinary team members, and specialists from relevant disciplines.
- Ask the patient how much information they want about their illness and what they have been told by other physicians.
- Briefly review the patient's condition.
- Physically sit down.
- Display empathy ("I can't imagine how hard this has been for you").
- Solicit questions.
- Develop a plan for patient care and/or a follow-up meeting.

Physician Tendencies in Addressing Difficult Topics

- Common physician tendencies: using too much technical detail, avoiding emotional topics, and dominating conversations
- Use understandable words, acknowledge emotion, and allow patients and families to speak.

Patient and Family Wishes About Communicating Prognosis

- Patients and families mostly want to know a prognosis, which is best given as a range estimate (e.g., hours to days, days to weeks, and weeks to months).

Frameworks for Communicating Difficult Information

- There are several formal frameworks and tools for communicating with patients.
  - One useful approach is the SPIKES framework, a six-step protocol for delivering bad news.
- Resuscitation discussions should be part of a larger discussion including overall condition and goals.
- Time-limited trials are agreements between physicians and patients/families to use a specified treatment for a defined period to determine if the patient improves.
  - The risks of the treatment trial and timeframe for improvement or reevaluation should be agreed to prior to initiating the trial.
- Few signs of imminent death are both sensitive and specific.
  - Mandibular movement with breathing, peripheral cyanosis, and Cheyne-Stokes respirations are specific for patient death within 3 days but occur in <60% of patients.

PERIOPERATIVE MANAGEMENT OF THE PALLIATIVE CARE PATIENT

The Management of Patients on Palliative Care

- Assess if the patient has decision-making capacity.
- Confirm the patient's surrogate decision-maker.
- Determine if the patient has an advance directive or do not resuscitate (DNR) order.
  - If so, discuss what limitations, if any, the patient wants during the perioperative period.
- Discuss any limitations on perioperative treatment with surgeon and surgical team.
- Consider involving spiritual care for patients with a high risk of perioperative death.
- Carefully plan postoperative pain control, especially for opioid-tolerant patients.
- Consider cachexia and poor skin integrity during positioning.
- Communicate timing of reversal of any treatment limitations to any oncoming or handoff providers.

Advance Directives

- Patients with advanced directives are more likely to receive care aligned with their preferences.
  - Advance directives are rarely unambiguous.
  - Many clinicians advocate for a surrogate decision-maker to be named.

Decision-Making Capacity

Criteria Used to Decide if a Patient Has Capacity

Defined as "the ability to communicate a choice, to understand the relevant information, to appreciate the medical consequences of the situation, and to reason about treatment choices"

- Asking questions like, "Can you tell me what surgery we are doing and why?" and "Can you tell me the risks of the procedure?" can help clarify whether a patient has decision-making capacity.

- A psychiatric consult can be helpful to make the determination.
- Patients without decision-making capacity need an identified surrogate decision maker.

Surrogate Decision Makers

- Surrogate decision makers make medical decisions on the patient's behalf.
  - Decisions should be in the patient's best interest and are the surrogate's best guess as to what the patient would want (which is not necessarily what the surrogate would choose).

How to Approach Perioperative DNR Conversations

Recommendations From the American Society of Anesthesiologists

- The American Society of Anesthesiologists (ASA) emphasizes that automatic and complete suspension of DNR orders (or other advance directives) may violate the patient's right to self-determination.
- A preprocedural discussion with the patient or surrogate is essential to determine one of the following approaches.
  - Full attempt at resuscitation
  - Limited attempt at resuscitation defined with regard to certain procedures
  - Limited attempt at resuscitation defined with regard to patient's goals and values
- Reinstating original advance directives and DNR orders usually occurs when the patient has recovered from the effects of anesthesia or when the patient leaves the PACU.

Recommendations From the American College of Surgeons and Association of periOperative Registered Nurses

- Similar to the ASA, these two societies also recommend a more tailored approach rather than automatic suspension.

Hospice Patients Who Present for Surgery

- Surgery may be to relieve suffering; risks, benefits, and the status of any advance directive orders should be discussed in advance.

QUESTIONS

INTRODUCTION

1. How are hospice and palliative care different?

WHAT DO PALLIATIVE CARE TEAMS DO?

2. Which members commonly comprise the interdisciplinary team in palliative care? What are their roles?

PALLIATIVE CARE AND PAIN

3. How does the ethical principle of double effect apply to palliative care?

CHALLENGES IN THE PALLIATIVE CARE PATIENT

4. What are the four main disease trajectories for dying?
5. What steps are in the SPIKES protocol for delivering bad news?

PERIOPERATIVE MANAGEMENT OF THE PALLIATIVE CARE PATIENT

6. How can an anesthesia provider determine if a patient has decision-making capacity?
7. The American Society of Anesthesiologists (ASA) has published guidelines for the care of patients with do not resuscitate (DNR) orders and limitations on treatment. Describe three scenarios for the care of these patients by completing the following table.

ASA Scenarios	Description
Full attempt at resuscitation	
Limited attempt at resuscitation defined with regard to specific procedures	
Limited attempt at resuscitation defined with regard to the patient's goals and values	

ANSWERS

INTRODUCTION

1. Palliative care is appropriate at any age, at any stage in a serious illness, and can be provided together with curative treatment. Services may be provided in the clinic, inpatient, or home settings. In contrast, hospice in the United States refers to an insurance benefit for patients with a life expectancy of ≤6 months. Hospice provides for a variety of medical and ancillary services with a focus on comfort rather than life-prolonging measures. Most hospice care is provided at home, with a small portion provided on an inpatient basis. (841)

WHAT DO PALLIATIVE CARE TEAMS DO?

2. Physicians, nurses, social workers, chaplains, and anesthesia providers commonly comprise the interdisciplinary team involved in palliative care. Roles may include symptom management and communication, assessment of psychosocial and spiritual needs of the patient and family, assistance with complex discharge needs, assisting patients and families in identifying and addressing spiritual distress and facilitating appropriate spiritual rituals, advanced pain management, and goals-of-care discussions. (842–843)

PALLIATIVE CARE AND PAIN

3. The ethical principle of double effect states that a physician can treat symptoms that may hasten death as a secondary effect, provided the doctor's intention is to have a good outcome (decreased pain and distress), rather than a bad outcome (death). In palliative care it applies to the fact that the primary goal of a treatment, for example, the treatment of pain with opioids, may also cause a secondary effect such as hastening the time to death. In this example, the intention of the provider is the titration of the medication (e.g., opioids) to the symptoms for a positive outcome, rather than to the secondary effect of death. (844)

CHALLENGES IN THE PALLIATIVE CARE PATIENT

4. The four main disease trajectories of dying are sudden death, terminal illness, organ failure, and frailty. In sudden death, a patient is healthy and functional, and then a catastrophic event, like a car accident, occurs. Terminal illness, in which a functional patient undergoes a decline over a period of weeks to months, occurs in patients with many types of cancer. Organ failure, in which patients have repeated decreases in functionality owing to illness and then improve but never get quite back to their previous baseline, occurs in illnesses like chronic obstructive pulmonary disease (COPD). Frailty, in which a patient with a long-term, chronic illness slowly loses function over a period of years, occurs in dementia. (847)

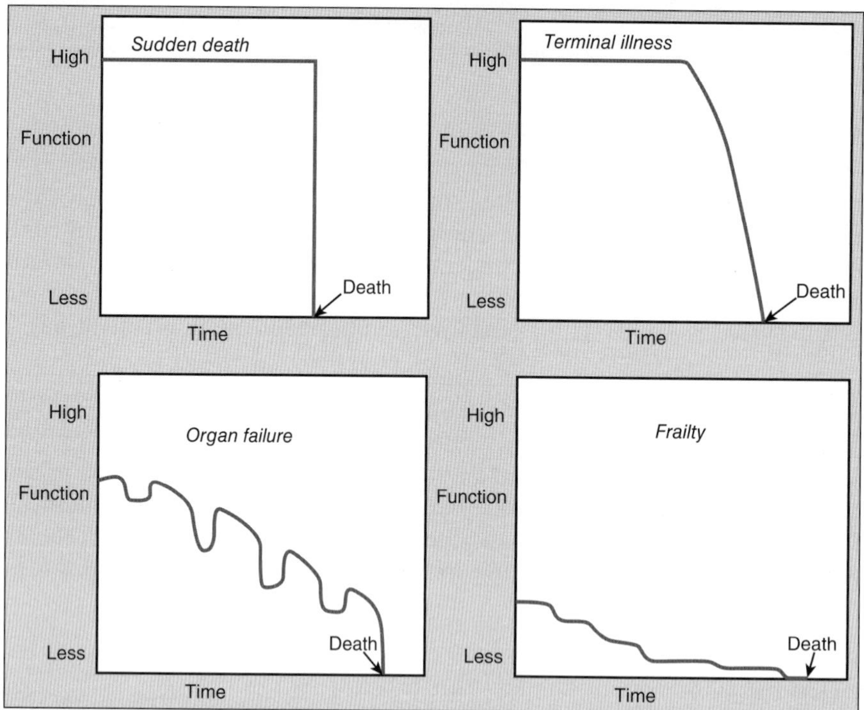

Redrawn from Lunney JR, Lynn J, Hogan C. Profiles of older Medicare decedents. J Am Geriatr Soc. 2002;50:1108–1112.

5. The SPIKES protocol was originally developed as a mnemonic to help physicians deliver bad news, but its steps can be used in a variety of situations. The first step, **S**etting, is a reminder to choose a quiet, private space with sufficient chairs for all those attending the meeting. During the second step, **P**erception, the physician asks about and assesses the patient's and family's understanding of the patient's condition. The third step, **I**nvitation, reminds the physician to ask how much detail the patient wants. The fourth step, **K**nowledge, is when the physician uses plain language to communicate medical information. The fifth step, **E**mpathy, emphasizes the importance of acknowledging emotions. During the sixth step, **S**equelae, all participants agree on next steps. (849)

PERIOPERATIVE MANAGEMENT OF THE PALLIATIVE CARE PATIENT

6. The capacity for patients to make decisions for themselves is defined as "the ability to communicate a choice, to understand the relevant information, to appreciate the medical consequences of the situation, and to reason about treatment choices." The anesthesia provider may ask the patient to explain their understanding of the surgery and its risks to determine if the patient has decision-making capacity. If the anesthesia provider remains uncertain, a psychiatric consult may be appropriate. A surrogate decision-maker may be necessary for patients who lack the capacity to give informed consent. (850-851)
7. The American Society of Anesthesiologists (ASA) published guidelines for the three possible scenarios for the care of patients with do not resuscitate (DNR) orders and limitations on treatment as illustrated in the following table. (851)

ASA Scenarios	Description
Full attempt at resuscitation	Full suspension of DNR The preexisting order is completely reversed and any procedures may be used.
Limited attempt at resuscitation defined with regard to specific procedures	The patient may request that interventions such as chest compressions, for example, not be used. The anesthesiologist and patient should agree on which procedures can and cannot be used during the anesthetic.
Limited attempt at resuscitation defined with regard to the patient's goals and values	The patient may give the physician authority to use clinical judgment to decide which resuscitation procedures are appropriate. Full resuscitation may be desirable for reversible events but not those that lead to an unwanted outcome.

Chapter

48 SLEEP MEDICINE AND ANESTHESIA

Mandeep Singh, Ameya Pappu, and Frances Chung

INTRODUCTION

- *Polysomnography* is a sleep study incorporating electroencephalography (EEG) and respiratory and cardiac measurements.

BASIC SLEEP PHYSIOLOGY

- *Sleep* is a state of reduced arousal actively generated by nuclei in the hypothalamus, brainstem, and basal forebrain.
- There are two control processes for sleep, which are additive.
  - *Circadian drive* (process C) regulates appropriate timing of sleep and wakefulness across the 24-hour day and is modulated by the hypothalamic suprachiasmatic nucleus.
    - Increases sleepiness according to accustomed sleep times
  - *Homeostatic drive* (process S) regulates sleep need and intensity according to time spent asleep and awake.
    - Increases sleepiness according to sleep deprivation
- Normal sleep is nonhomogeneous with dynamic architecture that is divided into nonrapid eye movement (NREM) and rapid eye movement (REM).
  - Cycle at 90- to 120-minute intervals, approximately
  - Consolidated in bouts of 6–8 hours.
- American Academy of Sleep Medicine (AASM) stages sleep based on characteristic EEG patterns

The AASM Classifications of Sleep and Wakefulness

- Wakefulness (Stage W)
  - Beta activity with eyes open (low amplitude, 12–40 Hz)
  - Alpha activity with eyes closed (low amplitude, 8–13 Hz)
- NREM sleep:
  - Stage N1: attenuation of alpha activity; low-amplitude, mixed-frequency signal (4–7 Hz) and vertex sharp waves
  - Stage N2: K-complexes and sleep spindles
  - Stage N3: higher-amplitude, lower-frequency (0.5–2 Hz) rhythms known as *delta waves*
- REM (stage R) sleep
  - Active high-frequency, low-amplitude rhythms

GENERAL ANESTHESIA

- General anesthesia is best described as a drug-induced coma.
  - Acts by altering neurotransmission at multiple sites in the cerebral cortex, brainstem, and thalamus
- Anesthesia-induced consciousness has three EEG patterns.
- Before *induction,* the patient has a normal, active EEG with prominent alpha activity (10 Hz) when eyes are closed.
  - Small doses of hypnotic agents acting at $GABA_A$ receptors induce sedation in which the patient is calm and easily arousable, with eyes generally closed.
  - A brief period of paradoxical excitation follows, characterized by an increase in beta activity on the EEG (13–25 Hz).
- During the *maintenance* period, there are four distinct phases.
  - Phase 1: light state of general anesthesia
    - Decrease in beta activity (13–30 Hz)
    - Increase in alpha activity (8–12 Hz) and delta activity (0–4 Hz)
  - Phase 2: the intermediate state
    - Decrease in beta activity
    - Increase in alpha and delta activity with anteriorization (a greater increase in alpha and delta activity in the anterior EEG leads relative to the posterior leads)
    - The EEG in phase 2 resembles that seen in stage 3, NREM sleep.
  - Phase 3: deeper state
    - Flat periods interspersed with periods of alpha and beta activity (burst suppression)
    - Amplitudes and time between alpha and beta activity lengthen as general anesthesia deepens.
  - Phase 4: most profound state of general anesthesia
    - Isoelectric EEG
- During the *emergence* from general anesthesia, EEG patterns reverse in order.

OTHER AROUSAL STATES

- EEG patterns during recovery from coma resemble EEG patterns during various arousal states.
  - Comatose resembles general anesthesia.
  - Vegetative state resembles sleep.
  - Minimally conscious resembles the awake state.

SLEEP AND ANESTHESIA STATES

Sleep states (natural) and anesthesia states (drug-induced) have similarities and differences.

Sleep States versus Anesthesia States

Sleep	Anesthesia
Nonhomogeneous state with distinct stages occurring in a cyclical pattern	Homogeneous state
Characterized by periodic arousals and variable body postures	The depth and duration are directly dependent on drug pharmacokinetics and pharmacodynamics.
Disrupted by significant psychological and environmental stimuli	Suppressed arousals; renders subject insensate to bodily injury
Spontaneous reversal after restorative function complete	Reversal requires voluntary stoppage of drug administration and effective drug elimination.

FUNCTIONAL NEUROANATOMY OF SLEEP AND AROUSAL PATHWAYS

- Anesthesia-induced loss of consciousness results from interactions of anesthetics with neural circuits regulating sleep and wakefulness states.
- Sleep state modulation is regulated by two groups of neural centers: those that promote wakefulness and those that promote sleep.
  - The wakefulness-promoting centers are the locus coeruleus (LC), dorsal raphe (DR), and tuberomammillary nucleus (TMN).
  - The sleep-promoting center is primarily the hypothalamic ventrolateral preoptic nucleus (VLPO).
- Mutual inhibition between the VLPO and LC produces switchlike, bistable states of wakefulness and sleep.

SLEEP-DISORDERED BREATHING OR SLEEP-RELATED BREATHING DISORDERS

- *Sleep-disordered breathing:* abnormal respiratory patterns during sleep

Types of Sleep-Disordered Breathing

- Obstructive sleep apnea (OSA)
- Central sleep apnea (CSA)
- Sleep-related hypoventilation
- Sleep-related hypoxemia

- Both OSA and CSA are characterized by a reduction (hypopnea) or cessation (apnea) of airflow but with different pathophysiologies.
  - OSA
    - Complete or incomplete upper airway (UA) closure during sleep
    - Presence of respiratory effort
  - CSA
    - Absent or reduced respiratory effort
    - Apnea may be cyclical, intermittent, or irregular (ataxic).

OBSTRUCTIVE SLEEP APNEA

- OSA involves episodes of apnea or hypopnea during sleep.
  - Varying severity of hypoxemia and/or hypercapnia
  - Terminated by EEG arousal

Pathophysiology of Upper Airway Collapse in Obstructive Sleep Apnea

- Awake patients have increased genioglossus muscle tone.
  - Pulls the tongue forward maintaining UA patency
- Several physiologic changes during sleep contribute to OSA.
  - Loss of upper airway dilating muscle tone
  - Impaired mechanoreceptor response to intrapharyngeal pressure
  - Ventilatory overshoot (high loop gain of the respiratory control system)
  - Increased arousal threshold
- Smaller upper airway cross-sectional area and higher critical closing pressures are seen in patients with OSA compared to those without OSA.
- General anesthesia magnifies this effect.
  - Profound decrease in tonic and phasic muscle activity
  - Loss of protective arousal response
  - Can lead to prolonged obstruction and severe oxygen desaturation

Clinical Diagnostic Criteria

- Gold standard for diagnosis is overnight polysomnography (PSG).

- AASM criteria for apnea or hypopnea
  - A reduction in airflow from intranasal pressure of at least 90% (*apnea*), or between 50% and 90% (*hypopnea*), for at least 10 seconds
  - Accompanied by either a 3% or 4% drop in oxygen saturation or an EEG arousal
- The *apnea-hypopnea index* (AHI) is defined as the average number of abnormal breathing events per hour.

Obstructive Sleep Apnea Diagnosis and Severity Based on Apnea-Hypopnea Index

The clinical diagnosis of OSA requires either:
- An AHI of ≥15
- AHI ≥5, with symptoms such as excessive daytime sleepiness, unintentional sleep during wakefulness, unrefreshing sleep, loud snoring reported by a partner, or observed obstruction during sleep

The severity of OSA is scored by:
- Mild: 5–15 events per hour
- Moderate: ≥15–30 events per hour
- Severe ≥30 events per hour

Polysomnography and Portable Devices

- Level 2 portable PSG (full unattended PSG with seven or more channels) has a diagnostic accuracy similar to standard PSG.
- Overnight oximetry is sensitive and specific for detecting OSA in high-risk surgical patients.
- Portable devices can be considered when there is high pretest likelihood for moderate to severe OSA without other substantial comorbidities.

Prevalence of OSA in the General and Surgical Populations

- The prevalence of moderate to severe OSA (AHI ≥15 events/hr) ranges from 6% to 17% in the adult population.
- Undiagnosed moderate to severe OSA
  - Nearly 80% of men and 93% of women in the community
  - In one large case series, it was 60% of surgical patients.

OSA and Comorbid Conditions

- There are multiple symptoms and comorbid conditions that accompany OSA.
- The anesthesia provider should be aware of the possible existence of these for risk stratification and optimization when indicated.

Symptoms and Clinical Features of Obstructive Sleep Apnea

Symptoms
- Daytime sleepiness
- Loud snoring
- Nonrestorative sleep
- Witnessed apneas by bed partner
- Awakening with choking
- Insomnia with frequent brief nocturnal awakenings
- Lack of concentration
- Cognitive deficits
- Changes in mood
- Morning headaches
- Sleep walking, confusional arousals (arousals from NREM sleep)
- Vivid, strange, or threatening dreams (arousals from REM sleep)
- Gastroesophageal reflux
- Nocturia
- Drowsy driving, and motor vehicle accidents

Comorbid Conditions
- Obesity
- Large neck circumference
- Craniofacial deformities (retrognathia, midfacial hypoplasia)
- Crowded pharynx
- Systemic hypertension
- Hypercapnia or high serum bicarbonate
- Cardiovascular disease
- Cerebrovascular disease
- Cardiac dysrhythmia
- Metabolic syndrome
- Pulmonary hypertension
- Obesity hypoventilation syndrome
- Cor pulmonale
- Polycythemia
- Floppy eyelid syndrome

Modified from Olson E, Chung F, Seet E. Surgical risk and the preoperative evaluation and management of adults with obstructive sleep apnea. In: Post TW, ed. *UpToDate*. https://www.uptodate.com/contents/surgical-risk-and-the-preoperative-evaluation-and-management-of-adults-with-obstructive-sleep-apnea. Accessed October 2021.

Surgery and OSA Severity

- A prospective study of postoperative OSA had several findings.
  - The AHI increases significantly on the first night.
  - The peak increase in AHI is on the third night.
  - Predictors of postoperative AHI include the preoperative AHI, age, and opioid use.
- Retrospective review of unexpected critical events in patients with OSA after anesthesia
  - Majority were within 24 hours of anesthesia.
  - About 97% received opioids within 24 hours before the event.

- Two-thirds also received sedatives.
- Death and brain damage were associated with
  - Unwitnessed events
  - No supplemental oxygen
  - Lack of respiratory monitoring
  - Coadministration of opioids and sedatives

OSA and Perioperative Complications

- OSA is a predictor of difficult intubation and impossible mask ventilation.
- Multiple studies have shown that patients with OSA are at increased risk for postoperative complications.
  - Unplanned reintubation
  - Myocardial infarction
  - Pulmonary aspiration
  - Acute respiratory distress syndrome
  - Pulmonary embolism (only after orthopedic surgery)
- OSA is an independent risk factor for postoperative cardiovascular morbidity and mortality.
  - Patients with severe OSA undergoing major noncardiac surgery
    - Increased postoperative risk for myocardial injury, cardiac death, congestive heart failure, thromboembolism, atrial fibrillation, and stroke
  - Patients with undiagnosed OSA compared to patients diagnosed with OSA and on prescribed continuous positive airway pressure (CPAP) therapy
    - May have threefold higher risk for postoperative cardiac arrest and shock

Clinical Pathways and Principles of Perioperative Management

- Multiple societies have published recommendations.
- General perioperative management
  - Screen patients for OSA.
  - Patients with OSA should be made aware of the increased risk.
  - Additional cardiopulmonary testing and optimization of comorbidities, if appropriate
  - Perioperative PAP therapy continued or instituted, as necessary

Preoperative Assessment

Patients With Diagnosed OSA

- History and physical examination
  - Focus on the nature and severity of symptoms and comorbidities, especially pulmonary hypertension.
- Laboratory studies
  - Serum bicarbonate level ≥28 mmol/L can indicate chronic hypercapnia.
- Transthoracic echocardiogram
  - May be useful for patients suspected of having severe pulmonary hypertension
- Positive airway pressure (PAP) devices
  - Review data to evaluate adherence to therapy and improvement in the AHI.
  - Recommend patients bring with them to the hospital to wear perioperatively during the appropriate times.
- Additional cardiopulmonary evaluation and initiation/adjustment of PAP therapy
  - Patients with significant comorbidities, an elevated serum bicarbonate, or resting hypoxemia in the absence of respiratory disease (see figure on p. 559.)

Patients With Suspected OSA

- PSG is the gold standard, but routine screening can be costly.
- STOP-BANG questionnaire screening tool
  - Useful and validated
  - High sensitivity and high negative predictive value

STOP-BANG Questionnaire

- **Snoring**? Do you Snore Loudly (loud enough to be heard through closed doors or your bed partner elbows you for snoring at night)?
- **Tired**? Do you often feel Tired, Fatigued, or Sleepy during the daytime (such as falling asleep during driving)?
- **Observed**? Has anyone Observed you Stop Breathing or Choking/Gasping during your sleep?
- **Pressure**? Do you have or are being treated for High Blood Pressure?
- **Body mass index** more than 35 kg/m^2?
- **Age** older than 50 years?
- **Neck size** large (measured around Adam's apple)? More than 40 cm?
- **Gender** = Male?

Scoring criteria for general population
Low risk of OSA: Yes to 0–2 questions
Intermediate risk of OSA: Yes to 3–4 questions
High risk of OSA: Yes to 5–8 questions
The sensitivity of the STOP-Bang score ≥3 to detect moderate to severe OSA (AHI >15) and severe OSA (AHI >30) is 93% and 100%, respectively.
The corresponding negative predictive values are 90% and 100%.
Proprietary to University Health Network, www.stopbang.ca

- Evaluate for uncontrolled disease and ventilatory or gas exchange problems.
  - If negative, elective surgery should proceed with perioperative risk-mitigation strategies.
  - If positive, additional cardiopulmonary evaluation can guide optimization and perioperative management planning.

- For patients with uncontrolled disease
  - A risk/benefit discussion of the surgery and its timing should take place including the patient, surgeon, and anesthesia provider.
  - A postoperative referral to a sleep medicine physician may be useful for follow-up (see figure on p. 560.)

Perioperative Risk Mitigation Strategies

- The Society of Anesthesia and Sleep Medicine has published guidelines for the intraoperative management of patients with OSA.

Principles of Perioperative OSA Management
▪ Avoid unmonitored use of sedative premedication. ▪ Regional techniques preferred ▪ Anticipate a difficult airway. ▪ Consider preoxygenation, head-up positioning, rapid sequence induction, and preoperative proton pump inhibitors. ▪ Short-acting drugs like remifentanil and propofol are preferred. ▪ Use benzodiazepines with caution. ▪ Minimize use/dose of neuromuscular blocking agents (NMBAs), monitor neuromuscular blockade, and completely reverse NMBA before extubation. ▪ Extubate when patient is awake, fully conscious, able to obey commands, and maintain a patent airway.

Principles of Perioperative OSA Management—Continued
▪ Recover in semi-upright or lateral position after extubation. ▪ Multimodal analgesia is strongly recommended to reduce opioid use (e.g., regional techniques, acetaminophen, nonsteroidal antiinflammatory drugs, dexamethasone, ketamine, gabapentin/pregabalin).

Postoperative Disposition of OSA Patients

- Postoperative disposition decision factors
  - Nature of the surgery
  - Severity of OSA
  - Requirement for postoperative parental opioids
- Discharge home if the following conditions are met
  - The patient has diagnosed mild or suspected low-risk OSA.
  - The surgery is minor.
  - Minimal or no opioids are needed for pain control.
- Postoperative continuous monitoring and/or PAP therapy
  - Suspected high-risk or intermediate-risk OSA
    - Recurrent respiratory events in the PACU
    - The need for postoperative parenteral opioids
  - Diagnosed moderate or severe OSA
    - Recurrent respiratory events in the PACU
    - The need for postoperative parenteral opioids
    - Significant comorbidities or noncompliance with PAP therapy (see figure on p. 560.)

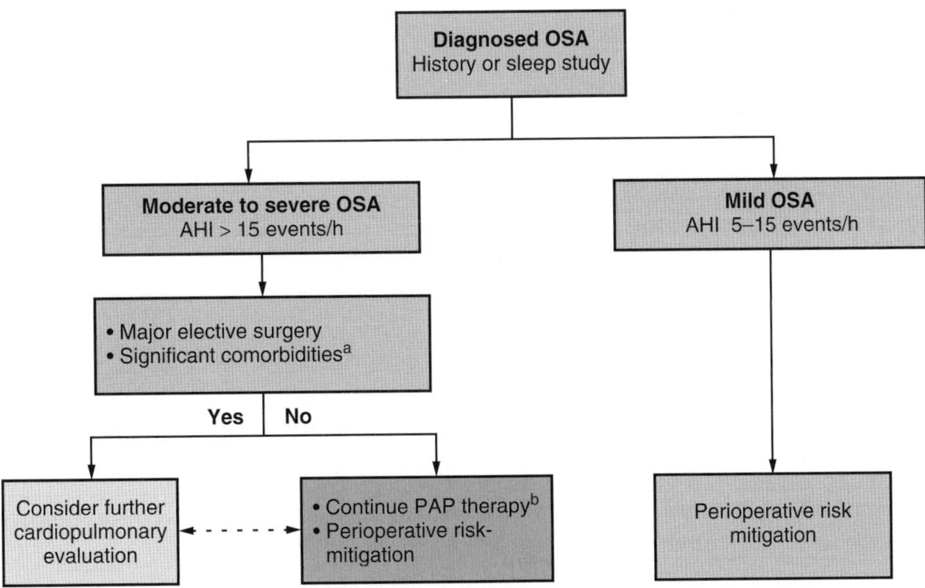

Preoperative evaluation of a person with diagnosed obstructive sleep apnea.

[a]Significant comorbidities: heart failure, arrhythmias, uncontrolled hypertension, cerebrovascular disease, metabolic syndrome, obesity (body mass index >35 kg/m^2), obesity hypoventilation syndrome, pulmonary hypertension.

[b]Positive airway pressure (PAP) therapy includes continuous PAP, bilevel PAP, and autotitrating PAP.

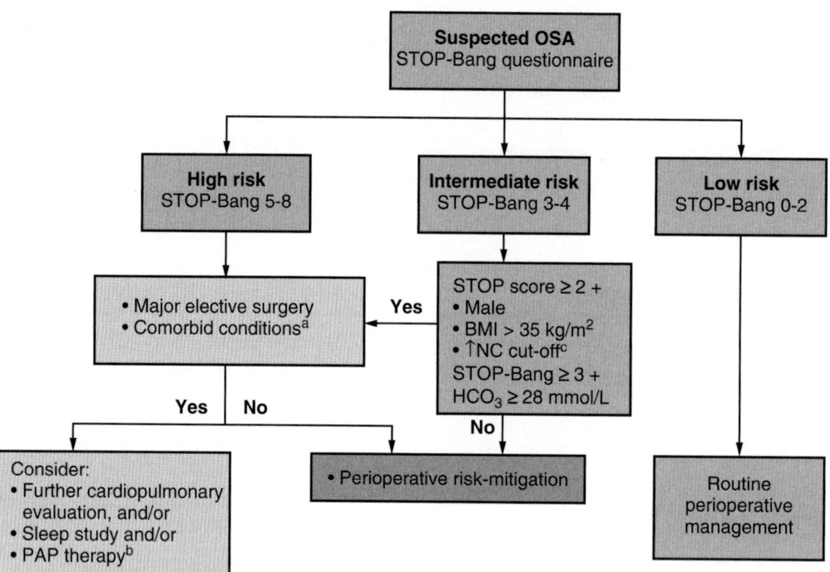

Preoperative evaluation of a person with suspected obstructive sleep apnea.

[a]Per the 2016 SASM guidelines, further cardiopulmonary evaluation may be indicated in patients with uncontrolled systemic disease or additional problems with ventilation or gas exchange, such as hypoventilation syndromes, severe pulmonary hypertension, and resting hypoxemia in the absence of other cardiopulmonary disease.
[b]Positive airway pressure (PAP) therapy includes continuous PAP, bilevel PAP, and auto-titrating PAP.
[c]Neck circumference (NC) cut-offs 17 inches/43 cm in male, 16 inches/41 cm in female.
(Modified from Vasu TS, Doghramji K, Cavallazzi R, et al. Obstructive sleep apnea syndrome and postoperative complications: clinical use of the STOP-BANG questionnaire. *Arch Otolaryngol Head Neck Surg*. 2010;136:1020–1024.)

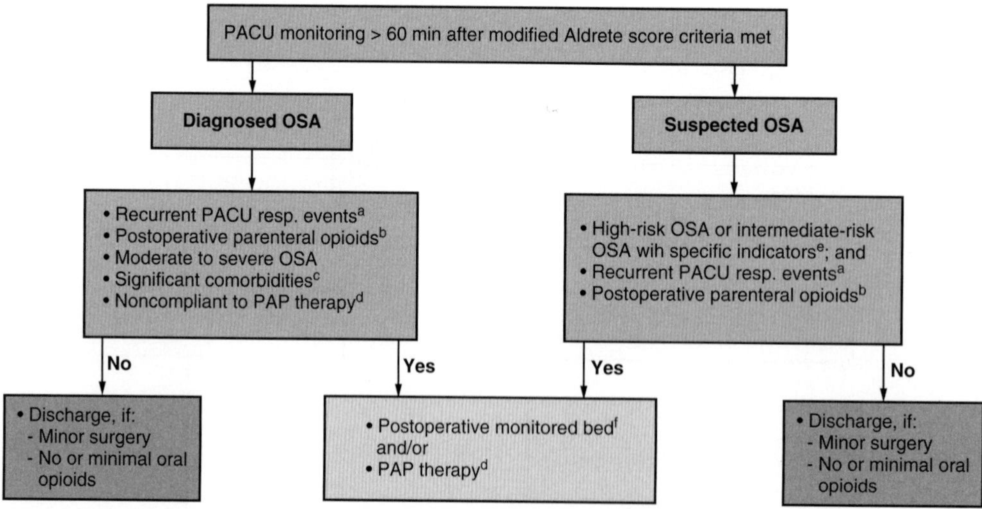

Postoperative management of a patient with known or suspected obstructive sleep apnea after general anesthesia.

[a]Recurrent postanesthesia care unit (PACU) respiratory event: repeated occurrence of oxygen saturation less than 90%, or bradypnea less than 8 breaths/min, or apnea 10 seconds and longer, or pain–sedation mismatch (high pain and sedation scores concurrently).
[b]Postoperative parenteral opioid requirement more than the usual standard of care such as multiple routes, long-acting preparations, or high-dose infusions.
[c]Per the 2016 SASM guidelines, uncontrolled systemic disease or additional problems with ventilation or gas exchange such as hypoventilation syndromes, severe pulmonary hypertension, and resting hypoxemia in the absence of other cardiopulmonary disease
[d]Positive airway pressure (PAP) therapy includes continuous PAP, bilevel PAP, or auto-titrating PAP.
[e]Intermediate-risk and specific indicators include STOP score ≥2 + male or BMI >35 kg/m^2 or ↑NC cutoff (where NC: neck circumference cut-offs 17 inches/43 cm in male, 16 inches/41 cm in female) and STOP-BANG ≥3 + HCO 3 ≥28 mmol/L.
[f]Monitored bed: environment with continuous oximetry and the possibility of early medical intervention (e.g., intensive care unit, step-down unit, or remote pulse oximetry with telemetry in surgical ward)

QUESTIONS

BASIC SLEEP PHYSIOLOGY

1. What distinguishes nonrapid eye movement (NREM) sleep from rapid eye movement (REM) sleep?

GENERAL ANESTHESIA

2. Describe the four distinct phases during the maintenance of general anesthesia. During which phase or phases is surgery usually performed? What is the EEG activity during phase 4?

SLEEP AND ANESTHESIA STATES

3. Is general anesthesia more similar to sleep or an induced coma? Explain.

FUNCTIONAL NEUROANATOMY OF SLEEP AND AROUSAL PATHWAYS

4. Are sedative drug requirements altered if a patient is sleep deprived?

SLEEP-DISORDERED BREATHING OR SLEEP-RELATED BREATHING DISORDERS

5. What are the characteristics and common types of sleep-disordered breathing?
6. What characterizes obstructive sleep apnea (OSA)?
7. What characterizes central sleep apnea (CSA)?

OBSTRUCTIVE SLEEP APNEA

Pathophysiology of Upper Airway Collapse in Obstructive Sleep Apnea

8. What is the pathophysiology of upper airway collapse in OSA?

Clinical Diagnostic Criteria

9. What test is the gold standard for the definitive diagnosis of OSA?
10. How are apneas and hypopneas defined by the American Academy of Sleep Medicine?
11. How is obstructive hypopnea distinguished from central hypopnea?
12. What is the apnea-hypopnea index (AHI)?
13. What defines severe, moderate, and mild OSA?
14. What are the clinical diagnostic criteria for OSA?

Polysomnography and Portable Devices

15. What is measured during laboratory polysomnography?
16. What are the various classes of home sleep testing devices currently available?

Prevalence of OSA in the General and Surgical Population

17. What is the prevalence of OSA in the general population?
18. What approximate percent of people in the general and surgical populations with moderate to severe OSA are undiagnosed?

OSA and Comorbid Conditions

19. What comorbid conditions are commonly found in patients with OSA?

Surgery and OSA Severity

20. What factors predict postoperative increased AHI from baseline, and on what postoperative day does the AHI peak?
21. According to the American Society of Anesthesiologists (ASA) Closed Claims Project database, on what postoperative day is opioid-induced respiratory depression most likely to occur? What are some contributory factors?
22. What are some factors associated with death and brain damage in patients with OSA following unexpected life-threatening critical respiratory events in the postoperative period?

OSA and Perioperative Complications

23. What are some causes of difficult airway management in patients with OSA?
24. What is the risk of postoperative complications in patients with diagnosed and undiagnosed OSA?

Preoperative Assessment

25. What are some of the principles of preoperative assessment of patients with OSA?
26. What are some types of positive airway pressure (PAP) devices used for treating patients with OSA?
27. What is the potential benefit of postoperative PAP therapy in patients with diagnosed or undiagnosed OSA?
28. Which patients may benefit from a preoperative assessment from a sleep medicine physician?
29. What are some tools that can be used for preoperative screening of patients for OSA?
30. What is the STOP-BANG questionnaire? What score indicates a high risk of OSA on the STOP-BANG questionnaire?
31. What is the best management strategy for a patient who scored a 7 when screened with the STOP-BANG questionnaire and is scheduled for an emergency laparotomy for a ruptured abdominal aortic aneurysm?
32. What is the best management strategy for a patient with OSA with significant daytime sleepiness who has been noncompliant with continuous positive airway pressure (CPAP) therapy for the past 10 years, has gained 20 kg in the past 2 years, has severe chronic obstructive pulmonary disease (COPD) requiring home oxygen at 2 L/min and moderate pulmonary hypertension? He is scheduled to undergo coronary artery bypass grafting for progressively worsening dyspnea.
33. What is the best management strategy for a patient with severe OSA with good CPAP compliance, no daytime sleepiness, and well-controlled hypertension who is scheduled for open reduction and internal fixation of radius and ulna fractures under axillary brachial plexus block?

Perioperative Risk Mitigation Strategies

34. What are some important perioperative strategies used to mitigate the risk of OSA?

Postoperative Disposition of OSA Patients

35. What are some factors that contribute to the postoperative disposition of the patient with OSA?
36. For how long should a patient with diagnosed or suspected OSA be monitored in the postanesthesia care unit (PACU) postoperatively?
37. What is the definition of recurrent respiratory events in the PACU?
38. What is pain–sedation mismatch?
39. How should patients with suspected OSA (i.e., scored as high risk on screening questionnaires) who develop recurrent respiratory events in the PACU be managed?
40. What is the proper management of a patient with a moderate risk of OSA (STOP-BANG score 4) who underwent knee arthroscopy under general anesthesia? Postoperatively, he is awake and breathing well with a respiratory rate of 16 breaths/min. His vital signs are stable, and the oxygen saturation is at 98% on room air. His pain score is 3/10 at rest and 4/10 on movement without the need for intravenous analgesics.
41. What is the proper management of a morbidly obese patient (body mass index of 45 kg/m^2) who underwent laparoscopic cholecystectomy under general anesthesia and is diagnosed with OSA, but noncompliant with CPAP therapy. The intraoperative course was uneventful. Postoperatively, she remained in the PACU for 2 hours. Her pain score is 8/10 at rest and 9/10 on movement despite treatment with hydromorphone 10 mg administered intravenously while in the PACU. She is drowsy and is noted to have repeated obstructive events that are associated with arousals terminating the events. Her respiratory rate is 7 breaths/min.
42. What is the proper management of a patient who underwent total knee replacement under spinal anesthesia with an adductor canal block and local infiltration analgesia? The patient was diagnosed with severe OSA and is noncompliant with her CPAP therapy. Postoperatively, she is awake and is breathing well with a respiratory rate of 14 breaths/min. Her oxygen saturation is at 96%, pain is well controlled, and she has only required hydromorphone 0.2 mg intravenously over the past 2 hours.

ANSWERS

BASIC SLEEP PHYSIOLOGY

1. Nonrapid eye movement (NREM) sleep has three distinct stages, with the last often referred to as "quiet" sleep. This stage of NREM sleep is associated with higher-amplitude, lower-frequency rhythms on the EEG also known as *delta* waves. During NREM there can also be decreased body temperature and heart rate. In contrast, rapid eye movement (REM) sleep is often referred to as "active" sleep and is associated with high-frequency, low-amplitude rhythms on the EEG. REM sleep is characterized by dreaming, irregular breathing and heart rate, and skeletal muscle hypotonia. (856–857)

GENERAL ANESTHESIA

2. There are four distinct EEG patterns, or phases, during the maintenance of general anesthesia. The first phase is light general anesthesia. Phase 2 has similar EEG patterns as stage 3, NREM sleep. Phase 3 is a deeper state, with flat periods interspersed with alpha and beta activity (burst suppression). Surgery is usually performed during phases 2 and 3. During phase 4 the EEG is completely flat, or isoelectric. This is consistent with induced coma or used for neuroprotection during neurosurgery. (857)

SLEEP AND ANESTHESIA STATES

3. General anesthesia can be described as drug-induced coma that is reversible. There are multiple distinguishing features between general anesthesia and sleep. General anesthesia is independent of any circadian rhythms, phases, or cycles; is not susceptible to interruption by environmental stimuli; renders the patient immobile and insensate; and requires the withdrawal of drug to reverse (i.e., does not reverse spontaneously). (857)

FUNCTIONAL NEUROANATOMY OF SLEEP AND AROUSAL PATHWAYS

4. Patients with circadian rhythm disruption or who are sleep deprived appear to have a decrease in sedative drug requirements. (857)

SLEEP-DISORDERED BREATHING OR SLEEP-RELATED BREATHING DISORDERS

5. Sleep-disordered breathing (SDB) is characterized by abnormalities of respiratory patterns during sleep. The abnormal patterns of breathing are broadly grouped into obstructive sleep apnea (OSA) disorders, central sleep apnea (CSA) disorders, sleep-related hypoventilation disorders, and sleep-related hypoxemia disorder. (860)
6. OSA is characterized by complete or incomplete upper airway closure during sleep in the presence of respiratory effort during some portion of the event. This results in varying severity of hypoxemia and hypercapnia. There are repeated episodes of complete or partial closure of the pharynx, associated hypoventilation and hypoxemia, and termination by EEG arousal. (860)
7. CSA disorders are characterized by reduction (hypopnea) or cessation (apnea) of airflow due to absent or reduced respiratory effort. Central apnea or hypopnea may occur in a cyclic, intermittent, or irregular (ataxic) fashion. (860)

OBSTRUCTIVE SLEEP APNEA

Pathophysiology of Upper Airway Collapse in Obstructive Sleep Apnea

8. Upper airway (UA) collapsibility and patency are dependent on a continuous balance between collapsing and expanding forces influenced by sleep-wake arousal. During sleep, UA collapse in patients with OSA is due to multiple factors such as loss of UA dilating muscle tone, impaired response to mechanoreceptors sensing intrapharyngeal pressures, ventilatory overshoot (high loop gain of the respiratory control system), and an increased arousal threshold. Moreover, patients with OSA have a UA that is predisposed to collapse due to the

presence of smaller UA cross-sectional area and higher critical closure pressures than patients without OSA. During NREM sleep and anesthesia, reduction of wakeful cortical influences, reflex gain, and ventilatory drive predisposes to UA collapse and hypoventilation. (860)

Clinical Diagnostic Criteria

9. Classically, the gold standard for the definitive diagnosis of OSA requires an overnight polysomnography (PSG) or sleep study. (860)
10. Based on the American Academy of Sleep Medicine (AASM), apneas and hypopneas are defined as a reduction in the rate of airflow from intranasal pressure of at least 90%, or between 50% and 90%, respectively, for at least 10 seconds accompanied by either a 3% or 4% decrease in oxygen saturation or EEG arousal. (860)
11. Obstructive hypopnea is present if thoracoabdominal motion is out of phase or if airflow limitation is observed on the nasal pressure signal. Central hypopnea is present if thoracoabdominal motion is in phase and there is no airflow limitation on the nasal pressure signal. Mixed apneas are events that begin as central for at least 10 seconds and end as obstructive, with a minimum of three obstructive efforts. (860)
12. The apnea-hypopnea index (AHI) is the average number of abnormal breathing events per hour of sleep. (861)
13. OSA severity is determined by the AHI as follows: mild is 5 to 15 events per hour; moderate is 15 to 30 events per hour; and severe is more than 30 events per hour. (861)
14. The clinical diagnosis of OSA requires either an AHI ≥15, or an AHI ≥5 with symptoms such as excessive daytime sleepiness, unintentional sleep during wakefulness, unrefreshing sleep, loud snoring reported by a partner, or observed obstruction during sleep. (861)

Polysomnography and Portable Devices

15. All laboratory PSG tests are performed using central, occipital, and frontal EEG; bilateral electro-oculography; electrocardiography; and chin and bilateral anterior tibialis muscle electromyography. Thoracoabdominal motion is usually monitored by respiratory inductance plethysmography, and airflow is monitored using either a nasal pressure transducer or nasal thermistor. Arterial oxygen saturation is monitored by pulse oximetry. Body position and snoring are recorded manually. (860)
16. Home sleep testing may be a viable alternative to standard PSG for the diagnosis of OSA when there is high pretest likelihood for moderate to severe OSA without other substantial comorbid conditions. The Portable Monitoring Task Force of the AASM has classified level 2 (full unattended PSG with seven or more recording channels), level 3 (devices limited to four to seven recording channels), and level 4 (monitors with one or two recording channels including nocturnal oximetry) devices. In particular, the level 2 portable PSG device has a diagnostic accuracy similar to that of standard PSG, whereas overnight oximetry is both sensitive and specific for detecting OSA in high-risk surgical patients. (861)

Prevalence of OSA in the General and Surgical Population

17. The prevalence of moderate to severe OSA ranges from 6% to 17% in the general population. The estimates are higher with increasing age and body mass index (BMI). (861)
18. In the general population, approximately 80% of men and 93% of women with moderate to severe OSA are undiagnosed. In one study, 60% of surgical patients with moderate to severe OSA were not diagnosed preoperatively. (862)

OSA and Comorbid Conditions

19. OSA is associated with long-term cardiovascular morbidity including myocardial ischemia, heart failure, hypertension, arrhythmias, cerebrovascular disease, metabolic syndrome, insulin resistance, gastroesophageal reflux, and obesity. It is important to be mindful of craniofacial deformities (e.g., macroglossia, retrognathia, midfacial hypoplasia), endocrine disorders (e.g., hypothyroidism, Cushing disease), demographic group (male, age over 50 years), and lifestyle factors (e.g., smoking, alcohol consumption) that are closely associated with OSA. (862)

Surgery and OSA Severity

20. Preoperative AHI, age, and opioid dosage are significant predictors of increased postoperative AHI. Although AHI significantly increases from baseline on the first night after surgery, peak increase occurs on the third postoperative night. These findings are clinically significant for surgical patients, as they are not monitored as closely during the second and third postoperative nights. It is well known that postoperative complications like myocardial infarction, congestive heart failure, and pulmonary embolus are more likely to occur during the second and third postoperative days, which is coincident with the increased AHI and decreased oxygen saturation. (862)
21. According to the American Society of Anesthesiologists (ASA) Closed Claims Project database, critical events involving postoperative opioid-induced respiratory depression in OSA patients is most likely to occur within the first 24 hours of surgery. Contributory factors include multiple prescribers, concurrent administration of nonopioid sedating medications, and inadequate nursing assessments or response. As many as 97% of these events were considered preventable. (863)

22. Death and brain damage associated with unexpected critical events in postoperative patients with OSA were more likely to occur with unwitnessed events, lack of supplemental oxygen, lack of respiratory monitoring, and coadministration of sedatives and opioids. (863)

OSA and Perioperative Complications

23. There are changes in UA anatomy associated with anesthesia that can make airway management difficult in the patient with OSA. These include augmented UA collapsibility, impaired capability of UA dilator muscles to respond to airway obstruction, disparities in hypoxemia and hypercarbia arousal thresholds, and unstable ventilatory control. (863)
24. Patients with OSA are more likely to have postoperative complications. There is a twofold higher risk of respiratory complications (including reintubation and mechanical ventilation); other pulmonary complications that were more likely in OSA were aspiration, acute respiratory distress syndrome, and pulmonary embolism. OSA is independently associated with atrial fibrillation. A prospective study revealed a significantly higher risk of postoperative cardiovascular events (myocardial injury, cardiac death, congestive heart failure, thromboembolism, atrial fibrillation, and stroke) in patients with undiagnosed severe OSA undergoing noncardiac surgery. Patients with undiagnosed OSA were found to have a threefold higher risk of postoperative cardiovascular complications, primarily cardiac arrest, and shock, compared to diagnosed OSA patients. (863)

Preoperative Assessment

25. A thorough history and physical examination are essential for assessing OSA preoperatively. Focused questions regarding the nature and severity of OSA symptoms should be asked. Previous consultations with a sleep physician and sleep reports should be reviewed. Patients may present with signs and symptoms of significant comorbid conditions including morbid obesity, metabolic syndrome, uncontrolled or resistant hypertension, arrhythmias, cerebrovascular disease, and heart failure. Preoperative assessment should also rule out the presence of significant nocturnal hypoxemia, hypercarbia, polycythemia, and cor pulmonale. Obesity hypoventilation syndrome (OHS) and pulmonary hypertension should be ruled out. A serum bicarbonate level of 28 mmol/L or more is indicative of chronic hypercapnia and is a useful screening tool for OHS. A preoperative transthoracic echocardiogram may be considered in patients suspected to have severe pulmonary hypertension and if intraoperative acute elevations in pulmonary arterial pressures (high-risk or long-duration surgery) are anticipated. (863)
26. A variety of positive airway pressure (PAP) devices are used for the treatment of OSA such as continuous positive airway pressure (CPAP), bilevel positive airway pressure (BiPAP), and auto-titrating positive airway pressure (APAP) machines. APAP devices provide upper airway stability while asleep based on airflow measurements, fluctuations in pressure, or airway resistance using internal algorithms and have the potential to account for night-to-night variability of OSA severity. (864)
27. The use of postoperative PAP therapy may reduce the postoperative AHI, improve oxygenation, and reduce hospital length of stay. Current guidelines recommend that surgical patients with moderate to severe OSA who are compliant with PAP therapy should bring the device to the hospital and continue its use. Patients who are noncompliant with the use of PAP therapy should be counseled at minimum to resume therapy preoperatively. (864)
28. Patients with diagnosed OSA and recent exacerbation of symptoms and those who were lost to follow-up care may benefit from a preoperative reassessment from a sleep medicine physician. Patients with significant comorbid conditions, a high serum bicarbonate level (indicating chronic hypercapnia), and preoperative hypoxemia in the absence of respiratory disease are also candidates for preoperative evaluation and possible initiation of PAP therapy. (866)
29. Overnight PSG is the gold standard diagnostic test for OSA, but routine screening with PSG can be costly and resource intensive. Preoperatively, the use of sensitive clinical criteria can identify and risk-stratify potential patients with OSA. The 2014 ASA guidelines recommend using a comprehensive checklist comprising physical characteristics, symptoms, and complaints related to OSA. Other tools that have been validated for screening surgical patients are the STOP-BANG questionnaire, the Berlin Questionnaire, and the Perioperative Sleep Apnea Prediction (P-SAP) score. (866)
30. The STOP-BANG questionnaire is a concise and easily used screening tool for OSA consisting of eight questions with the acronym STOP-BANG (www.stopbang.ca). This screening tool includes four "yes/no" questions with a mnemonic (*S* = snoring, *T* = tiredness, *O* = observed you stop breathing, *P* = blood pressure), and it combines demographic data of *B*MI (>35 kg/m^2), *A*ge (>50 years), *N*eck circumference (>40 cm), and *G*ender (male). Patients are deemed to be at low risk for OSA with scores of 0 to 2, intermediate risk with scores of 3 to 4, and high risk with scores of 5 to 8. In patients whose STOP-BANG scores are in the midrange (3 or 4), further criteria are required for classification. For example, a STOP score of ≥2 plus BMI criteria (BMI >35 kg/m^2 or male or neck circumference >43 cm in males, and >41 cm in females) or a

STOP-BANG score of ≥3 plus serum HCO_3 of ≥28 mmol/L would classify that patient as having a high risk of moderate to severe OSA. (866)

31. The patient scored a 7 when screened with the STOP-BANG questionnaire and is therefore at high risk of having undiagnosed moderate-to-severe OSA. However, the surgery is emergent so the sound management is to proceed with surgery, but with risk mitigation strategies through the entire perioperative period. After hospital discharge, this patient should be considered for referral to a sleep physician for assessment. (868)
32. The best management strategy for a patient with OSA who is noncompliant to CPAP therapy for the past 10 years, has significant weight gain, has oxygen-dependent chronic obstructive pulmonary disease (COPD), and has moderate pulmonary hypertension who is scheduled to undergo coronary artery bypass grafting for progressively worsening dyspnea is to refer the patient for preoperative assessment by a sleep physician. In this scenario, the patient is already diagnosed with moderate to severe OSA as evidenced by his daytime sleepiness. He has significant comorbid conditions (COPD, pulmonary hypertension, heart failure) and is scheduled for major elective surgery. This patient may benefit from preoperative institution of optimal PAP therapy to reduce his risk of perioperative adverse events. (867)
33. The best perioperative management strategy for a patient diagnosed with severe OSA who is compliant with CPAP and antihypertensive therapy is to proceed with elective surgery. This patient additionally benefits from regional rather than general anesthesia. (867)

Perioperative Risk Mitigation Strategies

34. To mitigate the risk of OSA, preoperative sedative premedication should be avoided. Intraoperatively, the anesthesia provider should be prepared for difficult mask ventilation, laryngoscopy, and endotracheal intubation. Adequate preoxygenation, head elevated body position, and measures to decrease the risk of aspiration of gastric acid should be considered. Short-acting agents such as propofol and remifentanil are preferred over long-acting agents. Multimodal analgesia with nonopioid analgesics should be used to decrease the opioid requirement. Extubation should take place when the patient is fully conscious, able to obey commands, has no residual neuromuscular blockade, and is able to maintain a patent airway. After extubation of the trachea, patients should be recovered in a semi-upright or lateral position. Local or regional anesthesia techniques may be of benefit as they avoid manipulation of the airway and reduce the postoperative requirement for sedating analgesic medication. Patients previously on PAP therapy at home may continue using their PAP devices during procedures under mild to moderate sedation. (866)

Postoperative Disposition of OSA Patients

35. Factors that contribute to the postoperative disposition of the patient with OSA include the nature of surgery, OSA severity, and requirement for postoperative parenteral opioids. The attending anesthesiologist is responsible for the final decision of patient disposition. (869)
36. Patients with diagnosed or suspected OSA should be monitored in the postanesthesia care unit (PACU) for an extended period of time. It is reasonable to observe these patients in the PACU for an additional 60 minutes in a quiet environment after criteria for discharge have been met. (870)
37. Recurrent respiratory events in the PACU are defined as (1) episodes of apnea for ≥10 seconds, (2) bradypnea (<8 breaths/min), (3) pain–sedation mismatch, and (4) repeated oxygen desaturation to <90%. (870)
38. Pain–sedation mismatch is the simultaneous occurrence of high pain scores and high sedation levels. The patient is found to be drowsy and, when aroused, complains of severe uncontrolled pain. In this scenario, it is important to be cautious with prescribing more sedating medications. Opioid-sparing techniques should be instituted for these patients, and arrangements should be made for postoperative monitoring after transfer from the PACU. (870)
39. Patients with suspected OSA (i.e., scored as high risk on screening questionnaires) who develop recurrent respiratory events in the PACU are at increased risk of postoperative respiratory complications. These patients should be monitored after transfer from the PACU with continuous pulse oximetry, and PAP therapy may be instituted for recurrent obstructive events associated with significant hypoxemia. Patients with preoperative PAP therapy should continue PAP therapy postoperatively. (870)
40. This postoperative patient with a moderate risk of OSA has no evidence of recurrent PACU respiratory events (normal respiratory rate and room air oxygen saturation) after an extended stay in the PACU. His pain is also well controlled without the need for significant doses of intravenous opioid analgesia. Since knee arthroscopy is a minor procedure, this patient may be discharged home safely. (870)
41. This clinical scenario describes a patient with diagnosed OSA who is noncompliant with her CPAP treatment. She has a significant comorbid condition (morbid obesity) and postoperatively she shows pain–sedation mismatch as evidenced by her high pain scores despite high-dose intravenous opioid analgesia and excessive sedation. She also exhibits recurrent PACU respiratory events (upper airway obstructive events associated

with arousals for termination and a respiratory rate of 7 breaths/min). All these factors call for PAP therapy as well as a postoperative monitored bed in the interest of patient safety. (870)

42. This patient with diagnosed severe OSA but noncompliant with CPAP therapy, who underwent major surgery needs a postoperative monitored bed. Because she shows no pain–sedation mismatch and no other PACU respiratory events, she does not need immediate treatment with PAP therapy in the PACU. However, she may require additional analgesics after transfer to the floor once the regional anesthetic recedes. In this setting, it is in the best interest of the patient to be monitored postoperatively. (870)

Chapter

49 ANESTHESIA AND ENVIRONMENTAL HEALTH

Hemra Cil and Seema Gandhi

HEALTH, HEALTHCARE, AND CLIMATE CHANGE

- Climate change represents a defining challenge of our times.
- Tackling climate change is the greatest public health opportunity of the 21st century.
- Healthcare is a leading cause of environmental pollution.
  - Overall, 4% to 5% of global warming can be attributed to healthcare.
  - U.S. healthcare contributes to 8% to 10% of national greenhouse gas (GHG) emissions.

ENVIRONMENTAL IMPACT OF ANESTHESIA GASES

- GHGs are defined as gases that trap heat in the atmosphere.
  - GHGs contribute to global warming by absorbing reflected heat and radiating it back to the earth's surface.
- Global warming potential (GWP) is a measure of how much a given mass of GHG contributes to global warming over a specified time (typically 20 or 100 years, i.e., GWP_{20} or GWP_{100}).
  - By definition, carbon dioxide (CO_2) has a GWP of 1.
- The commonly used volatile anesthetics sevoflurane, desflurane, and isoflurane, and the ozone-depleter nitrous oxide (N_2O) are potent GHGs with high GWP.
  - Volatile anesthetics are minimally metabolized in vivo.
  - Thus, direct release of these gases into the atmosphere is a major contributor to the environmental impact of anesthesia care.
- After CO_2 and methane, N_2O is the third leading contributor of GHG globally.
  - Among inhaled anesthetics, N_2O has the longest atmospheric lifetime of 114 years.
- The table below compares several aspects of the environmental impact of volatile anesthetics: atmospheric lifetime, GWP, and so-called driving equivalents of inhaled anesthetic agents in miles/hour.

			Driving Equivalent (miles/hr) at Fresh Gas Flow[c]			
Gas	Lifetime (years)	GWP[b,d]	0.5 L/min*	1.0 L/min*	2 L/min*	5 L/min*
N_2O	114	273	29	57	112	282
Sevoflurane	1.1	130	—	4	8	19
Desflurane	14	2540	93	190	378	939
Isoflurane	3.2	510	4	8	15	38
Halothane[a]	1.0	50	—	—	—	—

*0.6 Mac-hour for N_2O and 1 Mac-hour for sevoflurane, desflurane, and isoflurane.
[a]Halothane is no longer commercially available in the US but is available globally.
[b]GWP_{100} is the global warming potential of a greenhouse gas over a 100-year period compared with CO_2. Desflurane has a GWP_{100} of 2540, indicating that 1 kg of desflurane has the same global warming effect as 2540 kg of CO_2.
[c]The driving equivalent analogy provides a practical comparison to driving a typical passenger automobile, which emits approximately 400 grams of CO_2 per mile. For example, administering desflurane at fresh gas flow of 1 L/min for 1 hour at 1 MAC produces the same GHG emission as driving a car for 190 miles.
[d]The Intergovernmental Panel on Climate Change's Sixth Assessment Report, 2021, Working Group 1 contribution.

- For an individual anesthesia provider in daily practice, these are the most effective climate change mitigation strategies.
  - Avoid desflurane and N_2O.
  - Adopt low-flow and closed-circuit anesthesia when using volatile anesthetics.
  - Use neuraxial techniques, regional and total intravenous anesthesia when possible.

OCCUPATIONAL HAZARDS OF INHALED ANESTHETICS

- Inhaled anesthetic agents cause operating room (OR) pollution and can increase health risks for providers.
- Surveys from the 1970s noted increased risk of spontaneous abortion, genetic damage, and cancer in OR personnel.
  - Since then, waste anesthetic gas scavenging has improved, and waste gas regulations have been implemented.
- More recent studies have found little to no increase in adverse effects associated with waste anesthesia gases when they are scavenged effectively.

LOW-FLOW ANESTHESIA

- Inhaled anesthetics undergo very little metabolism in vivo; they are exhaled, scavenged, and released largely unchanged into the atmosphere as waste medical gases.
- The ecological impact is largely determined by the choice of gas used and the fresh gas flow (FGF) rate.
  - Lower FGF rates significantly reduce carbon emission and costs per case.
- Low-flow anesthesia (LFA) is defined as FGF <1 L/min, and minimal flow anesthesia as FGF <0.5 L/min.

CLOSED-CIRCUIT ANESTHESIA

- Closed-circuit anesthesia is a form of LFA that is rarely used but is attracting more interest because of its environmental and cost benefits.
- Two key principles of closed-circuit anesthesia
  - No gases are allowed to escape from the circuit.
  - All exhaled gases are returned to the patient after elimination of CO_2.
- Inhalational agents and carrier gases (O_2 and N_2O or air) are added to the circuit only in amounts equal to those eliminated and consumed.

CO_2 ABSORBENTS

- CO_2 absorbents have been used in anesthesia practice since 1924.
- Traditional soda lime absorbent contains the strong bases sodium hydroxide and potassium hydroxide.
  - Potassium hydroxide degrades sevoflurane to the nephrotoxin compound A.
  - Desiccated soda lime degrades desflurane, enflurane, and isoflurane to produce significant amounts of carbon monoxide.
- New-generation absorbents do not contain strong bases.
  - Litholyme (lithium hydroxide–based) and AMSORB Plus are examples.
  - These absorbents do not interact chemically with inhaled anesthetics and do not produce compound A.
  - Made of nonhazardous materials and suitable for landfill waste
- CO_2 absorbents are depleted more rapidly with LFA.
  - To maximize absorbent utilization (and decrease absorbent costs), closely monitor inspired CO_2 and wait until $FICO_2$ is $\geq$5 mmHg before replacing absorbent canister.

WASTE ANESTHETIC GAS SCAVENGING SYSTEMS

- Waste anesthetic gas scavenging systems decrease OR pollution by eliminating vented anesthetic gases.
  - These gases are emitted to the atmosphere largely unmetabolized and unregulated, causing environmental pollution.
  - Anesthesia scavenging systems entrain large air volumes using a heavy-duty continuously operating vacuum pump.
- Newer scavenging systems use technologies that capture, recycle/reuse, or destroy anesthetic gases.
  - One novel approach uses a low-flow scavenger interface with a one-way on-demand valve that reduces air entrainment; this also reduces the vacuum pump's duty cycle, which further reduces energy consumption.

ENVIRONMENTAL IMPACT OF PROPOFOL

- Total intravenous anesthesia (TIVA) refers to the administration of only intravenous agents (most frequently propofol) to induce and maintain general anesthesia.
- The GHG impact of propofol is less than that of inhaled anesthetics.

  - Propofol's environmental impact stems mainly from the electricity required for the syringe pump and not from drug production or direct release to the environment.
- Propofol is not biodegradable; improper disposal into landfill can contaminate water and aquatic life.
  - Propofol should be disposed of by incineration at >1000°C for more than 2 sec.

DRUG WASTE

- Drug waste has been linked to unnecessary healthcare costs and negative environmental impact.
- Several strategies can be used to reduce drug waste, including deciding which drugs should be opened and drawn into a syringe.

ENVIRONMENTAL IMPACT OF OPERATING ROOM PRACTICES

Waste

- The OR generates 20% to 30% of total hospital waste.
- Anesthesia care generates 25% of total OR waste, of which 60% could be recycled.
- Waste is divided into noncontaminated solid waste or regulated medical waste (e.g., infectious material, sharps, and certain medications).
  - Treatment and decontamination of regulated medical waste to enable safe handling and disposal is energy-intensive and expensive.
- The energy and cost of OR waste management can be reduced.
  - Appropriate classification of the waste (regulated medical waste vs. noncontaminated solids)
  - Recycling of paper, glass, and several types of plastics

Reusable versus Single-Use Equipment

- The environmental benefits of reusable medical equipment compared with single-use equipment have been repeatedly demonstrated.
  - For laryngoscopes, a single-use blade generates 5 to 6 times more CO_2 than a reusable alternative.
  - A single-use laryngoscope handle generates 16 to 18 times more CO_2 than a reusable alternative.
- Reprocessing allows for safe reuse of certain single-use devices to decrease waste, costs, and emissions while adhering to infection control guidelines.
  - Reprocessing is a Food and Drug Administration (FDA)-approved process that involves collecting, testing, packaging, and sterilizing single-use devices to meet the same standards as the original equipment manufacturer.
  - Many medical devices are approved for reprocessing, including invasive devices (e.g., surgical trocars, staplers, and angiography catheters) and noninvasive devices (e.g., blood pressure cuffs, sequential compression device sleeves, and patient transfer mattresses).

Reusable Breathing Circuits

- Reusable anesthesia breathing circuits with single-use airway filters can be safely used for up to 7 days without increasing bacterial/viral contamination risk.
  - Recommended frequency of anesthesia breathing circuits change varies from country to country (e.g., daily in the UK, weekly in Germany, but after each patient in the US).
  - Reusing anesthesia breathing circuits with single-use airway filters decrease waste, cost, energy and water use, as well as the carbon footprint.

Energy Efficiency

- Healthcare facilities provide round-the-clock care requiring energy-intensive equipment.
- The ORs use 3 to 6 times greater energy per square foot than the rest of the hospital.
  - Heating, ventilation, and air conditioning (HVAC) are responsible for 90% to 99% of energy consumption in the OR.
  - Energy-efficient technologies and practices like HVAC occupancy-based approaches may reduce the OR energy consumption without affecting patient care (e.g., reducing frequency of room air exchanges in an empty OR reduces energy consumption).

SUMMARY

- Healthcare professionals worldwide—including anesthesia providers—must show strong leadership in tackling climate change.
- Careful attention focused on environmental stewardship could decrease cost and resource utilization while providing the same quality of care.

QUESTIONS

HEALTH, HEALTHCARE, AND CLIMATE CHANGE

1. Describe at least three mechanisms by which climate change negatively affects public health.
2. List three ways that healthcare contributes to climate change.

ENVIRONMENTAL IMPACT OF ANESTHESIA GASES

3. Which anesthetic agents have the greatest environmental impact based on atmospheric lifetime and global warming potential?
4. What are the most effective strategies an individual anesthesia provider can take to decrease the environmental impact of anesthesia care?

OCCUPATIONAL HAZARDS OF INHALED ANESTHETICS

5. Describe the potential health hazards of cumulative exposure to waste anesthetic gases such as N_2O. How can these risks be minimized?

LOW-FLOW ANESTHESIA

6. What are the potential benefits of using low-flow anesthesia during maintenance of anesthesia?
7. List three disadvantages of low-flow anesthesia.
8. Describe the steps needed to conduct low-flow anesthesia, from induction of anesthesia to maintenance and emergence.

CLOSED-CIRCUIT ANESTHESIA

9. What are the principles of closed-circuit anesthesia?

CO_2 ABSORBENTS

10. How do new-generation CO_2 absorbents help to decrease the environmental impact of anesthesia?

WASTE ANESTHETIC GAS SCAVENGING SYSTEMS

11. How do newer waste anesthetic gas scavenging systems decrease the environmental impact of anesthesia care?

ENVIRONMENTAL IMPACT OF PROPOFOL

12. Compare the carbon footprint of total intravenous anesthesia (TIVA) and inhaled anesthetic agents.

DRUG WASTE

13. Describe the actions that an individual anesthesia provider can take to decrease drug waste in the OR.
14. How should propofol be disposed? What are the environmental consequences of propofol waste that is improperly disposed?

ENVIRONMENTAL IMPACT OF OPERATING ROOM PRACTICES

15. What is the environmental impact of the energy consumption related to OR use?
16. Describe three strategies to minimize the environmental impact of OR practices?

ANSWERS

HEALTH, HEALTHCARE, AND CLIMATE CHANGE

1. Manifestations of climate change include increased air pollution, variability in precipitation, and increased frequency and intensity of heat waves. Reduced air quality leads to increased risk of respiratory illnesses and cardiovascular disease. Increased variability in precipitation and increasing temperatures can lead to increases in vector-borne and water-borne diseases like malaria. Finally, extreme heat conditions increase the risk of morbidity and mortality and directly affect the outdoor workforce during heat waves. (874–875)
2. Healthcare contributes to climate change in different ways that include the following: greenhouse gas (GHG) emission, energy consumption, and healthcare waste generation. In terms of GHG emissions, US healthcare contributes 8% to 10% of the national GHG emissions. Healthcare facilities provide round-the-clock care requiring energy-intensive equipment and systems. Energy consumption in the OR is 3 to 6 times higher per square foot than in the hospital as whole. Healthcare facilities generate large amounts of waste, with the OR accounting for 20% to 30% of total hospital waste. (874–875, 880)

ENVIRONMENTAL IMPACT OF ANESTHESIA GASES

3. Nitrous oxide (N_2O), has a global warming potential (GWP) of 273. This means that 1 kg of N_2O has the same global warming effect as 273 kg of CO_2. Nitrous oxide is also a significant source of ozone depletion. Desflurane has the highest GWP of any volatile anesthetic, at 2540. In addition, both N_2O and desflurane have very long atmospheric lifetimes, approximately 114 years for N_2O and 14 years for desflurane. (875–876)
4. One strategy to reduce the environmental impact of anesthesia care is through the use of neuraxial or regional anesthesia instead of general anesthesia when feasible. When general anesthesia is planned, the administration of total intravenous anesthesia (TIVA) avoids volatile anesthetics altogether. If volatile anesthetics are used, avoiding desflurane and nitrous oxide administration and favoring use of sevoflurane will reduce greenhouse gas emissions. The use of low-flow anesthesia or closed-circuit anesthesia techniques will further decrease the environmental impact of anesthesia care. (875–878)

OCCUPATIONAL HAZARDS OF INHALED ANESTHETICS

5. The potential health hazards of cumulative exposure to waste anesthetic gases are due to spillage directly into the OR. This most commonly occurs after the induction of general anesthesia and prior to tracheal intubation—a period in which a high fresh gas flow rate is commonly used. Survey studies in the 1970s noted among healthcare providers an increased risk of spontaneous abortion, genetic damage, and cancer. However, during this time, the scavenging of inhaled anesthetics was poor compared with current standards. The most effective way to minimize these risks is to meet federal guidelines for exposure limits to inhaled anesthetics (N_2O and halogenated agents) and to maintain scavenging systems for waste anesthetic gases and ventilation systems in the OR and recovery areas. (875–876)

LOW-FLOW ANESTHESIA

6. The use of low-flow anesthesia (LFA) has environmental, economic, and physiological benefits. Environmental benefits include a decrease in GHG emission by decreasing anesthetic gas consumption. From an economic standpoint, LFA decreases the amount of total anesthetic used and thus the cost of volatile anesthetic per case. The physiologic benefits include reducing respiratory heat loss and preserving the humidity of inspired gases. (876–877)
7. Disadvantages of LFA include decreased ability to rapidly change the inspired anesthetic agent concentration and depth of anesthesia. The use of LFA causes more rapid consumption of CO_2 absorbents, leading to increased absorbent costs and increased risk of hypercarbia with exhausted absorbent. The decreased oxygen flow rate during LFA requires close attention to the inspired oxygen concentration to prevent delivery of a hypoxic gas mixture during long cases. (876–877)
8. Recommendations for managing fresh gas flow and anesthetic delivery during low-flow anesthesia are provided in the box below. (877)

Management of Low Fresh Gas Flow (FGF) During Anesthesia
Induction Set FGF close to minute ventilation during mask ventilation. Increase FGF if inspired oxygen (FIO_2) and gas concentration lower than set level. During intubation, turn off the FGF, leave the vaporizer at its set point. Set FGF to half of the minute ventilation after intubation. Then watch measured anesthetic concentration after intubation. Reduce FGF progressively based on gas concentration. If needed, increase/decrease vaporizer setting to maintain desired concentration. Move to anesthesia maintenance management if there is no significant difference between exhaled and inspired anesthetic gas concentration.
Maintenance First, set total oxygen flow (mL/min): Patient's estimated oxygen consumption (5 mL/kg per minute) Add 200 mL/min if side-stream gas analyzer sample gas does not return to the circuit. Add 100 mL/min for potential leaks. Decrease total oxygen flow in 50-mL/min increments until FIO_2 begins to decrease. Monitor exhaled anesthetic gas concentration to maintain desired MAC level. Monitor FIO_2.
Emergence Maintain low FGF until the vaporizer is off.

CLOSED-CIRCUIT ANESTHESIA

9. Closed-circuit anesthesia is the most extreme form of LFA. The two key principles of closed-circuit anesthesia are (1) no gases are allowed to escape from the circuit; all exhaled gases are returned to the patient after elimination of CO_2, and (2) inhalational agents and carrier gases (O_2 and N_2O or air) are added to the circuit only in amounts equal to those eliminated and consumed. Once steady state has been reached during anesthesia maintenance, the minimal fresh gas flow can be set based on the patient's predicted oxygen consumption plus the flow of gas into the expired gas monitor (unless that gas is returned to the circuit). (877–878)

CO_2 ABSORBENTS

10. Because new-generation CO_2 absorbents (e.g., Litholyme, AMSORB Plus) do not contain the strong alkali compounds sodium hydroxide or potassium hydroxide, they do not cause sevoflurane degradation to compound A, which allows their safe use with sevoflurane at low-flow rates. These newer absorbents are also made of nonhazardous materials and are suitable for landfill waste. (879)

WASTE ANESTHETIC GAS SCAVENGING SYSTEMS

11. Newer approaches to waste anesthetic gas scavenging include systems that can capture, recycle/reuse, or destroy anesthetic gases, thereby decreasing the amount of anesthetic gases vented into the atmosphere. Additionally, new systems that use a low-flow scavenger interface reduce both energy consumption and cost associated with operating a vacuum pump. (879)

ENVIRONMENTAL IMPACT OF PROPOFOL

12. Inhaled anesthetics are potent greenhouse gases with high global warming potential. The administration of TIVA, mostly used with propofol, has a lower carbon footprint than inhalation agents. However, propofol does have potentially adverse environmental impact as well. Propofol is not biodegradable; even a small amount that is improperly disposed can cause long term environmental contamination. Therefore proper disposal of propofol waste is necessary to maintain the environmental impact benefits of TIVA over inhalation agents. (879)

DRUG WASTE

13. Anesthesia providers can adopt several strategies to reduce drug waste in the OR. These approaches include (1) leaving emergency drugs unopened but easily available, (2) drawing up a minimal number of drugs at the start of a procedure, (3) choosing smaller vials whenever possible, and (4) using prefilled syringes for commonly used drugs. (879–880)
14. Because propofol is not biodegradable, it must be disposed of by incineration at >1000°C for more than 2 sec. Improper disposal can have deleterious effects on aquatic wildlife and terrestrial ecosystems. (879)

ENVIRONMENTAL IMPACT OF OPERATING ROOM PRACTICES

15. Energy consumption is the second largest source of GHG in the OR setting. Heating, ventilation, and air conditioning (HVAC) are responsible for 90% to 99% of energy consumption in the OR. Compared with other hospital locations, energy consumption in the OR is 3 to 6 times greater per square foot. Other energy-intensive processes in the OR include treatment and decontamination of regulated medical waste. (880–881)
16. Strategies to minimize the environmental impact of operating room practices include the proper management of waste and recycling, deployment of reusable equipment, and reducing energy waste. Appropriate classification of OR waste and recycling of paper, glass, and several types of plastic will reduce the requirement for energy-intensive treatment and decontamination of medical waste. The selection and purchasing of reusable medical equipment, textiles, and anesthesia breathing circuits can have tremendous environmental benefits compared with single-use, disposable items. For example, single-use textiles consume 200% to 300% more energy and 250% to 330% more water and generate 200% to 300% more CO_2 and sevenfold more waste than reusable ones. Approaches to reducing energy waste include utilization of energy-efficient HVAC systems, practices such as an HVAC occupancy-based approach, regular HVAC maintenance, and turning off all energy-intensive systems and equipment when they are not in use. (880–881)

INDEX

Note: Page numbers followed by "b", "f", and "t" indicate boxes, figures, and tables, respectively.

C

D

E

F

G

H

J

K

L

M

N

O

P

U

V

Patton/Bell/Thompson/Williamson
Structure & Function of the Body
17th Edition, Softcover Version

ISBN 978-0-323-871730

To address binding concerns after printing and ensure the quality and stability of our product, we have had to move the location of the ***Clear View of the Human Body*** insert, necessitating a revision of the page references printed within the book. We apologize for the inconvenience.

The revised references are as follows:

Front Matter, p. xiv: The reference to Chapter 1 should be Chapter 5.

Chapter 1, pp. 8, 10 (twice), 11: References to p. 8 should be p. 104.

Chapter 4, p. 84: Reference to p. 8 should be p. 104.

Chapter 5, pp. 93, 109: References to p. 8 should be p. 104.

Chapter 5, p. 115; Reference to p. 8 should be p. 104.

Chapter 7, p. 150: Reference to p. 8 should be p. 104.

Chapter 8, p. 176; Reference to p. 8 should be p. 104.

Chapter 9, p. 192: Reference to p. 8 should be p. 104.

Chapter 11, pp. 270, 277: References to p. 8 should be p. 104.

Chapter 13, pp. 303, 320: References to p. 8 should be p. 104.

Chapter 15, p. 364: Reference to p. 8 should be p. 104.

Chapter 16, p. 391: Reference to p. 8 should be p. 104.

Chapter 18, p. 439: Reference to p. 8 should be p. 104.

Chapter 21, pp. 493, 500; References to p. 8 should be p. 104.

Part Number: 7770001765